Register Now for O[...]
to Your Bo[...]

SPRINGER PUBLISHING COMPANY
C○NNECT™

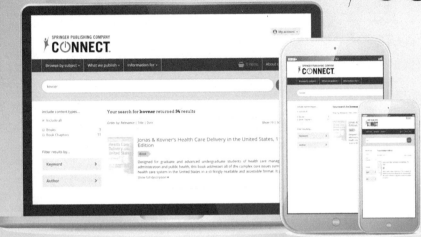

Your print purchase of *Multiple Sclerosis and Related Disorders: Clinical Guide to Diagnosis, Medical Management, and Rehabilitation, Second Edition*, **includes online access to the contents of your book**—increasing accessibility, portability, and searchability!

Access today at:
http://connect.springerpub.com/content/book/978-0-8261-2594-1 or scan the QR code at the right with your smartphone and enter the access code below.

Scan here for quick access.

17YUHKBRS

SPC

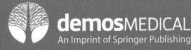

demosMEDICAL
An Imprint of Springer Publishing

View all our products at springerpub.com

Multiple Sclerosis and Related Disorders

Clinical Guide to Diagnosis, Medical Management, and Rehabilitation

Second Edition

EDITORS

Robert J. Fox, MD, MSc

Staff Neurologist
Mellen Center for MS Treatment and Research
Vice-Chair for Research
Neurological Institute
Cleveland Clinic Foundation
Cleveland, Ohio

Alexander D. Rae-Grant, MD, FRCP(C)

Staff Neurologist
Director of MS Education
Mellen Center for MS Treatment and Research
Cleveland Clinic Foundation
Cleveland, Ohio

Francois Bethoux, MD

Professor, Cleveland Clinic Lerner College of Medicine
Director of Rehabilitation Services
Mellen Center for MS Treatment and Research
Cleveland Clinic Foundation
Cleveland, Ohio

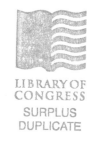
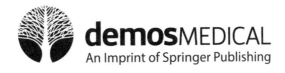

demosMEDICAL
An Imprint of Springer Publishing

Visit our website at www.springerpub.com

ISBN: 9780826125934
ebook ISBN: 9780826125941

Acquisitions Editor: Beth Barry
Compositor: diacriTech

Medicine is an ever-changing science. Research and clinical experience are continually expanding our knowledge, in particular our understanding of proper treatment and drug therapy. The authors, editors, and publisher have made every effort to ensure that all information in this book is in accordance with the state of knowledge at the time of production of the book. Nevertheless, the authors, editors, and publisher are not responsible for errors or omissions or for any consequences from application of the information in this book and make no warranty, expressed or implied, with respect to the contents of the publication. Every reader should examine carefully the package inserts accompanying each drug and should carefully check whether the dosage schedules mentioned therein or the contraindications stated by the manufacturer differ from the statements made in this book. Such examination is particularly important with drugs that are either rarely used or have been newly released on the market.

Library of Congress Cataloging-in-Publication Data
Names: Fox, Robert, 1969- editor. | Rae-Grant, Alexander, editor. | Bethoux,
  Francois, editor.
Title: Multiple sclerosis and related disorders : clinical guide to
  diagnosis, medical management, and rehabilitation / editors, Robert J.
  Fox, Alexander Rae-Grant, Francois Bethoux.
Other titles: Multiple sclerosis and related disorders (Rae-Grant)
Description: Second edition. | New York : Springer Publishing Company, [2018]
  | Alexander Rae-Grant's name appears first in the previous edition. |
  Includes bibliographical references and index.
Identifiers: LCCN 2018013748 | ISBN 9780826125934 (alk. paper) | ISBN 9780826125941 (e-book)
Subjects: | MESH: Multiple Sclerosis--diagnosis | Multiple Sclerosis--therapy
Classification: LCC RC377 | NLM WL 360 | DDC 616.8/34--dc23 LC record available at https://lccn.loc.gov/2018013748

Printed in the United States of America.
18 19 20 21 22 / 5 4 3 2 1

Thanks to Kathy for her precious friendship and bold partnership in life; to Brian for his inquisitive curiosity of the world around us; and to Kevin for reminding me of the truly important things in life. Thanks to the staff at the Mellen Center for pouring their lives into the care of people with multiple sclerosis and researching how better to manage this disease. And special thanks to all of the people living with multiple sclerosis and their care partners: you have taught me the true meaning of dedication, perseverance, and love.

Robert J. Fox

Thanks to my wife, Mary Bruce, for her encouragement and support. Thanks to my children Michael, Tucker, George, and Noah for making life complete. Thanks to my colleagues for their wisdom and particularly, to my patients for their courage and extraordinary resilience.

Alexander D. Rae-Grant

With all my gratitude to my wife Sandrine for putting up with me over the past 30 years; to my children Nicolas, Ambre, and Célina for all they have taught me; to my parents for allowing me to pursue a career in medicine; to my brother Stéphane for giving me important life lessons; and to all the patients and families I have had the privilege to interact with for reminding me to be humble.

Francois Bethoux

Contents

Contributors   ix
Foreword   J. Theodore Phillips, MD, PhD, FAAN   xv
Preface   xvii

PART I. Basics for Clinicians

1. **History of Multiple Sclerosis   1**
   T. Jock Murray

2. **Overview of Multiple Sclerosis   11**
   Alexander D. Rae-Grant and Robert J. Fox

3. **Pathology and Pathophysiology of Multiple Sclerosis   15**
   Kedar R. Mahajan and Don J. Mahad

4. **Epidemiology and Natural History of Multiple Sclerosis   22**
   Marcus W. Koch

5. **Multiple Sclerosis Genetics   28**
   Bruce A. C. Cree

PART II. Diagnosis

6. **Symptoms and Signs of Multiple Sclerosis   45**
   Marisa P. McGinley and Lael A. Stone

7. **Diagnosis of Multiple Sclerosis   52**
   Thomas Shoemaker and Scott D. Newsome

8. **Magnetic Resonance Imaging in Multiple Sclerosis   64**
   Christopher J. Karakasis, Aliye O. Bricker, and Stephen E. Jones

9. **Tools and Tests for Multiple Sclerosis   79**
   Robert A. Bermel

10. **Differential Diagnosis of Multiple Sclerosis   87**
    Megan H. Hyland and Jeffrey A. Cohen

PART III. Treatment

2018 American Academy of Neurology Guidelines for Multiple Sclerosis Disease-Modifying Therapy   94
Alexander D. Rae-Grant

11. **Approach to Disease-Modifying Therapy   97**
    Laura E. Baldassari and Jeffrey A. Cohen

12. **Relapse Management in Multiple Sclerosis   108**
    Andrew L. Smith and Robert J. Fox

13. **Treating Relapsing Forms of Multiple Sclerosis: Injection and Oral Therapies   116**
    Le H. Hua

14. **Treating Relapsing Forms of Multiple Sclerosis: Infusion Therapies   126**
    Jenny J. Feng and Daniel Ontaneda

15. **Treating Progressive Multiple Sclerosis   136**
    Carrie M. Hersh

16. **Emerging Therapies   149**
    Michael D. Kornberg and Peter A. Calabresi

PART IV. Rehabilitation and Symptom Management

17. **Overview of Rehabilitation in Multiple Sclerosis   159**
    Francois Bethoux

18. **Relationship-Centered Care in a Multiple Sclerosis Comprehensive Care Center   166**
    Adrienne Boissy and Claire Hara-Cleaver

19. **Fatigue in Multiple Sclerosis   173**
    Matthew Plow and Aaron Nicka

20. **Emotional Disorders in Multiple Sclerosis   183**
    Elias A. Khawam and Matthew Sacco

21. **Cognitive Dysfunction in Multiple Sclerosis** *191*
Stephen M. Rao

22. **Epilepsy, Sleep Disorders, and Transient Neurological Events in Multiple Sclerosis** *199*
Burhan Z. Chaudhry and Alexander D. Rae-Grant

23. **Eye Symptoms, Signs, and Therapy in Multiple Sclerosis** *208*
Collin M. McClelland and Steven L. Galetta

24. **Bulbar and Pseudobulbar Dysfunction in Multiple Sclerosis** *218*
Devon S. Conway

25. **Pain Management in Multiple Sclerosis** *225*
John F. Foley, Ryan R. Metzger, Kara Menning, Cortnee Roman, and Emily N. Stuart

26. **Upper Extremity Function in Multiple Sclerosis** *232*
Christine Smith and Kathleen M. Zackowski

27. **Bladder and Bowel Dysfunction in Multiple Sclerosis** *242*
Courtenay K. Moore

28. **Sexual Dysfunction and Other Autonomic Disorders in Multiple Sclerosis** *253*
Samantha Domingo and Carolyn Fisher

29. **Spasticity Management in Multiple Sclerosis** *259*
Francois Bethoux and Mary Alissa Willis

30. **Multiple Sclerosis and Mobility** *268*
Francois Bethoux, Jacob J. Sosnoff, and Keith McKee

31. **General Health and Wellness in Multiple Sclerosis** *279*
Mary R. Rensel, Brandon P. Moss, and Carrie M. Hersh

32. **Complementary and Alternative Medicine: Practical Considerations** *289*
Allen C. Bowling

PART V. Special Issues

33. **Pediatric Multiple Sclerosis** *296*
Amy T. Waldman

34. **Women's Issues** *310*
Megan E. Esch, Bridgette Jeanne Billioux, and Ellen M. Mowry

35. **Multiple Sclerosis and Associated Comorbidities** *324*
Yuval Karmon, Caila B. Vaughn, Shumita Roy, Svetlana Primma Eckert, and Bianca Weinstock-Guttman

36. **Work, Insurance, and Disability Issues in Multiple Sclerosis** *334*
Matthew H. Sutliff and Deborah M. Miller

37. **Caregiving in Multiple Sclerosis** *343*
Amy Burleson Sullivan

Part VI. Related Diseases

38. **Neuromyelitis Optica** *351*
Amanda L. Piquet and John R. Corboy

39. **Acute Disseminated Encephalomyelitis** *363*
Eliza Gordon-Lipkin and Brenda Banwell

40. **Transverse Myelitis** *372*
Isabella Strozzi and Michael Levy

41. **Autoimmune Encephalitis** *380*
Michel Toledano

42. **Neurosarcoidosis** *394*
Brandon P. Moss and Jinny Tavee

Index *405*

Contributors

Laura E. Baldassari, MD, MHS
Clinical Neuroimmunology Fellow
Mellen Center for MS Treatment and Research
Cleveland Clinic Foundation
Cleveland, Ohio

Brenda Banwell, MD, FRCPC, FAAN
Chief of Child Neurology
The Children's Hospital of Philadelphia
Professor of Neurology and Pediatrics
Perelman School of Medicine
University of Pennsylvania
Philadelphia, Pennsylvania

Robert A. Bermel, MD
Staff Neurologist and Director
Mellen Center for MS Treatment and Research
Neurological Institute
Cleveland Clinic Foundation
Cleveland, Ohio

Francois Bethoux, MD
Professor, Cleveland Clinic Lerner College of Medicine
Director of Rehabilitation Services
Mellen Center for MS Treatment and Research
Cleveland Clinic Foundation
Cleveland, Ohio

Bridgette Jeanne Billioux, MD
Neurology Chief Resident Physician
Department of Neurology
Johns Hopkins University School of Medicine
Baltimore, Maryland

Adrienne Boissy, MD, MA
Chief Experience Officer, Office of Patient Experience
Staff Neurologist
Mellen Center for MS Treatment and Research
Cleveland Clinic Foundation
Cleveland, Ohio

Allen C. Bowling, MD, PhD
Physician Associate
Colorado Neurological Institute
Englewood, Colorado
Clinical Professor of Neurology
Department of Neurology
University of Colorado
Aurora, Colorado

Aliye O. Bricker, MD
Clinical Assistant Professor
Department of Radiology
Cleveland Clinic Foundation
Cleveland, Ohio

Amy Burleson Sullivan, PsyD
Clinical Health Psychologist
Director of Behavioral Medicine, Research,
   Training
Mellen Center for MS Treatment and Research
Cleveland Clinic Foundation
Cleveland, Ohio

Peter A. Calabresi, MD
Professor of Neurology
Director of the Richard T. Johnson
   Division of Neuroimmunology and
   Neurological Infections
Director
Johns Hopkins Multiple Sclerosis Center
Johns Hopkins University School of Medicine
Baltimore, Maryland

Burhan Z. Chaudhry, MD
Assistant Professor, Neurology
Tulane University
New Orleans, Louisiana

Jeffrey A. Cohen, MD
Professor, Cleveland Clinic Lerner College of Medicine
Staff Neurologist
Mellen Center for MS Treatment and Research
Cleveland Clinic Foundation
Cleveland, Ohio

Devon S. Conway, MD, MS
Staff Neurologist
Mellen Center for MS Treatment and Research
Cleveland Clinic Foundation
Cleveland, Ohio

John R. Corboy, MD
Professor and Executive Vice-Chair of Neurology
Co-Chief of the Neuroimmunology/MS Division
Co-Director of the Rocky Mountain Multiple Sclerosis
    Center at Anschutz Medical Campus
University of Colorado School of Medicine
Aurora, Colorado

Bruce A. C. Cree, MD, PhD, MAS
Professor of Clinical Neurology
Clinical Research Director
UCSF Multiple Sclerosis Center
San Francisco, California

Samantha Domingo, PsyD
Psychologist, Internal Medicine
Samaritan Health Services
Corvallis, Oregon

Svetlana Primma Eckert, MD
Fellow
Department of Neurology
State University of New York at Buffalo
Buffalo, New York

Megan E. Esch, MD
Clinical Fellow, Neuroimmunology
Department of Neurology
Johns Hopkins University
Baltimore, Maryland

Jenny J. Feng, MD
Resident Physician
Department of Neurology
Cleveland Clinic Foundation
Cleveland, Ohio

Carolyn Fisher, PhD, BCB
Psychologist
Department of Psychiatry and Psychology
Cleveland Clinic Foundation
Cleveland, Ohio

John F. Foley, MD
Physician
Rocky Mountain MS Clinic
Salt Lake City, Utah

Robert J. Fox, MD, MSc
Staff Neurologist
Mellen Center for MS Treatment and Research
Vice-Chair for Research
Neurological Institute
Cleveland Clinic Foundation
Cleveland, Ohio

Steven L. Galetta, MD
Phillip K. Moskowitz, MD, Professor and Chair
Department of Neurology
NYU Langone Medical Center
New York, New York

Eliza Gordon-Lipkin, MD
Department of Neurology and Developmental Medicine
Kennedy Krieger Institute and Johns Hopkins School
    of Medicine
Baltimore, Maryland

Claire Hara-Cleaver, MSN, CNP
Neurological Nurse Practitioner
Mellen Center for MS Treatment and Research
Cleveland Clinic Foundation
Cleveland, Ohio

Carrie M. Hersh, DO, MSc
Staff Neurologist
Mellen Program for Multiple Sclerosis
Lou Ruvo Center for Brain Health
Cleveland Clinic Foundation
Las Vegas, Nevada

Le H. Hua, MD
Eric and Sheila Samson Chair for Multiple Sclerosis Research
Director, Mellen Program for Multiple Sclerosis
Lou Ruvo Center for Brain Health
Cleveland Clinic Foundation
Las Vegas, Nevada

Megan H. Hyland, MD, MS
Assistant Professor
Department of Neurology
University of Rochester Medical Center
Rochester, New York

Stephen E. Jones, MD, PhD
Assistant Professor
Department of Radiology
Cleveland Clinic Foundation
Cleveland, Ohio

Christopher J. Karakasis, MD
Clinical Assistant Professor
Department of Radiology
Cleveland Clinic Foundation
Cleveland, Ohio

Yuval Karmon, MD
Multiple Sclerosis and Neuroimmunology Clinic
Meir Medical Center
Kfar Saba, Israel

Elias A. Khawam, MD
Staff Psychiatrist
Cleveland Clinic Foundation
Cleveland, Ohio

Marcus W. Koch, MD, PhD
Assistant Professor
Department of Clinical Neurosciences
University of Calgary
Calgary, Alberta, Canada
Staff Neurologist
Calgary Multiple Sclerosis Clinic
Calgary, Alberta, Canada

Michael D. Kornberg, MD, PhD
Assistant Professor, Neurology
Richard T. Johnson Division of Neuroimmunology and
    Neurological Infections
Johns Hopkins University School of Medicine
Baltimore, Maryland

Michael Levy, MD, PhD
Associate Professor, Johns Hopkins University
Director, Neuromyelitis Optica Clinic
Department of Neurology
Johns Hopkins University School of Medicine
Baltimore, Maryland

Don J. Mahad, MD
Senior Clinical Lecturer
Centre for Clinical Brain Sciences
Anne Rowling Regenerative Neurology Clinic
Centre for Neuroregeneration
University of Edinburgh
Edinburgh, United Kingdom

Kedar R. Mahajan, MD, PhD
Clinical Neuroimmunology Fellow
Mellen Center for MS Treatment and Research
Cleveland Clinic Foundation
Cleveland, Ohio

Collin M. McClelland, MD
Department of Ophthalmology and Visual Neurosciences
University of Minnesota
Minneapolis, Minnesota

Marisa P. McGinley, DO
Associate Staff
Mellen Center for MS Treatment and Research
Cleveland Clinic Foundation
Cleveland, Ohio

Keith McKee, MD
Associate Staff
Mellen Center for MS Treatment and Research
Cleveland Clinic Foundation
Cleveland, Ohio

Kara Menning, FNP-C
Family Nurse Practitioner
Rocky Mountain MS Clinic
Salt Lake City, Utah

Ryan R. Metzger, PhD
Research Scientist
Rocky Mountain MS Clinic
Salt Lake City, Utah

Deborah M. Miller, PhD, LISW-S
Professor, Staff
Mellen Center for MS Treatment and Research
Cleveland Clinic Foundation
Cleveland, Ohio

Courtenay K. Moore, MD
Associate Professor of Surgery
Glickman Urological Institute, Section of Female Pelvic
    Medicine and Reconstructive Surgery
Cleveland Clinic Foundation
Cleveland, Ohio

Brandon P. Moss, MD
Neuroimmunology Fellow
Mellen Center for MS Treatment and Research
Cleveland Clinic Foundation
Cleveland, Ohio

Ellen M. Mowry, MD, MCR
Staff Clinical Health Psychologist
Mellen Center for MS Treatment and Research
Cleveland Clinic Foundation
Cleveland, Ohio

T. Jock Murray MD, FRCPC, MACP
Professor Emeritus
Dalhousie University
Halifax, Nova Scotia, Canada

Scott D. Newsome, DO, MSCS, FAAN
Associate Professor of Neurology
Director, Neurosciences Consultation and Infusion Center
  at Green Spring Station
Director, Stiff Person Syndrome Center
Johns Hopkins University School of Medicine
Baltimore, Maryland

Aaron Nicka, MS, OT
Occupational Therapist
Mellen Center for MS Treatment and Research
Cleveland Clinic Foundation
Cleveland, Ohio

Daniel Ontaneda, MD, MSc
Staff Neurologist
Mellen Center for MS Treatment and Research
Cleveland Clinic Foundation
Cleveland, Ohio

Amanda L. Piquet, MD
Assistant Professor of Neurology
University of Colorado School of Medicine
Aurora, Colorado

Matthew Plow, PhD
Associate Professor
Frances Payne Bolton School of Nursing
Case Western Reserve University
Cleveland, Ohio

Alexander D. Rae-Grant, MD, FRCP(C)
Staff Neurologist
Director of MS Education
Mellen Center for MS Treatment and Research
Cleveland Clinic Foundation
Cleveland, Ohio

Stephen M. Rao, PhD
Ralph and Luci Schey Endowed Chair
Director, Schey Center for Cognitive Neuroimaging
Lou Ruvo Center for Brain Health, Neurological Institute
Professor
Cleveland Clinic Lerner College of Medicine
Cleveland Clinic Foundation
Cleveland, Ohio

Mary R. Rensel, MD, FAAN
Director of Wellness, Assistant Professor of Medicine CCLCM
Mellen Center for MS Treatment and Research
Cleveland Clinic Foundation
Cleveland, Ohio

Cortnee Roman, FNP-C
Family Nurse Practitioner
Rocky Mountain MS Clinic
Salt Lake City, Utah

Shumita Roy, PhD
Department of Neurology
State University of New York at Buffalo
Buffalo, New York

Matthew Sacco, PhD
Associate Staff Psychologist, Behavioral Medicine
Cleveland Clinic Foundation
Cleveland, Ohio

Thomas Shoemaker, MD
Fellow
Johns Hopkins Multiple Sclerosis Center
Johns Hopkins University School of Medicine
Baltimore, Maryland

Andrew L. Smith, MD, MHA, MCRS
Staff Neurologist
University of Minnesota Multiple Sclerosis Center
Minneapolis, Minnesota

Christine Smith, OTR/L, MSCS
Coordinator of Occupational Therapy
Holy Name Medical Center
Teaneck, New Jersey

Jacob J. Sosnoff, PhD
Professor
Department of Kinesiology and Community Health
College of Applied Health Sciences
University of Illinois at Urbana-Champaign
Urbana, Illinois

Lael A. Stone, MD
Staff Neurologist
Mellen Center for MS Treatment and Research
Cleveland Clinic Foundation
Cleveland, Ohio

Isabella Strozzi, MD
Research Fellow
Neuromyelitis Optica Clinic
Department of Neurology
Johns Hopkins University School of Medicine
Baltimore, Maryland

Emily N. Stuart, BS
Clinical Research Coordinator
Rocky Mountain MS Clinic
Salt Lake City, Utah

Matthew H. Sutliff, PT, DPT, MSCS
Physical Therapist/Clinical Team Leader
Mellen Center for MS Treatment and Research
Cleveland Clinic Foundation
Cleveland, Ohio

Jinny Tavee, MD
Associate Professor
Medical Director, Neuromuscular Division
Department of Neurology
Northwestern University Feinberg School of
  Medicine
Chicago, Illinois

Michel Toledano, MD
Senior Associate Consultant, Neurology
Mayo Clinic
Rochester, Minnesota

Caila B. Vaughn, PhD
Clinical Assistant Professor
Department of Neurology
State University of New York at Buffalo
Buffalo, New York

Amy T. Waldman, MD, MSCE
Assistant Professor of Neurology (Pediatrics)
Perelman School of Medicine at the University of
  Pennsylvania
Children's Hospital of Philadelphia
Philadelphia, Pennsylvania

Bianca Weinstock-Guttman, MD
Professor
Department of Neurology
State University of New York at Buffalo
Buffalo, New York

Mary Alissa Willis, MD
Staff Neurologist
Mellen Center for MS Treatment and Research
Cleveland Clinic Foundation
Cleveland, Ohio

Kathleen M. Zackowski, PhD, OTR, MSCS
Senior Director, Patient Management, Care and
  Rehabilitation Research
National MS Society, New York, New York
Adjunct Associate Professor of Physical Medicine and
  Rehabilitation and Neurology
Johns Hopkins School of Medicine and Kennedy Krieger
  Institute
Baltimore, Maryland

Foreword

The second edition of *Multiple Sclerosis and Related Disorders: Clinical Guide to Diagnosis, Medical Management, and Rehabilitation* is a significant update and expansion of the first edition published in 2013. All of the original topics have been retained, along with the addition of four new topics covering upper extremity function in multiple sclerosis (MS), autoimmune encephalitis, transverse myelitis, and neurosarcoidosis. The previous chapter Disease Modifying Therapies in Relapsing Multiple Sclerosis is now divided into two new chapters covering injectable and oral options, and infusion options, separately. Also, two previous chapters regarding secondary and primary progressive MS have been combined into one new chapter concerning treatment of progressive forms of MS, reflecting recent advances in this area. Almost all of the original authors return in this edition; several new expert authors have been added as well. This makes for a highly cohesive, evolved, current (as of early 2018), and very readable collection of chapter materials covering virtually all aspects of comprehensive MS care. Editors Fox, Rae-Grant, and Bethoux's shared vision of "one readily readable volume [of] the core information that guides day-to-day care in a MS center" has once again been fulfilled, and exceeded.

The introductory five chapters cover the general history, description, pathology, epidemiology, natural history, and genetics of MS. This important section serves as a complete background and context within which subsequent chapters and topics are best considered.

Separate, topic-related keypoint summaries for clinicians and also for patients and families are included in each chapter. Chapters also include one or more patient case examples where appropriate.

The next five chapters concern the efficient and accurate diagnosis of MS. Importantly, the latest 2017 revisions of the McDonald diagnostic criteria are thoroughly covered in a practical and user-friendly fashion. The newer concept of disease phenotyping, determined by the presence or relative absence of disease activity, as an aid to disease-modifying treatment selection and prognosis in relapsing and progressive forms of MS is also reviewed. Advances in magnetic resonance imaging continue to contribute to our understanding of MS disease initiation and progression, and are fully updated, including discussions of MRI protocol standards and importance of MRI

in monitoring disease and treatment efficacy. Additional paraclinical diagnostic tests such as laboratory and serological testing, spinal fluid analysis, optical coherence tomography, and evoked potentials are reviewed. A separate, detailed chapter concerning potential diagnostic pitfalls leading to misidentification of MS is also included.

Six chapters, four completely new, follow that review disease-modifying therapies in relapsing and progressive forms of MS. Approved as well as investigational therapies are discussed, as monitoring and safety considerations.

Symptom management and rehabilitation are each arguably as important as effective disease-modifying therapy programs. Fifteen chapters extensively cover topics such as general health and wellness; cognitive and emotional dysfunction; fatigue; pain; spasticity; paroxysmal and sleep disorders; visual and bulbar dysfunction; bowel, bladder, and sexual dysfunction; autonomic disorders; upper extremity function, and ambulation issues. Complementary and alternative medical treatment approaches and their practical considerations are well reviewed.

Additional important chapters reviewing pediatric MS, women's issues, associated comorbidities, and insurance and disability issues are included, as well as two comprehensive reviews of relationship-centered care in comprehensive care centers, and caregiving in MS.

Finally, whereas the focus of this text is primarily MS, other related neuroimmunological or neuroinflammatory disorders such as acute disseminated encephalomyelitis, autoimmune encephalitis, neuromyelitis optica, neurosarcoidosis, transverse myelitis are each considered in separate chapters.

Running throughout the chapters of this text, as with the first edition, is a well-placed emphasis on MS as a chronic illness and process that extends substantially beyond accurate and timely diagnosis. This text effectively presents in one place not only the many aspects of MS evaluation and treatment, but also the no less important multifaceted aspects of comprehensive MS care.

In my view, this superb second edition does not replace the first, but rather updates, expands, and adds substantially to the first. As such, both editions will retain an important place side-by-side on my bookshelf.

J. Theodore Phillips, MD, PhD, FAAN
Santa Fe, New Mexico

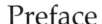

Preface

Findings from the multiple sclerosis (MS) prevalence initiative suggest that up to one million people in the United States are affected by MS and related neuroinflammatory disorders. These conditions, which include MS, neuromyelitis optica, acute disseminated encephalomyelitis, and other neuroimmunological conditions, are a leading cause of disability and work loss in young adults. In the past 25 years, advances in basic neuroimmunology, imaging, and clinical trials have led to a revolution in our understanding of these disorders and a dramatic change in the treatment options available to patients. With these advances comes added complexity in managing MS patients.

In this book, we have focused on key elements a healthcare practitioner needs to know to evaluate and manage MS and related neuroimmunological disorders. Information on disease history, pathophysiology, and biology are included to provide clinicians with a framework for understanding current diagnosis, monitoring, and treatment strategies for these disorders. In addition to reviewing disease-modifying treatments, we have focused on frequent symptoms of MS and their treatment options. Symptoms and functional limitations are the "face of the disease" for our patients and their loved ones, and present their own set of challenges. Assessment tools and treatment options for symptom management and rehabilitation have also evolved and become increasingly complex. An interesting recent development is the contribution of comorbidities to MS-related disability and symptoms, and the need to prevent and address these comorbidities as part of a comprehensive management plan. Wellness promotion and patient-centered care are among the growing care strategies than can and should be applied to the management of MS.

Our goal is to put together in one readily readable volume the core information that guides day-to-day care in an MS center. Each chapter is an amalgam of evidence-based data with experience-based guidance, combining the science and art of MS and related disease management. The authors present the approaches to care that they use in their centers.

Where applicable, the authors provide lists of "Key Points" for clinicians as well as "Key Points" for patients and families. These highlights make the "gist" of each chapter clear and immediately available, and also provide a short summary that can be shared with patients. Critical-to-know information and management pearls are pulled out from the text and boxed for quick reference throughout the book. Illustrative cases are included in chapters where appropriate to amplify clinical recommendations.

We have made every effort to update the most recent medication changes, recognizing that this is a very fast changing field and we anticipate new medications in the near future. With this edition we have completely revised chapters on disease-modifying therapies, since there has been tremendous progress in this area. We have added a chapter on upper extremity function and related activities of daily living, and expanded coverage of other neuroinflammatory disorders to include transverse myelitis, autoimmune encephalitis, and neurosarcoidosis. We have tried to show the great changes in our understanding of these conditions, while noting the long and eventful history of MS research and the great debt we owe to our predecessors. We have specifically focused on topics in rehabilitation, symptom management, and wellness for MS care as these become paramount when the patient progresses through the disease course, and there have been great advances in the past several years that provide many tools for clinicians to utilize to help patients.

We thank all of our authors for their generous gift of time and effort. Their chapters have been a great learning opportunity for the editors, and we hope this volume provides useful clinical guidance for the many clinicians caring for these neurological disorders. We thank the patients and their families for teaching us, case by case, what we need to know about their care, and for working with us in a collaborative way to guide the course of our future efforts.

Robert J. Fox, MD, MSc
Alexander D. Rae-Grant, MD, FRCP(C)
Francois Bethoux, MD

1

History of Multiple Sclerosis

T. Jock Murray

Multiple sclerosis (MS) is well known to the general public but was only defined as a separate disorder of the nervous system in the middle of the 19th century. Initially it was thought to be a rare disorder, but soon clinicians became aware that it was the most common serious neurological disorder that occurs in young adults. This brief introduction to the history of MS shows how ideas and knowledge developed and how it moved from a feeling of hopelessness to a now exciting and therapeutic era (1).

EARLY CASES OF MS

Perhaps the earliest case suggestive of multiple sclerosis (MS) was that of Saint Lidwina van Schiedam (1380–1433) who developed a relapsing and progressive neurological disease. She was documented by the Catholic Church when she was considered for canonization (1). The best described and most convincing case is that of Augustus d'Esté (1794–1848), the grandson of George III, documented over decades in his diary (2). It is a remarkable record of a man's struggle with the disease and the various therapies used by the physicians in the early 19th century. Margaret Gatty (1809–1873), a popular Victorian writer of children's books and a respected guide to British seaweeds, developed a "nervous disorder" at age 41, with weakness and incoordination in her hand, and intermittent and eventually progressive neurological illness, a painful facial tic, and leg weakness. Her physician described her case in *The Lancet* (3). Dealing with a long-standing and disabling medical condition that alters one's feelings and attitudes about life, self, and the future is a struggle known to many patients of MS. One who endured the battles, winning some and losing others to this relentless foe, was B. F. Cummings (1889–1919). In his diary, he documented a progressive form of MS and died at age 30, 10 years after the onset of his first symptoms (4). Cummings, who wrote under the pseudonym Barbellion, was referred to a well-known neurologist, "Dr. H.," undoubtedly Sir Henry Head, who "chased me around his consulting room with a drumstick tapping my tendons and cunningly working my reflexes." He thought he could sense his body deteriorating and he always wanted music playing, or he would lie in bed whistling so he would not hear the paralysis creeping and the feeling of gnawing at his spinal cord. His journal, *The Journal of a Disappointed Man* (4), is still in print.

EARLY DESCRIPTIONS OF MS

The first case of MS in the medical literature is described in the textbook on spinal cord diseases by Ollivier d'Angers in 1824 (5). Robert Carswell in 1838 and Jean Cruveilhier in 1842, working separately in the hospitals of Paris, prepared atlases of medical and neurological conditions and both illustrated examples of MS (6,7).

In 1849, Friedrich Theodor von Frerichs (1819–1885), a German clinician-pathologist, made the first clinical diagnosis in a living patient who presented with an acute spinal cord syndrome (8). Although some questioned his diagnosis, he was proven right when his student, Valentiner, did autopsies on some of his cases, demonstrating "the brilliant correctness of the diagnosis" (9).

Frerichs described the characteristics of the disease: (a) the condition is gradual with exacerbations and remissions; (b) one side of the body is involved, then the other; (c) paralysis of the legs occurs early and gets much worse; (d) motor changes are greater than sensory changes; (e) the seat of the disease is in the medulla with disturbances of the ninth, 10th, and 11th cranial nerves; (f) there are frequent psychic episodes and mental changes; (g) sclerosis of the nervous system is more frequent in the young; and (h) general health remains normal for a long time. It is surprising that Frerichs is never given credit for describing the disease, usually accorded later to Charcot. Other early descriptions came from the pathological observations of Ludwig Turck, Carl Rokitansky, Rindfleisch, and E. Leyden.

Although the long shadow of Charcot was prominent in French neurology of the day and he is accorded appropriate credit for making the disease well known, his colleague Edme Felix Alfred Vulpian (1826–1887) collaborated with Charcot and was the first author of the initial paper he and Charcot published on MS. Vulpian first used the term *sclérose en plaque disseminé* for the disorder in 1866. His contributions have been overlooked as the attention has been focused on Charcot's three published lectures on MS in 1868 (10).

DESCRIPTION BY CHARCOT

Charcot in the Salpêtrière hospital in Paris was an expert at documenting the clinical course of patients and correlating their condition with the pathology when they came to autopsy, a method he called the clinicopathological method, which enabled him to publish the initial descriptions of a number of conditions.

His Tuesday clinics and Friday lectures attracted admirers and students from abroad, enhancing the reputation of the Salpêtrière and French neurology. In 1868, he brought together all the clinical and pathological information that had been accumulated on MS by Vulpian and the 12 others who had made observations on the progressive neurological disease in young adults, and his own experience with cases, and gave three lectures on the clinical and pathological features of the condition, giving it a name. He showed the pathology with his own drawing of what he saw under the microscope. Once these were published, other clinicians around the world could recognize the disease and reports appeared in the medical literature of many countries over the next few decades. Charcot's observations were so complete that very little new information was added in the next few decades. Although he called it *sclérose en plaque*, in English-speaking countries it was called *insular sclerosis*, then *disseminated sclerosis*, and finally *multiple sclerosis*.

EARLY MONOGRAPHS

Although Charcot did not publish a great deal on MS—perhaps only 34 cases—his other views on the disease were probably expressed through the writings of his pupils Bourneville and Guérard (11) in the first monograph on the disease, and by Ordenstein (12). Marie, another of Charcot's students, presented 25 cases of MS in his monograph "Insular sclerosis and the infectious diseases" (13). Marie said the causes were well known—fever, overwork, exposure to cold, injury, and excess of every kind. But although these are common precipitants, he said he knew of another cause that is even more important—infection.

EARLY REPORTS

More and more cases of MS were being reported in the medical journals of the world. The first American report was presented by Dr. Morris in 1867 and published the next year, with the pathology by S. Weir Mitchell (14). The patient was a young physician, Dr. Pennock, who had symptoms of heaviness and numbness of his left and later his right leg that progressed so that he could no longer practice medicine and he died in 1867. Mitchell, often referred to as the father of American neurology, commented on the irregular gray translucent spots in the cervical and dorsal spinal cord, mainly in the white matter, and mainly in the lateral columns. Under the microscope he saw a total absence of the nerve tubes and nerve cells in these lesions, and small globules of fat and numerous degenerated fibers. Morris and Mitchell were not aware that they were describing the same disease reported by Charcot that same year, and they suggested no cause for the disease and had no references to other literature on similar conditions.

The first English description of MS appeared in four brief reports in *The Lancet* between 1873 and 1875. These were case reports from Guy's Hospital, and, although they were anonymous, three of the four were said to be under the care of Dr. Moxon. These same patients appeared in a later report by Moxon when he reported eight cases of what he called insular sclerosis, although he knew he was describing the disease published by Charcot (15).

Mitchell's colleague from the Civil War, Hammond, the former surgeon general, published a textbook in 1871 that contained chapters on "Multiple cerebral sclerosis" and "Multiple cerebro-spinal sclerosis" with descriptions of the pathology and referred to Charcot and other French authors on the subject. In his discussion, he mentioned that he had cared for 11 cases (16). Allan McLane Hamilton of New York City published a textbook on neurological conditions that described the picture of cerebrospinal sclerosis, referring to both Sclérose en Plaques Disséminées of Charcot and the insular sclerosis of Moxon (17). With the clear reports of Morris, Hammond, and Hamilton, it is surprising that the credit for the first report of MS in the United States was for many years given to Sequin (18). Other early reports came from Allan McLane in the United States, Samuel Wilks in England, H. MacLauren, Alfred K. Newman, and James Jamison in Australia, and William Osler in Canada (1).

THREE LANDMARK REVIEWS OF MS

Most advances in medicine are recorded by the date of publication of the discovery and remembered in association with the discoverer, but we normally do not recognize that the field can advance by an intelligent review of the state of the art by an expert or by a pivotal meeting. The understanding of MS was advanced significantly by the 1921 meeting of the Association for Research in Nervous and Mental Disease (ARNMD) (19), the reviews by Brain in 1930 (20), and the monograph by McAlpine, Compston, and Lumsden in 1955 (21). These clinicians had tremendous impact, and each clarified what was becoming a confusing state of affairs. Each stood back and looked at the array of ideas and observations and intelligently tried to put them in a reasonable context, emphasizing some views, questioning, or discarding others.

The ARNMD Report of 1922 was a landmark in the understanding of MS (22). It brought together individuals who summarized the state of knowledge at the time and consolidated views. The published report came from a meeting held in New York City, December 27 to 28, 1921. The many papers, some now classics, reviewed the pathology, epidemiology, etiology, and clinical features of the disease. In writing the conclusions to the meeting, the commissioners emphasized that MS was among the most common organic diseases that affected the nervous system. They concluded that there was no particular psychic disorder characteristic of the disease and euphoria was not present in most cases and mental deterioration was often absent. They concluded that there was no solid evidence for a bacteriological cause but expected further experiments on this. The commission took the middle road on the question of whether the disease was an inflammatory or degenerative disease and thought that it might be initially inflammatory and later degenerative.

Brain's remarkable review of the state of understanding of the disease in 1930 brought clarity to an increasingly confused field (20). This was not a consensus; this was the personal conclusion and perception of an outstanding physician about an increasingly confusing field.

Equally influential in summarizing the state of understanding of MS was the first major textbook of the disease, *Multiple Sclerosis* by McAlpine, Compston, and Lumsden in 1955 (21). The book was based on 1,072 cases accumulated by McAlpine, collated painstakingly by Compston, who wrote the first draft. Lumsden wrote the pathology section. In the last half of the 20th century, this was the major single reference about the disease (23).

THEORIES ABOUT CAUSATION

In the initial descriptions of this disease by Ollivier, Frerichs, Turck, and others, there was a limited speculation as to the cause, other than that it was sometimes associated with acute fevers or exposure to dampness and cold. Marie was adamant that this was due to infections. Lewellys F. Barker discussed the exogenous causes of MS at the 1921 ARNMD meeting and said that infection and heat were more likely aggravating factors rather than the cause. He added there was little support for Oppenheim's belief in an environmental toxin and he was skeptical about trauma as a cause.

By 1950, the list of possible etiological factors was narrowing. There was no longer a strong belief in factors such as stress, cold and dampness, trauma, heavy metal poisoning, or other external toxins. Reese summarized the thought in the mid-century by stating that there were two possibilities: a transmissible agent, either a virus or a chemical agent; or a particular reaction of the nervous system to many causes.

SEARCH FOR AN INFECTION

At the end of the 19th century, a belief in an infectious etiology of MS was widely held. Marie believed that the advances of Pasteur and Koch would eventually lead to a vaccine for the disease. Because there were limited specific medicines or therapies for infection at that time, general approaches to treatment were used. When the advances in therapy of syphilis were announced by Erlich, these approaches were applied to MS, not because physicians thought MS was syphilis (they would repeatedly point out that it was not) but because both diseases affected wide areas of the central nervous system (CNS) so it seemed logical to apply one's therapy to the other. Antisyphilitic therapies would be used

until World War II. Great discoveries were being made in the area of infectious disease around the turn of the century and many of the approaches were applied to MS.

One of the puzzling stories in MS research relates to transmission experiments, when attempts were made to transmit the disease to animals. W. E Bullock, L. Kuhn and G. Steiner, E. Siemerling, G. Marinesco, and J. Petit, all reported transmitting neurological disease like MS to animals using brain tissue or cerebrospinal fluid (CSF) from MS patients. But each time a report was made, others were unsuccessful in reproducing the same results. Dr. Teague of the New York Neurological Institute summarized this work at the 1921 ARNMD meeting on MS (24). At this point, five investigators concluded that it was an infectious transmissible disease, and four opposed this view on the basis of their negative findings. He concluded there was nothing convincing about the transmission experiments. Interest grew in a viral cause when two articles appeared in *The Lancet* in 1930. Chevassut, who worked under the supervision of Sir Purves-Stewart, claimed that she could recover a virus from 90% of MS patients (25). A companion paper by her mentor, Purves-Stewart, named the virus *Spherula insularis* and he announced the production of an autogenous vaccine that he had already given to 128 people with MS, 70 of whom were followed up long enough to yield results. Of the 70 cases, 40 had demonstrated improvement (26). It would seem that they had not only discovered the cause of MS but also developed a vaccine that produced clinical improvement. There was widespread quiet skepticism by the neurological community, and it became more vocal as they presented their work at medical meetings. Carmichael (27) was asked to investigate the research methods and results in their laboratory. He concluded there was nothing of merit in this, and later it was apparent that Miss Chevassut had been faking the results.

The story did not end easily as transmission reports continued until the 1950s (28,29).

When Gajdusek and others (30) formulated the concept of a slow virus in neurological disease, one that could infect cells and after a very long incubation period of years cause disease, MS was considered a prime suspect. However, all transmission experiments failed. The neurological community was disturbed to read in 1994 that a prominent German neurologist had carried out unethical experiments that involved the transmission of MS materials to humans during World War II (the Schaltenbrand experiments) (31). At present, many believe, as did Gowers a century earlier, that the virus, if present, is probably a triggering agent rather than the cause.

EPIDEMIOLOGY

It was apparent early on that the disease was not as rare as Charcot and others thought, as larger and larger numbers of patients were being accumulated in hospitals and clinics in Germany, France, Austria, and the United States. There was confusing information about gender distribution, as some investigators were reporting many more men, others equal numbers, and some more women. It is puzzling that a 1922 review of 26 studies of MS showed a consistent male predominance of 58% to 42% female (32). Six of the studies showed a slight female predominance but most showed a male predominance. Although there had been suggestions of MS occurring more in some occupations and social classes, this was not borne out in subsequent studies. By mid-century, Kurland concluded after reviewing the studies that the numbers of men and women with MS were equal (33). At present, we understand that the female-to-male ratio is 2.5:1 and in some recent studies 3:1. It remains to be determined if the early results are a reporting anomaly or if the demography is changing.

Bramwell (34) found a rate of 20 and later 32/1,000 neurological cases in Scotland. Rates varied from 27/1,000 patients in Manchester to 60/1,000 in a more rigidly selected group of neurological patients at the National Hospital for the Paralyzed and Epileptics in London. Repeatedly, it was commented that MS was much less frequent in the United States than in Europe. It was clear that Scandinavians had a higher incidence in many of the studies and that blacks had a low rate, although they were not immune, and the disease was less common in Japan.

Davenport gave an important review of geographical distribution in 1921 (32). He noted high rates in adjacent northern U.S. states, and wondered if that could be related to the many Swedes and Finns who live in that part of the country. He found higher rates in urban communities and in those with higher white to black populations, and in those who lived near the sea rather than the mountains. Since the 1950s it has been known that MS has an unusual geographical distribution. It increases in frequency with geographical latitude, both in the Northern and Southern hemispheres. Alter noted that the geographical distribution above and below the equator had a parabolic gradient that increased sharply with latitude, and that although the curve dramatically increased at increasing latitudes, it appeared to be lower or absent in very far north and south latitudes (35). In Europe, the incidence of MS was highest in the central European areas and lower both north and south of that area.

The highest rates have been recorded in the Shetland and Orkney Islands off the coast of Scotland. Perhaps the geographical distribution of MS in the world and the increasing prevalence farther away from the equator is related to where those with Nordic ancestry migrated. Those migrating from northern and central Europe were more likely to go to more temperate climes than warm or equatorial areas.

In all the studies, there was surprising uniformity in the clinical features of MS, regardless of the geography or the incidence of the area. Some variations were noticed, with a higher incidence of Devic's disease in India and Japan and higher rates of transverse myelopathy and optic neuropathy in the Orientals.

Whenever there are groups or clusters of MS cases, it is tempting to look for an association that might explain the occurrence. The Faroes are a small number of Danish islands between Iceland and Norway, settled by the Norse Vikings over a millennium ago. Intensive search for all cases on the Faroe Islands in the 1970s revealed 25 cases among native-born residents up to 1977 (36). All had the onset between 1943 and 1960 except for one case that had an onset in 1970. The 24 cases met the criteria for a point-source epidemic. Kurtzke, in 1979, suggested that this constituted an epidemic related to the introduction of British troops (or their baggage) and wondered if these were so, then MS was a transmissible disease and infection, with only one in 500 of the exposed individuals being affected.

GENETICS OF MS

Virtually all the early authors noted familial cases but thought it was rare, and each downplayed the importance of these occasional cases. Convincing evidence of a genetic factor had been noted by Curtius in Germany in 1933, showing that MS was 10 times more common in families with MS than in the general population (37). MacKay surveyed all such reports from 1896 to 1948 and demonstrated that this was not an occasional or unimportant factor (38). He documented all familial cases reported from Eichdorst's report in 1896 to the literature in 1948. He later showed a concordance rate of 23% in monozygotic twins, clearly indicating a genetic factor, later confirmed by Canadian and British studies.

VASCULAR THEORY

Early investigators such as Reinfleisch noted the presence of a vessel in the middle of most plaques. Marie believed that the vascular change was secondary to an infection, but others speculated that a thrombotic or vasospastic change might be the primary cause of the plaque. Following the discovery of effective anticoagulants a few years earlier, anticoagulants were used as a treatment for MS but interest in this approach rapidly declined. Speculation on a vascular basis for MS would again arise when Swank and others postulated a dietary factor in MS related to high fat intake affecting vascular flow (39). The treatment would logically be a diet low in animal fat (Swank diet). Putnam proposed anticoagulants for the treatment of MS on the basis of the possibility that there was a thrombosis in the vessel found in the center of a plaque. A vascular theory was again revived with the current interest in chronic cerebrospinal venous insufficiency (CCSVI) postulated by Dr. Paolo Zamboni in 2009.

THE IMMUNOLOGICAL THEORY

The possibility that MS could be due to a hypersensitivity reaction dates back to the observation of Glanzmann, who noted postinfectious CNS involvement in chicken pox, smallpox, and vaccinations (40). The creation of a model of experimental allergic encephalomyelitis (EAE) in 1933 by Rivers, Sprunt, and Berry seemed to strongly support the possibility that a similar process could be operating in MS (41). Variations on the EAE model are still used to assess possible changes and effects in MS and to assess the likelihood that drugs might be effective in the disease. For years there were arguments that EAE was not MS, but it has been an important and lasting model for the study of processes that probably occur in the human disease as well.

Research on the immunology of MS has been extensive over the years. Ebers, who recently reviewed the background and theory of immunology in MS, reported a comment of Helmut Bauer that more than 7,000 papers have been written on this topic. Much of the current therapy is based on modifying the immune system (42).

MS PLAQUE

Early writers speculated little on the nature of the gray softenings they saw and felt in the spinal cords of their patients and did not examine these areas with a microscope. Charcot, who used the microscope, believed that an overgrowth of glia was the specific abnormality and that the glia damaged the myelin sheaths and sometimes the axons. Local vascular changes were presumed to be secondary to the glial overgrowth and the breakdown of nerve tissue that was followed by macrophage removal of lipid products of myelin. His student, Joseph Babinski, also thought it was a demyelinating process, even though one of Charcot's drawings shows the appearance of remyelination, with thin layers of myelin surrounding the axon and fat granule cells removing the myelin debris. Dawson (43) believed that the process occurring in the shadow plaques was demyelination, but believed the vascular change shown earlier by Rindfleisch (44) was the primary pathology. Marie (13) admitted the importance of the vascular element but believed the cause to be an infection. Early on there was a significant focus on the glia; even Charcot considered the glia feature at first, with everything else being secondary to it. Rindfleisch (44) thought that the principal abnormality was a vascular abnormality, although he did acknowledge that the glia were involved. McDonald and his colleagues showed that the remyelinated axon had distinct morphological features and that these nerves had slowed conduction with a reduced safety factor (45). Later diagnostic tests (evoked potential studies) capitalized on the slowing of remyelinated central nerve fibers.

Once it was understood that nerves could demyelinate in MS, but could remyelinate again, it begged the question of why the disease progressed. Even if nerves had thin myelin and conducted slowly, reasonable function should continue. There must be some other factors that limit the process and cause the disease to eventually, and sometimes primarily, progress. The reason, noted by Charcot and others, is that not only myelin is damaged, but also axons are often damaged and lost.

INVESTIGATIONS

Despite the development of elegant investigative techniques for the confirmation of MS, the clinical history and examination continue to be the gold standard for the diagnosis. Early on, however, efforts were made to complement the clinical assessment. The first important advance was the identification of increased gamma globulin in the CSF of MS patients by Hinton in 1922 (46). The most characteristic change was the gold chloride test, with 50% of the fluids showing a paretic curve and 20% a luetic curve. Elvin Kabat used electrophoresis to look at MS CSF and suggested that the increased proportion of gamma globulin probably indicated immunological process occurring in MS (47).

Ventricular enlargement and cortical atrophy could be seen on pneumoencephalography, and myelography could demonstrate expansion of the cord in an area of transverse myelitis, but these were not useful diagnostic tests in most cases. Radionuclide scans occasionally showed evidence of breakdown in the blood–brain barrier. PET scanning showed some variations from a normal group, but this is not a helpful diagnostic method in MS.

With the advent of CT scanning in the 1970s, efforts were made to use this technique in MS (48). Studies showed that 9% to 75% of patients had enhancing lesions, depending on how selective the cases were, but the main advantage was the ability to rule out other conditions.

The major advance in diagnosis was made by the collaborative work of Isidor Rabi, Norman F. Ramsey, Edward M. Purcell, Felix Bloch, Nicholas Blomembergen, Richard R. Ernst, Raymond V. Damadian, and Paul C. Lauterbur, who were the pioneers of MRI. Damadian and Lauterbur were responsible for applying the technique clinically. Although arguments continue about who made the major contributions and who was the foremost pioneer, in the end it is the nature of modern innovations to be made by many individuals from many disciplines who ultimately remain anonymous (49).

In 1981, Young and his colleagues at the Hammersmith Postgraduate Hospital published the striking pictures of MS lesions seen by MRI (50). They showed the difference between the picture of CT and MRI in the same patient. The CT scan was normal but five lesions were clearly demonstrable on the MRI. He predicted "The technique may also prove a measure of the severity of disease … and thus be used to monitor the effectiveness of therapeutic regimens." A further study compared the lesions seen in 10 patients (eight definite and two possible MS patients) and saw 19 lesions on CT but 112 additional lesions more on MRI. Since then the characteristics of the lesions in MS have been better defined and the technology of MRI has improved year by year.

In 1986, Grossman showed that the enhancing agent gadolinium-DPTA caused some lesions to enhance while others did not (51). He indicated that the enhancement identified the breakdown of the blood–brain barrier, which indicated areas of inflammation. It then became an important technique to demonstrate new and active MS lesions, effectively monitoring the disease activity, which became important in subsequent clinical trials of new drugs for MS. The technology of MRI continues to improve and the next few years will see further advances.

Based on the increasing knowledge of the slower conduction in demyelinated and remyelinated nerves, the evoked potential technology was developed for the visual system, the auditory–brainstem system and the sensory–cortical system (52). These are useful, especially when they can demonstrate another area of involvement and confirm that there are lesions in different areas of the nervous system. In practice, only the visual evoked potential studies are of practical use, and are now infrequently used, replaced in many instances by ocular coherence tomography (OCT).

COGNITIVE CHANGES IN MS

Until recent times there was a tendency to suggest to MS patients that mental changes were not a feature of the disease, but cognitive and emotional changes have in fact been noted throughout the known history of the disease, noted by Cruveilhier, Vulpian, Frerichs, Valentiner, Charcot, Morris, Sequin, Wilks, Osler, Gowers, and others. There was controversy about how common this was, and whether it was a reaction to the emotional stress of the disease, due to the demyelinating lesions in the nervous system, or perhaps both.

Cottrel and Wilson evaluated the mental and emotional changes in MS (53). This was the first effort to address the methodology of performing such studies and used representative samples, successive cases, operational definitions, reliable data collection techniques, such as semi-structured interviews, and data analysis. They did not specifically measure cognitive changes, although they discussed these features in their patients. They discussed "spes sclerotica," "eutonia sclerotica," "euphoria sclerotica," and emotional lability as characteristic of MS. They believed that 70% had some degree of euphoria due to organic changes, but cognitive change was said to be rare. Ombredane attempted a systematic assessment of MS patients in Paris hospitals for his MD thesis (54), and although influential in shaping the thinking about cognitive changes in MS, an analysis of his results suggests that there were too many hidden factors in his data to make any conclusions of correlation of emotional change and intellectual change (55). In 1938, Arbuse reviewed the literature on psychiatric aspects of MS and concluded that mild euphoria was present in most people with MS and that inappropriate laughter and crying was not infrequent (56). Borberg and Zahle agreed that in their series of 330 patients "light euphoria" was the most common psychological symptom (57). A number of reviews of euphoria have suggested that it is a reflection of organic change, probably in the periventricular areas, but occurring in only 10% of patients (58).

Although better neuropsychometric techniques were developed, it was difficult to compare studies as they reflected different approaches and different schools of thought, and often were not based on a solid epidemiological approach. Since Charcot's descriptions, the observations about cognitive and emotional change have moved from broad case-based generalizations about the MS patient to detailed, specific studies of emotional trauma, memory, and depression. More recently, MRI has allowed speculation about the localization of specific mental changes.

Only in the last three decades have we seen more clarity of definition and approach in the use of various psychometric techniques, requiring specific tools which took into account timing of tasks and confounding factors such as depression and fatigue. Paradoxically, as we learn to separate and more effectively measure the cognitive changes and the affective changes, the separation has made it possible to learn how they are linked.

THERAPY

In a disease with fluctuation, recovery from attacks and spontaneous remissions, it is no surprise that any attempt at therapy might appear to work, when it may just be the natural history of the condition. In addition, there is a strong placebo effect in any chronic, distressing, threatening, and unpredictable disease. Although 19th century physicians were gloomy in their conclusions about therapy, they all had a list of remedies that they tried, often the same ones they would use in any chronic or serious disease. Some treatments were those applied to any serious neurological disease, and others were based on the current theory of what might be causing the disease. To a great extent, the belief changed with the major scientific medical interest at the time. In the late 19th century, it centered around the possibility of infection. Although this concept did not disappear, suspicion of a vascular cause, and later an immunological cause, and our current interest in a genetic cause, all reflect the major interest in medical science of the times.

The physician to Saint Lidwina in the 15th century thought the disease came from God so he advised against expensive therapies as it would just impoverish her father. Although his physicians were puzzled by his nervous condition, d'Esté in the early 19th century was treated with a continuing array of therapies such as leeches, purges, venesection, liniments, spa waters, and a long list of medications, including prescriptions containing mercury, silver, arsenic, iron, antimony, and quinine.

Charcot was similarly negative about the results of treating this disease. At the end of his lecture, when he came to the point of discussing therapy of MS, he said, "After what precedes need I detain you long … the time has not yet come when such a subject can be seriously considered." Marie used therapies that were suitable for sclerotics, such as iodide of potassium or sodium, and for infections, such as mercury.

The late 19th century was an era of polypharmacy and enthusiastic empirical therapies, so it is not surprising that a wide variety of treatments were aimed at improving people with MS. Sir Gowers was not convinced that any treatment worked but still had a list of recommended nerve tonics such as arsenic, nitrate of silver, and quinine in his textbook. He also recommended hydrotherapy, electricity, maintenance of general health, avoidance of depressing influences, and avoidance of pregnancy (59).

Beevor recommended rest and avoidance of worry, and treatments with nerve tonics, strychnine, quinine, iron, cod liver oil, and increasing doses of liquor arsenacalis (60). Russell advocated silver and arsenic, avoidance of stress, cold, and mental and physical fatigue, and limitation of indulgence in "wine and venery" (17).

One of the continuing themes in the writings of the 19th century was the similarities and differences between MS and syphilis. Even though clinicians were aware that MS was not a form of syphilis, all the therapies for syphilis, such as mercury, silver, and potassium iodide, were used on MS patients and in the early 20th century the new salvarsan for syphilis was added, especially when controversial transmission experiments reported a spirochete in the CSF of MS patients.

At the National Hospital, Queens Square, intravenous (IV) typhoid vaccine was given three times a week. If there were severe reactions, intramuscular milk injections were substituted. Denny-Brown said the results were poor and sometimes disastrous, which is not surprising (18). Oppenheim argued that the cause of MS was a toxin such as lead, copper, and zinc, and some unknown factor so he recommended silver nitrate and potassium iodide, mild galvanic current to the back of the head, spa baths at Oeynhausen or Nauheim, and leeches (61). Other therapies included iodides, colloidal silver preparations either by inunction or IV, and intramuscular injections of fibrolysin every 5 to 7 days.

In the 1930s, infection continued to be a primary concern, so tonsillectomy, adenoidectomy, and tooth extraction were commonly used. Tremor was treated with veronal and hyoscine. The most common treatment was arsenic given either by mouth or through injections of cacodylate of soda. Sodium nucleinate was considered helpful. Various spas, warm baths, massage, and methodical exercises were recommended. Constipation was treated with enemas, and incontinence with tincture of belladonna. Spasticity was treated with passive motion, warm baths, and baking, whereas ataxia was treated with Fraenkel exercises. For spastic contractures the Foerster operation was used, even though Foerster himself was not enthusiastic about it.

In the 1930s and 1940s, treatments for tuberculosis were also applied to MS. In the 1940s, immune globulins were used, and in the 1950s antibiotics, Russian vaccine (which appeared to be rabies vaccine), plasma and blood transfusions, and dietary changes were tried out. In the 1970s, antiviral agents and in the 1980s, interferons were assessed as treatments, all on the basis that MS might be an infection.

As well as recommended therapies, there were things to avoid. The ARNMD (1922) meeting recommended avoiding detoxification therapy on the basis of the rejected theories of Oppenheim which argued against the syphilis therapies applied to MS (19). Common recommendations were avoidance of extreme temperatures, stress, and the use of iodides, silver, mercury, neoarsphenamine, and farradic stimulation. Patients should also avoid pregnancy, stress, heavy exertion, and extremes of temperature.

Despite the array of possible treatments, Brain came to one sobering conclusion in 1930: "No mode of therapy is successful enough to achieve, at the most, a greater improvement than might have occurred spontaneously" (20).

When anticoagulants were discovered, Putnam became enthusiastic about the possibility that MS was due to embolic ischemia after some experiments he performed. For the next two decades, he treated his patients with warfarin (62). Denny-Brown said he was more impressed with the dangers of anticoagulants than with their benefits (18).

It is interesting to contemplate the approach to therapy of MS through the years. Therapy might be governed by the concept of etiology, the concept of pathology, the nature of the symptoms, or just the need to offer some kind of help. We also see intertwined the enthusiasm for anything new and the common tendency to extrapolate from a beneficial therapy to another disease.

Adrenocorticotropic Hormone

When steroids became available, they were tried in small doses in MS with unconvincing results, but the popularity of these wonder drugs caused them to persist as a therapy up to the present day. Oral steroids have been studied in repeated trials, without convincing results, since the early 1960s and only shown to have convincing benefit recently when the dosage paralleled the high IV dosage. One of the early proponents of adrenocorticotropic hormone (ACTH) therapy was Dr. Alexander of New York (63). Alexander was a prominent and widely published neurologist who had investigated Nazi medical experiments and helped draft the Nuremburg Code. The long-term therapy with ACTH, the "Alexander Regimen," was widely used even though the prolonged use of ACTH caused many steroid side effects.

ACTH was used extensively for acute attacks. One of the early well-controlled trials of this agent in MS was conducted in 1969 and demonstrated a positive but very modest improvement over placebo. Despite the marginal results, ACTH treatment became the standard for many years, replaced since the mid-1980s with high-dose IV methylprednisolone.

Immunosuppressant Therapy

It would seem logical in a disease that seems to be immunologically mediated to seek therapies that suppress the immune system, but inadequate understanding of the mechanisms led to empirical attempts with many treatments that affect the immune system, such as azathioprine, cyclophosphamide, cyclosporine, sulfinpyrazone, total lymphoid irradiation, and plasmapheresis. Except in very highly selected instances, these therapies have had more complications and side effects than benefit.

Interferons

The interferons were independently discovered by two groups in the 1950s, Issacs and Lindenmann (64) and Nagano and Kojima (65). It had been noted that during a viral infection in tissue culture, a soluble substance was released into the surrounding milieu, and that this tissue culture fluid could be harvested and used to protect other cells. Because this protection "interfered" with the process of the viral infection of the cells, the substance was named *interferon*. Soon after, it was noted that the interferon had antiproliferative and immunomodulatory properties. Three types were recognized, named after the primary cells of their origin: leukocyte interferon, fibroblast interferon, and immune interferon. The first two shared many properties and were later classified as type 1, and the distinct immune interferon was classified as type 2. Later, the type 1 was renamed alpha and beta interferon, whereas type 2 was named gamma interferon. A number of other interferons have subsequently been identified.

The antiproliferative property of the interferons led to an interest in them as a potential anticancer agent. Efforts were made to develop variations by cloning and development of recombinant forms of interferons in the 1970s and early 1980s. The initial promise did not play out, but the work continues and interest in its use in diseases such as MS developed at the same time.

In the early 1980s, Fog, Knobler and his associates, and Jacobs and his associates began to use interferons in the treatment of patients with MS. The early studies were with the Cantell preparation of interferon alpha made from human leukocytes prepared from the Finnish Red Cross Blood Donor Program. The popular press began to talk about a "breakthrough" when word got out that MS treatment trials studies were beginning at the Scripps Clinic in La Jolla, California, and the University of California, San Francisco. The first reports were disappointing because they did not reach statistical significance even though some patients reported feeling better. A third study was carried out by Jacobs and his colleagues in Buffalo, New York, using intrathecal injections of interferon beta (66). Although there were only 10 patients who received the drug and 10 placebo patients, there was a statistically significant reduction in exacerbations and disease severity (66). Limitations were the side effects and the need for intrathecal injections, but it increased the interest in the role of interferons in MS.

A number of important lessons were learned from these three pioneering studies: interferons were not useful in treating acute attacks but were of benefit in reducing the attacks; the side effects might be reduced by more purified recombinant forms; and IV injection was an acceptable method. Studies of different interferons demonstrated that interferon gamma worsened the disease, but evidence accumulated that interferon beta-1a and interferon beta-1b were beneficial.

When sufficient supplies of beta-interferons became available, a multiple sclerosis collaborative research group (MSCRG) was formed by Jacobs using Betaseron in a dose of 8 MIU every second day injected subcutaneously. This resulted in a 30% reduction in the frequency of acute attacks and a 50% reduction in moderate and severe attacks over a period of almost 5 years (67). Aside from the important clinical information, perhaps the most persuasive data came from the MRI data on these patients. Donald Paty had argued that the new technique of MRI should be a part of the study assessment, and this turned out to be the most convincing part of the study. There was a dramatic reduction both in new lesions and in the accumulated lesion burden, as confirmed by the frequent MRI subset analyses of 52 patients at the University of British Columbia.

A major event in the treatment of MS occurred on Friday, March 11, 1993 when the U.S. Food and Drug Administration met to approve Betaseron for marketing in the treatment of MS. Impressed by the clinical but particularly the MRI data, Betaseron was approved in August 1993 by a very rapid process. Berlex Laboratories, the company that produced Betaseron, decided to use a lottery to distribute the drug to those who wanted the new therapy because they initially could not meet the demand. This created a public relations disaster even though it did focus the therapy toward those who were expected to benefit from it. Treatment was initiated if patients had insurance to cover the high cost, or could afford it, and were selected by the lottery to receive it. Fortunately, the supply soon was adequate and the lottery was abandoned.

As commonly occurs in pharmacological research, clinical results were obtained only after more than four decades of painstaking laboratory and then clinical steps over four decades, from the development of interferons to its current demonstration of use in relapsing-progressive MS.

Glatiramer Acetate

Arnon (1996) related the 27-year saga of "persistent research effort, perseverance, and tenacity of purpose" that brought copolymer I, later named Copaxone, to the market (22). Following the production of random copolymers that resembled myelin basic protein in the laboratory of Professor Ephraim Katchalski at the Weitzman Institute in Israel, the team expected these agents to produce encephalitogenic activity, but were surprised that the drug had the capacity to protect against EAE. Dr. Oded Abramsky carried out the first clinical trial in MS patients, and Dr. Helmut Bauer and Dr. Murray Bornstein planned the others. Bornstein carried out three trials that showed a reduction of exacerbations of MS with remarkably few side effects. Production problems delayed availability of the drug but it was approved for the treatment of MS almost one quarter of a century after the drug was produced, a "designer drug" for MS patients.

New Developments in Therapy

Therapies for MS have changed dramatically over the last decade with new agents and increased experience (68). Mitoxantrone was approved for the treatment of MS but reserved for patients who progress rapidly or who fail on other medications. The risks of cardiac effects and leukemia have tempered initial hopes for this drug, and use must be accompanied by careful cardiac and hematological monitoring, and there is a limit to the amount of drug that can be given over the long term.

Natalizumab (Tysabri) has shown impressive results but, again, caution has increased because of cases of progressive multifocal leukoencephalopathy (PML), which has a risk of about one in 1,000 but increases if the person has previously been on an immunosuppressant therapy or is positive for John Cunningham virus (JCV). The risk also increases the longer the patient is on the drug. Use of the drug is now accompanied by testing for JCV and MRI monitoring.

Alternative Therapies: The Parallel System

Alternative medicine (complementary and alternative medicine [CAM]) has always been with us. Therapies that were once in the forefront of medical approaches to symptoms and diseases are now in the list of alternative or complementary therapies, and alternative therapies that are eventually shown to be beneficial enter the realm of medical therapy. Alternative medicine is a different system, based on belief and sometimes long-standing historical and cultural practices, rather than science.

Any chronic disease for which there is not an effective treatment tends to have a lot of alternative approaches to treatment, and MS is a good example. One need only consult the frequently updated *Therapeutic Claims in Multiple Sclerosis* (69) to see the long list of the most frequently used medical and alternative approaches to MS.

Many of these have a long history in conditions other than MS. For example, spa therapy, herbal preparations, stimulants, minerals, detoxification, and rest therapies have been used for over a century and a half in MS, and wax and wane in popularity. Therapy with hyperbaric oxygen was suggested by some early anecdotal reports and uncontrolled use of hyperbaric chambers occurred in many communities, even though subsequent trials showed no benefit in MS.

MULTIPLE SCLEROSIS SOCIETIES

An important impetus for change and encouragement for research in MS in the last half-century has been the formation of MS societies in each country. The first step was taken by Miss Sylvia Lawry, who was distressed about her brother who had been diagnosed with MS and she placed an advertisement in the *New York Times* on May 1, 1945, which stated:

> *Multiple Sclerosis. Will anyone recovered from it please communicate with the patient. T272 Times.*

From the responses it was apparent to Miss Lawry that there should be an organization to foster research into the cause, treatment, and eventual cure of MS. The organization was named the Association for the Advancement of Research into Multiple Sclerosis (AARMS) but a few months later it was changed to the Multiple Sclerosis Society. She then assisted in the organization of MS societies in Canada, Great Britain and Ireland, Australia, and other countries and then a Federation to link all these groups. Much of the research on MS over the last half-century has been sponsored by the MS societies.

REFERENCES

1. Murray TJ. *Multiple Sclerosis: The History of a Disease*. New York, NY: Demos Vermande; 2005.
2. Firth D. *The Case of Augustus d'Esté*. Cambridge, UK: Cambridge University Press; 1948.
3. Maxwell C. *Mrs. Gatty and Mrs. Ewing*. London, UK: Constable and Company Limited; 1949.
4. Barbellion WNP (pseudonym for Cummings BF). *The Journal of a Disappointed Man*. London, UK: Chatto & Windus; 1919.
5. Ollivier CP. *De La Moelle Epiniére et de ses maladies*. Paris, France: Crevot; 1824.
6. Carswell R. *Pathological Anatomy: Illustrations of the Elementary Forms of Disease*. London, UK: Longman, Orme, Brown, Green and Longman; 1938.
7. Cruveilhier J. *Anatomie Pathologique du Corps Humain*. Paris, France: JB Bailière; 1829–1842.
8. Frerichs FT. Ueber Hirnsklerose. *Arch für die Gesamte Medizin*. 1849;10:334–350.
9. Valentiner W. Ueber die Sklerose des Gehirns und Rückenmarks. *Deutsche Klin*. 1856;147–151, 158–162, 167–169.
10. Charcot JM. *Lectures on Diseases of the Nervous System*. G. Sigerson, trans. London, UK: The New Sydenham Society; 1877:158–222 (p. 221).
11. Bourneville DM, Guérard L. *De la sclérose en plaques disséminées*. Paris, France: Delahaye; 1869.
12. Ordenstein L. *Sur la paralysie agitante et la sclérose en plaques generalisées*. Paris, France: Delahaye; 1868.
13. Marie P. *Lectures on Diseases of the Spinal Cord*. Lubbock M, trans. London, UK: New Sydenham Society; 1895, 153:134–136.

14. Morris JC. Case of the late Dr. CW Pennock. *Am J Med Sci.* 1868;56:138–144.
15. Moxon W. Case of insular sclerosis of brain and spinal cord. *Lancet.* 1873;1:236.
16. Hammond WA. Multiple cerebro-spinal sclerosis. In: *A Treatise on Diseases of the Nervous System.* New York, NY: D. Appleton and Co.; 1871:637–653.
17. Russell JSR. Disseminate sclerosis. In: Albutt TC, ed. *A System of Medicine.* Vol. 7. London, UK: Macmillan & Co.; 1899:52–53, 90.
18. Denny-Brown D. Multiple sclerosis: the clinical problem. *Am J Med.* 1952;12:501–509.
19. Association for Research in Nervous and Mental Disease. *Multiple Sclerosis (Disseminated Sclerosis).* New York, NY: Paul B. Hoeber; 1922.
20. Brain WR. Critical review: disseminated sclerosis. *Q J Med.* 1930;23:343–391.
21. McAlpine D, Compston ND, Lumsden CE. *Multiple Sclerosis.* Edinburgh: E & S Livingstone; 1955.
22. Arnon R. The development of Cop I (Copaxone), an innovative drug for the treatment of multiple sclerosis: personal reflections. *Immunol Lett.* 1996;50:1–15.
23. Compston A. Reviewing multiple sclerosis. *Postgrad Med J.* 1992;68(801):507–515.
24. Teague O. Bacteriological investigation of multiple sclerosis. In: Dana CL, Jelliffe SE, Riley HA, Tilney F, Timme W, eds. *Multiple Sclerosis: Association for Research in Nervous and Mental Diseases.* Vol. 2. New York, NY: Paul B. Hoeber; 1922:121–131.
25. Chevassut K. Aetiology of disseminated sclerosis. *Lancet.* 1930;1:522–560.
26. Purves-Stewart J. A specific vaccine treatment in disseminated sclerosis. *Lancet.* 1930;1:560–564.
27. Carmichael EA. The aetiology of disseminate sclerosis: some criticisms of recent work especially with regard to the "Spherula insularis." *Proc R Soc Med.* 1931;34:591–599.
28. Steiner G, Kuhn L. Acute plaques in multiple sclerosis, their pathogenic significance and the role of spirochetes as etiological factors. *J Neuropath Exp Neurol.* 1952;11:343–373.
29. Ichelson RR. Cultivation of spirochetes from spinal fluids of multiple sclerosis cases and negative controls. *Proc Soc Exp Biol (NY).* 1957;95:57–58.
30. Gajdusek DC, Gibbs CJ Jr, Alpers M, eds. *Slow Latent and Temperature Virus Infections.* Washington, DC: U.S. Department of Health, Education and Welfare; 1965.
31. Shevell M, Evans BK. The "Schaltenbrand experiment"—Würzburg, 1940: scientific, historical, and ethical perspectives. *Neurology.* 1944;44:350–356.
32. Davenport C. Multiple sclerosis: from the standpoint of geographic distribution and race. *Arch Neur Psych.* 1922;8:51–58.
33. Kurland LT. Epidemiologic characteristics of multiple sclerosis. *Am J Med.* 1952;21:561–571.
34. Bramwell B. Disseminated sclerosis with special reference to the frequency and etiology of the disease. *Clin Stud.* 1904;2:193–210.
35. Alter M. Clues to the cause based on the epidemiology of multiple sclerosis. In: Field EJ, ed. *Multiple Sclerosis: A Clinical Conspectus.* Baltimore, MD: University Park Press; 1977:35–82.
36. Kurtzke JF, Hyllested K. Multiple sclerosis in the Faroe Islands. 1. Clinical and epidemiological features. *Ann Neurol.* 1979;5:6–21.
37. Curtius F. *Multiple Sklerose and Erbanlage.* Leipzig, Germany: G. Thieme; 1933.
38. MacKay RP. *Multiple Sclerosis and the Demyelinating Diseases. The Familial Occurrence of Multiple Sclerosis and Its Implications.* Baltimore, MD: Williams & Wilkins; 1950.
39. Swank RL. Multiple sclerosis: a correlation of its incidence with dietary fat. *Am J Med Sci.* 1950;220:421–430.
40. Glanzmann FL. Die nervosen komplikationen von varizellen, Variole Vakzine. *Schweiz med Wschr.* 1927;57:145.
41. Rivers TM, Sprunt DH, Berry GP. Observations on attempts to produce acute disseminated encephalomyelitis in monkeys. *J Exp Med.* 1933;58:39–53.
42. Ebers G. Immunology of MS. In: Paty DW, Ebers GC, eds. *Multiple Sclerosis.* Philadelphia, PA: FA Davis; 1999:403–426.
43. Dawson J. The history of disseminated sclerosis. *T Roy Soc Edin.* 1916;50:517–740.
44. Rindfleisch E. Histologische Detail zu der Grauen Degeneration von Gehirn and Rückenmark. *Virchow Arch Path Anat.* 1863;26:474–483.
45. McDonald WI. Pathophysiology of multiple sclerosis. *Brain.* 1974;97:179–196.
46. Hinton WA. CSF in MS. Studies in the cerebrospinal fluid and blood in multiple sclerosis. In: Ayer JB, Foster HE, eds. *Multiple Sclerosis: Association for Research in Nervous and Mental Diseases.* Vol 2. New York, NY: Paul B. Hoeber; 1922:113–121.
47. Kabat EA, Moore DH, Landow H. An electrophoretic study of the protein components in cerebrospinal fluid and their relationship to the serum proteins. *J Clin Invest.* 1942;21:571–577.
48. Cala LA, Mastaglia FL. Computerized axial tomography in multiple sclerosis. *Lancet.* 1976;1:689.
49. Mattson J, Merrill S. *The Pioneers of NMR and Magnetic Resonance in Medicine.* The story of MRI. Jericho, NJ: Bar-Ilan University Press/Dean Books Company; 1996.
50. Young IR, Hall AS, Pallis CA, et al. Nuclear magnetic resonance imaging of the brain in multiple sclerosis. *Lancet.* 1981;2:1063–1066.
51. Grossman RI, Conzales-Scarano F, Atlas SW, et al. Multiple sclerosis: gadolinium enhancement in MR imaging. *Radiology.* 1986;161:721–725.
52. Halliday AM, McDonald WI, Mushin J. Delayed visual evoked response in optic neuritis. *Lancet.* 1972;299:982–985.
53. Cottrell SS, Wilson SAK. The affective symptomatology of disseminated sclerosis. *J Neurol Psychopath.* 1926;7:1–30.
54. Ombredane A. *Sur les troubles mentaux de la sclérose en plaques* [thesis]. Paris, France: Les Presses Universitaires de France; 1929.
55. Berrios GE, Quemada JI, Andre G. Ombredane and the psychiatry of multiple sclerosis: a conceptual and statistical history. *Compr Psychiatry.* 1990;31(5):438–446.
56. Arbuse DI. Psychotic manifestations in disseminated sclerosis. *J Mt Sinai Hosp.* November/December 1938;4:403–410.
57. Borberg NC, Zahle V. On the psychopathology of disseminated sclerosis. *Acta Psychol Neurol.* 1946;21:75–89.
58. Rabins PV. Euphoria in multiple sclerosis. In: Jensen K, Knudsen L, Stenager LE, et al, eds. *Mental Disorders and Cognitive Deficits in Multiple Sclerosis.* London, UK: John Libbey; 1989:119–120.
59. Gowers WR. *A Manual of Diseases of the Nervous System.* Vol 2. 2nd ed. London, UK: J & A Churchill; 1893:544, 557–558.
60. Beevor CE. *Diseases of the Nervous System.* London, UK: H. K. Lewis; 1898:272–278.
61. Oppenheim H. *Textbook of Nervous Diseases for Physicians and Students.* Bruce A, trans. Edinburgh, Scotland: Otto Schulze & Co.; 1911:350 (translation of the 1908 German edition).
62. Putnam TJ, Chiavacci LV, Hoff H, et al. Results of treatment of multiple sclerosis with dicoumarin. *Arch Neurol.* 1947;57:1–13.
63. Alexander L. Minutes of the Medical Advisory Board, National Multiple Sclerosis Society, 1949.
64. Issacs A, Lindenmann J. Virus interference I: the interferon. *Proc Roy Soc Lond.* 1957;147:258–267.
65. Nagano Y, Kojima Y. Inhibition de l'infection vaccinale par un facteur liquide dans le tissu infect par le virus homologue. *C R Soc Biol.* 1958;152:1627–1627.
66. Jacobs L, O'Malley J, Freedman A, et al. Intrathecal interferon reduces exacerbations of multiple sclerosis. *Science.* 1981;214:1026–1028.
67. The IFNB Multiple Sclerosis Study Group. Interferon beta-1b is effective in relapsing-remitting-multiple sclerosis. *Neurology.* 1993;43:655–661.
68. Polman CH, Thompson AJ, Murray TJ, et al. *Multiple Sclerosis: The Guide to Treatment and Management.* 6th ed. New York, NY: Demos Vermande; 2006.
69. Sibley WA. *Therapeutic Claims in Multiple Sclerosis.* 4th ed. New York, NY. Demos Vermande; 1996.

2

Overview of Multiple Sclerosis

Alexander D. Rae-Grant and Robert J. Fox

KEY POINTS FOR CLINICIANS

- Multiple sclerosis (MS) is a continuously active disease with subclinical lesions occurring 5 to 10 times as often as clinical relapses.
- Gray matter demyelination occurs commonly and is an early component of MS pathology.
- New international criteria for diagnosis allow for an MS diagnosis at the time of the first clinical event in some patients.
- Monitoring of MS is becoming more important as we have more options for treatment for patients with different risks and monitoring protocols.
- Symptom management is critical in MS care.

In the past, students and trainees were taught that MS was a demyelinating white matter disease that spared the cortex and nerve axons, and had epochs of biological remission. Our concept of the disorder was one of episodes of activity (relapses) followed by disease quiescence. Relapses always resolved, so early treatment was not necessary. Even after the development of brain MRI, lesions correlated poorly with relapses so were frequently ignored. In terms of mechanism, we considered MS solely a disease of autoimmune T-cell activation. We did not think there were other diseases hiding under the umbrella of MS which might require substantially different treatment. Many thought that studying MS and ways of treating it was a waste of research time and effort.

Over the past 25 years, we have seen a revolution in our thinking about this disorder. This revolution has overturned the standard concepts of MS and has refocused our research and treatment approaches dramatically. Of any area in the neurosciences, the field of clinical neuroimmunology has seen the most dramatic change in terms of biological understanding, monitoring strategies, and therapeutic approaches. For those entering the field, this is a time of great promise but also challenge as we balance increasingly powerful medications and treatment against safety, tolerability, and ultimately cost. Despite these advances there is much work to be done, particularly to understand and address the causation and treatment of the progressive components of this disease.

NEW DIRECTIONS IN UNDERSTANDING MS

Prior to the application of MRI, the concept of MS was of a "punctuated equilibrium," that is, episodes of clinical worsening (relapses) interspersed with clinical and biological remission. Treatment was directed at relapse management, assuming that in between relapses the disease was quiescent. On this background, studies using sequential MRI in MS showed new MRI lesion formation 5 to 10 times as often as new clinical events. Progressive subclinical changes were observed in longitudinal studies, as shown by progressive brain and spinal cord atrophy, change in volume of T2 and T1 brain lesions, and other measures of brain degeneration. Clinical recovery after a relapse was therefore not due to resolution of the lesion per se, but based on a variety of factors including ion-channel redistribution, nitric oxide level modification, change in inflammatory cell populations, neural plasticity, and remyelination. The impact of these observations on our understanding of MS and our approach to its treatment cannot be overemphasized. The observation that much of MS was subclinical moved the philosophy of "treating for relapses" to a preventive strategy for ongoing disease management. Instead of, "treat the patient, not the MRI scan," we adopted "treat the disease, and use the MRI scan to understand the disease and its activity." In addition, the common observation that patients often had progression years after disease stability now made more sense, as new lesion formation would gradually erode the brain and spinal cord's ability to buffer injury.

Many other observations helped further our understanding of MS. For example, microscopic analysis of brain tissues in MS autopsy cases showed huge numbers of transected axons in acute MS lesions, averaging an astonishing 11,000 per cubic millimeter. Myelin and myelin-producing cells were reduced, too. Outside of focal lesions, axons were reduced in normal appearing white matter, indicating extensive injury beyond the visible lesion boundaries.

Observations from both autopsy and (more recently) brain biopsies have shown conclusively that the gray matter is targeted at least as much as the white matter in MS. While this observation had in fact been made on pathological specimens in the past, recent observations from biopsies of early MS cases emphasized the cortical component of MS and the concept that some immune activity may arise from the cerebrospinal fluid (CSF)/pial boundary into the brain, rather than as a purely blood-borne process. Conventional MRI sequences do not provide sufficient contrast to appreciate cortical demyelination, and so researchers are testing novel techniques to improve the characterization of cortical disease. The presence of early cortical disease may partially explain early cognitive dysfunction and the presence of seizures in a subset of patients with MS.

We have also seen the development of additional concepts regarding MS pathogenesis, among them a dying back oligodendrogliopathy, a complement-mediated inflammatory response, and other pathological and immunological concepts. We have begun to appreciate the importance not only of T cells, but of other immune effector systems such as B cells, macrophages, microglia, and mast cells in the MS cascade of injuries. Whether these observations will be confirmed as truly separate disorders with different treatment paradigms is unclear, but they open the door to potentially subsegment the group of patients we lump together as MS into more precise prognosis and treatment subsets.

The development of robust testing measures to segregate neuromyelitis optica from other neuroimmunological disease is, perhaps, the first of many such changes that will refine the understanding, monitoring, and treatment approaches to our patient population. At the same time, these concepts are allowing us to recognize that the degeneration of progressive MS is likely ongoing during the early, relapsing stage of MS, active inflammation is occurring in some patients in the progressive stage of MS, and the primary and secondary progressive forms of MS may be more similar than different. We have come to recognize that the gradually progressive manifestation of MS likely has a very different pathophysiology from the relapsing manifestation of MS. The underpinnings of progressive MS remain uncertain, but may involve neurodegenerative pathophysiologies such as mitochondrial dysfunction.

NEW DIRECTIONS IN DIAGNOSING MS

Before the widespread availability and use of MRI, the diagnosis of MS was more difficult than it is today. Over the past 15 years, the criteria for the diagnosis of MS have been revised in an attempt to meet two countervailing needs: first, to effectively reduce the number of patients diagnosed with MS who do not have this condition (specificity), and second, to increase the number of patients identified as having MS who have this disorder (sensitivity). In the past, we required either a second clinical event affected a different location of the central nervous system (CNS) to occur after an initial demyelinating event or a new MRI lesion to form before the diagnosis of MS was made. In addition, complex MRI diagnostic criteria were not easily applied in daily practice. In the current iteration of the International Panel Criteria for MS (also known as the McDonald Criteria), patients with a single clinical event who have both enhancing and nonenhancing demyelinating lesions (implying "dissemination in time") as well as lesions in two or more CNS regions (implying "dissemination in space") can meet the criteria for MS. These new criteria have sped up the time to diagnosis, reduced the waiting time to demonstrate dissemination in time, and simplified the diagnostic rules. All of these were common sources of frustration and confusion for patients and clinicians alike. Without a single test for MS, clinicians continue to be challenged by patients who have conditions mimicking MS; MS remains a clinical diagnosis, requiring clinical judgment and ongoing surveillance regarding alternative and additional diagnoses.

Another collateral benefit of more robust MRI measures is that CSF testing, at the best of times a distasteful pursuit for patients, is deemphasized in relapsing patients. We are moving to a more noninvasive, but no less scientifically grounded, approach to the diagnosis and monitoring of MS in most patients. However, the role of CSF testing has become more prominent in primary progressive MS, where confusion with other neurodegenerative disorders remains common. In contrast, the roles of evoked potentials have decreased over time, and the current diagnostic criteria do not include any evoked potentials (including visual evoked potentials).

NEW DIRECTIONS IN MONITORING MS

With the advent of multiple long-term therapies for MS, patient management has shifted toward methods to adequately monitor both the disease course and the treatment response. MRI provides a useful tool to monitor for new disease activity as indicated by new lesion formation and enhancing lesions. Conventional MRI also provides a general sense of brain atrophy, the end result of MS injury. As we shift to monitoring and testing treatments for the neurodegenerative component of MS, we will require more robust imaging measures that characterize smaller changes in brain volumes, lesion burden, and other tissue characteristics of both lesional and nonlesional brain tissue.

To this end, MRI appears to have promising utility. Volumetric lesion and atrophy measures are being used in clinical trials and longitudinal studies, and show progressive brain atrophy. Measures such as magnetization transfer ratio (MTR) and MRI spectroscopy may characterize the longitudinal change in tissue injury within both focal lesions and other areas of the brain that appear normal using conventional imaging. Diffusion tensor imaging is sensitive to changes in certain white matter tracts and may differentially characterize demyelination and axonal degeneration. Each of these tools may be beneficial in measuring neuroprotective or neurorestorative strategies as we move into new areas of therapeutic development.

Ocular coherence tomography (OCT) is a powerful tool to monitor the result of optic neuritis. Newer generation OCT machines using spectral domain technology have shown a reduction in retinal nerve fiber layer after optic neuritis, as well as injury to other retinal structures. Phase 2 trials of neuroprotective agents are now using OCT as a marker to measure axonal protection. OCT may provide another way of monitoring inflammation, axonal injury, and later degeneration in a quick, convenient, noninvasive, and relatively inexpensive fashion.

In the clinic, we are now using more quantitative measures to assist with the longitudinal monitoring of our patients. The timed 25-foot walk, nine-hole peg test, 6-minute walk, and the timed up and go test, all provide measurable continuous measures of function which can be charted over time. Some clinics are using computer-based measurement tools to track disease activity and measure physical function, depression, and cognitive capacities.

NEW DIRECTIONS IN TREATMENT OF MS DISEASE ACTIVITY

Prior to 1993, there were no Food and Drug Administration (FDA)-approved medicines for MS. Clinicians caring for patients with MS were often discouraged from "wasting their time" doing clinical trials in MS. In contract, currently there are over a dozen FDA-approved medicines for relapsing forms of MS, as well as FDA-approved medicines to increase walking speed in MS, improve bladder dysfunction, and lessen emotional incontinence. The immune targets of FDA-approved therapies have markedly expanded in the past several years and now include B cells and gamma/delta leukocytes. The first therapy for primary progressive MS was approved in 2017. Many more disease-modifying therapies and symptom therapies are currently in phase 2 and phase 3 trials.

It has become clear that an increased efficacy as measured by reduced relapses, short-term measures of disability on exam, and MRI activity can be achieved with some of the newer agents. However, higher efficacy may come with a price, as exemplified by the association of progressive multifocal leukoencephalopathy with several MS therapies. Nevertheless, we are now becoming more adept at risk-stratifying patients for natalizumab by assessing for John Cunningham virus (JCV) antibodies prior to and during therapy. Similar risk stratification is being used for the first oral agent available (fingolimod) by assessing for antibodies against varicella zoster and assessing cardiac rhythm disorders, medications, and baseline eye exam. Surprisingly, the goal of personalized treatment in MS has not been through personalizing efficacy, but through personalizing safety and mitigating risks.

A recently emerging theme in relapsing MS is the recognition that a subset of patients treated in clinical trials appears to be free of disease activity, as defined by stable clinical exam, lack of relapses, and stable MRI without new lesions or gadolinium enhancement. The proportion of patients free of disease activity (also called NEDA: No Evidence of Disease Activity) may become the new benchmark of success, both in clinical trials and in clinical populations. Of course, this simple definition begs the question of whether patients are truly free of disease activity or just lack changes that we can appreciate with current clinical and imaging monitoring methods. This will be a point of discussion particularly as we increase the number of trials in progressive MS, where robust measures of progression are urgently needed to guide treatment assessment and decision making.

NEW DIRECTIONS IN TREATMENT OF MS SYMPTOMS

While the search for newer disease-modifying therapies has been fruitful, other areas of MS management have also moved forward. We have an approved agent for pseudobulbar affect, a socially stigmatizing disorder seen in MS, amyotrophic lateral sclerosis, head injury, and some dementing disorders. A long-acting form of 4-aminopyridine is approved to increase walking speed in MS. Botulinum toxin has been approved for the management of limb spasticity and bladder dysfunction. Additional agents are available for the treatment of neurogenic bladder symptoms. Implanted baclofen pumps provide a management tool for patients with severe spasticity and have seen useful application in both ambulatory and nonambulatory patients. Now, the challenge has become identifying who to treat with what and when, a challenge to be met with better training and careful patient selection.

GREATER RECOGNITION OF THE IMPORTANCE OF OTHER HEALTH MEASURES IN MS

In the past, neurologists typically confined themselves to the diagnosis and sometimes treatment of MS alone. They did not provide care for (or indeed cared about) other medical issues in their MS population. Over the past 10 years, we have come to recognize how comorbid conditions such as obesity, smoking, and vascular disease require attention in the MS population and how they accelerate progression of MS owing to secondary injury. We are seeing a greater focus on the potential role of vitamin D deficiency in the pathogenesis of MS. We are learning that depression, sleep disorders, and pain are not only common in MS, but also drivers of health-related quality of life and even employment in affected patients. We need to treat the whole patient and attend the patient's social surroundings, rather than just seeing them as relapses and brain lesions.

EMBRACING A TEAM APPROACH TO MS

It has become clear that a neurologist alone cannot meet the needs of this challenging patient population. A team approach, where many healthcare practitioners with different competencies aid the patient through their disease course, works better than a solo act. New research has supported the concept that wellness approaches, cognitive behavioral therapies, exercise, rehabilitation, and a host of other interventions are not only beneficial but also critical in enhancing function and improving the lot of patients and their families. As we move into newer healthcare systems, a more comprehensive approach to all the factors which go into MS care needs to be taken so that we can effectively and efficiently help this group of people through their long-term disease.

ONGOING CHALLENGES AND FUTURE PROMISE

Despite great successes in so many areas of MS—successes in understanding its pathogenesis, diagnosis, treatment, and monitoring—many challenges still remain. Perhaps no challenge is more prominent than that of treating progressive MS. Although symptomatic therapies in progressive MS have emerged, there still is a fundamental lack of understanding regarding progressive MS pathobiology, methods for phase 2 proof-of-concept trials, and optimal clinical outcomes for phase 3 trials. These holes in our understanding have inhibited the development of an effective therapy for progressive MS. We also need better clinical and imaging tools to monitor the evolution of MS disease beyond just foci of inflammation. These tools will better characterize disease progression over time and the potential impact of disease-modifying and symptomatic therapies.

At the present time, we are at crossroads in MS. If we catch patients early enough in their relapsing course, intervene, monitor treatment response, and alter treatment accordingly, then we feel we can substantively alter the course of their disease. Admittedly, definitive long-term evidence of this success is still limited, but preliminary clinical trial and innovative propensity-weighted virtual trials suggest this is the case. However, we want to provide more protection from neurological worsening, and optimally to provide for improvement or restoration of function where it has been permanently injured in the past. The continued significant unmet needs and challenges in MS call for an active MS research enterprise, clinically astute and forward-thinking treatment strategies, as well as targeted advocacy and fundraising. The last two decades of tremendous progress in MS need to be leveraged toward the remaining significant unmet needs of this disease.

Finally, there is more to CNS neuroimmunology than just MS. Acute disseminated encephalomyelitis, neuromyelitis optica spectrum disorder, autoimmune encephalitis, and neurosarcoidosis all share somewhat similar immune pathophysiologies, but have different manifestations, diagnostic criteria, and treatments. Recognizing these entities is important as these patients are often seen by the same providers who care for MS.

KEY POINTS FOR PATIENTS AND FAMILIES

- Because MS is active even when you are not having symptoms, treatment is important to reduce the disease before you have major problems.
- Treating MS is like treating high blood pressure in that treatment is preventive.
- Monitoring MS is important to tell clinicians whether the medicines are working for you, are safe, and whether they need to be modified.
- The symptoms of MS are usually treatable and treating them is an important part of maintaining a good quality of life.

3

Pathology and Pathophysiology of Multiple Sclerosis

Kedar R. Mahajan and Don J. Mahad

KEY POINTS FOR CLINICIANS

- Demyelinating lesions are present in both gray and white matter, occurs early in the disease course, and increase over time.
- Resident glia (microglia and astrocytes), peripheral mononuclear cells (B and T cells) and macrophages contribute to inflammation in lesions.
- Inflammation and neurodegeneration also occurs in white and gray matter that appear normal on conventional MRI.
- Neurodegeneration, including axonal and neuronal loss, is prevalent and can be an early feature.
- Neurodegeneration may occur independent of demyelination and contributes to regional and global atrophy as well as clinical disability.

INTRODUCTION

There has been considerable attention to immune dysregulation and inflammation in driving the pathology and pathophysiology of multiple sclerosis (MS), leading to advances in developing disease-modifying therapies (DMTs). Although MS lesions are heterogenous, T cell, macrophage, immunoglobulin (Ig), and complement infiltration and deposition are features of many lesions. Infiltrating cells gain entry into the central nervous system (CNS) via the choroid plexus, leptomeningeal vessels, and parenchymal capillaries/postcapillary venules (1). Resident glia including astrocytes and macrophages are activated. Intrathecal production of Igs by clonally expanded B cells in cerebrospinal fluid (CSF) is also a feature that can also aid in the diagnosis of MS. Despite the development of 15 DMTs now targeting aspects of immune disregulation, little progress has been made in combating progressive MS. Here, we provide an overview of the role of inflammation and neurodegeneration in MS, which can impact both white matter (WM) and gray matter (GM) early in MS. Examples of advanced MRI techniques and postmortem validation are also mentioned.

WM LESIONS

WM lesions are identified on gross pathology as hyperpigmented plaques, and by the loss of myelin (demyelination) and axons using immunohistochemistry. They are commonly distributed in the following regions: periventricular, corpus callosum, centrum semiovale, juxtacortical, and spinal cord (2–4).

Inflammatory demyelinating plaques (also called active plaques) are more prevalent early in the relapsing course, likely reflecting disease activity and clinical relapses, and are less common in later chronic progressive stages. Table 3.1 describes characteristics of WM plaque patterns distinguished as either "active" or "chronic" by cellular (microglia/macrophage, mφ) and myelin protein contents. Table 3.2 describes characterization of active plaques by myelin features of the lesion border, myelin protein loss, Ig and complement deposition, and loss of oligodendrocytes (OLs).

Four distinct demyelination patterns are described by the extent of their inflammation and cellular characteristics (5). Pattern I is noted in acute MS with active demyelination, sharply demarcated borders, perivascular infiltrating T cells, activated microglia, and myelin laden macrophages. Pattern II also includes T cell infiltration with myelin laden macrophages but also includes deposition of Igs and complement. Pattern III lesions have ill-defined borders, dying OLs, vessels with inflammation but a rim of spared myelin with early loss of myelin-associated glycoprotein (MAG)/2',3'-cyclic-nucleotide 3'-phosphodiesterase (CNPase), decreased macrophages expressing CCR5, and increased undifferentiated macrophages expressing CCR1. Pattern IV are noted in patients with a primary progressive course and have T-cell

TABLE 3.1 Lesion Classification by Microglia/Macrophage (mφ) Infiltration and Myelin Protein Phagocytosis

PLAQUE PATTERNS	PATHOLOGICAL HALLMARKS
Acute	
Early active	mφ containing minor and major myelin proteins
Late active	mφ containing only major myelin proteins
Chronic active, smoldering, slowly expanding	Hypocellular center of lesion with rim of activated mφ
Chronic inactive	Demarcated demyelinated hypocellular lesion and border with sparse mφ

infiltration, perilesional OL loss, and activated microglia/macrophages. Completely remyelinated areas have been described as "shadow plaques." As patients tend to favor one particular lesion pattern (5), the implications for their etiology, prognosis, and response to therapy may differ.

The amount of WM lesion burden accumulates with advanced stages of MS as evidenced by accrual of T2 lesions on MRI. However, not all microstructural injury or inflammation is evident on clinical MRI sequences. These limitations are responsible for the "clinico-radiological paradox," where WM and GM that appear normal using conventional imaging (called normal-appearing WM and GM), demonstrate significant abnormalities detectable only by more advanced techniques. These abnormalities may contribute to clinical deficits. Additionally, not all WM lesions seen on conventional T2-weighted images depict demyelination. Normal myelin content is observed in up to 30% of lesions that are seen on T2-weighted, T1-weighted, and magnetization transfer imaging (6).

Advanced MRI methods hope to bridge the clinical and radiological gap by improved characterization of in vivo cellular and microstructural changes in normal appearing and lesional tissue. For example, PET ligands have been tested to identify microglial activation (e.g., ^{11}C-PK11195 (7), ^{11}C-PBR28 (8)), or astrocytes (^{11}C-acetate (9)).

Also, identifying central veins in lesions with susceptibility-weighted imaging may help discriminate T2/fluid-attenuated inversion recovery (FLAIR) lesions due to ischemic small vessel (microvascular) disease from MS (10).

GM LESIONS

GM lesions have been recognized since the 1800s by Charcot and involve both cortical and deep GM. Cortical GM lesions have been classified into three types based on their anatomical location by Brownell and Hughes in the 1960s (3). Type I (leukocortical) lesions span the interface between WM and cortical GM and have glial, neuronal, and synaptic loss (11). Type II (intracortical) lesions are perivascular and restricted to the cortical GM with minimal lymphocytic infiltration (12). Type III (subpial) lesions appear on the surface of the cortex and extend variably downward—either to layers III/IV or the entire width of the cortex (the latter sometimes referred to as type IV cortical lesions). Subpial lesions can transverse multiple gyri, involve a significant proportion of the cortical ribbon (13), and favor deep cortical sulci.

GM involvement was largely unappreciated given conventional MRI limitations, but with advanced techniques such as ultra-high field 7 T and double inversion recovery, lesions have been more readily detectible. 7 T MRI with postmortem validation is able to detect 100% of leukocortical lesions, 11% of intracortical lesions, 32% of subpial lesions, and 68% of subpial lesions which extend the entire width of the cortex (types I–IV, respectively) (14).

Cortical demyelination can occur early (15) and independent of WM lesions (13,16). It also involves multiple regions, including the hippocampus, occipital lobe, cerebellum, primary motor cortex, and spinal cord (17–19). Deep GM nuclei are also susceptible to demyelination and involve the thalamus, hippocampus, caudate, putamen, pallidum, amygdala, hypothalamus, and substantia nigra (20). Together, cortical and deep GM pathology exceed the contribution of WM lesion in correlations with disability, disease progression, and cognitive impairment (21–23).

TABLE 3.2 Pathological Lesion Classification of Active Lesions

PATTERN	DEMYELINATING LESION BORDER	MYELIN PROTEIN LOSS	IG/COMPLEMENT DEPOSITION	OLS
I	Sharp, perivenular	Minor and major	–	Inactive plaque center – present
II	Sharp, perivenular	Minor and major	+	Active lesion border – variable loss
III	III defined, not perivenular. Preservation of myelin rim along inflamed vessels	Minor	–	Inactive center – absent. Active lesion border – pronounced loss
IV	Sharp, perivenular	Minor and major	–	Inactive center and active lesion border – near complete loss

Ig, immunoglobulin.
Source: Adapted from Lucchinetti C, Brück W, Parisi J, et al. Heterogeneity of multiple sclerosis lesions: implications for the pathogenesis of demyelination. *Ann Neurol.* 2000;47(6):707–717.

INFLAMMATION

Peripheral immune cells, resident glia, as well as secreted factors all play a role in inflammation in normal appearing and lesional tissue at various stages of the disease course in both WM and GM. DMTs modulating lymphocyte proliferation, migration, and function have remarkably decreased disease activity and subsequent disability progression (see Chapter 11) and support an "outside-in" model for MS pathogenesis. Innate immune cells, including pro-inflammatory activated M1 microglia are present in preactive lesions preceding blood–brain barrier (BBB) breakdown. These cells contribute to demyelination and may trigger BBB breakdown secondarily, supporting an "inside-out" process. Additionally, differences in gut microbiota in patients with MS correlate with differences in expression of genes responsible for the adaptive and innate immune systems.

Genetic predisposition from human leukocyte antigen (HLA) alleles expressed on innate immune cells either increase (class I A3; class II DRB1*1501, DRB1*0301 and DRB1*1303) or decrease (class I A2) risk for MS (24). Large-scale genome-wide association studies have identified over 150 single nucleotide polymorphisms affecting cytokines and their receptors, transcription factors, and adhesion/costimulatory molecules (see Chapter 5). An example of the influence of genetics with pathology is the increased spinal cord demyelination seen with patients harboring the HLA-DRB1 *15 risk allele (25). A greater understanding of genetic traits will shed light on aberrations of the immune system, vitamin D metabolism, and other potential mechanisms that increase risk of developing MS.

The complexity of the interaction between multiple cell types, soluble mediators, gut microbiota, and genetic and environmental factors, present an opportunity for a multitude of approaches for potential therapeutic targets but lends singling one approach to address various mechanisms difficult to fathom. Many therapies with promising mechanism of actions and positive effects in animal models have failed in clinical trials either due to toxicity (roquinimex—inhibitor of interferon [IFN] gamma and tumor necrosis factor [TNF] alpha), worsening of disease severity or MRI outcomes (TNF alpha [infliximab] or TNF alpha receptor [lenercept] inhibitors), or potential failure in crossing the BBB (ustekinumab— targeting p40 subunit of IL12 and IL23 but with a molecular weight of 150 kDa). Conversely, the marked attenuation of disease activity by potent but relatively well-tolerated intravenous monoclonal antibody therapies either depleting (rituximab, ocrelizumab, ofatumumab, or alemtuzumab) or limiting infiltration (natalizumab) of lymphocytes, is informative to appreciating pathophysiology of MS by highlighting the importance of inflammation. Table 3.3 summarizes

TABLE 3.3   Overview of Inflammatory Mediators in MS

Adaptive immune system	CD52 expressed on T and B lymphocytes; depleted by alemtuzumab
T cells	
CD4⁺	
Th1	Pro-inflammatory. Promoted by IL12. Secrete IFNγ, TNFα/β, IL2. ↓ by IFNβ.
Th2	Anti-inflammatory. Promoted by IL4. Secrete IL3, IL4, IL5, IL6, IL10, IL13, TGFβ. ↑ by IFNβ.
Th17	Pro-inflammatory. Promoted by IL23, IL1, IL6, IL21, TGFβ. ↑ with relapses. Secrete IL9, IL17, IL21, IL22, TNFα.
Treg (natural)	Limit autoimmunity by promoting tolerance to self-antigens. Express CD25 and FOXP3.
Treg (adaptive)	Attenuate immune system via IL10 (Treg-1) and TGFβ (Th3)
CD8⁺	Release of perforin ↑ permeability of BBB and axonal damage by promoting ion influx.
Treg (adaptive)	Attenuate immune system
B cells (depleted by anti-CD20 monoclonal antibody therapies thereby **↓IL6 and B-cell mediated Ag presentation**—rituximab, ocrelizumab, ofatumumab)	
Secrete Igs to process antigen for T-cell activation and macrophage phagocytosis	
Present antigen to autoreactive T cells	
Secrete pro-inflammatory (IL6, IL12, TNF) and anti-inflammatory cytokines	
Innate immune system	
DCs	↑ expression of pro-inflammatory cytokines. Promote Th1 phenotype.
γδ T cells	↑ correlates with disease activity and progression. Present in lesions and intestinal epithelium.
Mast cells	↑ expression of inflammatory cytokines. Promote BBB disruption. Present myelin antigens to T cells. Activate and promote T cell differentiation.
Microglia/	Antigen presenting cells. Release cytokines and trophic factors.
macrophages	M1 microglia (pro-inflammatory): release TNFα, IFNγ, ROS, IL6, proteinases, complement M2 microglia (anti-inflammatory): release NGF, BDNF, IGF-1, IL10, TGFβ
NK cells	(**CD56**^bright **population**) stimulated by IL2 and cytotoxic toward autologous activated CD4⁺ cells. ↑ by daclizumab (anti-IL2 receptor α agonist); *taken off market due to adverse effects*.
Astrocytes	Secrete IL8, CCL2, CCL5, CXCL10. Interact with mast cells. Can present antigen. Attract/activate T-cells.

(continued)

TABLE 3.3 Overview of Inflammatory Mediators in MS (*continued*)

Adhesion molecules and integrins	
ICAM-1	↑ on luminal surface of brain endothelial cells in lesions
ICAM-3	Expressed on lymphocytes and monocytes in perivascular cuffs and lesion edges. ↓ on monocytes during maturation into macrophages
LFA-1	Expressed on activated microglia in lesions. Mediate lymphocyte-microglial interaction by binds ICAM-3 on lymphocytes in lesions
VCAM-1	Expressed on lymphocytes and monocytes in perivascular spaces, lipid filled macrophages in active lesion cores and borders, and activated OLs in perilesional WM
VLA-4	Dimer of α4 and β1 integrins. Binds VCAM-1 on perivascular perivascular lymphocytes and monocytes in chronic active lesions
	<u>Natalizumab</u> binds α4 integrin and blocks interaction with VCAM-1 thereby limiting migration of T and B cells and macrophages into the CNS.
Chemokines, chemokine receptors, miRNAs	
MCP1/CCL2	Expressed in acute lesions on hypertrophic astrocytes. Attracts monocytes and memory T cells, DCs, NK cells, and microglia
MIP1-α/β/CCL3/4	Expressed on lesional microglia/macrophages. Chemo-attractant for primarily monocytes/macrophages
RANTES/CCL5	Expressed on perivascular cells, blood vessel endothelial cells, and perivascular astrocytes. Promotes glial proliferation and survival.
CXCL10/IP-10	Expressed on reactive astrocyte cell bodies and foot processes in active lesions and NAWM endothelium. Potent lymphocyte chemoattractant. Coexpressed with CXCR3+ perivascular cells. CSF levels correlate with disease activity and CSF WBC count
miRNAs	Regulate innate and adaptive immunity. Up/down-regulated in lesional and normal appearing tissue associated with glia and peripheral lymphocytes.

↑, increased/upregulated; ↓, decreased/downregulated; BBB, blood–brain barrier; BDNF, brain-derived neurotrophic factor; CCL, chemokine ligand; CD, cluster of differentiation; DC, dendritic cell; ICAM, intracellular adhesion molecule; IFN, interferon; IGF, insulin-like growth factor; Ig, immunoglobulin; LFA, leukocyte adhesion molecule; MCP, monocyte chemo-attractant protein; MIP, macrophage inflammatory protein; miRNAs, micro-ribonucleic acid molecules; MS, multiple sclerosis; NAWM, normal appearing white matter; NGF, nerve growth factor; NK, natural killer; OL, oligodendrocyte; RANTES, regulated on activation, normal T cell expressed and secreted; ROS, reactive oxygen species; TNF, tumor necrosis factor; Treg, T regulatory cells; VCAM, vascular cell adhesion molecule; VLA, very late activation antigen; WBC, white blood cell; WM, white matter.

components of the innate and adaptive immune system, adhesion molecules, integrins, chemokines and their receptors, and potential-approved therapies.

GM Inflammation

Early cortical lesions in tumefactive MS biopsy specimens exhibit CD3+ and CD8+ T-cell infiltration in subpial, leukocortical, and intracortical perivascular lesions (15). In postmortem tissue, cortical lesions have abundant microglia but lymphocytic infiltration was minimal compared to WM lesions (12). There are conflicting data regarding the presence of inflammation in chronic cortical lesions in progressive MS. Studies utilizing tissue from patients with secondary progressive MS from a UK tissue bank identified B-cell follicle-like structures associated with meningeal inflammation and subpial demyelination (26–28). A study using tissues from a Dutch tissue bank failed to confirm these findings, as it did not identify any follicle-like structures in chronic MS patients or meningeal inflammation associated with demyelination (29). Deep GM structures such as the thalamus are also noted to have activated microglia/macrophages in normal appearing and lesional WM and GM (30). Furthermore, in vivo imaging of microglia with PET (PK11195 ligand) has identified extensive regional

microglial activation, predominantly in secondary progressive cases compared to relapsing–remitting (31).

NEURODEGENERATION

MS has the potential to be the prototypic disease to study neurodegeneration and evaluate neuroprotective therapies. Loss of GM volume occurs even in pediatric MS, correlates with cognitive impairment and fatigue, and increases risk for clinically definite MS in patients presenting with clinically or radiologically isolated syndromes (32–34). Fundamentally, neurodegeneration in MS can be conceptualized as occurring (a) as a direct result of inflammation, (b) related but independent of inflammation, or (c) as a primary neurodegenerative disorder where inflammation is secondary (35).

Axonal Loss

Axonal damage or loss can be the result of several mechanisms: (a) inflammatory axonal transection, (b) chronic demyelination–related axonal transection and degeneration, (c) Wallerian degeneration, and (d) ischemia- or pressure-related mechanical damage from surrounding edema. The extent of axonal loss correlates with disability, particularly in eloquent areas such as the spinal cord. Roughly 2/3 of axonal counts and density is lost in chronic-inactive spinal cord lesions (36), notably in the cervical region. Neuronal and axonal loss can be evaluated in vivo by magnetic resonance spectroscopy, an advanced MRI technique that detects N-acetyl aspartate (NAA) (found in neurons and their processes).

Inflammatory axonopathy in active and chronic active lesions is possibly mediated by perforin secretion by CD8+ T cells and pro-inflammatory mediators by microglia/macrophages (nitric oxide, proteolytic enzymes, cytokines, and free radicals). Activated microglia surrounds axonal ovoids in normal appearing white matter (NAWM) and damaged neurites in GM lesions. Chronically demyelinated axons in chronic active and inactive lesions contain axonal avoids indicating ongoing injury from recent transection (37–39). Wallerian degeneration follows axonal transection and entails breakdown of the distal portion of the axon and the removal of the corresponding myelin sheath. Activation of proteases and increase in intracellular calcium is thought to damage the axonal cytoskeleton (40). Once transected, the axon may continue to conduct for up to a week. In the CNS, axonal loss due to Wallerian degeneration may occur within days with immediate functional consequences, whereas the loss of myelin may occur over months or years following the initial axonal transection (41).

Neuronal Loss

Neurons loss is a component of GM volume. Cortical and deep GM atrophy correlates with disability and disease progression more significantly than WM lesion burden. GM atrophy exceeds WM volume in progressive stages of MS (42–44). Lesions in the hippocampus (19), thalamus (45), neocortex (11), and the spinal cord ventral horns (46,47) demonstrate neuronal loss. Thalamic atrophy, however, appears to correlate with extra-thalamic injury rather than

thalamic lesions (30). Neuronal pathology is comprised of neuronal injury, apoptosis, and synaptic loss in subpial and hippocampal lesions (11,12,15).

Energy Failure

Axons, particularly when demyelinated, are susceptible to mitochondrial dysfunction (48). Oxidative injury from reactive oxygen species cause loss of respiratory chain complex IV thereby compromising adenosine triphosphate (ATP) and is toxic to mitochondrial DNA. Chronically demyelinated axons have increased mitochondrial content, size, activity, and motile mitochondria likely as a compensatory mechanism (49). Meanwhile, there is robust evidence from seven independent studies implicating mitochondrial dysfunction and decreased capacity to produce ATP within neuronal cell bodies in progressive MS (50–56). In chronic progressive courses, impaired energy reserves and compensatory mechanisms likely lead to axonal and neuronal loss. There is robust evidence of a compromised bioenergetics status involving mitochondria within neurons in cortical lesions as well as in nonlesional GM (57).

SUMMARY

Previous research that elucidated the role the immune system in MS has greatly impacted the development of highly efficacious therapies, which attenuate new inflammatory lesions. Unfortunately, our understanding of the mechanisms underlying the neurodegeneration that contributes to cortical and deep GM loss of axons, neurons, and synapses is greatly lacking. Efforts to meet this need will be necessary in developing effective therapies for progressive forms of MS and evaluating the efficacy of neuroprotective strategies in clinical trials.

KEY POINTS FOR PATIENTS AND FAMILIES

- Lesions with loss of myelin (demyelination) occur in both white and gray matter in the brain and spinal cord throughout the course of MS.
- New MS lesions are comprised of inflammatory cells that are found in the brain and spinal cord and have migrated in from the blood.
- Apart from demyelination, MS also causes neurodegeneration, loss of neurons, and damage to axons. Neurodegeneration can occur early in the disease and become prominent in individuals with a progressive course.
- Neurodegeneration may occur independently of demyelination and correlates stronger with clinical disability than lesions alone.
- Clinical MRI scans are not able to detect all lesions or appreciate neurodegeneration as well as more advanced imaging techniques.

REFERENCES

1. Ransohoff RM, Kivisakk P, Kidd G. Three or more routes for leukocyte migration into the central nervous system. *Nat Rev Immunol.* 2003;3(7):569–581.
2. Raine CS. The Dale E. McFarlin Memorial Lecture: the immunology of the multiple sclerosis lesion. *Ann Neurol.* 1994;36:S61–S72.
3. Brownell B, Hughes JT. The distribution of plaques in the cerebrum in multiple sclerosis. *J Neurol Neurosurg Psychiatry.* 1962;25:315–320.
4. Filli L, Hofstetter L, Kuster P, et al. Spatiotemporal distribution of white matter lesions in relapsing-remitting and secondary progressive multiple sclerosis. *Mult Scler.* 2012;18(11):1577–1584.
5. Lucchinetti C, Brück W, Parisi J, et al. Heterogeneity of multiple sclerosis lesions: implications for the pathogenesis of demyelination. *Ann Neurol.* 2000;47(6):707–717.
6. Fisher E, Chang A, Fox RJ, et al. Imaging correlates of axonal swelling in chronic multiple sclerosis brains. *Ann Neurol.* 2007;62(3):219–228.
7. Debruyne JC, Versijpt J, Van Laere KJ, et al. PET visualization of microglia in multiple sclerosis patients using [11C]PK11195. *Eur J Neurol.* 2003;10(3):257–264.
8. Oh U, Fujita M, Ikonomidou VN, et al. Translocator protein PET imaging for glial activation in multiple sclerosis. *J Neuroimmune Pharmacol.* 2011;6(3):354–361.
9. Takata K, Kato H, Shimosegawa E, et al. 11C-acetate PET imaging in patients with multiple sclerosis. *PLOS ONE.* 2014;9(11):e111598.
10. Sati P, Oh J, Constable RT, et al. The central vein sign and its clinical evaluation for the diagnosis of multiple sclerosis: a consensus statement from the North American Imaging in Multiple Sclerosis Cooperative. *Nat Rev Neurol.* 2016;12(12):714–722.
11. Wegner C, Esiri MM, Chance SA, et al. Neocortical neuronal, synaptic, and glial loss in multiple sclerosis. *Neurology.* 2006;67(6):960–967.
12. Peterson JW, Bö L, Mörk S, et al. Transected neurites, apoptotic neurons, and reduced inflammation in cortical multiple sclerosis lesions. *Ann Neurol.* 2001;50(3):389–400.
13. Kutzelnigg A, Lucchinetti CF, Stadelmann C, et al. Cortical demyelination and diffuse white matter injury in multiple sclerosis. *Brain.* 2005;128(pt 11):2705–2712.
14. Kilsdonk ID, Jonkman LE, Klaver R, et al. Increased cortical grey matter lesion detection in multiple sclerosis with 7 T MRI: a postmortem verification study. *Brain.* 2016;139(pt 5):1472–1481.
15. Lucchinetti CF, Popescu BF, Bunyan RF, et al. Inflammatory cortical demyelination in early multiple sclerosis. *N Engl J Med.* 2011;365(23):2188–2197.
16. Bo L, Geurts JJ, van der Valk P, et al. Lack of correlation between cortical demyelination and white matter pathologic changes in multiple sclerosis. *Arch Neurol.* 2007;64(1):76–80.
17. Bo L, Vedeler CA, Nyland HI, et al. Subpial demyelination in the cerebral cortex of multiple sclerosis patients. *J Neuropathol Exp Neurol.* 2003;62(7):723–732.
18. Geurts JJ, Bö L, Roosendaal SD, et al. Extensive hippocampal demyelination in multiple sclerosis. *J Neuropathol Exp Neurol.* 2007;66(9):819–827.
19. Papadopoulos D, Dukes S, Patel R, et al. Substantial archaeocortical atrophy and neuronal loss in multiple sclerosis. *Brain Pathol.* 2009;19(2):238–253.
20. Vercellino M, Masera S, Lorenzatti M, et al. Demyelination, inflammation, and neurodegeneration in multiple sclerosis deep gray matter. *J Neuropathol Exp Neurol.* 2009;68(5):489–502.
21. Geurts JJ, Calabrese M, Fisher E, et al. Measurement and clinical effect of grey matter pathology in multiple sclerosis. *Lancet Neurol.* 2012;11(12):1082–1092.
22. Roosendaal SD, Moraal B, Vrenken H, et al. In vivo MR imaging of hippocampal lesions in multiple sclerosis. *J Magn Reson Imaging.* 2008;27(4):726–731.
23. Louapre C, Govindarajan ST, Giannì C, et al. The association between intra- and juxta-cortical pathology and cognitive impairment in multiple sclerosis by quantitative T2* mapping at 7 T MRI. *Neuroimage Clin.* 2016;12:879–886.
24. Sawcer S, Hellenthal G, Pirinen M, et al. Genetic risk and a primary role for cell-mediated immune mechanisms in multiple sclerosis. *Nature.* 2011;476(7359):214–219.
25. DeLuca GC, Alterman R, Martin JL, et al. Casting light on multiple sclerosis heterogeneity: the role of HLA-DRB1 on spinal cord pathology. *Brain.* 2013;136(pt 4):1025–1034.
26. Howell OW, Reeves CA, Nicholas R, et al. Meningeal inflammation is widespread and linked to cortical pathology in multiple sclerosis. *Brain.* 2011;134(pt 9):2755–2771.
27. Magliozzi R, Howell O, Vora A, et al. Meningeal B-cell follicles in secondary progressive multiple sclerosis associate with early onset of disease and severe cortical pathology. *Brain.* 2007;130(pt 4):1089–1104.
28. Magliozzi R, Howell OW, Reeves C, et al. A Gradient of neuronal loss and meningeal inflammation in multiple sclerosis. *Ann Neurol.* 2010;68(4):477–493.
29. Kooi EJ, Geurts JJ, van Horssen J, et al. Meningeal inflammation is not associated with cortical demyelination in chronic multiple sclerosis. *J Neuropathol Exp Neurol.* 2009;68(9):1021–1028.
30. Mahajan K, Nakamura K, Vignos M, et al. S2—Neuroimaging in MS: thalamic MRI and histopathologic correlations in advanced multiple sclerosis. In: *American Academy of Neurology.* Boston, MA; 2017. http://tools.aan.com/annualmeeting/search/?fuseaction=home.detail&id=5725
31. Politis M, Giannetti P, Su P, et al. Increased PK11195 PET binding in the cortex of patients with MS correlates with disability. *Neurology.* 2012;79(6):523–530.
32. Hyncicova E, Vyhnálek M, Kalina A, et al. Cognitive impairment and structural brain changes in patients with clinically isolated syndrome at high risk for multiple sclerosis. *J Neurol.* 2017;264(3):482–493.
33. Azevedo CJ, Overton E, Khadka S, et al. Early CNS neurodegeneration in radiologically isolated syndrome. *Neurol Neuroimmunol Neuroinflamm.* 2015;2(3):e102.
34. Till C, Ghassemi R, Aubert-Broche B, et al. MRI correlates of cognitive impairment in childhood-onset multiple sclerosis. *Neuropsychology.* 2011;25(3):319–332.
35. Trapp BD, Nave KA. Multiple sclerosis: an immune or neurodegenerative disorder? *Annu Rev Neurosci.* 2008;31:247–269.
36. Bjartmar C, Kidd G, Mörk S, et al. Neurological disability correlates with spinal cord axonal loss and reduced N-acetyl aspartate in chronic multiple sclerosis patients. *Ann Neurol.* 2000;48(6):893–901.
37. Bitsch A, Schuchardt J, Bunkowski S, et al. Acute axonal injury in multiple sclerosis. Correlation with demyelination and inflammation. *Brain.* 2000;123 (pt 6):1174–1183.
38. Ferguson B, Matyszak MK, Esiri MM, et al. Axonal damage in acute multiple sclerosis lesions. *Brain.* 1997;120 (pt 3):393–399.
39. Trapp BD, Peterson J, Ransohoff RM, et al. Axonal transection in the lesions of multiple sclerosis. *N Engl J Med.* 1998;338(5):278–285.
40. Stys PK. General mechanisms of axonal damage and its prevention. *J Neurol Sci.* 2005;233(1-2):3–13.
41. Bjartmar C, Kinkel RP, Kidd G, et al. Axonal loss in normal-appearing white matter in a patient with acute MS. *Neurology.* 2001;57(7):1248–1252.
42. Chard DT, Griffin CM, Parker GJ, et al. Brain atrophy in clinically early relapsing-remitting multiple sclerosis. *Brain.* 2002;125 (pt 2):327–337.
43. Fisher E, Lee JC, Nakamura K, et al. Gray matter atrophy in multiple sclerosis: a longitudinal study. *Ann Neurol.* 2008;64(3):255–265.
44. Fisniku LK, Chard DT, Jackson JS, et al. Gray matter atrophy is related to long-term disability in multiple sclerosis. *Ann Neurol.* 2008;64(3):247–254.
45. Cifelli A, Arridge M, Jezzard P, et al. Thalamic neurodegeneration in multiple sclerosis. *Ann Neurol.* 2002;52(5):650–653.
46. Schirmer L, Albert M, Buss A, et al. Substantial early, but nonprogressive neuronal loss in multiple sclerosis (MS) spinal cord. *Ann Neurol.* 2009;66(5):698–704.
47. Vogt J, Paul F, Aktas O, et al. Lower motor neuron loss in multiple sclerosis and experimental autoimmune encephalomyelitis. *Ann Neurol.* 2009;66(3):310–322.

48. Mahad DH, Trapp BD, Lassmann H. Pathological mechanisms in progressive multiple sclerosis. *Lancet Neurol.* 2015;14(2): 183–193.

49. Kiryu-Seo S, Ohno N, Kidd GJ, et al. Demyelination increases axonal stationary mitochondrial size and the speed of axonal mitochondrial transport. *J Neurosci.* 2010;30(19):6658–6666.

50. Dutta R, McDonough J, Yin X, et al. Mitochondrial dysfunction as a cause of axonal degeneration in multiple sclerosis patients. *Ann Neurol.* 2006;59(3):478–489.

51. Campbell GR, Ziabreva I, Reeve AK, et al. Mitochondrial DNA deletions and neurodegeneration in multiple sclerosis. *Ann Neurol.* 2011;69(3):481–492.

52. Broadwater L, Pandit A, Clements R, et al. Analysis of the mitochondrial proteome in multiple sclerosis cortex. *Biochim Biophys Acta.* 2011;1812(5):630–641.

53. Witte ME, Nijland PG, Drexhage JA, et al. Reduced expression of PGC-1alpha partly underlies mitochondrial changes and correlates with neuronal loss in multiple sclerosis cortex. *Acta Neuropathol.* 2013;125(2):231–243.

54. Kim JY, Shen S, Dietz K, et al. HDAC1 nuclear export induced by pathological conditions is essential for the onset of axonal damage. *Nat Neurosci.* 2010;13(2):180–189.

55. Hares K, Kemp K, Rice C, et al. Reduced axonal motor protein expression in non-lesional grey matter in multiple sclerosis. *Mult Scler.* 2014;20(7):812–821.

56. Haile Y, Deng X, Ortiz-Sandoval C, et al. Rab32 connects ER stress to mitochondrial defects in multiple sclerosis. *J Neuroinflammation.* 2017;14(1):19.

57. Dutta R, Trapp BD. Mechanisms of neuronal dysfunction and degeneration in multiple sclerosis. *Prog Neurobiol.* 2011;93(1):1–12.

4

Epidemiology and Natural History of Multiple Sclerosis

Marcus W. Koch

KEY POINTS FOR CLINICIANS

- The incidence and prevalence of multiple sclerosis (MS) varies between different geographical regions and ethnicities.

- MS is a lifelong disease; the overall survival of patients with MS is about 6 years shorter than that of the general population.

- The environmental risk factors, vitamin D (deficiency), and smoking influence the risk of developing MS, as well as the disease course.

- Sex, age at onset, and onset symptoms cannot reliably predict the disease course.

- The times to landmark disability have recently been found to be longer than initially reported, with a time to Expanded Disability Status Scale (EDSS) 6.0 of about 30 years overall and about 15 years in primary progressive MS. There is a significant interindividual variation in the time to reach this landmark.

EPIDEMIOLOGY, SURVIVAL, INCIDENCE, AND PREVALENCE OF MULTIPLE SCLEROSIS

Compared to other diseases of the central nervous system such as stroke, epilepsy, and traumatic brain injury, MS is a relatively uncommon disease. MS has a protracted disease course, with often long periods of clinical stability, and can be viewed as a lifelong condition; the overall survival of patients with MS is about 6 years less than that of the general population (1).

> *People with MS die about 6 years earlier than the general population.*

MS is newly diagnosed in about one in 20,000 people per year (incidence) and affects about one in 1,000 people (prevalence) (2). The incidence and prevalence of MS are, however, highly variable between different geographical areas. The prevalence of MS increases with latitude, such that the countries farthest from the equator have the highest prevalence of MS, whereas countries closer to the equator have a lower prevalence. For example, MS affects about one in 400 people in Canada (3), but only one in 5,000 people in Brazil (4). Several factors are believed to contribute to this latitudinal difference.

The influence of increased vitamin D production due to a greater exposure to sunlight in countries closer to the equator is one explaining factor (see following discussion on environmental risk factors). Ethnic differences between countries could also contribute. It has classically been thought that people of European descent may be especially susceptible to MS, whereas those of Asian and African descent may be less susceptible. This is illustrated best by epidemiological studies from around the world, which compare the prevalence of MS among different ethnic groups living together in the same area: one study in Israel, for instance, showed that Jews of European extraction had a much higher prevalence of MS (68 per 100,000) than Arabs (11 per 100,000). A South African study showed that whites had a much higher prevalence (26 per 100,000) than both Indians (8 per 100,000) and blacks (0.22 per 100,000) (5). Similar findings were also seen in New Zealand, where the prevalence of MS among people of European descent was much higher (103 per 100,000) than that among the Maoris (16 per 100,000) (6). MS is rare in Southeast Asia, with prevalence in the range of 1.4 per 100,000 in Shanghai, China (7) to 3.6 per 100,000 in South Korea (8). More recent research into the influence of ethnicity on MS incidence in the United States, however, has challenged these classical population-based studies. Two large studies based on an investigation of a large population of members of a health insurance in southern California showed that the incidence of MS and other demyelinating diseases was higher in blacks than in other ethnic groups in both adults and children (9,10). One reason for this difference in MS incidence may lie in the differences in vitamin D levels among ethnicities, as the National Health and Nutrition Examination Survey, a U.S. study tracking nutritional status, including vitamin D levels, in the U.S. population since 1988, has consistently shown blacks to have lower levels of vitamin D compared to other ethnic groups (11,12). The reason for the influence of ethnicity on MS incidence and prevalence across many populations, however, is not fully understood.

> *The prevalence of MS differs between geographical locations and ethnicities. For example, MS affects about one in 400 people in Canada, but only one in 5,000 people in Brazil.*

In the vast majority of patients, MS presents with a relapse, and the subsequent disease course is characterized by relapses and remissions: relapsing–remitting MS (RRMS). In about 10% of all patients with MS, the disease begins with a slow and relentless accumulation of disability, usually without any relapses. This form of the disease is called primary progressive MS (PPMS). In the longer term, most patients with RRMS experience a change in their disease course from the period with relapses and remissions to a more uniform and slow worsening of symptoms. This is called secondary progressive MS (SPMS). SPMS patients may continue to have relapses or cease having relapses, but the relapse rate tends to be less later in the disease course.

The median age at disease onset is around 30 years in RRMS and around 40 years in PPMS, the conversion to SPMS also occurs around a median age of 40 years. Women have a slightly, up to several years, earlier onset than men.

RRMS occurs more commonly in women, with a female-to-male ratio that was classically given as about 2. Recently, it has been found that this sex ratio of MS has changed in the last decade, so that it is now even more common in women, with the ratio of women-to-men with MS increasing from 1.4 in 1955 to 2.3 in 2000 (13). The reason for this increase is unknown. PPMS affects men and women equally.

> *RRMS occurs about twice as often in women than in men. PPMS affects men and women equally.*

ENVIRONMENTAL RISK FACTORS FOR MS

While research on environmental risk factors for MS is ongoing and many possible risk factors are being investigated, three environmental risk factors, vitamin D, Epstein–Barr virus (EBV) infection, and smoking, currently have the most convincing evidence to support them.

Vitamin D has recently been found to influence the risk of developing MS. The best evidence for this comes from an investigation of routine blood samples in U.S. military personnel. Routine medical examinations for U.S. military personnel include the drawing of a blood sample, which is then stored. One study investigated 25-hydroxy-vitamin D levels in these blood samples and related the vitamin D level to the subsequent risk of developing MS in a nested case-control study. This included 257 people who developed MS and two matched controls per case drawn from over 7 million people registered in the U.S. Department of Defense Serum Repository. In the study, it was found that the risk of developing MS decreases with rising serum vitamin D levels (odds ratio 0.59 per 50 nmol/L increase in vitamin D serum level) (14). Further studies suggest an association of vitamin D levels and the risk of developing MS with exposure to ultraviolet light: a retrospective Australian study showed that actinic skin damage (which occurs as a consequence of too much exposure to ultraviolet light), as well as the (remembered) time spent in the sun during childhood were associated with a lower risk of developing MS (15). The reason for the latitudinal variation in MS risk is most likely the lower exposure to ultraviolet light at higher latitudes, and the subsequent lower levels of vitamin D.

> *A low serum level of vitamin D is a risk factor for MS.*

Studies on the influence of infections with EBV on MS risk are made difficult by the fact that the great majority (around 95%) of adults is seropositive for EBV, which makes for large required sample sizes. A recent meta-analysis on EBV and MS risk including 1,779 people with MS and 2,526 control persons showed that seronegativity for EBV is associated with a very low risk of developing MS (odds ratio of 0.06) (16). Another large meta-analysis showed that a history of infectious mononucleosis (symptomatic EBV) was associated with a roughly doubled risk of developing MS (relative risk 2.17) (17). An analysis from a clinical trial cohort showed no important impact of EBV antibody levels on the risk of developing MS in a cohort of patients with clinically isolated syndrome (CIS). The BENEFIT study included 468 people with CIS, 448 were positive for EBV antibodies. In this study, the EBV-positive patients were divided into quartiles by the height of their EBV antibody titer, and there were no significant differences between these quartiles with regard to the risk of developing clinically definite MS during the 5-year follow-up period, or to clinical or MRI disease activity. Interestingly, the two patients who were consistently found to be EBV antibody negative, though they were not included in the analyses, did not go on to develop MS (18).

> *The reason for the latitudinal variation in MS risk is most likely the exposure to ultraviolet light at higher latitudes and the subsequent lower levels of vitamin D.*

Good evidence for the influence of smoking on the risk of developing MS comes from the two Nurses' Health Studies, each including more than 100,000 women. An analysis of these studies showed an increased risk of MS among current (relative incidence rate compared to non-smokers: 1.6) as well as former smokers (relative incidence rate: 1.2). There also was a suggestion of dose dependency, with the relative incidence increasing with increasing pack years (19). Further studies have since shown that second-hand smoke is associated with a higher risk of MS among children (20) and adults (21). The aforementioned analysis of the BENEFIT trial cohort, however, failed to show an important impact of cigarette smoking on the risk of developing clinically definite MS in a cohort of people with CIS. In this study, elevated blood levels of cotinine, a nicotine metabolite and reliable marker of current or recent tobacco use, were unrelated to the risk of developing clinically definite MS, or to the clinical or MRI disease activity during the 5-year follow-up period (18).

> *Smoking and secondhand smoke are risk factors for MS.*

THE NATURAL HISTORY OF MS

Studies on the natural history of MS have usually investigated how certain risk factors are related to the arrival at certain landmark disability levels. Typically, the time to a landmark disability score (such as EDSS 6.0, when patients need a cane for walking) was measured from disease onset. Early studies reported a relatively quick progression from disease onset to EDSS 6.0, with a median time from disease onset of RRMS in the range of 15 (22) to 20 (23) years, but newer studies have corrected these estimates to a median time from onset of around 30 years (24,25). Early studies on the natural history of PPMS reported very short median times to EDSS 6.0 of less than 10 years (22,23). More recent

studies have corrected these to a median time from disease onset of around 15 years (26). It should be noted that there is a very wide interpersonal variation in the progression of MS. Even within PPMS, which is thought to be the most uniform of the disease courses, the time to EDSS 6.0 ranged from around 8 years in 25% of patients with the quickest progression to more than 25 years in the 25% with the slowest progression (26).

> *The accumulation of disability in MS is slower than previously thought and varies widely between individuals.*

The classical epidemiological studies on risk factors for disease progression suggested that factors such as female gender and an early age at disease onset were associated with a better prognosis, although more recent studies show that the influence of risk factors is more complex. In studies that measure the time from disease onset to landmark disability, women and patients with an early disease onset take longer to reach landmark disability scores, such as EDSS 6.0. If we consider the age at which a landmark disability score is reached, this changes: men and women reach an EDSS score of 6.0 at a similar age (24). Patients with an early disease onset seem to be at an advantage, as their time to EDSS 6.0 is significantly longer than that of patients with a late disease onset. On the other hand, if the age at EDSS 6.0 is considered, these patients are actually at a considerable disadvantage as they reach this outcome at a younger age (24,27). These studies suggest that disability accumulation in MS is at least partly dependent on age, rather than on gender or the age at onset. Onset symptoms are not clearly and consistently related to the overall MS prognosis.

> *Estimates of progression to EDSS 6.0 show a median time from onset of around 30 years.*

Ethnic differences in MS are not well researched to date. There is some indication that ethnic differences are not only associated with the risk of developing MS (see earlier paragraph) but also with the disease course. Two retrospective studies from the United States showed that adult blacks required a cane at a shorter time from onset than whites (28), and that black children with MS had a higher relapse rate than white children (29).

> *Disability accumulation in MS occurs in two phases.*

Another important issue that can be learned from natural history studies is the fact that risk factors affect the early rather than the late disease phase. One large population-based study showed that the time from onset to the landmark disability scores of EDSS 4.0, 6.0, and 7.0 was influenced by such risk factors as sex, age at onset, and number of relapses in the first years from onset, but that none of these factors influences the time from EDSS 4.0 to EDSS 6.0 or 7.0 (30). This suggests that these risk factors only exert their influence at disability levels below EDSS 4.0, but that beyond this point the disease follows a more uniform course independent of any of these factors. Another epidemiological study from a different cohort confirmed these findings, and showed that the influence of risk factors already ended at a disability level of EDSS 3.0 (31). This last study also showed that the time between disease onset and the assignment of EDSS 3.0 was highly variable, whereas the time from EDSS 3.0 to EDSS 6.0 was much more uniform. Taken together, these studies suggest that MS is a disease with two phases of disability accumulation: an early phase of variable duration, which is partly influenced by such risk factors as sex and the age at onset, and a late phase with a more uniform duration, that proceeds independent of any of the known risk factors.

> *Time to progress from EDSS 4.0 to 6.0 is consistent no matter what prior course or type of MS the patient has.*

> *The known risk factors influence the disease course only up to a disability level of EDSS 3.0 or 4.0.*

ENVIRONMENTAL RISK FACTORS AND THE NATURAL HISTORY OF MS

The previously discussed environmental risk factors for MS of smoking and vitamin D status not only influence the risk of developing MS, but also influence the disease course (the role of EBV infection in the course of MS is less clear). Smoking leads to an increase in EDSS scores in the short term (32), and is associated with a faster increase in T2 MRI lesions, and faster brain atrophy (33). The role of smoking for the longer term outcomes, however, is less clear: one study suggested that smoking was neither associated with the risk of secondary progression, nor with that of reaching EDSS 4.0 or EDSS 6.0 (34), whereas other studies showed a greater risk of smokers to progress to secondary progression (33,35). While more research is needed to determine

the role of smoking in the different stages of MS, patients should clearly be encouraged to stop smoking, not only because of the general health benefits that will bring them, but also because of the particular negative influence smoking has on MS. Studies on vitamin D status and the disease course of MS showed that lower vitamin D levels are associated with higher levels of disability (36) and that higher levels of vitamin D are associated with a lower risk of relapse in adults and children (37,38). Recent good evidence for the impact of vitamin D levels on disease activity in established MS, finally, comes from a prospective analysis in a large randomized controlled trial cohort. Fitzgerald and coworkers examined the association between vitamin D levels and MRI activity, brain atrophy, and disability progression over a follow-up period of 2 years in a cohort of 1,482 patients with RRMS enrolled in the BEYOND study. They found a significant association of vitamin D levels and MRI activity, with patients with higher vitamin D levels developing fewer new active MRI lesions. Patients with vitamin D levels above 100 nmol/L had the lowest rate of new MRI lesions (39). In light of these findings, it would appear wise to at least avoid vitamin D deficiency in patients with MS. Treatment trials with vitamin D supplementation are continuing.

BENIGN MS

Several "rules of thumb" have been proposed to help advise patients about their prognosis. We have previously described that having a particular onset symptom, sex, or age at onset cannot be used to accurately predict the prognosis.

The concept of "benign MS" reflects the idea that people with a slow disease progression in the beginning of the disease often remain at a low level of disability later. It was proposed that a disability level of EDSS 3.0 or lower 10 years after disease onset were indicative of an overall mild disease course. Such patients with "benign MS" constitute about 20% of the MS population and were believed to have very little risk of further worsening in the later disease course. One study followed up patients for up to 20 years and showed that patients with an EDSS score of 2.0 or lower at 10 years had more than a 90% chance of remaining below a score of EDSS 4.5 at 20 years (25). Recently, this idea has been challenged by a larger study examining patients with a disability level of EDSS 3.0 or lower at 10 years. Of these patients, a little more than one-half had progressed beyond EDSS 3.0 at 20 years' follow-up, and about 20% had progressed beyond EDSS 6.0 (40). However, with around 80% of the initial cohort still not requiring the use of a cane at 20 years follow-up, it would appear that the concept of benign MS still has some merit.

Another reason to object to the idea of benign MS lies in the fact that the studies describing this concept rely on the EDSS as an outcome marker. While the EDSS is a useful scale for estimating physical disability, especially over long periods of follow-up, it falls short in measuring cognitive and behavioral symptoms and fatigue. It is important to realize that patients with little physical disability may still be impacted by less visible MS symptoms, which may well impact their ability to function. For example, a study in Norway showed that among patients with benign MS, depressive symptoms were associated with not being employed, even if these symptoms were mild (41). Sayao and coworkers reassessed a group of patients with a 20-year history of benign MS at 25 to 30 years of disease duration, and found that around 40% of this group had progressed in physical disability, fatigue, and cognitive function after all (42). Taken together, these studies highlight the uncertainty of predicting the long-term MS disease course.

KEY POINTS FOR PATIENTS AND FAMILIES

- The overall prognosis of MS is difficult to predict in individual patients.
- Patient characteristics such as sex, age at onset, or onset symptoms cannot reliably predict the future disease course.
- Recently, environmental risk factors, vitamin D (deficiency), and smoking have been shown to influence the risk of developing MS, as well as the disease course.
- Patients with MS should not smoke, not only because of the general ill health effects, but also because there is good evidence to support a negative influence of smoking on the disease course of MS.
- A low serum level of vitamin D is associated with a worse disease course of MS, and vitamin D supplementation should be considered if patients are found to be deficient.
- The overall prognosis of MS, as expressed in time to landmark disability, has recently been found to be better than initially reported, with a time to EDSS 6.0 of about 30 years overall, and about 15 years in PPMS.

REFERENCES

1. Kingwell E, van der Kop M, Zhao Y, et al. Relative mortality and survival in multiple sclerosis: findings from British Columbia, Canada. *J Neurol Neurosurg Psychiatr*. 2012;83:61–66.
2. Koch-Henriksen N, Sørensen PS. The changing demographic pattern of multiple sclerosis epidemiology. *Lancet Neurol*. 2010;9:520–532.
3. Beck CA, Metz LM, Svenson LW, et al. Regional variation of multiple sclerosis prevalence in Canada. *Mult Scler*. 2005;11:516–519.
4. Callegaro D, Goldbaum M, Morais L, et al. The prevalence of multiple sclerosis in the city of São Paulo, Brazil, 1997. *Acta Neurol Scand*. 2001;104:208–213.
5. Bhigjee AI, Moodley K, Ramkissoon K. Multiple sclerosis in KwaZulu Natal, South Africa: an epidemiological and clinical study. *Mult Scler*. 2007;13:1095–1099.
6. Taylor BV, Pearson JF, Clarke G, et al. MS prevalence in New Zealand, an ethnically and latitudinally diverse country. *Mult Scler*. 2010;16:1422–1431.
7. Cheng Q, Miao L, Zhang J, et al. A population-based survey of multiple sclerosis in Shanghai, China. *Neurology*. 2007;68:1495–1500.
8. Kim NH, Kim HJ, Cheong HK, et al. Prevalence of multiple sclerosis in Korea. *Neurology*. 2010;75:1432–1438.
9. Langer-Gould A, Zhang JL, Chung J, et al. Incidence of acquired CNS demyelinating syndromes in a multiethnic cohort of children. *Neurology*. 2011;77(12):1143–1148. doi:10.1212 WNL.0b013e31822facdd.
10. Langer-Gould A, Brara SM, Beaber BE, et al. Incidence of multiple sclerosis in multiple racial and ethnic groups. *Neurology*. 2013;80(19):1734–1739. doi:10.1212/WNL.0b013e3182918cc2.
11. Yetley EA. Assessing the vitamin D status of the US population. *Am J Clin Nutr*. 2008;88(2):558S–564S.
12. Schleicher RL, Sternberg MR, Lacher DA, et al. The vitamin D status of the US population from 1988 to 2010 using standardized serum concentrations of 25-hydroxyvitamin D shows recent modest increases. *Am J Clin Nutr*. 2016;104(2):454–461. doi:10.3945/ajcn.115.127985.
13. Alonso A, Hernán MA. Temporal trends in the incidence of multiple sclerosis: a systematic review. *Neurology*. 2008;71:129–135.
14. Munger KL, Levin LI, Hollis BW, et al. Serum 25-hydroxyvitamin D levels and risk of multiple sclerosis. *JAMA*. 2006;296:2832–2838.
15. van der Mei IAF, Ponsonby AL, Dwyer T, et al. Past exposure to sun, skin phenotype, and risk of multiple sclerosis: case-control study. *BMJ*. 2003;327:316.
16. Ascherio A, Munger KL. Environmental risk factors for multiple sclerosis. Part I: the role of infection. *Ann Neurol*. 2007;61:288–299.
17. Handel AE, Williamson AJ, Disanto G, et al. An updated meta-analysis of risk of multiple sclerosis following infectious mononucleosis. *PLOS ONE*. 2010;5:ii.
18. Munger KL, Fitzgerald KC, Freedman MS, et al. No association of multiple sclerosis activity and progression with EBV or tobacco use in BENEFIT. *Neurology*. 2015;85(19):1694–1701. doi:10.1212/WNL.0000000000002099.
19. Hernán MA, Olek MJ, Ascherio A. Cigarette smoking and incidence of multiple sclerosis. *Am J Epidemiol*. 2001;154:69–74.
20. Mikaeloff Y, Caridade G, Tardieu M, et al. Parental smoking at home and the risk of childhood-onset multiple sclerosis in children. *Brain*. 2007;130:2589–2595.
21. Hedström A, Bäärnhielm M, Olsson T, et al. Exposure to environmental tobacco smoke is associated with increased risk for multiple sclerosis. *Mult Scler*. 2011;17:788–793.
22. Weinshenker BG, Bass B, Rice GP, et al. The natural history of multiple sclerosis: a geographically based study. I. Clinical course and disability. *Brain*. 1989;112(pt 1):133–146.
23. Confavreux C, Vukusic S, Moreau T, et al. Relapses and progression of disability in multiple sclerosis. *N Engl J Med*. 2000;343:1430–1438.
24. Tremlett H, Paty D, Devonshire V. Disability progression in multiple sclerosis is slower than previously reported. *Neurology*. 2006;66:172–177.

25. Pittock SJ, Mayr WT, McClelland RL, et al. Change in MS-related disability in a population-based cohort: a 10-year follow-up study. *Neurology*. 2004;62:51–59.
26. Koch M, Kingwell E, Rieckmann P, et al. The natural history of primary progressive multiple sclerosis. *Neurology*. 2009;73:1996–2002.
27. Confavreux C, Vukusic S. Age at disability milestones in multiple sclerosis. *Brain*. 2006;129:595–605.
28. Cree BA, Khan O, Bourdette D, et al. Clinical characteristics of African Americans vs Caucasian Americans with multiple sclerosis. *Neurology*. 2004;63:2039–2045.
29. Boster AL, Endress CF, Hreha SA, et al. Pediatric-onset multiple sclerosis in African-American Black and European-origin White patients. *Pediatr Neurol*. 2009;40:31–33.
30. Confavreux C, Vukusic S, Adeleine P. Early clinical predictors and progression of irreversible disability in multiple sclerosis: an amnesic process. *Brain*. 2003;126:770–782.
31. Leray E, Yaouang J, Le Page E, et al. Evidence for a two-stage disability progression in multiple sclerosis. *Brain*. 2010;133:1900–1913.
32. Pittas F, Ponsonby AL, van der Mei IAF, et al. Smoking is associated with progressive disease course and increased progression in clinical disability in a prospective cohort of people with multiple sclerosis. *J Neurol*. 2009;256:577–585.
33. Healy BC, Ali EN, Guttmann CR, et al. Smoking and disease progression in multiple sclerosis. *Arch Neurol*. 2009;66:858–864.
34. Koch M, van Harten A, Uyttenboogaart M, et al. Cigarette smoking and progression in multiple sclerosis. *Neurology*. 2007;69:1515–1520.
35. Hernán MA, Jick SS, Logroscino G, et al. Cigarette smoking and the progression of multiple sclerosis. *Brain*. 2005;128:1461–1465.
36. Smolders J, Menheere P, Kessels A, et al. Association of vitamin D metabolite levels with relapse rate and disability in multiple sclerosis. *Mult Scler*. 2008;14:1220–1224.
37. Simpson S, Taylor B, Blizzard L, et al. Higher 25-hydroxyvitamin D is associated with lower relapse risk in multiple sclerosis. *Ann Neurol*. 2010;68:193–203.
38. Mowry EM, Krupp LB, Milazzo M, et al. Vitamin D status is associated with relapse rate in pediatric-onset multiple sclerosis. *Ann Neurol*. 2010;67:618–624.
39. Fitzgerald KC, Munger KL, Köchert K, et al. Association of vitamin D levels with multiple sclerosis activity and progression in patients receiving interferon beta-1b. *JAMA Neurol*. 2015;72(12):458–465. doi:10.1001/jamaneurol.2015.2742.
40. Sayao AL, Devonshire V, Tremlett H. Longitudinal follow-up of "benign" multiple sclerosis at 20 years. *Neurology*. 2007;68:496–500.
41. Glad SB, Nyland H, Aarseth JH, et al. How long can you keep working with benign multiple sclerosis? *J Neurol Neurosurg Psychiatry*. 2011;82(1):78–82. doi:10.1136/jnnp.2010.210732.
42. Sayao A, Bueno A, Devonshire V, et al. The psychosocial and cognitive impact of longstanding 'benign' multiple sclerosis. *Mult Scler*. 2011;17(11):1375–1383. doi:10.1177/1352458511410343.

5

Multiple Sclerosis Genetics

Bruce A. C. Cree

KEY POINTS FOR CLINICIANS

- Family aggregation and twin studies indicate that heredity contributes to multiple sclerosis (MS) risk.

- The primary MS susceptibility locus is within the major histocompatibility complex and encodes a protein, HLA-DRB1*15, that has a critical function in presenting antigens to T cells.

- Over 200 other genetic loci throughout the genome contribute to MS susceptibility.

- Many of these loci are associated with other autoimmune diseases suggesting sharing of a biological pathway, or pathways, in autoimmunity.

- The majority of identified MS susceptibility loci thus far are noncoding polymorphisms, that is, common genetic alleles also found in healthy individuals that do not directly influence protein structure. These polymorphisms could influence expression of over 500 MS associated genes.

- Genetic variants in the vitamin D enzymatic pathway are associated with MS susceptibility and underscore the importance of vitamin D's role in MS.

RACE AND GEOGRAPHY

Race and geography are known to influence MS prevalence. This suggests that heritable factors may contribute to MS pathogenesis (1). The risk of MS is much higher in populations of Northern European ancestry than in other ethnic groups residing at the same latitudes (2–5). It follows that this increased susceptibility might be due to genetic differences between ethnic groups. MS is approximately 50% less common in African Americans compared to whites (6,7). MS is still less common in both native Japanese and Japanese Americans (five per 100,000) compared to Northern European populations (100–150 per 100,000) (8). Similarly, MS is relatively less common among Native Americans in both the United States and Canada (9–12). These observations lead to the hypothesis that genetic traits for MS risk may be enriched in certain populations and occur less frequently in others thereby contributing to these racial patterns. However, despite a generally shared environment, ethnic factors that can track with race such as diet might also account for such differences.

FAMILIAL AGGREGATION

Although first described as a sporadic disease, the familial occurrence of MS was recognized in the late 19th century (13,14). Systematic studies of familial aggregation in MS support a genetic contribution to the disease (15–21). These studies found that approximately 15% to 20% of MS patients reported a family history of MS, a proportion that is significantly higher than what would be expected based on the relatively low prevalence of MS in these populations. The ratio of the relative risk of disease in siblings of affected individuals compared to the relative risk of disease in the overall population is referred to as λ_s (22). For MS, this risk ratio is approximately 15 to 40 indicating a moderately strong familial influence on MS risk (23). To help place the relevance of this value in the context of other heritable complex diseases heritable, the λ_s ratio for MS is higher than that for schizophrenia (9) similar to that for type 1 diabetes (15) and less than that for autism (59) (24). However, commonly shared environmental factors might also explain such familial aggregation (25).

> *Systematic studies of familial aggregation in MS support a genetic contribution to the disease.*

Twin Studies

Perhaps the most compelling observation indicating that MS susceptibility has a genetic component comes from twin studies that demonstrate concordance rates of approximately 30% in monozygotic twins and 3% to 5% in dizygotic twins (26–31). This rate for fraternal twins is similar to that of first-degree relatives of MS patients. Conjugal pair studies also show that the risk of MS increases substantially if both parents are affected by MS, again implying a heritable component to MS susceptibility (32–34) (Table 5.1). Taken together, familial and population-based studies indicate that some component of MS risk is heritable; however, that the majority of MS patients have no family history indicates either that environmental factors may outweigh genetic risks or that genetic risk can be attributed to the influence of multiple traits that by themselves have low disease penetrance. The concept that MS risk may be inherited as a complex trait rather than following simple Mendelian inheritance patterns, as is the case for recessive mutations such as cystic fibrosis or dominant mutations like Huntington's disease, is essential for understanding the genetic contributions to MS risk (Figure 5.1) (35).

> *Perhaps the most compelling observation indicating that MS susceptibility has a genetic component comes from twin studies that demonstrate concordance rates of approximately 30% in monozygotic twins and 3% to 5% in dizygotic twins.*

THE FIRST MOLECULAR MARKERS FOR MS: THE HUMAN LEUKOCYTE ANTIGENS

The first studies that identified a link between MS heredity and genetic variation compared human leukocyte antigen (HLA) protein polymorphisms between MS cases and healthy controls. These early studies found that cell surface antigens present on the membranes of peripheral blood mononuclear cells were more frequent in MS patients compared to unaffected controls. The first such antigens were HLA-A3 (36–38), followed by HLA-B7, and then HLA-DRw2 (39–43). These HLA associations were in fact not independent but rather reflected a common shared haplotype as a consequence of linkage disequilibrium. Linkage disequilibrium refers to the observation that alleles of certain neighboring genes tend to be inherited together as a consequence of natural selection, although the driving factors for such selection may be obscure. Thus the molecules HLA-A3, HLA-B7, and HLA-DRw2 are closely associated especially in European descended populations. Further elucidation as to which, or possibly more than one, of these linked genes contributes to MS genetics required development of improved molecular techniques.

LINKAGE ANALYSIS

In the 1980s, new DNA based technology was developed for studying Mendelian patterns of inheritance first with restriction fragment length polymorphisms (RFLPs) followed by microsatellite repeats (44,45). Using RFLPs to dissect the molecular contributions of the HLA locus to MS susceptibility, it became clear that alleles of HLA-DR2 are the major contributors to MS risk (46). These new molecular techniques not only allowed for dissection of linked genes at HLA but also made possible the ability to screen for other associations with MS found at many other positions across the genome. By studying the linkage between an inherited trait and DNA markers in families with some members affected by a heritable disease, it was possible to identify the chromosomal location of disease-causing genes (Figure 5.2). Markers that were physically near the disease-causing gene were likely to be inherited along with the disease trait because recombination between genetic loci occurs less frequently between neighboring genes relative to genes at greater distances. Thus the phenomenon of linkage disequilibrium that confounded efforts to discern between alleles of genes at HLA could be exploited to identify previously unknown disease-related genes. These new techniques were first applied to Mendelian inherited diseases and culminated in identification of many single gene mutations, such as those for cystic fibrosis and Huntington's disease.

TABLE 5.1 Familial Risks for MS

RELATIONSHIP TO PATIENT	RECURRENCE RISK (%)	RISK RELATIVE TO POPULATION	PROPORTION OF GENETIC SHARING (%)
Adopted first degree relative	0.2	Identity	0
Sibling with MS	3.0–5.0	15–25 fold increase	50
Dizygotic twin	3.0–5.0	15–25 fold increase	50
Monozygotic twin	34.0	170 fold increase	100
One parent with MS	3.0–5.0	15–25 fold increase	50
Two parents with MS	6.0–10.0	30–50 fold increase	50 with each parent

Note: Assumes lifetime population prevalence of 0.2% (33).
MS, multiple sclerosis.

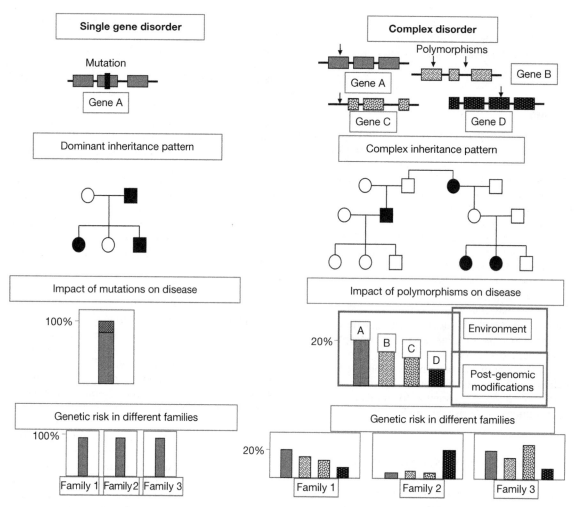

FIGURE 5.1 The inheritance pattern of a dominantly transmitted single gene mutation is contrasted with that of a complex polygenic disorder in which polymorphisms, as well as environmental factors and postgenomic modifications, contribute to the disease phenotype. Unlike the dominantly inherited trait that has high penetrance (the likelihood of developing the phenotype associated with the genotype) whose phenotype can be traced from one generation to the next, the inheritance pattern of a complex polygenic disorder may not be readily apparent from studying the family tree. Furthermore, unlike single gene disorders, polygenic traits could have different phenotypes across families.

Source: Modified from Peltonen L, McKusick VA. Dissecting human disease in the postgenomic era. *Science*. 2001;**291**:1224–1229.

> *Alleles of HLA-DR2 are the major contributors to MS risk.*

MS AS A COMPLEX TRAIT

The linkage-based approach had the potential to also be applied not only to single gene disorders but also to complex multigenic traits. However, the hurdles for identifying such traits would be considerably higher because the penetrance of each trait would be far less than for disease causing mutations (47). Penetrance refers to the likelihood that a particular genotype will manifest as a phenotype. For Mendelian inherited mutations such as those for dominant diseases such as Huntington's disease, the penetrance is very high, meaning that nearly all individuals who carry the disease-causing genotype will develop the disease. However, for complex traits, the penetrance is low and polymorphisms associated with the complex trait could be common in the overall population. This was clearly the case for the HLA locus. None of the HLA alleles associated with MS by themselves are disease-causing mutations. All these alleles were commonly found in healthy controls but were overrepresented among MS patients. The importance of this observation initially was perhaps not fully appreciated. Investigators assumed that because heritable MS risk could be found in families in whom the MS-associated HLA alleles were not carried that other loci, perhaps with

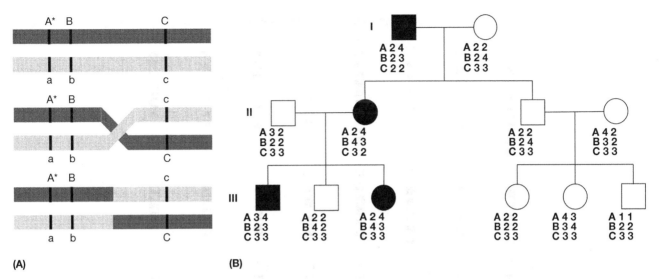

FIGURE 5.2 Meiotic recombination is the underlying genetic principle of linkage analysis. Paternal (dark gray) and maternal (light gray) chromosomes are aligned in a germ cell (cells that give rise to sperm or ova). Sequence A* is a disease-causing allele, whereas a is the normal allele. Alleles for nearby DNA sequences on the same chromosome are depicted as B and C. Paternal alleles are represented in capital letters and maternal alleles are represented in lower case. During meiotic recombination, paired chromosomal DNA strands crossover. The crossover event results in a break in the paternal DNA strand that is recombined with the maternal DNA strand resulting in recombined chromosomes. The mixed chromosomes are passed to the sperm or ova. If the disease gene is A*, then recombination is more likely to occur between the disease gene and alleles of C than alleles of B. By following the segregation of the disease gene in families along with the segregation of genetic markers, the disease causing gene A* can be mapped relative to the markers B and C (A). Pedigree analysis showing segregation of markers with a dominantly inherited trait. In the second generation, the marker combination A4 B3 C2 is inherited by the affected daughter. Owing to recombination between markers B and C, in the third generation affected individuals carry the marker combination A4 B3 C3 showing that the trait is linked to the A4 B3 haplotype. Although these markers are linked to the trait, they can also be found in the general population. Linkage analysis relies on segregation of markers that are linked to a trait taking into account family structure (B).

even stronger effects than that of HLA, must be present elsewhere in the genome. If this was the case, then systematic study of the genome in families affected by MS would surely identify these other loci.

GENOMIC LINKAGE SCREENS

The first series of genome-wide screens using several hundred microsatellite DNA markers across in approximately 100 affected sib pairs were undertaken in the 1990s (48–50). Assuming that other loci in the genome would have had similar effects on MS risk as that of, or even greater than, the major histocompatibility complex (MHC), these studies would have been expected to identify at least a few novel loci. However, no statistically significant additional loci were identified. Furthermore, one of these studies was unable to detect a signal from the MHC (48). Follow-up studies using multiply affected families also failed to detect any convincing new MS susceptibility loci (51–55). Adding more microsatellite markers to the initial genome screens also failed (56–58). Pooling data for meta-analysis similarly failed to identify loci other than the MHC (59,60). It became clear that identification of the effects of genetic variation on MS susceptibility would require not only

better markers but also substantially increased numbers of families for statistical power. The way forward required a much larger number of affected families to which any single group had access. The International Multiple Sclerosis Genetics Consortium (IMSGC) was thus founded in 2003 and brought together previously competing investigators in a collaborative effort to decode MS heritability (61) (www .neurodiscovery.harvard.edu/research/imsgc.html).

The first large-scale linkage study with sufficient statistical power to detect loci with effects similar to that of the MHC across the genome in populations from Australia, Scandinavia, the United Kingdom, and the United States identified a definite association between the MHC and MS susceptibility (Figure 5.3) (62). However, other loci whose associations with MS had been proposed from smaller studies were not replicated. This study was an important milestone in the study of MS genetics because for the first time, an adequate number of markers and MS-affected families were brought together through an international collaborative effort. Furthermore, the markers used were sufficiently numerous and evenly spaced across the genome that there was confidence that the majority of the genome was adequately represented for linkage analysis. Perhaps most importantly, 730 families were studied, thus providing

2005 genome-wide linkage screen

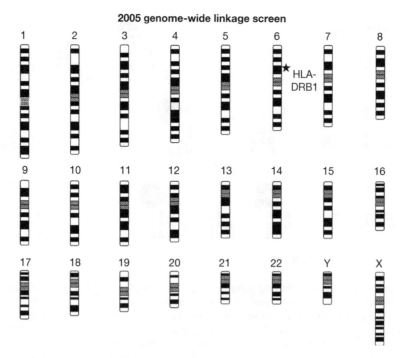

FIGURE 5.3 MS genomic regions of interest identified by linkage.
MS, multiple sclerosis.

Source: From Sawcer S, Ban M, Maranian M, et al. A high-density screen for linkage in multiple sclerosis. *Am J Hum Genet*. 2005;77(3):454–467.

adequate power to detect genetic effects that increased the odds of MS risk by more than twofold. Only MHC was found to increase risk of MS, which indicated that other possible loci that might influence MS risk must have more modest individual effects. Identification of such loci was effectively not possible using linkage analysis unless tens of thousands of families were analyzed. (63) This inherent limitation of linkage methodology potentially could be overcome by a different approach genetic analysis: the genome-wide association screen (GWAS).

Genome-Wide Association Screen

Further technological innovation led to identification of single nucleotide polymorphisms (SNPs). SNPs are genetic variants that occur at a single base pair position within the genome (Figure 5.4). The remarkable achievement of sequencing of the human genome in conjunction with mapping hundreds of thousands of these SNP variants led to the realization that 99.9% of the human genome is invariant (64,65). Nevertheless, there are still billions of genetic variations, many of which are exceedingly rare whereas others are more common. By focusing on the variants that are more commonly found, for example, SNP alleles that are present in at least 5% of the overall population, it would be possible to map traits that are linked to common SNP variants. By coupling such potentially informative SNP variants with microchip-based miniaturization, it became

possible to map hundreds of thousands of SNP variants from thousands of individuals (Figure 5.4). If heritable traits such as MS susceptibility are linked to commonly identified variants, then genotyping these common SNP variants could map the loci of the heritable trait. This hypothesis is referred to as the common disease–common variant hypothesis.

Unlike linkage analysis that required relatively large effect sizes for tracking heritable traits in families, the newer SNP-based technology was capable of detecting smaller individual genetic effects by increasing the numbers of affected individuals and unaffected controls. With a sufficiently large enough number of samples, association testing that compares the prevalence of any given SNP marker between two populations has the capability to detect modest or small genetic effects as long as the numbers of affected and unaffected individuals are sufficient. Moreover, the samples for association screens did not necessarily require DNA from family members because although family structure could be taken into account in GWAS statistics, it did not have to be taken into account. In essence, this approach simply compares the prevalence of any given SNP marker in cases and controls, which is similar to a chi-square statistic. As long as the controls are from the same genetic background as the cases, then statistically significant differences in the prevalence of a particular SNP allele would presumably be due to a disease-related trait.

Case-control design compare single nucleotide
polymorphisms (SNPs) in two populations

Non-affected individuals
(controls)

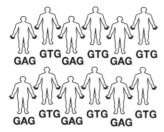

Affected individuals
(cases)

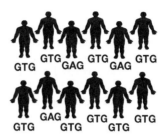

50% of controls carry the
GAG genotype and 50% carry
the GTG genotype (A→T SNP)

75% of cases carry the
GAG genotype and 25% carry
the GTG genotype (A→T SNP)

FIGURE 5.4 Association analysis comparing the prevalence of markers in two populations. In this example, the marker of interest, an SNP at position 2, is present in 75% of cases and 25% of controls. The odds ratio for the association of this marker with the disease state is therefore 3.0.

SNP, single nucleotide polymorphisms.

GWAS Identifies the First Genes Outside the MHC

MS was one of the first diseases to be studied using this new GWAS technique. The IMSGC conducted the first GWAS in 2007 using over 334,923 SNPs in 930 MS trio families (a trio family is a MS patient and both parents) with a replication of datasets consisting of another 609 family trios and an additional 2,322 case subjects and 789 unrelated controls (66). It was hoped that this massive and costly effort would finally determine the genetic architecture of MS especially in regard to the much sought after non-MHC contributions. As anticipated, the MHC was definitively associated with MS susceptibility; however, beyond the MHC only two other loci were identified with a statistically significant level of confidence. These loci encoded genes involved in immune regulation: the interleukin 2 receptor (IL2Rα) and the interleukin 7 receptor (IL7Rα). Associations with MS susceptibility for both loci were subsequently validated in other populations (67–72).

> *Alleles of the interleukin 2 and the interleukin 7 receptors were the first non–major MHC loci that were definitely associated with MS risk.*

The landmark achievement of identifying two non-HLA loci established that genes outside the MHC contributed to MS susceptibility. However, variations at these alleles, along with those of the MHC, could not account for all MS heritability. Moreover, the alleles identified were, by definition, common alleles (the SNPs genotyped from most GWAS have minor allele frequencies [MAFs] of at least 5% meaning that the SNPs are present in at least 5% of the population). However, the commonality of MS susceptibility–associated SNPs in both MS cases and controls were surprising. For example, the IL2Rα variant was present in 85% of controls and 88% of cases. IL7Rα variant results were similar: the MS-associated variant was present in 78% of MS patients and 75% of controls. The presence of these variants in the majority of controls had two very important implications. First, these variants are not mutations but instead are the most common polymorphisms of each receptor. Therefore, the consequence to the protein associated with the polymorphism is normal function as opposed to loss of function or gain of an abnormal function associated with either recessive or dominant mutations, respectively. Second, because there was only a very slight overrepresentation of these polymorphisms in MS cases, the effect that this polymorphism has on MS risk is miniscule. Indeed, the odds ratios for these alleles were less than 1.5. If other non-HLA MS risk alleles were linked to common SNP variants, then sample size calculations showed that variants associated with a 1.1 fold or higher odds of MS risk would require at least 10,000 MS cases and a similar number of controls (47,73).

Although this GWAS identified only two non-HLA loci with a genome wide level of statistical significance, there may be many other loci associated with MS susceptibility that missed the statistical cutoff for definite association. GWAS performed by other groups, as well as meta-analyses that combined GWAS data from different studies, identified multiple other MS susceptibility loci (74–82).

In order to expand the statistical power needed for the next round of GWAS, the IMSGC expanded its membership ultimately involving 23 research groups from 15 countries. The IMSGC also partnered with the Welcome Trust Case Control Consortium 2 (WTCCC2) to make use of the most up-to-date GWAS technology (83). Ultimately, 9,772 MS cases and 17,376 control DNA samples passed stringent quality control assessments. 441,547 autosomal SNPs were genotyped in this massive dataset. During analysis, it became clear that an important problem might bias the study: population stratification. Because this GWAS did not use a family based approach, the comparison of cases to controls was predicated on the assumption that cases and controls shared a common genomic structure except at the MS susceptibility loci. However, if cases and controls had somewhat different genomic structures due to differential sampling, then the differences identified between cases and controls could be due to either disease-causing loci or irrelevant differences in genomic structure introduced by sampling bias. When cases and controls from a single country, such as the United Kingdom, were compared, there was no evidence of population stratification. However, because cases and controls were not perfectly matched by country of origin, the entire dataset showed evidence of genomic inflation, meaning that because cases and controls were not perfectly matched there was a systematic difference for genomic markers between these two groups that would bias the GWAS results due to population stratification. Several methods to control for genomic inflation were employed but ultimately a novel approach (variance component method) was able to effectively adjust for the genomic inflation bias.

The IMSGC and WTCCC2's MS GWAS identified 52 loci that were definitively associated with MS susceptibility. This study not only replicated the known MHC, IL2Rα, and IL2Rα associations but also found 20 loci that had been implicated in MS risk through other GWAS studies as well as meta-analyses. Furthermore, 29 novel loci were identified. All non-MHC loci had minor influences on MS susceptibility with odds ratios ranging from 1.07 to 1.21. Perhaps the most important observation from this study was that the majority of SNPs identified were located near genes encoding immune functions. This observation supported the hypothesis that MS is indeed an autoimmune disease. Furthermore, many of the implicated genes share common pathways involved in immune regulation, providing important clues as to how normal immune function might become dysregulated in MS. Moreover, 23 of the identified loci are known to be involved in other autoimmune diseases indicating that common mechanisms, at least in part, underlie autoimmune diseases. However, the identification of these common loci did not lead immediately to an understanding as to why the central nervous system (CNS) is the primary target of autoimmune injury, although several possible genes are expressed in the CNS and some, such as GALC, encode proteins that were previously implicated in MS (84).

> The IMSGC and WTCCC2 MS GWAS identified 52 loci that were definitively associated with MS susceptibility.

In the most recent iteration of the IMSGC's efforts to create a complete genomic map of MS, data from 15 separate GWAS were integrated into a single discovery dataset consisting of 14,802 subjects and 26,703 controls (85). Data from the 1000 Genomes European panel was used to impute 8.6 million SNPs with MAF of at least 1%. An additional dataset consisting of 20,822 MS subjects and 18,956 controls was genotyped using a custom designed MS chip of some 4,842 non-MHC SNPs identified in the discovery cohort. A second replication cohort of 12,267 MS subjects and 22,625 controls was used for validation. This effort yielded identification of 200 non-MHC loci with genome-wide statistically significant associations that contribute to MS susceptibility with odds ratios between 1.06 and 2.06. Interestingly, the risk allele frequencies ranged from 2.1% to 98.4% in the European population. MS-associated SNPs were identified on every chromosome except for the Y chromosome. This study also found the first convincing X-linked locus.

Nearly all of the genetic loci map to noncoding areas of the genome, meaning that the polymorphisms are not associated with structural changes to an expressed protein's primary sequence. Some SNPs are intragenic and therefore could relate to splicing, for example, producing different ratios of splice protein products. However, the majority of the MS-associated SNPs are intergenic meaning that they are not immediately found near any known genes. These areas may contain transcriptional regulatory elements such as promoters or enhancers, open chromatin, histone modification sites, or even transcribed regulatory ribonucleic acids (RNAs) that are not translated into proteins. The recent ENCODE project's remarkable discovery that 80% of the human genome contains elements linked to biological processes underscores that DNA regions without open reading frames can be biologically important and in fact do not contain what previously had been disregarded as "junk" DNA (86,87).

The observation that the majority of the MS genomic map involves noncoding areas suggests that MS susceptibility may be a disorder of networks involved in gene regulation rather than structural alteration in gene products. If this is the case, then understanding MS risk will need to be refined by revealing the different patterns of gene expression between MS patients and unaffected controls in relevant cell types. As a first effort to understand the influence of these loci on MS susceptibility atlases of gene expression based on cell type were consulted for expression of mRNAs linked to the MS-associated loci. In this data mining study, gene expression profiles from various available cell types were analyzed for expression of mRNAs that are genetically linked to the MS-associated SNPs. Not surprisingly, significant enrichment of mRNAs linked to MS-associated loci was present in cells of the adaptive immune system (both T cells and B cells). Interestingly, cells of the innate immune system such as natural killer cells and dendritic cells also showed enrichment of mRNAs linked to the MS-associated loci, underscoring a potential role of both adaptive and innate immunity in MS susceptibility. Thymic tissue also showed upregulation of gene transcripts potentially linked to MS susceptibility loci. Data generated from examining the expression profiles of differentiated neuronal lineage cells derived human induced pluripotent stem cells as well as purified primary human microglia and astrocytes found enrichment of mRNAs from MS-associated loci in microglial cells. This observation suggests that gene regulation within microglia, the CNS's resident immune cells, might also influence MS susceptibility. Taken together these data suggest that MS susceptibility loci possibly could alter gene expression profiles in diverse cells of the peripheral adaptive and innate immune systems as well as microglia, the resident innate immune cells of the nervous system.

With 200 loci potentially influencing the expression of an even larger number of neighboring message and or regulatory RNAs that could have both cis and trans effects on expression patterns of other RNAs, understanding the genetic basis for MS susceptibility will require a completely different way of thinking about genetics than what is traditionally associated with Mendelian disorders. To begin to understand whether the MS-associated SNPs can alter gene expression, gene expression profiles from peripheral blood mononuclear cells (PBMCs) from MS patients and unaffected controls were analyzed to determine whether the MS-associated SNPs were associated with alterations in mRNA transcripts. In this preliminary experiment in MS PBMCs, 30% of the 200 non-MHC MS associated SNPs were found to be cis-acting expression quantitative trait loci (cis-eQTLs) for 92 genes. This experiment provides primary evidence for the hypothesis that genetic basis for MS susceptibility acts through altering gene expression in at least some cells of the peripheral immune system (in this experiment CD4 naïve T cells and monocytes).

That genetic MS-related loci are involved in gene regulation in lymphoid cells comes as little surprise given the overwhelming evidence indicating that MS is an immune-mediated disorder. However, why the brain and spinal cord are selectively targeted in MS remains unknown. One hope of genetic studies is to elucidate why the CNS is apparently targeted by the immune system. To this end, an analysis of eQTLs from brain-derived tissues was also undertaken to see if the alterations in gene expression in the target organ contribute to MS susceptibility. Here the results were less clear with some MS loci potentially influencing expression of neuron-associated transcripts but also simultaneously potentially influencing expression of B cell transcripts. This observation illustrates a challenge with this type of analysis: identification of disease-associated SNPs is not synonymous with identification of the causative problem. It is important to understand that for the majority of the identified loci, multiple neighboring genes are also linked to the MS-associated SNP. Therefore, with the current level of resolution of GWAS, the exact genetic variant involved in MS susceptibility cannot be determined. Although it is possible that the MS-associated variants are the SNPs identified by the GWAS, it is also possible that the identified SNPs are in linkage disequilibrium with the true MS-associated alleles. Additional SNPs or resequencing of regions of interest will be necessary to refine the map and identify the causal variant.

Although the expression profile analysis of brain tissue did not clearly identify a pattern of CNS expressed genes that explain why the brain and spinal cord are targeted in MS, this analysis provided another line of evidence implicating microglial in MS susceptibility. A previously identified MS susceptibility gene *CLECL1* was expressed at low levels in cortical tissue. However, this transcript is found in microglia that compose only a small amount of cortical tissue. In purified microglia, *CLECL1* is expressed at levels 20-fold higher than in cortical slices. That this MS susceptibility gene is expressed in microglial cells provides another line of evidence indicating that these CNS cells could participate in in MS susceptibility.

That, there are a 200 loci associated with MS risk and that many of these loci could potentially modulate gene expression of a large number of genes poses a major challenge for understanding the heritable aspects of MS. One strategy to try to integrate the function of the many genes plausibly involved in MS is to cluster the genes by established function within established cellular pathways. This approach leverages bioinformatics to help reduce a large amount of complex data into gene/protein networks that functionally linked through canonical prior knowledge and subsequently structured in the form of pathways diagrams. A prioritized list of 551 genes were selected based on the eQTL data described earlier, along with genes that had at least one exonic variant, genes that have high regulatory potential and genes that exhibit similar tissue-specific coexpression patterns. Additional modeling efforts exploring potential protein–protein interactions found that about 1/3 of the 551 prioritized genes were connected and could be organized into 13 communities or subnetworks that have higher levels of connectivity. These in silico modeling efforts found that many of the potential MS-related genes map to pathways with known functions in immune cells including processes involved in lymphoid development, maturation, and differentiation. However, neurons and astroglial cells repurpose at least some of the genes involved in immune signaling such as tumor necrosis factor alpha, ciliary neurotrophic factor, nerve growth factor, and neuregulin, leading to an interesting and potentially important ambiguity as to in which tissue or tissues these genes exerts their effect in promoting MS susceptibility. Much work is needed to further understand the contextual basis in which MS susceptibility genes exert their influence.

The analysis of MS GWAS data has not only lead to the identification of a large number of genetic loci involved in MS susceptibility but also fundamentally changed the way in which MS heritability is conceived. Simple Mendelian concepts of heritability or even quantitative traits arising from multiple loci (polygenic) apply only in part to the complex genomics at work in MS. With 200 loci across the genome and more than 500 potential genes involved in multiple biological pathways, understanding the genetic basis of MS susceptibility requires development of new ways to understand how alterations in transcriptional levels of multiple genes influence molecular functions within cell types. Many other human complex diseases share similar genomic features. For example, Mendelian alleles that have large effect sizes do not contribute to Crohn's disease, rheumatoid arthritis, or schizophrenia. In each of these disease states, GWAS studies have found multiple risk alleles that individually contribute only fractionally to genetic risk but in aggregate appear to influence the disease phenotype through effects on cellular regulatory networks. In this "omnigenic" model of heritability, alterations in core genes that have biologically interpretable roles in a disease contribute only partially to the disease trait. Most of the susceptibility arises from alterations of secondary genes that are interconnected to the core genes through networks (88). In the case of MS, the "core" genes are likely composed of the antigen presenting genes within the MHC associated with MS risk nearly 50 years ago. These genes exert the strongest individual effects in terms of MS risk. Secondary loci, which by themselves contribute only minute fractional risks, exert a greater overall impact on MS susceptibility by virtue of the shear number of genes involved in secondary pathways that indirectly connect back to the core genetic pathway.

MISSING HERITABILITY

Despite the remarkable achievement of the IMSGC, the estimate of the total contribution to MS heritability by these, the MHC and non-MHC 200 loci is only 39% (48% if suggestive effects that did not meet genome wide levels of statistical significance in the replication datasets are included). Given that the MHC itself accounts for 20% of MS heritability, the total contribution of the other 200 genetic loci to MS risk is only ~20%. This suggests that 50% to 60% of MS genetic risk will be accounted for by variants that cannot be identified using SNP chips

designed to test the common allele–common variant hypothesis. Identification of rare disease causative alleles that have individually weak or modest effects poses additional challenges for genetic analysis. First, the number of potential rare variants is much greater than the number of common variants. Second, the majority of rare variants have not yet been described in publicly available databases. Identification and cataloguing these rare variants will require sequencing many more genomes. Finally, optimal methods for typing an individual's DNA for rare variants are still being developed.

> *The MHC itself accounts for 20% of MS heritability, the total contribution of the other 200 genetic loci to MS risk is only ~20%. This suggests that 50% to 60% of MS genetic risk will be accounted for by variants that cannot be identified using SNP chips designed to test the common allele–common variant hypothesis.*

VITAMIN D GENETICS

Vitamin D deficiency is a risk factor for MS susceptibility and likely accounts for some of the differences in MS's geographic prevalence. Multiple studies showed that 25-OH vitamin D levels are lower in MS cases compared to controls in both European descended and African American populations (89–92). The IMSGC–WTCC2 GWAS identified two genes involved in vitamin D metabolism as conferring increased susceptibility to MS. CYP27B1 encodes an enzyme that catalyses the synthesis of 1,25-dihydroxy vitamin D (1,25 dihydroxyvitamin D is the biologically active form of the vitamin). CYP24A1 encodes and enzyme that degrades 1,25-dihydroxyvitamin D. Given that vitamin D deficiency is a risk factor for MS and that two genes (CYP27B1 and CYP24A1) that regulate the Vitamin D synthesis and degradation confer susceptibility to MS, these genes may contribute to MS risk by decreasing levels of active vitamin D. CYP27B1 was also shown to influence MS risk in MS families with multiply affected individuals (93). By systematically sequencing all genomic protein-encoding regions in 43 MS patients from multiplex families, a nonsynonymous variant of CYP27B1 (R389H) was identified segregating in one family with an incompletely penetrant dominant inheritance pattern. This variant leads to complete loss of CYP27B1 activity and therefore causes low levels of 1,25-dihydroxyvitamin D. The R389H CYP27B1 variant was genotyped in 3,000 parent-affected trios and was transmitted from parent to affected offspring in 19 trios. Applying whole-genome sequencing to a study of 2,619 individuals, a low frequency (MAF = 2.5%)

synonymous coding variant in the *CYP2R1* gene was associated with vitamin D levels (94). CYP2R1 is a hepatic enzyme that catalyzes 25-hydroxylation of vitamin D (95). The A allele of this SNP increases the risk of vitamin D insufficiency by twofold. In a case-control study of 5,927 cases and 5,599 controls, individuals carrying this SNP were found to be at increased risk for MS with an odds ratio of 1.4. These results underscore the important role of vitamin D in MS and show that not only environmental factors but also genetic factors influence vitamin D levels.

Given that vitamin D deficiency is a risk factor for MS and that two genes *(CYP27B1 and CYP24A1) that regulate the Vitamin D synthesis and degradation confer susceptibility to MS, these genes may contribute to MS risk by decreasing levels of active vitamin D.*

Vitamin D itself has important regulatory roles in gene expression. RNA expression level of the major MS susceptibility gene HLA-DRB1*15:01 is regulated by vitamin D, albeit somewhat paradoxically (i.e., expression of the allele is upregulated by vitamin D) (96). Vitamin D receptor binding elements have been identified in the majority of MS-associated genes, implying that expression of many of these genes could also be controlled by vitamin D (97). Although the details of the network of interactions between genes that regulate vitamin D synthesis and MS susceptibility genes, whose expression is in turn regulated by vitamin D, have yet to be established, these studies illustrate the importance of vitamin D in MS pathogenesis. Low levels of vitamin D, either because of environmental factors such as decreased sunlight exposure or low dietary intake of vitamin D, or because of genetic traits that reduce levels of 1,25-dihydroxyvitamin D, clearly contribute to MS susceptibility and may also contribute to disease activity (98–101).

Vitamin D itself has important regulatory roles in gene expression. RNA expression level of the major MS susceptibility gene *HLA-DRB1*15:01 is regulated by vitamin D.*

A ROLE FOR B CELLS IN MS SUSCEPTIBILITY

In addition to the recent IMSGC efforts that identified potential involvement for all cells of the innate and adaptive immune response in MS susceptibility, including B cells, a recent case-control study in Sardinians found

that a polymorphism in the *TNFSF113B* gene encoding the cytokine B-cell activating factor (BAFF) (102). BAFF is expressed by B cells and activates and differentiates B cells. Recent clinical trials found that depletion of B cells using monoclonal antibodies significantly suppress relapsing activity in MS suggesting a prominent role for B cells in MS (103). The genetic variant (BAFF-var) associated with MS is also associated with SLE and is thought to give rise to a shorter transcript that escapes miRNA inhibition, thereby resulting in increased production of BAFF. Whether the BAFF-var will be associated with an attenuated response to B cell depleting antibodies due to increased B cell activation by BAFF remains to be determined.

EXOME AND GENOME SEQUENCING

A second example of exome sequencing's power to detect rare alleles of MS susceptibility genes is the discovery of a missense mutation in the *TYK2* gene (104). An allele of the *TYK2* gene was previously found to be protective in genome-wide association scans (80,105,106). In contrast, the missense allele identified by exome sequencing modestly increases the risk of MS. Similar to the study of CYP27B1, the rare allele of TYK2 (rs557627444) was first identified in a multiply-affected large MS pedigree and then replicated in 2,104 trios.

The studies of *CYP27B1*, *CYP2R1*, and *TYK2* showcase the powerful advantage of exome and whole genome sequencing. Unlike the SNP chip based technology that is restricted by the genetic variants imprinted on the chip, sequencing the exome has the potential to identify any variant present within an individual's coding DNA. Therefore, exome sequencing technology has the potential to identify rare coding variants that would not be present on SNP chips.

Individual genome sequencing is also now possible. The cost of high throughput sequencing has dramatically decreased since the first human genome was sequenced (~1 billion U.S. dollars) and currently runs approximately $1,500/genome. It is anticipated that in the next few years, the price will fall further to less than $100/genome. The advantage of genome sequencing over exome sequencing is that the entire genome is sequenced, which includes all the noncoding DNA that may contain important regulatory elements in addition to the sequences used to encode specific proteins. Not accounted for by the relatively low cost of sequencing is the added cost of data management and analysis for the additional noncoding sequences.

Although the technology for determining genetic sequences has rapidly progressed such that it will soon be commercially feasible to sequence any individual's entire genome, the analytic techniques for interpreting the massive amounts of data are still being developed. The technology for deriving the primary sequence has temporarily outpaced the technology for genomic data analysis. Both software and hardware computational technologies are being developed that will enable desktop analysis of the human genome's 3 billion base pairs.

Preliminary studies suggest that every individual's DNA contains over 50,000 SNP variants and over 5,000 insertion/deletion polymorphisms (107). Importantly, 42% of the SNPs and 86% of the insertion/deletion polymorphisms are novel, meaning that they had not been previously been recorded in publicly available databases. Given the very large numbers of rare polymorphisms contained in every individual's DNA, assigning disease causative roles for these variants poses considerable methodological challenges. The identification of the rare R389H CYP27B1 allele was made possible by the additional information imparted by the multiplex family structure and was validated by large-scale trio analysis. It is likely that additional rare coding variants will be identified by this approach.

THE MHC AND MS SUSCEPTIBILITY

The MHC is 3.5 millions bases (Mb) of DNA located on the short arm of chromosome 6. It is the most genetically dense area of the human genome and encodes over 3,000 genes. The HLA genes are grouped into three structurally related classes from the telomere to the centromere: class I, class III, and class II (Figure 5.5). The HLA genes encode for glycoproteins that are expressed on the cell surface and play critical roles in recognition of self-antigens by the immune system. Many of these genes are highly polymorphic, adding additional complexity of this locus. Multiple autoimmune diseases have risk alleles that map to this region, thereby underscoring its importance in regulation of immune function (108).

As a consequence of selective pressures, the MHC is characterized by extensive linkage disequilibrium that can span the MHC and confounds mapping studies. Thus, alleles of class I genes can be genetically linked to distant alleles of class II genes. Many of the HLA alleles were first identified serologically and gave rise to a complex and often inconsistent nomenclature. Recent extensive efforts were made at mapping the serological types to DNA sequences and the genetic architecture of the MHC is now much better understood (109–113). As a consequence, the genetic basis of the serotypes is now understood and a consistent nomenclature has finally come into focus that will help advance further study of the MHC (hla.alleles.org/).

As described earlier, the first genetic associations identified in MS were found for HLA class I alleles using serological typing of HLA antigens on leukocytes (36–40). When HLA class II alleles were also associated with MS susceptibility, it was proposed that the class I associations were accounted for by linkage disequilibrium with the class II loci (41–43). Clarifying the associations of HLA loci with MS susceptibility was ultimately made possible

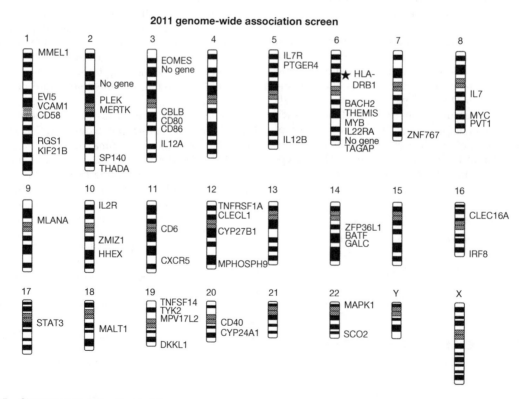

FIGURE 5.5 Chromosome 6 position in Mb.
Mb, millions bases.

by DNA-based typing of HLA polymorphisms in multiple datasets.

It is now clear that the primary MS susceptibility signal at HLA stems from the MHC class II locus. In European descended populations, the primary risk allele is HLA-DRB1*15:01, that is part of a haplotype: DRB1*15:01, DQA1*01:02, DQB1*0602. This haplotype encodes for cell surface glycoprotein genes that can present antigens and peptides to T cells. Together, these genes correspond to the serological markers known as HLA-DR2, DQ6.

> In European descended populations, the primary risk allele is HLA-DRB1*15:01, that is part of a haplotype: DRB1*15:01, DQA1*01:02, DQB1*0602.

Fine mapping studies indicate that the most important contributors to MS susceptibility are polymorphisms in the DRB1 gene (114). Neighboring polymorphisms in the DQB1 gene, although tightly linked to DRB1, do not contribute to MS risk, thus establishing a centromeric boundary for MS risk at HLA-DRB1.

Multiple polymorphisms within HLA-DRB1 influence MS susceptibility in populations (Figure 5.5). HLA-DRB1*1501 contributes to MS susceptibility with a dominant, dose-dependent effect (115). In African descended populations, the closely related HLA-DRB1*15:03 allele contributes to MS risk (114,116). HLA-DRB1*03 contributes to MS risk as a recessive trait (96).

HLA-DRB1*13:03 also contributes to MS risk (83). In the presence of HLA-DRB1:15, the HLA-DRB1*08 allele further increases MS risk (117–119), whereas the HLA-DRB1*14 and HLA-DRB1*10 alleles attenuate the risk of MS transmitted by HLA-DRB1*15 (Figure 5.6). To add to the complexity, certain alleles seem to contribute to MS in some, but not all, populations. In Sardinia, in addition to HLA-DRB1*15 and HLA-DRB1*03, HLA-DRB1*04 alleles contribute to MS susceptibility (120–123). Although the allelic interactions at this class II MHC locus are remarkably complex similar principals will likely apply to other risk loci.

Fine mapping studies of the telomeric boundary of MS susceptibility found that the MHC class I locus independently contributes to MS susceptibility, although the exact risk gene, or genes, in this region have not been precisely mapped (83,124–126). Alleles of the class I gene HLA-A are proposed to have a protective effect for MS susceptibility. However, as with the class II locus, extensive linkage disequilibrium is present in the class I region and therefore the class I signal might stem from linked alleles of neighboring genes including HLA-B (127), HLA-C (125), and HLA-G (126). Alleles of these genes form a linked haplotype that spans the MHC: HLA-A*02:01--HLA-B*44:02--HLA-C*05:01--HLA-DRB1*04:01. Thus far no study to date has definitively established the precise location of the class I MS susceptibility signal. The MHC class I signal implies a role for the innate immune system in MS and is consistent with other genome-wide effects showing that MS susceptibility arises from both adaptive and innate immunity. The most recent IMSGC effort found 32 loci within the MHC that contribute statistically significant independent effects with genome-wide levels of significance (85). Interestingly, one

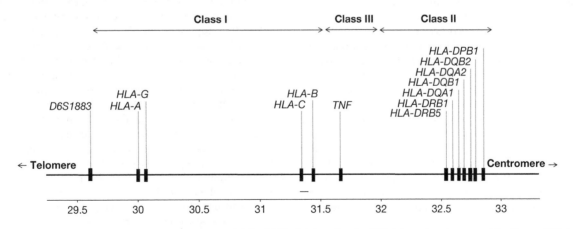

FIGURE 5.6 Combinations of *HLA-DRB1* alleles and risk of MS. Odds ratios for MS risk and various combinations of *HLA-DRB1* alleles are depicted graphically. The *y*-axis shows the log of the odds ratio with positive values increasing the risk of MS and negative values decreasing the risk of MS. The highest odds ratios are for *HLA-DRB1*15* homozygotes and for *HLA-DRB1*15/HLA-DRB1*08* heterozygotes. In contrast, *HLA-DRB1*14* and *HLA-DRB1*10* alleles are associated with a lower risk of MS in *HLA-DRB1*15* heterozygotes. The graph depicts that the impact of the *HLA-DRB1*08* allele on increasing MS risk is proportionally as strong as that of *HLA-DRB1*10* in lowering MS risk in *HLA-DRB1*15* heterozygotes.
HLA, human leukocyte antigen; MS, multiple sclerosis.

Adapted from data presented in Dyment DA, Herrera BM, Cader MZ, et al. Complex interactions among MHC haplotypes in multiple sclerosis: susceptibility and resistance. *Hum Mol Genet.* 2005;14(14):2019–2026.

third of these effects mapped to intergenic regions or in long-range haplotypes containing nonclassical HLA genes, underscoring the complexity of this locus in MS susceptibility.

> *Fine mapping studies of the telomeric boundary of MS susceptibility found that the MHC class I locus independently contributes to MS susceptibility, although the exact risk gene, or genes, in this region have not been precisely mapped.*

In addition to influencing MS risk, HLA alleles may contribute to the MS phenotype. The most consistent effect of HLA on MS phenotype is for the HLA-DRB1*15:01 allele on the age of onset. Several studies showed that this allele decreases the age of onset and does so in a dose-dependent manner (83,116,128–131). HLA-DRB1*15:01 may also contribute to the radiographic burden of disease on T2 weighted brain MRI and impact cognitive performance (132). In contrast, the HLA-B*44:02 allele, which is proposed to be protective for MS susceptibility, may reduce the radiographic burden of disease on T2 weighted brain MRI (127). Interestingly, a spontaneously occurring null allele of the HLA-DRB5 gene located telomeric to HLA-DRB1 might contribute to MS severity (133). Using a summary score of the known HLA alleles that influence MS susceptibility (the cumulative HLA genetic burden score or HLAGB), a single-center study of genotype–phenotype correlation found that a higher HLAGB score was associated with a younger age of onset and greater atrophy of subcortical gray matter in women with relapsing onset MS (134). These observations were accounted for primarily by the *HLADRB1*15:01* haplotype with a protective effect conferred by the *HLA-B*44:02* allele. Taken together, these studies show a consistent effect of the HLA locus on conferring a younger age of onset and may influence radiographic measures of disease severity, both in terms of focal lesion formation as well as diffuse gray matter injury. However, a consistent effect of HLA on disability progression has not been found (120,135). A potential impact of HLA on long-term disability either may be too small to detect in the modestly sized genotype–phenotype studies performed to date.

CURRENT DIRECTIONS AND LIMITATIONS

Rare variants with low MAFs are being examined by GWAS and exome and genome sequencing studies in multiplex families to identify novel rare variants. The success of exome sequencing in identifying rare variants of *CYP27B1* and *TYK2* illustrates the limitations of the common variant hypothesis. These rare alleles may be the proverbial tip of the iceberg and many more rare MS variants might be found by exploiting this strategy. However, these rare variants were identified in families with multiply affected members. Multiply affected families are relatively uncommon in MS and not all such families have informative structures for identification of rare variants. Furthermore, risk alleles in multiply affected families might be expected to have stronger effect sizes than variants that contribute to sporadic MS. At this time, no solution is apparent that does not require extremely large samples sizes using the case-control approach.

In non-European descended populations, genetic association studies have replicated some but not all non-MHC SNPs (136,137). It is encouraging that at least some MS risk alleles identified in European descended populations replicate in other racial groups and further substantiates that such risk alleles are genuine. Several explanations for lack of replication in diverse populations are possible and include relatively smaller sample sizes resulting in lack of power, inadequate control for population stratification, nonadditive gene–gene (epistatic) interactions, and gene–environment interactions. For example, different geographic locations could be associated with varying prevalence of environmental factors required to interact with an individual's genome and hence modify an individual's risk. European descended alleles are also present in the control groups for non-European populations indicating that genetic diversity alone does not exclusively account for racial differences in MS prevalence.

As impressive as the advances in recent years have been for MS risk gene discovery, several limitations of genetic research in MS have become clear. First, it is highly unlikely that genotyping will yield clinically meaningful diagnostic tools. The effect sizes for genetic effects on MS risk are far too small to find application in diagnosing MS patients. Second, in as much as very large sample sizes became necessary for identifying the genetic differences between MS cases and controls, it seems likely that equally large sample sizes will become necessary for identifying genetic factors that influence the MS clinical phenotype, including rate of disease progression. As intriguing as the preliminary studies of MS risk genes on MRI and clinical correlates may be, the studies performed to date are underpowered and reported results carry a risk of being falsely positive (much as was the case for early studies of MS risk). Given that multiple factors influence the MS phenotype, including disease duration as well as widespread use of disease-modifying therapies, future studies of genotype–phenotype correlations may face even greater challenges than studies of MS risk. Similarly, although use of genetics as a tool for individualizing treatment selection holds intrinsic appeal, proof that a genetic marker is associated with a particular outcome will require careful study of large populations given that the contribution of genetics to the overall effect of highly potent immune therapies is likely to be small. These daunting challenges raise the question as to whether genetic study in MS has value. Although MS genetics is unlikely to yield concrete clinical utility in the near future, genetics remains an invaluable tool for defining the key constituents underlying the complex biology of the disease. The most recent genetic map of MS that defines some 200 loci that could regulate over 500 genes illustrates that MS susceptibility arises from involvement of multiple biological pathways within every cell of the adaptive and innate immune system. Methods to characterize this level of biological complexity are not currently available but will likely be needed to understand the fundamental biology of not only MS but also likely many other human illnesses with polygenic origin. Only through identifying the variants involved in determining MS susceptibility and the expression patterns of the genes these variants are associated with in the relevant cells and tissue types can we hope to understand the role of heritability in the disease pathogenesis. A deeper understanding of the fundamental biology in MS is currently absent. However, if such an understanding were attained it would likely point to new therapeutic opportunities.

KEY POINTS FOR PATIENTS AND FAMILIES

- While most patients with MS do not have a family history, about one out of five patients will have family members who have MS.
- Children of a parent with MS have about a 3% to 5% lifetime risk of MS. Although this is higher than the general population, still they are unlikely to develop MS.
- There are no predictive genetic tests for MS.
- An identical twin of an MS patient has about a 30% chance of getting MS, showing that MS is related to multiple genetic factors and not any specific gene.

MS, multiple sclerosis.

REFERENCES

1. Davenport CB. Multiple sclerosis from the standpoint of geographic distribution and race. *Arch Neurol.* 1922;8:51–58.
2. Dean GH, McLoughlin H, Brady R, et al. Multiple sclerosis among immigrants in Greater London. *Br Med J.* 1976;1(6014):861–864.
3. Pugliatti M, Sotgiu S, Rosati G. The worldwide prevalence of multiple sclerosis. *Clin Neurol Neurosurg.* 2002;104(3):182–191.
4. Alter M, Kahana E, Zilber N, et al. Multiple sclerosis frequency in Israel's diverse populations. *Neurology.* 2006;66(7):1061–1066.
5. Smestad C, Sandvik L, Holmoy T, et al. Marked differences in prevalence of multiple sclerosis between ethnic groups in Oslo, Norway. *J Neurol.* 2008;255(1):49–55.
6. Kurtzke JF, Beebe GW, Nagler B, et al. Studies on the natural history of multiple sclerosis—8. Early prognostic features of the later course of the illness. *J Chronic Dis.* 1977;30(12):819–830.
7. Wallin MT, Page WF, Kurtzke JF. Multiple sclerosis in US veterans of the Vietnam era and later military service: race, sex, and geography. *Ann Neurol.* 2004;55(1):65–71.
8. Detels R, Visscher BR, Malmgren RM, et al. Evidence for lower susceptibility to multiple sclerosis in Japanese-Americans. *Am J Epidemiol.* 1977;105(4):303–310.
9. Oger JF, Arnason BG, Wray SH, et al. A study of B and T cells in multiple sclerosis. *Neurology.* 1975;25(5):444–447.
10. Kurtzke JF, Beebe GW, Norman JE, Jr. Epidemiology of multiple sclerosis in U.S. veterans: 1. Race, sex, and geographic distribution. *Neurology.* 1979;29(9 pt 1):1228–1235.
11. Hader WJ. Prevalence of multiple sclerosis in Saskatoon. *Can Med Assoc J.* 1982;127(4):295–297.
12. Svenson LW, Woodhead SE, Platt GH. Regional variations in the prevalence rates of multiple sclerosis in the province of Alberta, Canada. *Neuroepidemiology.* 1994;13(1–2):8–13.
13. Gowers WR. *A Manual of Diseases of the Nervous System.* 2nd ed. London, England: Churchill; 1893.
14. Eichorst H. Über infantile und heriditare multiple Sklerose. *Virchow's Arch Pathologie Anat Berl.* 1896;146:173–192.
15. Curtius FSH. Multiple sklerose und erbanlage. *Z Gesamte Neurol Psychiatr.* 1938;160(1):226–245.
16. McAlpine D. The problem of disseminated sclerosis. *Brain.* 1946;69:233–250.
17. Pratt RT, Compston ND, McAlpine D. The familial incidence of disseminated sclerosis and its significance. *Brain.* 1951;74(2):191–232.
18. Millar JH, Allison RS. Familial incidence of disseminated sclerosis in Northern Ireland. *Ulster Med J.* 1954;23(suppl 2):29–92.
19. Sadovnick AD, Baird PA, Ward RH. Multiple sclerosis: updated risks for relatives. *Am J Med Genet.* 1988;29(3):533–541.
20. Robertson NP, Fraser M, Deans J, et al. Age-adjusted recurrence risks for relatives of patients with multiple sclerosis. *Brain.* 1996;119(pt 2):449–455.
21. Carton H, Vlietinck R, De Keyser J, et al. Risks of multiple sclerosis in relatives of patients in Flanders, Belgium. *J Neurol Neurosurg Psychiatry.* 1997;62(4):329–333.
22. Risch N. Linkage strategies for genetically complex traits. I. Multilocus models. *Am J Hum Genet.* 1990;46(2):222–228.
23. Compston A. Genetic epidemiology of multiple sclerosis. *J Neurol Neurosurg Psychiatry.* 1997;62(6):553–561.
24. Merikangas KR, Risch N. Genomic priorities and public health. *Science.* 2003;302(5645):599–601.
25. Guo SW. Sibling recurrence risk ratio as a measure of genetic effect: caveat emptor! *Am J Hum Genet.* 2002;70(3):818–819.
26. Ebers GC, Bulman DE, Sadovnick AD, et al. A population-based study of multiple sclerosis in twins. *N Engl J Med.* 1986;315(26):1638–1642.
27. Mumford CJ, Wood NW, Kellar-Wood H, et al. The British Isles survey of multiple sclerosis in twins. *Neurology.* 1994;44(1):11–15.
28. Willer CJ, Dyment DA, Risch NJ, et al. Twin concordance and sibling recurrence rates in multiple sclerosis. *Proc Natl Acad Sci U S A.* 2003;100(22):12877–12882.
29. Hansen T, Skytthe A, Stenager E, et al. Risk for multiple sclerosis in dizygotic and monozygotic twins. *Mult Scler.* 2005;11(5):500–503.
30. Islam T, Gauderman WJ, Cozen W, et al. Differential twin concordance for multiple sclerosis by latitude of birthplace. *Ann Neurol.* 2006;60(1):56–64.
31. Ristori G, Cannoni S, Stazi MA, et al. Multiple sclerosis in twins from continental Italy and Sardinia: a nationwide study. *Ann Neurol.* 2006;59(1):27–34.
32. Robertson NP, O'Riordan JI, Chataway J, et al. Offspring recurrence rates and clinical characteristics of conjugal multiple sclerosis. *Lancet.* 1997;349(9065):1587–1590.

33. Ebers GC, Yee IM, Sadovnick AD, et al. Conjugal multiple sclerosis: population-based prevalence and recurrence risks in offspring. Canadian Collaborative Study Group. *Ann Neurol.* 2000;48(6):927–931.

34. Dyment DA, Ebers GC, Sadovnick AD. Genetics of multiple sclerosis. *Lancet Neurol.* 2004;3(2):104–110.

35. Peltonen L, McKusick VA. Dissecting human disease in the postgenomic era. *Science.* 2001;291:1224–1229.

36. Bertrams J, Kuwert E. HL-A antigen frequencies in multiple sclerosis. Significant increase of HL-A3, HL-A10 and W5, and decrease of HL-A12. *Eur Neurol.* 1972;7(1):74–78.

37. Bertrams J, Kuwert E, Liedtke U. HL-A antigens and multiple sclerosis. *Tissue Antigens.* 1972;2(5):405–408.

38. Naito S, Namerow N, Mickey MR, et al. Multiple sclerosis: association with HL-A3. *Tissue Antigens.* 1972;2(1):1–4.

39. Jersild C, Svejgaard A, Fog T. HL-A antigens and multiple sclerosis. *Lancet.* 1972;1(7762):1240–1241.

40. Jersild C, Fog T, Hansen GS, et al. Histocompatibility determinants in multiple sclerosis, with special reference to clinical course. *Lancet.* 1973;2(7840):1221–1225.

41. Winchester R, Ebers G, Fu SM, et al. B-cell alloantigen Ag 7a in multiple sclerosis. *Lancet.* 1975;2(7939):814.

42. Compston DA, Batchelor JR, McDonald WI. B-lymphocyte alloantigens associated with multiple sclerosis. *Lancet.* 1976;2(7998):1261–1265.

43. Terasaki PI, Park MS, Opelz G, et al. Multiple sclerosis and high incidence of a B lymphocyte antigen. *Science.* 1976;193(4259):1245–1247.

44. Botstein D, White RL, Skolnick M, et al. Construction of a genetic linkage map in man using restriction fragment length polymorphisms. *Am J Hum Genet.* 1980;32(3):314–331.

45. Weber JL, May PE. Abundant class of human DNA polymorphisms which can be typed using the polymerase chain reaction. *Am J Hum Genet.* 1989;44(3):388–396.

46. Cohen D, Cohen O, Marcadet A, et al. Class II HLA-DC beta-chain DNA restriction fragments differentiate among HLA-DR2 individuals in insulin-dependent diabetes and multiple sclerosis. *Proc Natl Acad Sci U S A.* 1984;81(6):1774–1778.

47. Sawcer S. The complex genetics of multiple sclerosis: pitfalls and prospects. *Brain.* 2008;131(pt 12):3118–3131.

48. Ebers GC, Kukay K, Bulman DE, et al. A full genome search in multiple sclerosis. *Nat Genet.* 1996;13(4):472–476.

49. Haines JL, Ter-Minassian M, Bazyk A, et al. A complete genomic screen for multiple sclerosis underscores a role for the major histocompatability complex. The Multiple Sclerosis Genetics Group. *Nat Genet.* 1996;13(4):469–471.

50. Sawcer S, Jones HB, Feakes R, et al. A genome screen in multiple sclerosis reveals susceptibility loci on chromosome 6p21 and 17q22. *Nat Genet.* 1996;13(4):464–468.

51. Kuokkanen S, Gschwend M, Rioux JD, et al. Genomewide scan of multiple sclerosis in Finnish multiplex families. *Am J Hum Genet.* 1997;61(6):1379–1387.

52. Coraddu F, Sawcer S, D'Alfonso S, et al. A genome screen for multiple sclerosis in Sardinian multiplex families. *Eur J Human Genet.* 2001;9(8):621–626.

53. Akesson E, Oturai A, Berg J, et al. A genome-wide screen for linkage in Nordic sib-pairs with multiple sclerosis. *Genes Immun.* 2002;3(5):279–285.

54. Ban M, Stewart GJ, Bennetts BH, et al. A genome screen for linkage in Australian sibling-pairs with multiple sclerosis. *Genes Immun.* 2002;3(8):464–469.

55. Eraksoy M, Hensiek A, Kurtuncu M, et al. A genome screen for linkage disequilibrium in Turkish multiple sclerosis. *J Neuroimmunol.* 2003;143(1–2):129–132.

56. Hensiek AE, Roxburgh R, Smilie B, et al. Updated results of the United Kingdom linkage-based genome screen in multiple sclerosis. *J Neuroimmunol.* 2003;143(1–2):25–30.

57. Dyment DA, Sadovnick AD, Willer CJ, et al. An extended genome scan in 442 Canadian multiple sclerosis-affected sibships: a report from the Canadian Collaborative Study Group. *Hum Mol Genet.* 2004;13(10):1005–1015.

58. Kenealy SJ, Babron MC, Bradford Y, et al. A second-generation genomic screen for multiple sclerosis. *Am J Hum Genet.* 2004;75(6):1070–1078.

59. Ligers A, Dyment DA, Willer CJ, et al. Evidence of linkage with HLA-DR in DRB1*15-negative families with multiple sclerosis. *Am J Hum Genet.* 2001;69(4):900–903.

60. International HapMap Consortium. The international HapMap project. *Nature.* 2003;426(6968):789–796.

61. Sawcer SJ, Maranian M, Singlehurst S, et al. Enhancing linkage analysis of complex disorders: an evaluation of high-density genotyping. *Hum Mol Genet.* 2004;13(17):1943–1949.

62. Sawcer S, Ban M, Maranian M, et al. A high-density screen for linkage in multiple sclerosis. *Am J Hum Genet.* 2005;77(3):454–467.

63. Risch N, Merikangas K. The future of genetic studies of complex human diseases. *Science.* 1996;273(5281):1516–1517.

64. GAMES; Transatlantic Multiple Sclerosis Genetics Cooperative. A meta-analysis of whole genome linkage screens in multiple sclerosis. *J Neuroimmunol.* 2003;143(1–2):39–46.

65. International Human Genome Sequencing Consortium. Finishing the euchromatic sequence of the human genome. *Nature.* 2004;431(7011):931–945.

66. Hafler DA, Compston A, Sawcer S, et al. Risk alleles for multiple sclerosis identified by a genomewide study. *N Engl J Med.* 2007;357(9):851–862.

67. Matesanz F, Fedetz M, Collado-Romero M, et al. Allelic expression and interleukin-2 polymorphisms in multiple sclerosis. *J Neuroimmunol.* 2007;119(1):101–105.

68. Gregory SG, Schmidt S, Seth P, et al. Interleukin 7 receptor alpha chain (IL7R) shows allelic and functional association with multiple sclerosis. *Nat Genet.* 2007;39(9):1083–1091.

69. Lundmark F, Duvefelt K, Hillert J. Genetic association analysis of the interleukin 7 gene (IL7) in multiple sclerosis. *J Neuroimmunol.* 2007;192(1–2):171–173.

70. Lundmark F, Duvefelt K, Lacobaeus E, et al. Variation in interleukin 7 receptor alpha chain (IL7R) influences risk of multiple sclerosis. *Nat Genet.* 39(9):1108–1113.

71. Rubio JP, Stankovich J, Field J, et al. Replication of KIAA0350, IL2RA, RPL5 and CD58 as multiple sclerosis susceptibility genes in Australians. *Genes Immun.* 2008;9(7):624–630.

72. Weber F, Fontaine B, Cournu-Rebeix I, et al. IL2RA and IL7RA genes confer susceptibility for multiple sclerosis in two independent European populations. *Genes Immun.* 2008;9(3):259–263.

73. Sawcer S. Bayes factors in complex genetics. *Eur J Hum Genet.* 2010;18(7):746–750.

74. Burton PR, Clayton DG, Cardon LR, et al. Association scan of 14,500 nonsynonymous SNPs in four diseases identifies autoimmunity variants. *Nat Genet.* 2007;39(11):1329–1337.

75. Comabella M, Martin R. Genomics in multiple sclerosis—current state and future directions. *J Neuroimmunol.* 2007;187(1–2):1–8.

76. Australia and New Zealand Multiple Sclerosis Genetics Consortium (ANZgene). Genome-wide association study identifies new multiple sclerosis susceptibility loci on chromosomes 12 and 20. *Nat Genet.* 2009;41(7):824–828.

77. Baranzini SE, Wang J, Gibson RA, et al. Genome-wide association analysis of susceptibility and clinical phenotype in multiple sclerosis. *Hum Mol Genet.* 2009;18(4):767–778.

78. De Jager PL, Jia X, Wang J, et al. Meta-analysis of genome scans and replication identify CD6, IRF8 and TNFRSF1A as new multiple sclerosis susceptibility loci. *Nat Genet.* 2009;41(7):776–782.

79. Jakkula E, Leppa V, Sulonen AM, et al. Genome-wide association study in a high-risk isolate for multiple sclerosis reveals associated variants in STAT3 gene. *Am J Hum Genet.* 2010;86(2):285–291.

80. Nischwitz S, Cepok S, Kroner A, et al. Evidence for VAV2 and ZNF433 as susceptibility genes for multiple sclerosis. *J Neuroimmunol.* 2010;227(1–2):162–166.

81. Sanna S, M Pitzalis M, Zoledziewska, M, et al. Variants within the immunoregulatory CBLB gene are associated with multiple sclerosis. *Nat Genet.* 2010;42(6):495–497.

82. IMSGC. Genome-wide association study of severity in multiple sclerosis. *Genes Immun.* 2011;12(8):615–625.

83. Sawcer S, Hellenthal G, Pirinen M, et al. Genetic risk and a primary role for cell-mediated immune mechanisms in multiple sclerosis. *Nature*. 2011;476(7359):214–219.

84. Menge T, Lalive PH, von Büdingen HC, et al. Antibody responses against galactocerebroside are potential stage-specific biomarkers in multiple sclerosis. *J Allergy Clin Immun*. 2005;116(2):453–459.

85. IMSGC. The Multiple Sclerosis Genomic Map: Role of peripheral immune cells and resident microglia in susceptibility. 2017. Available at: https://www.biorxiv.org/content/biorxiv/early/2017/07/13/143933.full.pdf.

86. Djebali S, Davis CA, Markel A, et al. Landscape of transcription in human cells. *Nature*. 2012;489(7414):101–108.

87. Dunham I, Kundaje A, Aldred SF, et al. An integrated encyclopedia of DNA elements in the human genome. *Nature*. 2012;489(7414):57–74.

88. Boyle EA, Li YI, Pritchard JK. An expanded view of complex traits: from polygenic to omnigenic. *Cell*. 2017;169(7):1177–1186.

89. Munger KL, Levin LI, Hollis BW, et al. Serum 25-hydroxyvitamin D levels and risk of multiple sclerosis. *JAMA*. 2006;296(23):2832–2838.

90. Islam T, Gauderman WJ, Cozen W, Mack TM. Childhood sun exposure influences risk of multiple sclerosis in monozygotic twins. *Neurology*. 2007;69(4):381–388.

91. Gelfand JM, Cree BA, McElroy J, et al. Vitamin D in African Americans with multiple sclerosis. *Neurology*. 2011;76(21):1824–1830.

92. Ramagopalan SV, Handel AE, Giovannoni G, Rutherford Siegel S, Ebers GC, Chaplin G. Relationship of UV exposure to prevalence of multiple sclerosis in England. *Neurology*. 2011;76(16):1410–1414.

93. Ramagopalan SV, Dyment DA, Cader MZ, et al. Rare variants in the CYP27B1 gene are associated with multiple sclerosis. *Ann Neurol*. 2011;70(6):881–886.

94. Manousaki D, Dudding T, Haworth S, et al. Low-frequency synonymous coding variation in CYP2R1 has large effects on vitamin D levels and risk of multiple sclerosis. *Am J Hum Genet*. 2017;101(2):227–238.

95. Cheng JB, Levine MA, Bell NH, et al. Genetic evidence that the human CYP2R1 enzyme is a key vitamin D 25 hydroxylase. *Proc Natl Acad Sci U S A*. 2004;101(20):7711–7715.

96. Ramagopalan SV, Maugeri NJ, Handunnetthi L, et al. Expression of the multiple sclerosis-associated MHC class II Allele HLA-DRB1*1501 is regulated by vitamin D. *PLOS Genet*. 2009;5(2):e1000369.

97. Ramagopalan SV, Heger A, Berlanga AJ, et al. A ChIP-seq defined genome-wide map of vitamin D receptor binding: associations with disease and evolution. *Genome Res*. 2010;20(10):1352–1360.

98. Smolders J, Menheere P, Kessels A, et al. Association of vitamin D metabolite levels with relapse rate and disability in multiple sclerosis. *Mult Scler*. 2008;14(9):1220–1224.

99. Soilu-Hanninen M, Laaksonen M, Laitinen I, et al. A longitudinal study of serum 25-hydroxyvitamin D and intact parathyroid hormone levels indicate the importance of vitamin D and calcium homeostasis regulation in multiple sclerosis. *J Neurol. Neurosurg Psychiatry*. 2008;79(2):152–157.

100. Mowry EM, Krupp LB, Milazzo M, et al. Vitamin D status is associated with relapse rate in pediatric-onset multiple sclerosis. *Ann Neurol*. 2010;67(5):618–624.

101. Simpson S Jr, Taylor B, Blizzard L, et al. Higher 25-hydroxyvitamin D is associated with lower relapse risk in multiple sclerosis. *Ann Neurol*. 2010;68(2):193–203.

102. Steri M, Orrù V, Idda L, et al. Overexpression of the cytokine BAFF and autoimmunity risk. *N Engl J Med*. 2017;376(17):1615–1626.

103. Gelfand JM, Cree BA, Hauser SL. Ocrelizumab and other CD20+ B-cell-depleting therapies in multiple sclerosis. *Neurotherapeutics*. 2017;14:835–841.

104. Dyment DA, Cader MZ, Chao MJ, et al. Exome sequencing identifies a novel multiple sclerosis susceptibility variant in the TYK2 gene. *Neurology*. 2012;79(5):406–411.

105. Ban M, Goris A, Lorentzen AR, et al. Replication analysis identifies TYK2 as a multiple sclerosis susceptibility factor. *Eur J Hum Genet*. 2009;17(10):1309–1313.

106. Mero IL, Lorentzen AR, Ban M, et al. A rare variant of the TYK2 gene is confirmed to be associated with multiple sclerosis. *Eur J Hum Genet*. 2010;18(4):502–504.

107. Baranzini SE, Mudge J, van Velkinburgh JC, et al. Genome, epigenome and RNA sequences of monozygotic twins discordant for multiple sclerosis. *Nature*. 2010;464(7293):1351–1356.

108. Rioux JD, Goyette P, Vyse TJ, et al. Mapping of multiple susceptibility variants within the MHC region for 7 immune-mediated diseases. *Proc Natl Acad Sci U S A*. 2009;106(44):18680–18685.

109. Allcock RJ, Atrazhev AM, Beck S, et al. The MHC haplotype project: a resource for HLA-linked association studies. *Tissue Antigens*. 2002;59(6):520–521.

110. Stewart CA, Horton R, Allcock RJ, et al. Complete MHC haplotype sequencing for common disease gene mapping. *Genome Res*. 2004;14(6):1176–1187.

111. Miretti MM, Walsh EC, Ke X, et al. A high-resolution linkage-disequilibrium map of the human major histocompatibility complex and first generation of tag single-nucleotide polymorphisms. *Am J Hum Genet*. 2005;76(4):634–646.

112. de Bakker PI, McVean G, Sabeti PC, et al. A high-resolution HLA and SNP haplotype map for disease association studies in the extended human MHC. *Nat Genet*. 2006;38(10):1166–1172.

113. Horton R, Gibson R, Coggill P, et al. Variation analysis and gene annotation of eight MHC haplotypes: the MHC Haplotype Project. *Immunogenetics*. 2008;60(1):1–18.

114. Oksenberg JR, Barcellos LF, et al. Mapping multiple sclerosis susceptibility to the HLA-DR locus in African Americans. *Am J Hum Genet*. 2004;74(1):160–167.

115. Barcellos LF, Oksenberg JR, Begovich AB, et al. HLA-DR2 dose effect on susceptibility to multiple sclerosis and influence on disease course. *Am J Hum Genet*. 2003;72(3):710–716.

116. Cree BA, Reich DE, Khan O, et al. Modification of Multiple Sclerosis Phenotypes by African Ancestry at HLA. *Arch Neurol*. 2009;66(2):226–233.

117. Dyment DA, Herrera BM, Cader MZ, et al. Complex interactions among MHC haplotypes in multiple sclerosis: susceptibility and resistance. *Hum Mol Genet*. 2005;14(14):2019–2026.

118. Barcellos LF, Sawcer S, Ramsay PP, et al. Heterogeneity at the HLA-DRB1 locus and risk for multiple sclerosis. *Hum Mol Genet*. 2006;15(18):2813–2824.

119. Chao MJ, Barnardo MC, Lui GZ, et al. Transmission of class I/II multi-locus MHC haplotypes and multiple sclerosis susceptibility: accounting for linkage disequilibrium. *Hum Mol Genet*. 16(16):1951–1958.

120. Marrosu MG, Muntoni F, Murru MR, et al. Sardinian multiple sclerosis is associated with HLA-DR4: a serologic and molecular analysis. *Neurology*. 1988;38(11):1749–1753.

121. Marrosu MG, Murru MR, Costa G, et al. DRB1-DQA1-DQB1 loci and multiple sclerosis predisposition in the Sardinian population. *Hum Mol Genet*. 1998;7(8):1235–1237.

122. Marrosu MG, Murru MR, Murru MR, et al. Dissection of the HLA association with multiple sclerosis in the founder isolated population of Sardinia. *Hum Mol Genet*. 2001;10(25):2907–2916.

123. Brassat D, Salemi G, Barcellos LF, et al. The HLA locus and multiple sclerosis in Sicily. *Neurology*. 2005;64(2):361–363.

124. Brynedal B, Duvefelt K, Jonasdottir G, et al. HLA-A confers an HLA-DRB1 independent influence on the risk of multiple sclerosis. *PLOS ONE*. 2007;2(7):e664.

125. Yeo TW, De Jager PL, Gregory SG, et al. A second major histocompatibility complex susceptibility locus for multiple sclerosis. *Ann Neurol*. 2007;61(3):228–236.

126. Cree BA, Rioux JD, McCauley JL, et al. A major histocompatibility Class I locus contributes to multiple sclerosis susceptibility independently from HLA-DRB1*15:01. *PLOS ONE*. 2010;5(6):e11296.

127. Healy BC, Liguori M, Tran D, et al. HLA B*44: protective effects in MS susceptibility and MRI outcome measures. *Neurology.* 2010;75(7):634–640.

128. Celius EG, Harbo HF, Egeland T, et al. Sex and age at diagnosis are correlated with the HLA-DR2, DQ6 haplotype in multiple sclerosis. *J Neurol Sci.* 2000;178(2):132–135.

129. Masterman T, Ligers A, Olsson T, et al. HLA-DR15 is associated with lower age at onset in multiple sclerosis. *Ann Neurol.* 2000;48(2):211–219.

130. Hensiek AE, Sawcer SJ, Feakes R, et al. HLA-DR 15 is associated with female sex and younger age at diagnosis in multiple sclerosis. *J Neurol Neurosurg Psychiatry.* 2002;72(2):184–187.

131. Smestad C, Brynedal B, Jonasdottir G, et al. The impact of HLA-A and -DRB1 on age at onset, disease course and severity in Scandinavian multiple sclerosis patients. *Eur J Neurol.* 2007;14(8): 835–840.

132. Okuda DT, Srinivasan R, Oksenberg JR, et al. Genotype-Phenotype correlations in multiple sclerosis: HLA genes influence disease severity inferred by 1HMR spectroscopy and MRI measures. *Brain.* 2009;132(pt 1):250–259.

133. Caillier SJ, Briggs F, Cree BA, et al. Uncoupling the roles of HLA-DRB1 and HLA-DRB5 genes in multiple sclerosis. *J Immunol.* 2008;181(8):5473–5480.

134. Isobe N, Keshevan A, Gourraud PA, et al. Association of HLA genetic risk burden with disease phoentypes in multiple sclerosis. *JAMA Neurol.* 2016;73(7):795–802.

135. Romero-Pinel L, Pujal JM, Martínez-Yélamos S, et al. HLA-DRB1: genetic susceptibility and disability progression in a Spanish multiple sclerosis population. *Eur J Neurol.* 2011;18(2):337–342.

136. Johnson BA, Wang J, Taylor EM, et al. Multiple sclerosis susceptibility alleles in African Americans. *Genes Immun.* 2010;11(4): 343–350.

137. Isobe N, Madireddy L, Khankhanian P, et al. An ImmunoChip study of multiple sclerosis in African Americans. *Brain.* 2015;138(pt 6):1518–1530.

6 Symptoms and Signs of Multiple Sclerosis

Marisa P. McGinley and Lael A. Stone

KEY POINTS FOR CLINICIANS

- Multiple sclerosis (MS) may present with a myriad of symptoms affecting the central nervous system (CNS).
- Careful history-taking is required to distinguish MS-related symptoms that are helpful for diagnosis from less specific complaints.
- It is important to look for confirmation of symptoms on neurological examination, for example, increased reflexes or tone on exam support a complaint of stiffness and/or cramping.
- Pattern recognition is important in distinguishing MS symptoms and signs.
- Specific symptoms of demyelinating events (e.g., unilateral visual loss, diplopia, gait ataxia, motor weakness, focal paresthesias, Lhermitte's phenomenon) are useful in diagnosis. However, nonspecific symptoms that are sometimes seen in MS (fatigue, headache, depression, back pain) are less helpful as they are seen in many conditions.

INTRODUCTION

The Nature of the Problem

MS may present in a multitude of ways and many times the initial symptom of MS is not recognized until the occurrence of a second symptom. The medical literature is replete with case reports of unusual presentations of MS, as lesions can be found in virtually any area of the CNS and therefore cause a variety of symptoms (1–5). This chapter confines itself to the so-called primary symptoms of MS, that is, those caused by direct damage to the CNS, whether it is acute and inflammatory or progressive and degenerative, or a combination of the two, rather than secondary symptoms which may occur because of the primary symptom. Examples of primary symptoms causing secondary symptoms would be bladder dysfunction (primary) causing repeat urinary tract infections (secondary); increased motor tone, that is, spasticity (primary) causing fatigue due to sleep disturbance (secondary). A few symptoms can be both primary and secondary symptoms of MS such as depression and fatigue.

The most common presenting symptoms for MS are related to acute optic neuritis (6,7), usually visual loss and accompanying pain in 90% of cases. However, when lumped together in broader categories, the most

common system affected is likely the somatosensory system, with over 70% of patients having sensory complaints at some point in their disease course (8,9). Motor complaints would likely be the next most common with nearly the same percentage of patients affected. While some symptoms are more common in younger, relapsing–remitting patients (e.g., visual symptoms, paresthesias) and others are more common in older patients at a more progressive phase (e.g., muscle weakness, spasticity), some symptoms can occur at any point in the disease course.

Because symptoms of MS can affect so many areas of the CNS, MS may present in a multitude of ways. Patients who have multiple or somewhat odd symptoms are frequently told by non-MS clinicians, as well as lay people or even Internet search engines, that their symptoms "sound like MS." Differentiating true MS symptoms from a "laundry list" of complaints, therefore, can be an exercise in fine-tuned pattern recognition. That is to say, a clinician who is attuned to and very familiar with typical descriptions of neurological symptoms by patients who turn out to have MS may hear and interpret symptoms somewhat differently from those who hear only a one- or two-word description from a list of possibly neurological symptoms, particularly in the context of nonspecific white matter changes on cranial MRI. Vague symptoms appear to take on more import to the patient and primary care clinician in this context as discussed by Corboy's study of this phenomenon (10). This chapter attempts to lead the history-taker through the steps that MS clinicians take in sorting out the symptoms which are most likely to be MS, from those which are least likely to be MS, and then turn to how one can find confirmation for these symptoms on neurological examination. More detailed information on the pathophysiology, consequences, and treatment of the most common and disabling MS symptoms can be found in other chapters.

EVALUATION OF SYMPTOMS

Part 1: History

The first pieces of information that we learn about a patient are the demographics, which are only moderately useful to decide if symptoms are MS related or not. While MS is certainly most common in white females from 20 to 50 years old, classic symptoms can occur in any age or ethnic group. The main exception to this would be unilateral visual loss, where age is a distinguishing factor in helping to decide if this symptom is MS (more likely to be an optic neuritis in younger patients and an ischemic optic neuropathy in older patients) (6,7). A second exception may be progressive myelopathy (more likely due to MS in younger individuals and cervical spondylosis in older ones). Speaking in broad generalization, history-takers should attempt to place demographical information at the back of their minds when listening to histories of possibly MS symptoms.

Probably the most important piece to deciphering if a symptom is MS related or not would be the quality of the symptom combined with the location. Localization should clearly match the CNS only, for example, hemibody, or band around the torso, or unilateral visual loss; or alternatively be so peculiar sounding that the patient often prefaces the description with "I know this sounds crazy but ..." as in a patch of skin which feels wet or itching in the absence of any apparent skin change. Sensory or motor symptoms involving the whole body, or just hands and feet, are rarely related to MS. See Tables 6.1 and 6.2 and Figure 6.1 for symptoms that are suggestive of CNS syndromes that can occur in MS.

Timing of the occurrence of symptoms is critical. For example, symptoms may occur a few days after a known trigger of demyelination, such as infection, or during the postpartum period (a time of increased relapse activity). Timing in the sense of how long the symptom lasts is also critical, as MS-related symptoms tend to occur in two types: longer lasting, that is, at least 48 to 72 hours up to several weeks, and brief repetitive symptoms known as transient neurological events or paroxysmal symptoms, lasting a few seconds to minutes, but occurring in a stereotypical manner. Paroxysmal symptoms can occur frequently in MS patients and are often mistaken for seizures although alteration in consciousness is rare. These generally involve transient face, arm, and leg, or only arm and leg sensory and/or motor

TABLE 6.1 Some Symptom Descriptions Which Suggest MS Due to CNS Symptomatology

"I woke up with loss of vision in 1 eye and pain with moving that eye"

"When I bend my neck down I get an electric feeling through my body"

"I developed tingling in both feet which over a couple of days went up to just under the bra line on both sides"

"I developed double vision with 2 images one above the other"

"I got a patch of itching over my shoulder blade with no rash"

"I notice that when I exercise or take a hot shower my leg gets weaker"

"I find I now have to go to the bathroom right away when I get the signal"

CNS, central nervous system; MS, multiple sclerosis.

TABLE 6.2 Red Flags of MS Symptoms and Signs

- Age of patient >60
- Total body complaints, e.g., total body weakness or numbness
- Excessive fatigue or depression in the absence of neurological signs on examination
- Absence of visual complaints other than presbyopia
- Absence of bladder complaints other than cough and sneeze incontinence
- Diarrhea rather than constipation
- Sudden, i.e., seconds to minutes onset of symptoms
- Positional symptoms other than Lhermitte's phenomenon
- Absence of investigation of comorbidities such as diabetes, sleep apnea, depression, and cervical spondylosis
- Prominent systemic manifestations (fever, weight loss, rash, arthritis, etc.)

symptoms. Most MS symptoms though, last greater than 48 to 72 hours, and many, such as those consistent with progressive myelopathy, may take years to become apparent. On occasion, this chronicity makes clinicians think of orthopedic causes such as ankle or knee injuries, which are actually the result rather than the cause of the gait abnormality, before they consider CNS disorders.

Another important clue is to find out if heat and exertion worsen symptoms. Heat is a well-known trigger for temporary worsening of MS symptoms, but this should again be approached with caution in taking the history, as descriptions of complete exhaustion or generalized heat intolerance may be due to many conditions. More useful are individual symptoms worsening in the heat such as graying of vision with heat or exertion, that is, Uhthoff's phenomenon (increased symptoms occurring with increased body temperature). Very typical of CNS dysfunction related to MS would be descriptions of foot drop, sometimes described as making a slapping sound, after long walks, particularly if the distance needed to bring out the foot drop decreases with the passage of years, for example, the description that "2 years ago I was able to walk 1 mile before the foot drop occurred, but now I can only walk 2 blocks before it occurs." Some MS patients have no heat sensitivity at all, and many become stiffer in cold weather, or have increased bladder urgency upon encountering cold

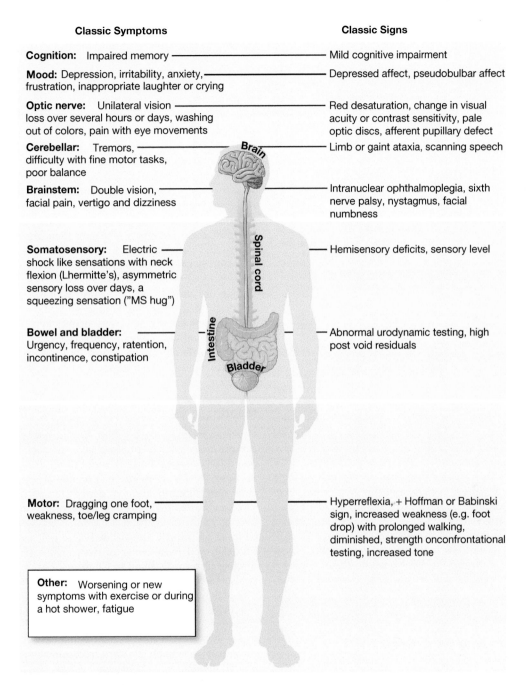

Classic Symptoms

Cognition: Impaired memory

Mood: Depression, irritability, anxiety, frustration, inappropriate laughter or crying

Optic nerve: Unilateral vision loss over several hours or days, washing out of colors, pain with eye movements

Cerebellar: Tremors, difficulty with fine motor tasks, poor balance

Brainstem: Double vision, facial pain, vertigo and dizziness

Somatosensory: Electric shock like sensations with neck flexion (Lhermitte's), asymmetric sensory loss over days, a squeezing sensation ("MS hug")

Bowel and bladder: Urgency, frequency, ratention, incontinence, constipation

Motor: Dragging one foot, weakness, toe/leg cramping

Other: Worsening or new symptoms with exercise or during a hot shower, fatigue

Classic Signs

Mild cognitive impairment

Depressed affect, pseudobulbar affect

Red desaturation, change in visual acuity or contrast sensitivity, pale optic discs, afferent pupillary defect

Limb or gaint ataxia, scanning speech

Intranuclear ophthalmoplegia, sixth nerve palsy, nystagmus, facial numbness

Hemisensory deficits, sensory level

Abnormal urodynamic testing, high post void residuals

Hyperreflexia, + Hoffman or Babinski sign, increased weakness (e.g. foot drop) with prolonged walking, diminished, strength onconfrontational testing, increased tone

FIGURE 6.1   Classic symptoms and signs.

MS, multiple sclerosis.

air. Worsening with change in position is rarely typical for MS symptoms. The main exceptions would be Lhermitte's phenomenon and severe spasticity when change of position causes spasms. While Lhermitte's may be caused by many abnormalities affecting the cervical spine, patients who describe a "zinging" electrical sensation down their backs with neck flexion should undergo cervical cord imaging. Spasticity generally worsens with prolonged sitting or laying down and may present with complaint of calf tightness or pain, toe/foot cramps, or involuntary leg jerking/ flexing mostly at night. As with any disease, it is of utmost importance to document a detailed history of the patient's symptoms, commenting on characteristics, duration, severity, aggravating and alleviating factors, prior diagnostic workup and treatments, and the overall impact on the patient's function.

Part 2: Confirming the Symptoms With Signs on Examination

After completing the history, the examination should be geared toward strengthening the evidence that MS is the cause of the symptoms, or discovering alternative explanations. For example, if the patient complains of pain in the legs, increased reflexes and/or Hoffman or Babinski sign may confirm the suspicion that this is spasticity. Questionable histories of visual loss may be corroborated by red desaturation, altered visual acuity or contrast sensitivity, and/or pale optical discs. Patients will often complain of unilateral sensory or motor changes, but on an exam if the abnormalities are actually bilaterally, but asymmetric, this may be more consistent with MS. Conversely, if the exam is truly unilateral this does not exclude MS, but other vascular or radicular etiologies should be investigated. Whenever possible, the examination of the possible MS patient should begin with the evaluation of gait. Ideally, the patient should walk far enough to see subtle changes consistent with foot drop or decreased arm swing. Having the patient stand and hop on one foot will help confirm complaints of decreased strength on one side of the body, and also elicit these complaints from individuals who may have not noticed, or were reluctant to mention weakness. Spasticity and ataxia can also be ascertained with observation of gait. The presence of various sorts of functional gaits such as astasia–abasia can also be evaluated. In proceeding through the rest of the neurological exam, it is interesting to note that eye signs may not produce symptoms noticeable to the patient although they are classic for MS, such as an intranuclear opthalmoplegia (INO) (11). Alternative explanations for symptoms may be found on examination such as dystonia, muscle fasciculations, or cogwheeling, all leading to other diagnoses. Unfortunately, some patients, even those with MS, may elaborate their symptoms, with inconsistent or nonphysiological exam features. Ideally, some of the symptoms reported by the patient will be supported by examination findings (Figure 6.1).

SYMPTOM REVIEW BY SYSTEM

Cognition

Changes in cognition and affect are common in MS, although generally not as the presenting symptom. Before invoking MS as the potential cause for memory change or cognitive change, it is critical to distinguish this from delirium or acute worsening in mental functioning due to infection, such as an indolent urinary tract infection, or side effect of medication. Particularly, if the mental decline is less than a month in duration and there are any symptoms referable to the urinary tract such as retention/hesitation, a urinalysis should be obtained. Similarly, a careful review of the medications, both prescribed and over-the-counter supplements, should be conducted, and potentially cognitively altering medications, such as statins, benzodiazepines, and narcotics, should be eliminated wherever possible.

Poorly controlled diabetes as well as hypothyroidism and low vitamin B_{12} are remarkably common in the same population that is susceptible to MS and should therefore be screened for as part of the cognitive evaluation. Cognitive changes due to MS must also be distinguished from general overload, as when individuals are trying to do too much, or are fatigued because of poor sleep quantity or quality. Anxiety and depression can similarly adversely affect both mood and fatigue, and many patients with depression say that their memory is impaired (12,13). MS patients may suffer from cognitive changes at any time during the disease course and statistics regarding incidence range from 20% to 50% (14,15). On formal neuropsychological testing, domains of verbal memory and attention/speed of information processing are most affected. Neuropsychological testing can assist with both distinguishing cognitive change in patients suspected of having MS from anxiety and depression and also assist individuals with knowing which areas of cognition are relatively retained, and thus can be utilized more fully (16).

Mood

Depression and anxiety can be primary or secondary symptoms of MS. Depression as a comorbidity has been noted to be associated with more rapid decline of MS (17). Because the MS population also has a high risk for suicide, rapid identification of depression as well as aggressive treatment and follow-up is recommended. There are several helpful screening tools for depression, which can be integrated into clinical practice to help with both identification and monitoring of depression. These scales are discussed in more detail in Chapter 20 of this book. There is also likely an increased incidence of bipolar disease in MS patients. Mania has been reported as well as frank psychosis (18–20). Steroid-induced affective changes are common in MS patients and should be considered when using these medicines. Pseudobulbar affect or emotional incontinence is likely an underrecognized symptom in MS as well (21,22).

Cranial Nerves

VISUAL SYSTEM

As previously stated, the most common, single presenting symptom in MS is optic neuritis, which generally involves unilateral visual loss (6,11). Ninety percent of patients present with pain on moving the eye, and often describe their visual loss as "like looking through a screen or petroleum jelly." Decreased color vision is common, and patients may be checked for red desaturation possibly indicating a previous asymptomatic optic neuritis as well. INO, which is due to a disturbance in the medial longitudinal fasciculus of the brainstem, may present as double vision, or may be completely asymptomatic for reasons that are unclear given the significant nature of the disturbance. Since MS is the most common cause of INO, imaging should be obtained in these cases unless MS is known to be present. Nystagmus is also common in MS, and patients may complain of "jumpy" vision, particularly if they are tired or overheated. Various types of nystagmus and ocular movements have been reported and depend on which location or locations in the central neuraxis are affected.

Other cranial nerves may also show evidence of dysfunction in MS. Disturbances of facial sensation are common with or without pain. Trigeminal neuralgia, in particular, can be troubling to patients, and MS should certainly be considered as a potential cause in young female patients presenting with this condition, particularly if it is bilateral (23). Atypical facial pains as well as ear pain may occur as well, but it is useful to have patients seen for dental evaluation to exclude temporomandibular joint (TMJ) disorders and other pathologies, as well as ears, nose, and throat (ENT) evaluation. Hearing loss may also occur in MS, although it is recommended to exclude other central (e.g., Susac's syndrome) and peripheral causes of hearing loss. Vertigo and dizziness may be seen in MS patients, but in the vast majority of the time MS is not the sole cause for the dizziness, given the significant number of patients who have cervicogenic dizziness which responds to effective physical therapy. Recent reports have indicated that many patients with MS and vertigo actually have benign positional vertigo, which is readily treated with exercises such as the modified Epley (24).

Likewise, while swallowing problems certainly can occur in later stages of MS, ambulatory patients with MS who complain of swallowing problems generally point to the lower throat as the sticking point, and swallowing evaluation and gastrointestinal (GI) workup reveals other more treatable causes of the difficulty. Dysfunction in articulation may occur in MS, usually in association with other lower cranial nerve difficulties. The staccato rhythms of cerebellar speech are occasionally seen in MS patients as well.

Somatosensory Pathways

Disturbances in sensory pathways in MS patients are very common, and most often involve hemibody complaints. Other typical complaints are patches of odd sensations, particularly the feeling of wetness or itching or something crawling (formication) in the absence of anything being on the skin. Spinal cord lesions may present with the so-called "MS hug," which is a band- or belt-like sensation often involving the thoracic region. Hemibanding sensations can also occur, and may lead to superfluous cardiac workups. Severe abdominal girdling sensation can occur as well, often associated with difficult-to-manage constipation. Patients may or may not have evidence of sensory dysfunction on examination, although loss of vibratory sensation is common in MS patients.

While many physicians are taught in training that pain does not occur in MS, unfortunately this is not true, and many of the sensory symptoms in MS are indeed painful, particularly those generated from spinal cord lesions as well as trigeminal neuralgia (25). However, complaints of total body pain, like total body weakness, are not typical of MS. A distribution of the pain in an area consistent with CNS localization, as opposed to radicular or joint or fibromyalgia type pain, would be the most reliable way of distinguishing MS-related pain from other causes. Paroxysmal symptoms may also cause brief but excruciating pain, usually involving the face, arm, and leg, or only the arm and the leg in a repetitive manner. Other head pains may be found in MS, for example in optic neuritis, particularly when bilateral, or severely swollen cervical cord lesions, which may cause pain in the back of the head and upper neck associated with stiffness and difficulty with movement. Increases in tone, such as that found with spasticity or spasms, may also be perceived as painful, particularly in the calf, but sometimes also in the thigh and/or toes.

Motor Pathways

The dysfunction of motor pathways in MS follows an upper motor neuron distribution. Face, arm, and leg, or just arm and leg distribution of weakness is typical, although the patient may or may not be aware of the arm weakness particularly if it is on the nondominant side. Patients may not complain of spasticity per se, but complaints of calf or toe cramping at night, particularly unilateral or asymmetrical, may be related to MS, particularly in the context of increased reflexes on examination. Cold or prolonged inactivity such as sitting may worsen spasticity. Muscle weakness associated with MS occurs with increased tone and would only be associated with muscle atrophy in very late stages. Weakness from MS is often accompanied by altered autonomic function in the affected limb, causing swelling and dependent cyanosis, which may lead to a fruitless search for deep vein thrombosis or arterial insufficiency. Foot dragging can occur frequently, and is often brought out by heat or exertion. Pattern of progression of weakness of one foot, which then progresses to weakness on the corresponding rest of the body, is relatively common and may occur over days, weeks, or even years or decades. Sudden or acute onset of weakness would be much more likely to indicate a vascular cause rather than MS.

Cerebellum and Cerebellar Connections

Limb and gait ataxia are some of the most disabling symptoms that can occur in MS. Unfortunately, once the cerebellum and its connections are involved, symptoms tend to progress through time. Patients rarely complain of the scanning pattern which can occur with cerebellar speech, but family members will acknowledge the change in speech on questioning. However, patients are very much aware of and troubled by dysmetria, cerebellar tremors, and truncal ataxia when present.

Bowel and Bladder Pathways

MS patients frequently complain of bowel and bladder issues. Constipation is the most common bowel complaint, and bowel incontinence is often overflow incontinence. Constipation may be relatively mild to begin with, but is then exacerbated by symptomatic medications, and the tendency of MS patients to consciously or unconsciously reduce fluid intake in an attempt to control bladder problems. Diarrhea is not typically associated with MS, and if not medication- or food-related, should be investigated. Bladder complaints are also common in MS (26), and certainly are exacerbated by constipation as well as medications used for symptom management. MS patients may also have structural or non-MS-related bladder complaints, such as cough and sneeze (stress) incontinence, but the true complaints consistent with neurogenic bladder are more likely to be difficulty emptying (hesitancy), increased urge to void (urgency), and urge or overflow incontinence. History is very helpful in distinguishing structural and functional bladder complaints, but it is necessary to perform a postvoid residual volume measurement or more extensive urological testing to diagnose and recommend treatment for the various types of neurogenic bladder dysfunction.

NONSPECIFIC VERSUS SPECIFIC SYMPTOMS

Frequently, patients are sent for MS evaluation because of nonspecific symptoms. These include fatigue, myalgias, headache, memory impairment, depression, and diffuse paresthesias. These symptoms are seen commonly in a variety of syndromes (e.g., rheumatic disorders, somatization disorders, fibromyalgia, depression) and are not helpful in the diagnosis of MS. When taking a history of the symptoms of MS, focusing on more specific symptoms that suggest demyelination may be key. These include symptoms such as the Lhermitte's phenomenon (electrical feelings when flexing the neck), unilateral visual loss suggesting optic neuritis, focal paresthesias in a CNS distribution, diplopia particularly vertical, and spinal cord symptoms such as a combination of paresthesias below a level, motor weakness below a level, and bowel and bladder disruption. When we diagnose MS, we use the specific symptoms for diagnosis. When we treat MS, we also need to attend to the nonspecific symptoms in terms of management.

ILLUSTRATIVE CASE

Jenny Penny is a 23-year-old right-handed white female. Six months ago she developed a painful sensation behind her left eye, which was worse with movement. Over 3 days she developed a progressive loss of central vision in that eye with impaired color vision and decreased light brightness. This spontaneously resolved over 3 weeks. Three months ago she noticed a tingling sensation in the toes of both feet which ascended to the bra line over 4 days. This was associated with some sense of unsteadiness with walking and also trouble initiating urination. She now notices that when she flexes her neck forward she gets a tingling sensation in both arms and legs. She has also been much more tired than usual since this all began. When she was evaluated in the office she had a left afferent pupillary defect (APD), diminished vibratory sensation and proprioception in her bilateral feet, and mild gait ataxia. This case illustrates several characteristic symptoms and signs along. Her episode of vision loss was consistent with an episode of optic neuritis, which was supported by the evidence of an ADP on exam. The second episode of numbness with a sensory level, unsteadiness, urination trouble, and Lhermitte's is consistent with transverse myelitis, which was also supported by her exam findings of sensory loss and mild gait ataxia. She also has several nonspecific symptoms of fatigue and urinary difficulty, which when put into the larger clinical picture are also consistent with MS. It is the combination of her gender, race, clinical events, and exam findings that make MS the most likely diagnosis based on signs and symptoms.

CONCLUSION-FINDING PATTERNS WHICH FIT TOGETHER

As illustrated, MS has truly protean manifestations, which can affect virtually every area controlled by the CNS. Distinguishing MS symptoms can often be best done by history, and then confirmed on examination, and then focused testing, as covered in other chapters. Pattern recognition and the abilities to listen carefully and observe are key in this endeavor.

KEY POINTS FOR PATIENTS AND FAMILIES

- While the list of potential MS symptoms is long, actual MS symptoms can and must be distinguished from generic categories such as "bladder problems" or "visual symptoms."

- It is often more important to distinguish what is not due to MS, that is, a symptom is due to MS only if all other possibilities have been eliminated.

- Symptoms involving the entire body, for example, total body pain or weakness or fatigue severe enough to cause someone to actually fall asleep while sitting, are unlikely to be due to MS.

- MS symptoms can cause pain in some circumstances, much of which can be improved with appropriate diagnosis and management.

- MS symptoms often worsen with increased body temperature from fever or exercise, but may worsen with inactivity or cold in some cases.

- The symptoms of MS vary from patient to patient. Most people with MS have one or more of the following during their course: numbness or tingling, weakness, double vision, loss of vision in one eye, bladder difficulty, and trouble with walking or balance.

- Not all symptoms are due to MS even when you have MS, and you may need to check with your primary doctor or neurologist whether new symptoms are due to something else.

- The symptoms help diagnose MS. However, the diagnosis of MS is not based solely on symptoms as they may have many causes.

REFERENCES

1. Sponsler JL, Kendrick-Adey AC. Seizures as a manifestation of multiple sclerosis. *Epileptic Disord.* 2011;13:401–410.
2. Chanson JB, Kremer S, Blanc F, et al. Foreign accent syndrome as a first sign of multiple sclerosis. *Mult Scler.* 2009;15:1123–1125.
3. Aguirregomozcorta M, Ramió-Torrentà L, Gich J, et al. Paroxysmal dystonia and pathological laughter as a first manifestation of multiple sclerosis. *Mult Scler.* 2008;14:262–265.
4. Özünlü A, Mus N, Gulhan M. Multiple sclerosis: a cause of sudden hearing loss. *Audiology.* 1998;37:52–58.
5. De Santi L, Annunziata P. Symptomatic cranial neuralgias in multiple sclerosis: clinical features and treatment. *Clin Neurol Neurosurg.* 2012;114:101–107.
6. Chan JW. Early diagnosis, monitoring, and treatment of optic neuritis. *Neurologist.* 2012;18:23–31.
7. Sakai RE, Feller DJ, Galetta KM, et al. Vision in multiple sclerosis: the story, structure-function correlations, and models for neuroprotection. *J Neuroophthalmol.* 2011;31:362–373.
8. Rae-Grant AD, Eckert NJ, Bartz S, et al. Sensory symptoms of multiple sclerosis: a hidden reservoir of morbidity. *Mult Scler.* 1999;5:179–183.
9. Osterberg A, Boivie J. Central pain in multiple sclerosis—sensory abnormalities. *Eur J Pain.* 2010;14:104–110.
10. Carmosino MJ, Brousseau KM, Arciniegas DB, et al. Initial evaluations for multiple sclerosis in a university multiple sclerosis center: outcomes and role of magnetic resonance imaging in referral. *Arch Neurol.* 2005;62:585–590.
11. Pula JH, Reder AT. Multiple sclerosis. Part I: neuro-ophthalmic manifestations. *Curr Opin Ophthalmol.* 2009;20:467–475.
12. Mills RJ, Young CA. The relationship between fatigue and other clinical features of multiple sclerosis. *Mult Scler.* 2011;17:604–612.
13. Brown RF, Valpiani EM, Tennant CC, et al. Longitudinal assessment of anxiety, depression, and fatigue in people with multiple sclerosis. *Psychol Psychother.* 2009;82(pt 1):41–56.
14. Staff NP, Lucchinetti CF, Keegan BM. Multiple sclerosis with predominant, severe cognitive impairment. *Arch Neurol.* 2009;66:1139–1143.
15. Langdon DW. Cognition in multiple sclerosis. *Curr Opin Neurol.* 2011;24:244–249.
16. Foley R, Benedict R, Gromisch E, et al. The need for screening, assessment, and treatment for cognitive dysfunction in MS: results of a multidisciplinary CMSC consensus conference, September 24, 2010. *Int J MS Care.* 2012;14:58–64.
17. Marrie RA, Horwitz R, Cutter G, et al. The burden of mental comorbidity in multiple sclerosis: frequent, underdiagnosed, and undertreated. *Mult Scler.* 2009;15:385–392.
18. Feinstein A. Neuropsychiatric syndromes associated with multiple sclerosis. *J Neurol.* 2007;254(suppl 2):II73–II76.
19. Agan K, Gunal DI, Afsar N, et al. Psychotic depression: a peculiar presentation for multiple sclerosis. *Int J Neurosci.* 2009;119:2124–2130.
20. Iacovides A, Andreoulakis E. Bipolar disorder and resembling special psychopathological manifestations in multiple sclerosis: a review. *Curr Opin Psychiatry.* 2011;24:336–340.
21. Work SS, Colamonico JA, Bradley WG, et al. Pseudobulbar affect: an under-recognized and under-treated neurological disorder. *Adv Ther.* 2011;28:586–601.
22. Ghaffar O, Chamelian L, Feinstein A. Neuroanatomy of pseudobulbar affect: a quantitative MRI study in multiple sclerosis. *J Neurol.* 2008;255:406–412.
23. Cruccu G, Biasiotta A, Di Rezze S, et al. Trigeminal neuralgia and pain related to multiple sclerosis. *Pain.* 2009;143:186–191.
24. Frohman EM, Kramer PD, Dewey RB, et al. Benign paroxysmal positioning vertigo in multiple sclerosis: diagnosis, pathophysiology and therapeutic techniques. *Mult Scler.* 2003;9:250–255.
25. Nurmikko TJ, Gupta S, MacIver K. Multiple sclerosis-related central pain disorders. *Curr Pain Headache Rep.* 2010;14:189–195.
26. Stoffel JT. Contemporary management of the neurogenic bladder for multiple sclerosis patients. *Urol Clin North Am.* 2010;37:547–557.

7

Diagnosis of Multiple Sclerosis

Thomas Shoemaker and Scott D. Newsome

KEY POINTS FOR CLINICIANS

- The diagnosis of multiple sclerosis (MS) remains dependent on evidence of dissemination of central nervous system lesions in time and space.

- The diagnostic criteria for MS continues to evolve over time with increasing integration of paraclinical testing including MRI and spinal fluid analysis in order to help achieve a diagnosis earlier in the disease course without sacrificing accuracy.

- Application of the 2017 McDonald Criteria can help confirm a diagnosis in patients presenting with clinically isolated syndromes (CIS) suggestive of MS, as long as there remains no better explanation for the patients presentation. Misapplication of the criteria may lead to misdiagnosis.

- The most recently revised 2017 McDonald Criteria has incorporated a few important changes including: (a) allowing typical CIS patients to fulfill dissemination in time criteria with the presence of cerebrospinal-fluid-specific oligoclonal bands; (b) symptomatic lesions can be used to demonstrate dissemination in space and/or time; (c) cortical lesions can be used for dissemination in space.

As there has yet to be a single gold standard test for establishing a diagnosis of MS, the clinician's role remains central to the diagnosis of MS. A meticulous clinical history supplemented by a thoughtful neurologic examination and paraclinical testing (i.e., MRI, and sometimes spinal fluid analysis) help form the foundation for achieving an accurate diagnosis. The diagnosis of MS is often straightforward with demonstration of central nervous system (CNS) demyelination with both dissemination in time (DIT) and dissemination in space (DIS). This simplicity belies the real world difficulty that can arise when establishing a new diagnosis of MS.

CURRENT CLINICAL PHENOTYPES OF MS

In 2013, an international group of experts reexamined the MS phenotypes that were established in 1996 to determine if clinical course descriptors and types needed updating based on new insights and progress in MS research and care. It was ultimately determined that the basic features of the original 1996 phenotype description be maintained with some modifications in the recognized phenotypes (see the following section) and the incorporation of specific modifiers

relevant to disease activity and progression. The clinical phenotypes/subtypes recognized are the following (1):

CIS: CIS is recognized as the first clinical presentation of MS and most commonly manifest as acute optic neuritis (AON), transverse myelitis, or brainstem syndrome. Interestingly, CIS was not recognized in the initial clinical course descriptors partly because CIS can occur in a variety of conditions other than MS. However, natural history studies and clinical trials in MS have demonstrated that the majority of patients with CIS will go on to fulfill McDonald Criteria for relapsing–remitting MS (RRMS), especially when more typical demyelinating lesions coexist on neuraxial imaging.

RRMS: RRMS is the most common subtype of MS (approximately 85%) and presents with well-defined, discrete relapses (described later). Patients with RRMS can experience complete recovery from a relapse or have residual neurological dysfunction/disability. By definition, patients with RRMS should not experience disease progression in-between relapses and when this occurs one has to consider the transition to secondary progressive MS (SPMS).

SPMS: SPMS is typically diagnosed retrospectively and is considered within the spectrum of relapsing MS.

There is no clear clinical or paraclinical marker that determines exactly when patients transition from RRMS to SPMS. Clinicians typically will consider a diagnosis of SPMS when patients experience ongoing clinical disability progression for at least a year that is not attributed to a relapse. SPMS patients can experience occasional relapses and new MRI lesions, but these are few in number.

Primary progressive MS (PPMS): PPMS remains a separate clinical course than relapse onset MS and incorporates different criteria for diagnosis (discussed later). PPMS patients do not experience relapses and from the onset experience gradual clinical disability progression. Similar to SPMS, patients with PPMS can experience occasional plateaus in their accumulation of disability (without progression) and represent approximately 15% of patients with MS.

Clinical relapses can occasionally be seen in patients with established PPMS. The prior category of progressive relapsing MS is no longer recognized as an MS phenotype with the inclusion of disease activity as a modifier (discussed later) in the revised clinical phenotypes. These patients are now considered as having primary progressive disease with "activity present."

A less straightforward situation is radiologically isolated syndrome (RIS), where patients have findings on MRI typical for demyelination, but have no clinical history suggestive of either RRMS or PPMS. This syndrome is covered in more detail later in this chapter since it is currently not considered as a distinct MS phenotype, but deserves recognition since some patients with RIS are at risk for MS.

EVOLUTION OF MS DIAGNOSTIC CRITERIA

To aide in the diagnosis of MS, a number of formal and informal criteria have been used since Jean Marie Charcot termed the condition *sclerosis en plaque* in the late 1860s. His clinical observations led to the formulation of Charcot's triad of MS: intention tremor, scanning speech, and nystagmus.

The first formal diagnostic criteria in MS were the Schumacher Committee Criteria, which was established in 1965 (2). These criteria were put forth in an effort to better define MS in hopes of creating a more standard patient population for therapeutic trials. The committee that formed the Schumacher Criteria cautioned that "the diagnosis in most cases, even when termed 'clinically definite,' must remain one merely of high probability because of the lack of specific diagnostic tests." The Schumacher Criteria were entirely based on clinical findings and required DIS as defined as evidence of involvement of two or more separate regions of the CNS (3). Moreover, the CNS involvement must have occurred temporally in one of the following patterns: (a) In two or more episodes of worsening, separated by a period of 1 month or more, with each episode lasting at least 24 hours; (b) Slow or step-wise progression of signs and symptoms, over a period of at least 6 months.

In 1983, the Poser Criteria expanded upon the Schumacher Criteria by adding paraclinical testing, cerebrospinal fluid (CSF) and evoked potentials (4). These additions allowed clinicians to garner a higher level of confidence in diagnosing MS and provided the guidance necessary for differentiating definite MS from probable MS and not MS (see the following).

- Clinically definite MS: At least two clinical episodes are required with either neurological dysfunction demonstrable by neurological examination or paraclinical evidence of the existence of a nonclinical lesion in the CNS. At least one event should be of clinical evidence;
- Laboratory supported definite MS: At least one attack and oligoclonal bands (OCBs) in addition to fulfilling one of the following criteria;
  - Two attacks, and one clinical or paraclinical evidence
  - One attack and two clinical evidences
  - One attack, one clinical and one paraclinical evidence
- Clinically probable MS: At least one clinical episode with one of the following criteria fulfilled;
  - Two attacks and one clinical evidence
  - One attack and two clinical evidences
  - One attack, one clinical and one paraclinical evidence
- Laboratory supported probable MS: Two attacks with no other evidence;
- No MS—There is no clinical evidence of having MS

After the advent of MRI, several clinicians proposed that neuraxial imaging should be incorporated into the MS diagnostic criteria. In 2000, a meeting with international experts under the chairmanship of Professor Ian McDonald was convened in order to explore and incorporate MRI into the diagnostic criteria. This meeting ultimately led to the establishment of the original McDonald Criteria (Table 7.1) and served as a foundation for future revisions in the diagnostic criteria (2005, 2010, and 2017) (3,5,6). The initial imaging criteria were based upon research of Barkhof and Tintoré, which required the detection of characteristic lesions that were larger than 3 mm in cross section and with lesions fulfilling three of four of the following (7,8):

1. One gadolinium-enhancing lesion, or nine T2-hyperintense lesions if there is no gadolinium-enhancing lesion
2. At least one infratentorial lesion
3. At least one juxtacortical lesion
4. At least three periventricular lesions

A note was made that a spinal cord lesion could be substituted for a brain lesion.

The initial McDonald Criteria enabled earlier diagnosis of MS than either the Schumacher Criteria or Poser Criteria and proved to have both a higher specificity and sensitivity for diagnosis. Patients could be diagnosed with MS following a single clinical attack if they had evidence of DIS and DIT, which was achieved by a follow-up MRI with or without spinal fluid (see bottom of Table 7.1).

The McDonald Criteria were revised in 2005 to allow fulfillment of DIS and DIT by allowing spinal cord

TABLE 7.1   2001 McDonald Criteria Diagnostic Scheme

CLINICAL PRESENTATION	ADDITIONAL DATA REQUIRED
Two or more attacks and one objective clinical evidence of two or more lesions	None
Two or more attacks and one objective clinical evidence of one lesions	One of three of the following • DIS, demonstrated by MRI • Two or more MRI-detected lesions consistent with MS plus positive CSF • Await further clinical attack implicating a different site
One attack; objective clinical evidence of one lesion (monosymptomatic presentation; clinically isolated syndrome)	DIS, demonstrated by MRI or Two or more MRI-detected lesions consistent with MS plus positive CSF And DIT, demonstrated by MRI or second clinical attack

CSF, cerebrospinal fluid; DIS, dissemination in space; DIT, dissemination in time; MS, multiple sclerosis.

enhancing and nonenhancing lesions to substitute for brain lesions and new T2 lesions developing only 1 month or more after a baseline scan. Previous criteria required at least 3 months between scans.

These revised imaging criteria required a complicated system of lesion counting and excluded some symptomatic lesions from DIS criteria, together which proved to be challenging for clinicians to correctly implement in their daily clinical practice. Utilizing the findings from additional research these criteria were further refined in the 2010 McDonald Criteria. The DIS criteria required only ≥1 T2 lesion in at least two of four characteristic MS locations (juxtacortical, periventricular, infratentorial, and spinal cord), and no symptomatic lesion was excluded from fulfilling DIS criteria. Additionally, a single MRI could now fulfill DIT criteria as long as there was simultaneous co-occurrence of an asymptomatic enhancing lesion and nonenhancing lesion. These revised criteria for DIT allowed a diagnosis of MS to be made based upon a single clinical attack and one MRI, which allowed for even earlier diagnosis. One notable change in the 2010 criteria was the removal of CSF testing as a part of the diagnostic criteria. CSF findings could be supportive of a diagnosis of MS but it did not influence the fulfillment of criteria as in the 2001 and 2005 McDonald Criteria.

PRESENT DIAGNOSTIC CRITERIA FOR RELAPSING MS

The McDonald Criteria were revised again in 2017. These revisions aimed to simplify the diagnostic process, facilitate earlier diagnosis than the 2010 criteria, preserve the specificity and sensitivity of the diagnosis, and promote appropriate application of the criteria to minimize misdiagnoses (9).

Notable changes in the 2017 McDonald Criteria for Relapsing MS:

- *Cortical lesions are now included in dissemination in space MRI criteria.*
- *Symptomatic and asymptomatic lesions can be used to demonstrate dissemination in space and/or time.*
- *The presence of oligoclonal bands in CSF can be used to fulfill DIT criteria.*

In order to appropriately apply the criteria, the Panel emphasized that it should be applied to individuals who present with a typical clinical presentation suggestive of MS. The panel felt that a significant amount of misdiagnoses results from misapplication of the criteria (reviewed further in the following section). The central tenets of DIT and DIS remain the foundation of diagnosis. A diagnosis can be made in individuals with a single clinical episode (or multiple episodes) as long as there is supportive clinical and/or paraclinical evidence of dissemination of demyelination in time and space and there is no better explanation for the patient's presenting clinicoradiological syndrome. This goal can be accomplished in a number of ways as outlined in Table 7.2.

If the criteria described earlier are satisfied and there is no better explanation for the clinical presentation, then an MS diagnosis is substantiated. If there is high concern for an acquired demyelinating disorder but the abovementioned criteria are not sufficiently fulfilled, the diagnosis is CIS (see the following section), which can be further stratified into high or low risk CIS (usually based on MRI findings). If a more plausible explanation for the clinical signs and symptoms is uncovered during an evaluation for MS (or even after establishing the diagnosis of MS), then the diagnosis is "not MS." These criteria should be applied with caution in individuals who have coexisting conditions that could cause their current symptoms and disability.

The statement "no better explanation" has been interpreted in differing ways. For some, it implies the need to engage in an effort to rule out all potential mimickers of MS, which may lead to additional laboratory testing, imaging, and consultations. Another approach is to only seek out mimicking conditions when the 2017 McDonald Criteria are not sufficiently fulfilled and there are either red flags or a discrepancy between the provided clinical history, paraclinical testing, and neurological exam. Regardless of the clinician's approach, it remains essential to apply the "no better explanation" clause during an evaluation for MS. Following publication of the 2005 McDonald Criteria, an international task force generated a consensus approach to the differential diagnosis of MS, which focused on the classification of clinical presentations into typical and/or suggestive for MS versus those

TABLE 7.2   The 2017 McDonald Criteria for Diagnosis of Multiple Sclerosis With an Attack at Onset; Clinically Isolated Syndrome and Relapsing Remitting Multiple Sclerosis

CLINICAL EPISODES SUGGESTIVE OF CNS DEMYELINATION	CLINICAL EVIDENCE OF CNS LESIONS	ADDITIONAL CRITERIA TO FULFILL DIAGNOSIS
≥2	≥2 lesions OR Objective clinical evidence of one lesion with clear-cut historical evidence of a prior attack in a distinct anatomic location	None
≥2	Objective clinical evidence of one lesion	**Dissemination in space demonstrated by:** A second clinical attack in a distinct CNS anatomic location OR ≥1 T2-hyperintense lesion in ≥2 of four MS-typical regions of the CNS (periventricular, cortical/juxtacortical, infratentorial, or spinal cord)
1	Objective clinical evidence of ≥2 lesions	**DIT, demonstrated by:** A second clinical attack OR Simultaneous presence of asymptomatic gadolinium-enhancing and nonnhancing lesions at any time* OR A new T2 and/or gadolinium-enhancing lesion(s) on follow-up MRI, irrespective of its timing with reference to a baseline scan OR Demonstration of OCBs in CSF *No distinction between symptomatic and asymptomatic lesions
1	Objective clinical evidence of one lesion	**DIS and DIT, demonstrated by:** For DIS: A second clinical attack OR ≥1 T2 lesion in at least two of four MS-typical regions of the CNS (periventricular, cortical/juxtacortical, infratentorial, or spinal cord) AND For DIT: A second clinical attack OR Simultaneous presence of asymptomatic gadolinium-enhancing and nonenhancing lesions at any time OR A new T2 and/or gadolinium-enhancing lesion(s) on follow-up MRI, irrespective of its timing with reference to a baseline scan OR Demonstration of OCBs in CSF

CNS, central nervous system; CSF, cerebrospinal fluid; DIS, dissemination in space; DIT, dissemination in time; MS, multiple sclerosis; OCB, oligoclonal band.

that are atypical for MS (10). Included in their approach was identification of major red flags (fairly definitively not supportive of MS diagnosis) and minor red flags (may be consistent with MS or an alternative diagnosis). These red flags are primarily clinical and radiographic, signifying that much of the evaluation for alternative diagnoses is accomplished with a thorough history, examination, and review of appropriate imaging. Red flags and alternate diagnoses are discussed in more detail below and later in this chapter.

In the 2017 McDonald Criteria publication, more attention was given to neuromyelitis optica spectrum disorders (NMOSDs) as the authors felt strongly about

considering this condition in any patient being evaluated for MS, especially given the considerable clinical and sometimes radiological overlap between these two conditions (9). Testing for aquaporin-4 IgG (AQP4-IgG) is recommended in patients with features suggestive of NMOSD including bilateral optic neuritis, longitudinally extensive transverse myelitis, area postrema syndromes, large cerebral lesions, normal brain imaging at symptom onset, and in groups with a known increased risk for NMOSD (i.e., African Americans, Asians, Latin Americans, etc.). See Chapter 38 for further discussion of NMOSD.

Once the diagnosis of relapsing remitting MS has been established, further delineation of relapsing MS into

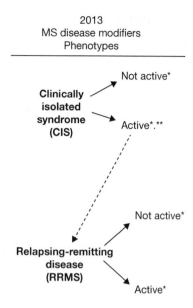

2013
MS disease modifiers
Phenotypes

Clinically isolated syndrome (CIS)

Not active*

Active*.**

Relapsing-remitting disease (RRMS)

Not active*

Active*

FIGURE 7.1 Relapsing multiple sclerosis phenotypes.

specific phenotypes is advised to aide in prognostication and selection of disease-modifying therapies (1). The phenotypes are determined based on the presence or absence of disease activity and disease progression. The phenotypic subdivisions include "active" or "not active." *Active* disease is defined as MS with clinical relapses or new lesions on MRI. *Not active* disease is essentially the absence of these clinical and imaging findings (Figure 7.1).

PUTTING THE 2017 MCDONALD CRITERIA INTO PRACTICE

Population of Interest

The previous interations of the McDonald Criteria were derived largely based upon young adult Caucasian populations in Europe and North America with syndromes consistent with MS. Following the publication of the 2010 McDonald Criteria, subsequent studies supported the applicability of the criteria in diverse ethnic and racial populations. Nevertheless, the international panel stressed vigilance in excluding other diagnoses in diverse populations that are at high risk for other conditions (i.e., NMOSD) including children, older adults, and patients of less typical ethnic backgrounds for MS including Asian, Latin American, Middle Eastern, and African. With evidence of DIT and DIS of at least two demyelinating lesions and attacks, a clinician may make a diagnosis of MS without any additional testing.

Clinical Criteria for DIS

Patients presenting with typical MS symptoms often have findings on examination suggesting additional areas of demyelination. For example, a patient experiencing a Lhermitte's phenomenon with an incomplete sensory level

on examination may also have a relative afferent pupillary defect with accompanying red color desaturation or other findings that are picked up on routine neurological exam. These signs on exam indicate lesions in at least two separate sites in the neuraxis (spinal cord and optic nerve), which could satisfy DIS by clinical grounds alone.

Clinical Criteria for DIT

Obtaining a complete and thorough history is critical, especially since many patients experience prior symptoms consistent with MS that are initially dismissed as a "pinched nerve," migraine, or positional vertigo. On initial presentation with AON, a patient may reveal a prior episode of horizontal diplopia that lasted several weeks which was previously attributed to needing a new glasses prescription. However, if a corresponding internuclear ophthalmoplegia is found on examination, then criteria are met for DIT from a clinical perspective. Indeed, specific findings are not required if the clinical history is classic for demyelination. Alternatively, if a patient presents with an episode of AON without a prior neurological history, then DIT is not fulfilled clinically. If the patient goes on to develop a second clinical demyelinating episode (such as a partial transverse myelitis), then clinical DIT will have been fulfilled. Clinical judgment should be employed in the interpretation of these historical events, as the true nature of historical events is often unclear.

MRI Criteria for DIT and DIS

MRI remains the most sensitive tool available to aid in the diagnosis of MS. MRI activity is most robust early on in the disease course, which allows in some cases an early diagnosis of MS by demonstrating DIT. Moreover, MRI can help rule out non-MS related conditions (i.e., spinal stenosis). In a patient presenting with typical CIS, the MRI can prove helpful in demonstrating evidence for DIS and DIT (Table 7.3).

TABLE 7.3 2017 McDonald Criteria for Demonstration of Dissemination in Space and Time by MRI in a Patient With CIS

DIS can be demonstrated by ≥1 T2 lesion in at least two of four areas of the CNS:[a]
- Periventricular
- Cortical/Juxtacortical
- Infratentorial
- Spinal cord

DIT can be demonstrated by either of the following:
- Simultaneous presence of gadolinium-enhancing and nonenhancing lesions at any time (without distinction between symptomatic and asymptomatic lesions)
- OR
- A new T2-hyperintense and/or gadolinium-enhancing lesion on a follow-up MRI, with reference to a baseline scan (irrespective of the timing of the baseline MRI)

[a]There is no distinction between symptomatic and asymptomatic MRI lesions.
CIS, clinically isolated syndrome; CNS, central nervous system; DIS, dissemination in space; DIT, dissemination in time.

If there is a history and neurological findings supporting multiple clinical episodes that are suggestive of MS, fulfillment of DIT and DIS with MRI is not required to fulfill the diagnostic criteria for MS. However, the diagnosis of MS should be made very cautiously in a patient with normal or nonspecific findings on MRI.

Other Paraclinical Evidence for DIT: CSF-Specific OCBs

With the 2017 revised McDonald Criteria, CSF testing was reincorporated into the formal diagnostic criteria for relapsing MS and remains a part of the criteria for diagnosing PPMS (9). The CSF evaluation can be instrumental when the diagnosis is not straightforward, like when the clinical history is atypical, or MRI findings are suggestive of possible demyelination. CSF evaluation can be helpful not only by identifying CNS-specific OCBs but also by ensuring the overall CSF profile is consistent with MS and not more suggestive of other neuroinflammatory/neuroinfectious conditions.

Typical CSF findings in MS may include a mild pleocytosis, mildly increased protein, intrathecal synthesis of immunoglobulin G (IgG index or IgG synthesis rate), and OCBs. The cell count is often normal to modestly elevated ($<5 \times 10^6$/L) (11). If the CSF pleocytosis is greater than 5×10^6/L, then an alternative diagnosis should be considered, although, a robust CSF pleocytosis may occur in the setting of an acute relapse ($>5 \times 10^6$/L) (12). In MS, lymphocytes comprise up to 90% of the spinal fluid composition with polymorphonuculear cells less than 5% (13). Total CSF protein tends to stay within reference range but there may be modest elevations in some individuals (14). CSF protein levels of over 100 mg/dL suggest an alternative diagnosis. In addition, CSF glucose levels are typically normal in MS or mildly elevated (i.e., if steroid treatment is ongoing for an acute relapse). If a patient has hypoglycorachia (low glucose), then it is strongly suggested to consider other conditions (i.e., neurosarcoidosis, infections, neoplastic process). The presence of OCBs unique to the CSF is the CSF finding most specific to MS and the one spinal fluid test that has been reincorporated back into the 2017 McDonald Criteria. The presence of OCBs is best evaluated with isoelectric focusing followed by immunoblotting or immunofixation of IgG with a simultaneous comparison of paired CSF and serum samples. The term OCBs specifically refers to the finding of IgG bands in the CSF without corresponding bands in the serum. This is inferred to represent an isolated CNS inflammatory process leading to the development of intrathecal antibody production. The number of unique bands required to be diagnostic (positive) varies between laboratories, but a general rule of thumb is that when tested as described earlier, the presence of two or more unique bands is present in nearly 90% of patients with definite MS (15). The caveat is that OCBs can be found in other disorders affecting the CNS including herpes encephalitis, HIV,

Rasmussen encephalitis, and occasionally in Alzheimer's disease and amyotrophic lateral sclerosis (16–18). Fortunately, there is little clinical and imaging overlap with most of these conditions and MS.

In addition to qualitative assessment of OCBs, quantitative IgG analysis (e.g., IgG index and IgG synthesis rate) may serve as a complementary test but may not be used to fulfill DIT criteria because it is only an assessment of blood–brain barrier integrity, and thus is not sufficiently specific for MS.

Additional Paraclinical Investigations: Visual Evoked Potentials and Optical Coherence Tomography

Diagnosing MS requires that at least one clinical attack must be corroborated by objective findings. While neurological examination and MRI typically fulfill this role, findings on visual evoked potential (VEP) and optical coherence tomography (OCT) may be used in patients reporting prior visual disturbances. The VEP P100 latency may be prolonged after demyelination of the anterior or posterior visual pathways. VEP abnormalities can persist for many years and are regarded as sensitive to previous optic neuritis but are not specific. OCT is a noninvasive high-resolution office based imaging technology that uses low-coherence interferometry to generate quantitative and qualitative images of retinal structures, including the retina nerve fiber layer (RNFL) (19). As such, OCT can be useful in finding objective evidence of anterior visual pathway injury. In patients who describe episodes concerning for optic neuritis, thinning of RNFL can be observed as early as 3 months after symptom onset (20). Moreover, retinal thinning on OCT correlates with visual function, global disability, and brain atrophy. Similarly, MS patients with RNFL thinning at baseline have a higher risk of disability worsening over time (21).

DIAGNOSIS OF PPMS

Similar to the approach for diagnosing relapsing MS, the criteria for PPMS have evolved over time and now use a combination of clinical examination, MRI, and/or CSF findings. The most recent iteration focuses on simplification of the imaging criteria and allowing DIT/DIS to be fulfilled by a symptomatic lesion (9).

In contrast to relapsing MS, where clinical relapses are the basis of diagnosis, PPMS requires at least 1 year of disease progression in addition to two of the paraclinical findings outlined below. According to the McDonald Criteria, the year of progression may be either retrospectively or prospectively determined. The diagnosis may be established during the initial patient encounter if there is a suitable history with corroborative exam findings. Progression in PPMS is defined as a continuous clinical deterioration from disease onset in the absence of distinct relapses (22). Minor fluctuations are permitted during this period, including occasional plateaus and transient minor improvements, but the overall trajectory should be continuous worsening of neurologic function. Additionally, the rate of progression may fluctuate between gradual and rapid decline. A common presentation in PPMS is progressive lower extremity monoparesis/paraparesis. The patient may describe a steady worsening of leg strength and ambulation over time.

In addition to ≥1 year of clinical progression, two of the following three criteria must be fulfilled to make a diagnosis of PPMS:

1. Evidence of DIS in the brain based on one or more T2 lesions in the characteristic MS regions (periventricular, cortical/juxtacortical, or infratentorial)
2. Evidence of DIS in the spinal cord based on two or more T2 lesions in the cord
3. Positive CSF (OCBs)

As in RRMS, the revised 2017 McDonald Criteria now allow for inclusion of symptomatic lesions (which were previously excluded) and cortical lesions to fulfill DIS. Moreover, gadolinium enhancement of lesions is not required.

The assessment of suspected PPMS in a patient necessitates careful attention as the diagnosis may be more difficult than RRMS to establish and there are several mimicking conditions to consider and exclude prior to making a PPMS diagnosis. As with relapsing MS, often the passage of time reveals the underlying diagnosis.

Similar to relapsing MS, once progressive MS has been diagnosed further phenotype designation should be attempted based upon clinical course (1). These phenotypes include "Active and with progression," "Active but without progression," "Not active but with progression," and "Not active and without progression (stable disease)" (Figure 7.2). Although uncommon, clinical relapses can be seen in patients PPMS.

> *Diagnosing PPMS requires a year of progressive neurologic decline. This can be determined either prospectively or retrospectively.*

DEFINING A RELAPSE

Relapsing MS is defined by the presence of clinical relapses. As such, it is important for both clinicians and patients to have a firm understanding of what is and what is not a relapse. The term "relapse" has several synonyms including exacerbations, attacks, bouts, and episodes, all of which confer the same meaning. A relapse is the initial occurrence or the marked worsening of

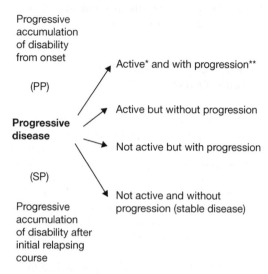

FIGURE 7.2 Progressive multiple sclerosis phenotypes.

symptoms *typical of an acute inflammatory demyelinating event in the CNS* which represents neurological dysfunction and typically presents with a subacute cadence. The symptoms must not occur in the setting of a fever or concurrent infection and need a duration of at least 24 hours to be determined a relapse (the "24 hour rule"). The typical relapse has a duration of days to weeks and should be separated from the preceding relapse by at least 30 days. New symptoms that develop within the 30-day window are considered part of the same relapse. Objective neurologic findings are not required to substantiate historical relapses. The 2017 McDonald Criteria panel acknowledged that, "some historical events with symptoms and evolution characteristic for MS, but for which no objective neurological findings are documented, can provide reasonable evidence of a prior demyelinating event" (Figure 7.3A and B).

While relapses are often temporary, all temporary MS symptoms are not relapses. Recurrence of established symptoms in the setting of a stressor (either physiologic or emotional) are recognized as pseudorelapse, which is discussed in greater detail in the following section. Similarly, Uhthoff's phenomenon is a temperature (heat)-related worsening of symptoms that results from established demyelination and does not represent new inflammatory activity. Paroxysmal symptoms such as trigeminal neuralgia and dysarthria ataxia syndrome pose more of a complex issue and may require further evaluation as they may represent either new inflammatory disease activity or progression of established lesions.

Features of a Relapse
Neurological disturbance of kind seen in MS(CIS)
indicating inflammatory/demyelinating pathology.
Subjective report or objective observation
24 hours duration minimum.
Excludes pseudorelapses
(A) and single paroxysmal episodes.
Separate relapses: at least 30 days between *onset* of event 1 and *onset* of event 2.

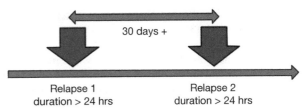

If a historical event and no abnormal clinical signs of that event:
Example (below): patient presents with brainstem symptoms and signs, as well as history 6 years ago
Lhermitte's phenomenon lasting > 24 hours, If possible, the previous Lhermitte's episodes should be
Corroborate MRI cervical cord (see arrowed lesions).

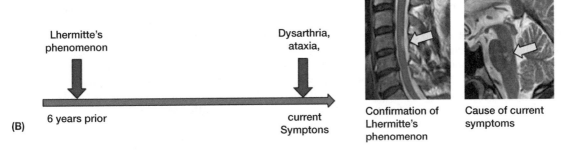

FIGURE 7.3 Clinical features defining a relapse. In particular: (A) for two episodes to be considered distinct relapses, there must be at least 30 days between the onset of the first relapse and the onset of the second relapse; (B) for relapses reported by history without corresponding examination findings, attempt to confirm the historical relapse by MRI. In this example, the history of Lhermitte's phenomenon was confirmed by MRI of the cervical cord, which showed a focal, posterior column lesion (arrowed).

> *The "24 hour rule": An MS relapse requires at least 24 hours of continuous neurologic symptoms/dysfunction in the absence of fever, infection, or other exogenous stressors.*

PSEUDO-RELAPSES

Pseudo-relapses (also termed pseudo-exacerbations or recrudescence) are defined as the recurrence of previously experienced signs and symptoms sustained for 24 hours in the setting of a trigger. They may have a stereotypic quality and will resolve when the offending trigger is removed or treated. Pseudo-relapses may be provoked by various triggers including infections, medications, emotional stress, and menses (23–26). Pseudo-relapses are distinct from true MS relapses due to the lack of new CNS inflammatory demyelination. Rather, the symptoms produced are secondary to transient conduction blocks occurring at the level of the axon leading to reversible electrophysiological dysfunction (27). As a consequence of the pathophysiology, the intervention

in a pseudo-exacerbation should be focused on identifying the provoking trigger and addressing it. Steroids or other MS-specific therapies are not necessary for pseudo-relapses.

RADIOLOGICALLY ISOLATED SYNDROME

With the widespread adoption and regular use of brain MRI in clinical practice and medical research, incidental findings have become common and occur in up to 18% in some healthy populations (28–30). Asymptomatic white matter abnormalities on MRI can be attributed to a number of different causes including congenital abnormalities, migraines, or small vessel ischemic disease. However, some changes may be consistent with preclinical MS based on the morphology and distribution of the lesions. These changes can occur in almost 1% of patients in some cohorts (31). These patients are frequently encountered by MS clinicians as they are often referred to MS centers. Such MRI findings have recently been termed RIS, which Okuda and colleagues defined as MRI lesions highly suggestive of demyelinating pathology, not better acounted for by another disease process. Proposed diagnostic criteria for RIS include the following (32):

A. The presence of incidentally identified CNS white matter anomalies meeting the following MRI criteria:
   1. Ovoid, well-circumscribed, and homogeneous foci with or without involvement of the corpus callosum
   2. T2 hyperintensities measuring greater than 3 mm and fulfilling Barkhof criteria (at least three out of four) for DIS
   3. CNS white matter anomalies not consistent with a vascular pattern
B. No historical accounts of remitting clinical symptoms consistent with neurologic dysfunction
C. The MRI anomalies do not account for clinically apparent impairments in social, occupational, or generalized areas of functioning
D. The MRI anomalies are not due to the direct physiologic effects of substances (recreational drug abuse, toxic exposure) or a medical condition
E. Exclusion of individuals with MRI phenotypes suggestive of leukoaraiosis or extensive white matter pathology lacking involvement of the corpus callosum
F. The CNS MRI anomalies are not better accounted for by another disease process

RIS is important to recognize because those patients who meet criteria of RIS are at increased risk of developing MS. In a retrospective cohort, individuals who met RIS criteria had a 34% risk of developing clinical manifestations of a demyelinating event after 5 years including 2% who went on to develop PPMS (33). The individuals most likely to go on to develop demyelinating events were younger and had cervical and thoracic cord lesions on MRI. Patients who fit the criteria for RIS may require further imaging, paraclinical investigations, and clinical follow-up.

> *RIS refers to MRI findings suggestive of MS in individuals without clinical evidence of MS.*

MISDIAGNOSIS OF MS AND "UNDIAGNOSING" MS

Informing patients regarding the diagnosis of MS is rarely an easy discussion, especially since it often triggers worries about a lifelong illness that can lead to permanent disability and potentially early death (34). However, informing patients that they do not have MS after previously being told they do can be even more difficult. A recent study found that 66.4% of surveyed clinicians found this task more difficult than informing an individual of a new diagnosis (35).

Estimates for the rate of misdiagnosis of MS vary depending on the setting but appear to range from 6% to 13% (36–42). Of those referred to an MS center specifically for a second opinion regarding the diagnosis of MS, misdiagnosis rates appear higher. One study reported that 33% of those referred did not have MS whereas another study reported a 35% rate of misdiagnosis (40,41). In a study of four academic MS centers, 110 patients were identified over 13 months as being incorrectly diagnosed with MS (42). The most common alternative diagnoses (accounting for two-thirds of these misdiagnosed patients) included fibromyalgia, nonspecific or nonlocalizing neurologic symptoms with nonspecific T2 hyperintensities on MRI, conversion or psychogenic disorder, and NMOSD. Other studies identified psychiatric conditions and migraine as prominent alternative diagnoses (38,40). One study observed that many of those misdiagnosed had proposed the diagnosis themselves or had either a medical background or family members with the condition (38).

It is important to recognize not only which conditions are frequently mistaken for MS but also to recognize the factors leading to these misdiagnoses. Solomon and Weinshenker described three main reasons for the misdiagnosis of MS: (a) misinterpretation and misapplication of clinical symptoms and exam findings; (b) misinterpretation and misapplication of radiographic criteria and terminology; (c) lack of reconsideration of an established diagnosis (43). The increased application of MRI in clinical care has subsequently led to over diagnosis secondary to misapplication of imaging criteria meant for patients with clinical syndromes suggestive of CNS demyelination (44). More frequent CSF testing has been suggested to aide in decreasing misdiagnosis of MS given its high specificity and the absence of OCBs in the commonly cited alternative diagnoses. Certain red flags have also been suggested that, when present, should give clinicians pause prior to making the diagnosis of MS. These red flags include the following:

1. Nonspecific or nonlocalizing symptoms despite multifocal MRI abnormalities
2. Historical neurological episodes without current objective corroborative findings
3. Apparent "new" lesions observed on interval MRI examinations which are secondary to different image acquisitions over time rather than truly new lesions
4. Normal spinal fluid analysis

Additional clinical red flags may include a normal neurological examination, no evidence of MRI dissemination over time and space, onset of symptoms before age 10 or after age 55, a progressive course before age 35, localized disease/symptoms, normal bladder/bowel function, impaired level of consciousness, prominent uveitis, peripheral neuropathy, early dementia, seizures, aphasia, extrapyramidal features, fever, headache, abrupt hemiparesis, abrupt hearing loss, and prominent pain. Furthermore, there are several specific clinical signs and symptoms that are more suggestive of non-MS diagnoses (Table 7.4) (53).

Reversing a diagnosis of MS ("undiagnosing" MS) is a difficult task for clinicians, especially when there is concern about patients experiencing psychological or economic consequences from losing the diagnosis of MS. Nonetheless, a recent survey found that the majority of clinicians who encountered a misdiagnosis feel compelled to inform their patients of this misdiagnosis. These clinicians cited the need to allow patients to make safe healthcare decisions and avoid potential harms (35).

THE FUTURE OF DIAGNOSING MS

The diagnosis of MS has evolved considerably to incorporate imaging technology, which has allowed for an earlier and more accurate diagnosis. Future developments in MS diagnosis will likely see further refinements of the current approach, but seem unlikely to change dramatically.

In forthcoming iterations of the diagnostic criteria, we may see the addition of newer assessment techniques and biomarkers. For example, a reliable and accurate diagnostic biomarker from either the CSF or serum has been long sought but has not yet been identified. While there has been a number of exploratory biomarkers, none have been clinically validated to date (45–47). The discovery of such a test would simplify the diagnostic process. Alternatively, imaging advances may further the diagnostic process. For example, ultra-high-field strength MRI scanners can detect highly specific MS characteristics such as a central vein within MS lesions (central vein sign) or paramagnetic rims at the margin of lesions (48–50). Other emerging techniques include genetic and metabolomic profiling (51,52).

Even with advancing technology, the diagnosis of MS will likely always fundamentally rely on a clinical picture consistent with multifocal demyelination: a clinical history, examination, and paraclinical tests to elicit evidence of multifocal demyelination that is DIT and DIS.

TABLE 7.4   Clinical Red Flags to Consider and Associated Diagnoses

CLINICAL RED FLAGS	POSSIBLE DIAGNOSIS
General	
Hyperacute presentation	Ischemia, haemorrhage seizure, syncope
Fevers, weight loss, night sweats, alopecia, synovitis	Infection, vasculitis, systemic lupus erythematosus
Livedo reticularis, early trimester abortions, and thrombotic history	Antiphospholipid syndrome
Cerebral hemispheres	
Encephalopathy	ADEM, PRES, encephalitis
Hemianopsia and cortical blindness	Ischemic stroke, PRES, neoplasm, PML
Insidious cognitive decline	Neurodegenerative, genetic leukoencephalopathy and leukodystrophy
Optic nerve	
Progressive vision loss	Neoplasm, sarcoidosis, LHON
Altitudinal deficit and monocular blindness	Ischemic optic neuropathy
Clinically severe or simultaneous bilateral ON	NMOSD and LHON
Neuroretinitis and uveitis	NMOSD
Spinal cord	
Anterior spinal syndrome	Ischemia
Complete transverse myelitis	NMOSD, idiopathic myelitis, ADEM, ischemia
Radiculitis	Infection, sarcoidosis, lymphomatosis, carcinomatosis, anti-MOG NMOSD
Progressive spastic paraparesis	HTLV-1, HIV, cobalamin deficiency, PLS, CSM, dAVF

ADEM, acute disseminated encephalomyelitis; CSM, cervical spondylotic myelopathy; dAVF, dural arteriovenous fistula; HTLV, human T-Cell Lymphotropic virus; LHON, Leber's hereditary optic neuropathy; MOG, myelin oligodendrocyte glycoprotein; NMOSD, neuromyelitis optica spectrum; ON, optic nerve; PLS, primary lateral sclerosis; PML, progressive multifocal encephalopathy syndrome; PRES, posterior reversible encephalopathy syndrome.
Source: Adapted from Toledano M, Weinshenker BG, Solomon AJ. A clinical approach to the differential diagnosis of multiple sclerosis. *Curr Neurol Neurosci Rep*. 2015;15(8):57. doi:10.1007/s11910-015-0576-7.

KEY POINTS FOR PATIENTS AND FAMILIES

- The diagnosis of MS is made using a combination of history, neurologic examination, MRI, and sometimes additional tests. The diagnosis can sometimes be made after the first attack but may require a period of observation to confirm (or exclude) the diagnosis.

- Additional testing such as OCT, VEP, and CSF sampling via lumbar puncture may assist in supporting the diagnosis.

- There are many conditions that cause symptoms like MS and some can cause white matter lesions on MRI. Therefore, it is prudent for MS mimics to be considered when making a diagnosis of MS, especially if red flags are present.

- Misdiagnosis of MS can happen and the diagnosis may need to be changed as new information is revealed.

REFERENCES

1. Lublin FD, Reingold SC, Cohen JA, et al. Defining the clinical course of multiple sclerosis. *Neurology*. 2014;83(3):278–286. doi:10.1212/WNL.0000000000000560.
2. Schumacher GA, Beebe G, Kibler RF, et al. Problems of experimental trials of therapy in multiple sclerosis: report by the panel on the evaluation of experimental trials of therapy in multiple sclerosis. *Ann N Y Acad Sci*. 1965;122(1):552–568. doi:10.1111/j.1749-6632.1965.tb20235.x.
3. Polman CH, Reingold SC, Banwell B, et al. Diagnostic criteria for multiple sclerosis: 2010 revisions to the McDonald criteria. *Ann Neurol*. 2011;69(2):292–302. doi:10.1002/ana.22366.
4. Poser CM, Paty DW, Scheinberg L, et al. New diagnostic criteria for multiple sclerosis: guidelines for research protocols. *Ann Neurol*. 1983;13(3):227–231. doi:10.1002/ana.410130302.
5. Polman CH, Reingold SC, Edan G, et al. Diagnostic criteria for multiple sclerosis: 2005 revisions to the "McDonald Criteria." *Ann Neurol*. 2005;58(6):840–846. doi:10.1002/ana.20703.
6. McDonald WI, Compston A, Edan G, et al. Recommended diagnostic criteria for multiple sclerosis: guidelines from the international panel on the diagnosis of multiple sclerosis. *Ann Neurol*. 2001;50(1):121–127. doi:10.1002/ana.1032.
7. Barkhof F, Filippi M, Miller DH, et al. Comparison of MRI criteria at first presentation to predict conversion to clinically definite multiple sclerosis. *Brain J Neurol*. 1997;120(Pt 11):2059–2069.
8. Tintoré M, Rovira A, Martínez MJ, et al. Isolated demyelinating syndromes: comparison of different MR imaging criteria to predict conversion to clinically definite multiple sclerosis. *Am J Neuroradiol*. 2000;21(4):702–706.
9. Thompson AJ, Banwell B, Barkhof F, et al. Diagnosis of multiple sclerosis: recommended 2017 revisions of the "McDonald" criteria. *Lancet Neurol*. 2018;17(2):162–173.
10. Miller D, Weinshenker B, Filippi M, et al. Differential diagnosis of suspected multiple sclerosis: a consensus approach. *Mult Scler*. 2008;14(9):1157–1174. doi:10.1177/1352458508096878.
11. Freedman MS, Thompson EJ, Deisenhammer F, et al. Recommended standard of cerebrospinal fluid analysis in the diagnosis of multiple sclerosis: a consensus statement. *Arch Neurol*. 2005;62(6):865–870. doi:10.1001/archneur.62.6.865.
12. Eisele P, Szabo K, Griebe M, et al. Cerebrospinal fluid pleocytosis in multiple sclerosis patients with lesions showing reduced diffusion. *Mult Scler*. 2014;20(10):1391–1395. doi:10.1177/1352458513515083.
13. Compston A, Confavreux C, Lassmann H, et al. *McAlpine's Multiple Sclerosis*. 4th ed. Philadelphia, PA: Churchill Livingstone; 2006.
14. Rammohan KW. Cerebrospinal fluid in multiple sclerosis. *Ann Indian Acad Neurol*. 2009;12(4):246–253. doi:10.4103/0972-2327.58282.
15. Dobson R, Ramagopalan S, Davis A, et al. Cerebrospinal fluid oligoclonal bands in multiple sclerosis and clinically isolated syndromes: a meta-analysis of prevalence, prognosis and effect of latitude. *J Neurol Neurosurg Psychiatry*. 2013;84(8):909–914. doi:10.1136/jnnp-2012-304695.
16. Chu AB, Sever JL, Madden DL, et al. Oligoclonal IgG bands in cerebrospinal fluid in various neurological diseases. *Ann Neurol*. 1983;13(4):434–439. doi:10.1002/ana.410130410.
17. Frankel EB, Greenberg ML, Makuku S, et al. Oligoclonal banding in AIDS and hemophilia. *Mt Sinai J Med*. 1993;60(3):232–237.
18. Sinclair AJ, Wienholt L, Tantsis E, et al. Clinical association of intrathecal and mirrored oligoclonal bands in paediatric neurology. *Dev Med Child Neurol*. 2013;55(1):71–75. doi:10.1111/j.1469-8749.2012.04443.x.
19. Huang D, Swanson EA, Lin CP, et al. Optical coherence tomography. *Science*. 1991;254(5035):1178–1181.
20. Syc SB, Saidha S, Newsome SD, et al. Optical coherence tomography segmentation reveals ganglion cell layer pathology after optic neuritis. *Brain*. 2012;135(2):521–533. doi:10.1093/brain/awr264.
21. Martinez-Lapiscina EH, Arnow S, Wilson JA, et al. Retinal thickness measured with optical coherence tomography and risk of disability worsening in multiple sclerosis: a cohort study. *Lancet Neurol*. 2016;15(6):574–584. doi:10.1016/S1474-4422(16)00068-5.
22. Lublin FD, Reingold SC. Defining the clinical course of multiple sclerosis: results of an international survey. National Multiple Sclerosis Society (USA) Advisory Committee on Clinical Trials of New Agents in Multiple Sclerosis. *Neurology*. 1996;46(4):907–911.
23. Wingerchuk DM, Rodriguez M. Premenstrual multiple sclerosis pseudoexacerbations: role of body temperature and prevention with aspirin. *Arch Neurol*. 2006;63(7):1005–1008. doi:10.1001/archneur.63.7.1005.
24. Case AM, Reid RL. Effects of the menstrual cycle on medical disorders. *Arch Intern Med*. 1998;158(13):1405–1412. doi:10.1001/archinte.158.13.1405.
25. Villoslada P, Arrondo G, Sepulcre J, et al. Memantine induces reversible neurologic impairment in patients with MS. *Neurology*. 2009;72(19):1630–1633. doi:10.1212/01.wnl.0000342388.73185.80.
26. Burns MN, Nawacki E, Siddique J, et al. Prospective examination of anxiety and depression before and during confirmed and pseudo-exacerbations in patients with multiple sclerosis. *Psychosom Med*. 2013;75(1):76–82. doi:10.1097/PSY.0b013e3182757b2b.
27. Smith KJ, McDonald WI. The pathophysiology of multiple sclerosis: the mechanisms underlying the production of symptoms and the natural history of the disease. *Philos Trans R Soc Lond B Biol Sci*. 1999;354(1390):1649–1673. doi:10.1098/rstb.1999.0510.
28. Bos D, Poels MMF, Adams HHH, et al. Prevalence, clinical management, and natural course of incidental findings on brain MR

images: the population-based Rotterdam Scan Study. *Radiology.* 2016;281(2):507–515. doi:10.1148/radiol.2016160218.

29. Hartwigsen G, Siebner HR, Deuschl G, et al. Incidental findings are frequent in young healthy individuals undergoing magnetic resonance imaging in brain research imaging studies: a prospective single-center study. *J Comput Assist Tomogr.* 2010;34(4):596–600. doi:10.1097/RCT.0b013e3181d9c2bb.

30. Katzman GL. Incidental findings on brain magnetic resonance imaging from 1000 asymptomatic volunteers. *JAMA.* 1999;282(1):36. doi:10.1001/jama.282.1.36.

31. Lyoo IK, Seol HY, Byun HS, et al. Unsuspected multiple sclerosis in patients with psychiatric disorders: a magnetic resonance imaging study. *J Neuropsychiatry Clin Neurosci.* 1996;8(1):54–59. doi:10.1176/jnp.8.1.54.

32. Okuda DT, Mowry EM, Beheshtian A, et al. Incidental MRI anomalies suggestive of multiple sclerosis: the radiologically isolated syndrome. *Neurology.* 2009;72(9):800–805. doi:10.1212/01.wnl.0000335764.14513.1a.

33. Okuda DT, Siva A, Kantarci O, et al. Radiologically isolated syndrome: 5-year risk for an initial clinical event. *PLoS ONE.* 2014;9(3):e90509. doi:10.1371/journal.pone.0090509.

34. Burkill S, Montgomery S, Hajiebrahimi M, et al. Mortality trends for multiple sclerosis patients in Sweden from 1968 to 2012. *Neurology.* July 2017;89(6):555–562. doi:10.1212/WNL.0000000000004216.

35. Solomon AJ, Klein EP, Bourdette D. "Undiagnosing" multiple sclerosis. *Neurology.* 2012;78(24):1986–1991. doi:10.1212/WNL.0b013e318259e1b2.

36. Engell T. A clinico-pathoanatomical study of multiple sclerosis diagnosis. *Acta Neurol Scand.* 1988;78(1):39–44. doi:10.1111/j.1600-0404.1988.tb03616.x.

37. Herndon RM, Brooks B. Misdiagnosis of multiple sclerosis. *Semin Neurol.* 1985;5(02):94–98. doi:10.1055/s-2008-1041505.

38. Murray TJ, Murray SJ. Characteristics of patients found not to have multiple sclerosis. *Can Med Assoc J.* 1984;131(4):336–337.

39. Pelidou S-H, Giannopoulos S, Tzavidi S, et al. Neurological manifestations of connective tissue diseases mimicking multiple sclerosis. *Rheumatol Int.* 2007;28(1):15–20. doi:10.1007/s00296-007-0384-8.

40. Carmosino MJ, Brousseau KM, Arciniegas DB, et al. Initial evaluations for multiple sclerosis in a University Multiple Sclerosis Center: outcomes and role of magnetic resonance imaging in referral. *Arch Neurol.* 2005;62(4):585–590. doi:10.1001/archneur.62.4.585.

41. Poser CM. Misdiagnosis of multiple sclerosis and β-interferon. *The Lancet.* 1997;349(9069):1916. doi:10.1016/S0140-6736(05)63920-7.

42. Solomon AJ, Bourdette DN, Cross AH, et al. The contemporary spectrum of multiple sclerosis misdiagnosis: a multicenter study. *Neurology.* 2016;87(13):1393–1399. doi:10.1212/WNL.0000000000003152.

43. Solomon AJ, Weinshenker BG. Misdiagnosis of multiple sclerosis: frequency, causes, effects, and prevention. *Curr Neurol Neurosci Rep.* 2013;13(12):403. doi:10.1007/s11910-013-0403-y.

44. Nielsen JM, Korteweg T, Barkhof F, et al. Overdiagnosis of multiple sclerosis and magnetic resonance imaging criteria. *Ann Neurol.* 2005;58(5):781–783. doi:10.1002/ana.20632.

45. Srivastava R, Aslam M, Kalluri SR, et al. Potassium channel KIR4.1 as an immune target in multiple sclerosis. *N Engl J Med.* 2012;367(2):115–123. doi:10.1056/NEJMoa1110740.

46. Petzold A. The prognostic value of CSF neurofilaments in multiple sclerosis at 15-year follow-up. *J Neurol Neurosurg Psychiatry.* 2015;86(12):1388–1390. doi:10.1136/jnnp-2014-309827.

47. Sellebjerg F, Börnsen L, Khademi M, et al. Increased cerebrospinal fluid concentrations of the chemokine CXCL13 in active MS. *Neurology.* 2009;73(23):2003–2010. doi:10.1212/WNL.0b013e3181c5b457.

48. George IC, Sati P, Absinta M, et al. Clinical 3-tesla FLAIR* MRI improves diagnostic accuracy in multiple sclerosis. *Mult Scler.* 2016;22(12):1578–1586. doi:10.1177/1352458515624975.

49. Filippi M, Rocca MA, Ciccarelli O, et al. MRI criteria for the diagnosis of multiple sclerosis: MAGNIMS consensus guidelines. *Lancet Neurol.* 2016;15(3):292–303. doi:10.1016/S1474-4422(15)00393-2.

50. Gaitán MI, Sati P, Inati SJ, et al. Initial investigation of the blood-brain barrier in MS lesions at 7 tesla. *Mult Scler.* 2013;19(8):1068–1073. doi:10.1177/1352458512471093.

51. Reinke S, Broadhurst D, Sykes B, et al. Metabolomic profiling in multiple sclerosis: insights into biomarkers and pathogenesis. *Mult Scler.* 2014;20(10):1396–1400. doi:10.1177/1352458513516528.

52. De Jager PL, Jia X, Wang J, et al. Meta-analysis of genome scans and replication identify CD6, IRF8 and TNFRSF1A as new multiple sclerosis susceptibility loci. *Nat Genet.* 2009;41(7):776–782. doi:10.1038/ng.401.

53. Toledano M, Weinshenker BG, Solomon AJ. A clinical approach to the differential diagnosis of multiple sclerosis. *Curr Neurol Neurosci Rep.* 2015;15(8):57. doi:10.1007/s11910-015-0576-7.

8

Magnetic Resonance Imaging in Multiple Sclerosis

Christopher J. Karakasis, Aliye O. Bricker, and Stephen E. Jones

---

KEY POINTS FOR CLINICIANS

- MRI remains a mainstay for diagnosis and disease monitoring for multiple sclerosis (MS), with the goal of therapy to achieve no evidence of disease activity (NEDA).

- Current trends are to standardize MS imaging protocols, reporting, and acquisition and analysis of quantitative data, in particular incorporating volumetric sequences, such as T1 and fluid-attenuated inversion recovery (FLAIR).

- 7 T MRI is useful for delineation and evaluation of perivenous lesions, while the analysis paradigm of these lesions continues to evolve. Magnetic resonance fingerprinting (MRF) is a recently invented technique that may further advance MS imaging in the near future.

- Progressive multifocal leukencephalopathy (PML) may be monitored in the setting of monoclonal antibody therapies for MS.

Like many diseases, MS was well known long before the introduction of MRI in the early 1980s. Although MS is fundamentally a clinical diagnosis supported by detailed history, careful neurological examination, and often additional bloodwork and sometimes cerebrospinal fluid (CSF) assessment, MRI has had a growing impact on accurate and early diagnosis. It is also now an integral part of monitoring disease activity (1,2). MRI of the central nervous system (CNS) can support, supplement, or even replace some clinical criteria necessary for the diagnosis (3–6). MRI can clearly demonstrate multiple aspects of known MS pathology, such as dissemination in time (DIT) and dissemination in space (DIS). The former is shown by changes in serial MRI imaging, or the simultaneous appearance of lesions with different ages (e.g., some enhancing with gadolinium and some not enhancing). The latter is shown by multiple and widespread lesions. For example, estimates show more than 95% of patients with clinically definite MS having multifocal cerebral white matter lesions on brain MRI (1). MS is known to have an early inflammatory phase, which is shown by enhancement after intravenous administration of gadolinium contrast, resulting from breakdown of the blood–brain barrier. Subsequent to the acute phase, localized loss of oligodendrocytes and axonal fibers manifests on MRI as chronic white matter lesions, which slowly accumulate over time. In addition, the disease enters a degenerative phase, causing volume loss of both white and gray matter.

Although MS is classically considered as a demyelinating disease involving white matter of the brain and spinal cord, gray matter involvement is also prevalent but more difficult to image. Newer imaging techniques including postprocessing and high field strength imaging may help in demonstrating this involvement. In addition, the growing development of volumetric brain measurement techniques may reveal the subtle progressive volume loss associated with the degenerative phase, which is not readily detected on routine visual inspection.

RELEVANT MRI PHYSICS

The strong magnetic field created by an MRI scanner causes hydrogen nuclei throughout the body's water molecules to align. By perturbing the magnetic field using the application of magnetic field gradients and radiofrequency electromagnetic radiation, whose orchestration is termed a "sequence," the alignments of these hydrogen nuclei can be altered in subtle ways to produce a detectable signal. Sophisticated analysis algorithms can use these signals to reconstruct images, where the grayscale contrast takes on different meanings depending on the details of the sequence. Furthermore, different tissue types such as fat, fluid, muscle, and the gray and white matter in the brain, all have different hydrogen nuclei concentrations and relaxation properties. These influence the depicted MRI image, for example, ranging from dark to bright signal intensity. MRI is sensitive to the details of water concentration and is an exquisitely sensitive modality for detecting focal abnormalities, particularly in the white matter.

Different MRI sequences have been developed to best emphasize certain tissue characteristics. For example, T1-weighted sequences cause water to be dark, or have low signal intensity, while fat demonstrates bright signal. Conversely, T2-weighted sequences cause water and tissues with high water concentration to show bright signal intensity. The fluid-attenuated inversion recovery (FLAIR) sequence is a variant of a T2-weighted sequence in which free water, such as CSF, is suppressed and becomes dark. The FLAIR technique is valuable as it improves the visibility of T2 bright lesions located near bright CSF structures, such as sulci and ventricles. Proton density (PD) sequences display a grayscale that is directly proportional to the concentration of hydrogen nuclei (the higher the number of protons in a given unit of tissue, the brighter the signal). This allows for excellent contrast between the central deep gray nuclei of the brain and brain stem (which have fewer protons and therefore darker signal) and inflammatory lesions containing higher proton content and therefore bright signal. PD sequence images are also particularly valuable in evaluating the cerebellum.

CHARACTERIZATION OF MS ON CONVENTIONAL MRI

The standard MRI protocol for detection of MS lesions and disease activity includes axial T2-weighted images (sometimes including PD images obtained using a dual echo sequence), as well as both axial and sagittal FLAIR images to better identify callosal and pericallosal lesions. Precontrast T1-weighted images (usually axial) identify T1 dark signal intensity lesions or "black holes." Postcontrast T1-weighted images identify areas of enhancement thought to correspond to areas of active demyelination. MRI protocol has continued to evolve, with the most recent recommendations for a standardized MRI protocol of the brain described in Table 8.1 (7). Note that newer three-dimensional (3D) FLAIR sequences obtained in sagittal plane have near-isotropic voxels that can be reformatted into any plane, including axial. In addition, the utilization of 3D sequences permits quantitative analysis of lesions, with the prospect of automated processing. However, newer sequences may not be available on all scanners. There are differences across different vendors, relative to field strength (i.e., 1.5 vs 3 T), and with specific sequence parameters. For these reasons, it is best, if possible, to consistently perform follow-up imaging with the same MRI machine and imaging protocol if possible to allow the most accurate comparison.

Central to the diagnosis and management of patients with MS is the concept of lesions disseminated in both space and time. When the first disease-modifying treatments for MS were introduced in the 1990's, the primary goals of treatment were the reduction of relapse rate and the attenuation of disease progression. Today however, with the availability of new

TABLE 8.1 Revised Standardized MS Protocol Brain MRI Sequences

SEQUENCE	PLANE	FEATURES
FLAIR	3D Sagittal	Axial reconstruction: Supratentorial lesions Sagittal reconstruction: Callosal/pericallosal lesions
T2	Axial or 3D	Helpful for infratentorial lesions
DWI	Axial	To assess for PML
T1 precontrast	Axial or 3D	Black holes; necessary to compare with postcontrast
T1 postcontrast	Axial or 3D	Active lesions
PD (optional)	Axial	Helpful for infratentorial lesions or subtle lesions
SWI (optional)	Axial	To identify central vein associated with T2 lesions

3D, three-dimensional; DWI, diffusion weighted image; FLAIR, fluid-attenuated inversion recovery; PD, proton density; PML, progressive multifocal leukencephalopathy; SWI, susceptibility weighted imaging.

effective MS therapies, the goal of treatment moves toward "no evidence of disease activity" (NEDA) (8). This concept encompasses clinical parameters such as absence of relapse or progression on expanded disability status scale (EDSS), psychological and cognitive factors, with the pertinent imaging data being new T2/FLAIR lesions or postcontrast enhancing lesions. Imaging also allows for the detection of clnically silent lesions.

MS lesions can be located anywhere throughout the brain and spinal cord. Since MRI lesions can be nonspecific, or rather that many non-MS forms of neuropathology also produce similar lesions, it is important to classify lesions in terms of their signal characteristics, location, and morphology. Imaging criteria for MS diagnosis using recent

TABLE 8.2 2010 International MRI Criteria for Demonstration of DIS

DIS can be demonstrated by one or more T2 lesions in at least two of four areas of the CNS:

Periventricular
Juxtacortical
Infratentorial
Spinal cord

Gadolinium enhancement of lesions is not required for DIS

If a patient has a brain stem or spinal cord syndrome, the symptomatic lesions are excluded from the criteria and do not contribute to the lesion count.

CNS, central nervous system; DIS, dissemination in space.
Source: Polman CH, Reingold SC, Banwell B, et al. Diagnostic criteria for multiple sclerosis: 2010 revisions to the McDonald Criteria. *Ann Neurol.* 2011;69:292–302.

guidelines are seen in Table 8.2. Note that older criteria requiring lesion counting are no longer used, and the criteria for DIT and DIS have both been simplified.

MRI Signal Characteristics and Morphology

Lesions within the brain are generally small, 5 to 10 mm, with a rounded or ovoid shape. Signal characteristics of the lesions can be divided into early or acute, and late or chronic (see Figure 8.2).

Acute lesions have borders that are somewhat fluffy and ill defined on T2 and FLAIR sequences (Figure 8.3), while chronic lesions have sharply defined borders (Figure 8.4). For both acute and chronic lesions, the signal intensity is bright on T2, FLAIR, and PD sequences. Regarding T1 sequences, acute lesions may be the same or darker than the adjacent normal white matter. Occasionally, hyperacute lesions may even show a thin rim of bright signal on T1 images. Chronic lesions on T1 sequences show well-defined dark regions (so-called "black holes") with associated volume loss (Figure 8.5), likely representing long-standing disease with axonal destruction, and show some correlation with overall disease progression or disability (9,10).

In the acute setting, an actively demyelinating lesion typically enhances following intravenous contrast administration, reflecting inflammation-related localized breakdown of the blood–brain barrier. Enhancement patterns are often initially solid, subsequently enlarging radially and developing a classic, "incomplete ring" pattern (Figure 8.6), before dissipating after 2 to 6 weeks. The natural time course of enhancement of an acute MS lesion can be rapidly altered with treatment by steroids or immunosuppressants, specifically with the rapid resolution of enhancement, often within days (9). These acute, actively demyelinating lesions are often bright on diffusion weighted images (DWIs), likely reflecting high cellularity due to infiltrative inflammatory cells. Typically, MS lesions show minimal mass effect on the adjacent brain, or at least the degree of mass effect is disproportionately low compared to the size of the lesions, as might be expected for a glioma, for example. Note that large "mass-like" lesions can also occur, although infrequently, with an imaging appearance termed *tumefactive MS* (Figure 8.7).

Location

The classical pattern of MS disease shows multiple lesions that are bilaterally scattered along periventricular margins, mostly elongated and oriented perpendicular to the ventricles (Figure 8.8). Lesions are commonly located within the corpus callosum or at the "callososeptal junction" along the midline at the septum pelucidum. The elongated periventricular lesions correspond to the classic description of "Dawson's fingers" representing collections of inflammatory cells clustered around perpendicularly oriented small veins or venules (11). When viewed in the sagittal plain, the characteristic appearance of rounded and ovoid white

matter lesions scattered along the ependymal margin or "under-surface" of the corpus callosum and extending into the pericallosal white matter and calloseptal junction has been coined as the "dot-dash" sign, shown to have 90% to 95% sensitivity and specificity for the diagnosis of MS (12,13) (see Figures 8.1 and 8.8). Other common lesion locations in the brain include the juxtacortical white matter, anterior temporal lobes, brachium pontis, and cerebellum (Figure 8.8).

Although the typical MS patient will have relatively fewer lesions in the spinal cord compared to the brain, likely reflecting the relatively large volume of the brain compared to the cord volume, spinal cord lesions are usually more symptomatic. In fact, as many brain lesions can be clinically silent, cord lesions often cause the initial symptoms that persuade a patient to seek medical care. Thus, any cervical MRI demonstrating a spinal cord lesion with features suspicious for MS should prompt follow-up imaging of the brain. As in the brain, these lesions are bright on T2 or PD images, often located in the periphery of the cord, are generally less than two vertebral body segments in length, and encompass less than one-half of the cross-sectional area of the cord (Figure 8.8I). Also similar to the brain, acute or actively demyelinating lesions typically show enhancement following contrast administration. In addition, acute cord lesions can be mildly to moderately expansile, enlarging the overall diameter of the spinal cord at that level. In distinction, chronic cord lesions are associated with focal volume loss, or myelomalacia. This may impart a scalloped shape to the surface of the cord visible on sagittal images. In addition, cord lesions not uncommonly disappear entirely on imaging after months or years.

DISSEMINATION IN SPACE

Dissemination of lesions in space can be demonstrated on MRI by identifying one or more T2 bright lesions in at least two of four locations considered characteristic for MS: periventricular white matter, juxtacortical white matter, posterior fossa, or in the spinal cord (5) (see Figure 8.8).

DISSEMINATION IN TIME

DIT can be demonstrated in its simplest form by identifying new lesions on consecutive follow-up MRI (see Figure 8.9). Fulfillment of DIT on a single MRI examination is the simultaneous presence of lesions of different ages. Specifically, the criterion requires the presence of an asymptomatic gadolinium-enhancing (or lesions with an acute pattern of imaging characteristics) *and* nonenhancing lesions (or lesions with chronic imaging pattern) simultaneously on a single MRI study in a patient with typical clinical presentation, provided there is no non-MS pathology (5,14,15).

With progression of disease, there is an accumulation and coalescence of chronic lesions, many containing frank axonal destruction. Long-standing MS patients typically demonstrate a pattern of brain parenchymal volume loss that bears the stigmata of recurrent inflammatory

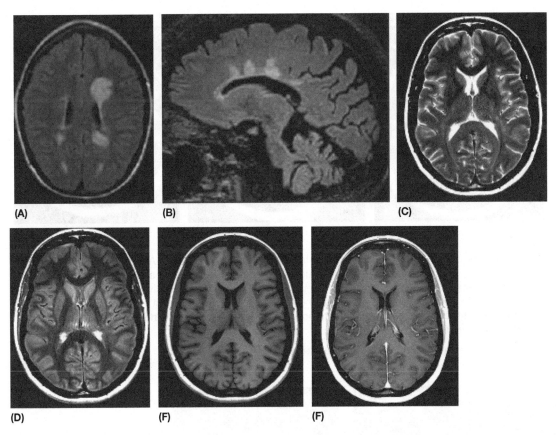

FIGURE 8.1   Example of typical MS protocol. Axial FLAIR (A) and sagittal FLAIR (B) images both demonstrate callosal and pericallosal lesions with a perpendicular orientation along the callososeptal margin more conspicuous on the sagittal plane image (B). Axial T2-weighted image (C) demonstrates additional periventricular and deep white matter lesions in both hemispheres—slightly less obvious than on the FLAIR. Bottom row: axial PD image (D) is useful to identify central deep white matter lesions. Axial precontrast T1-weighted (E) and axial postcontrast T1-weighted (F) images are used to identify areas of enhancement correlating to areas of active demyelination.

FLAIR, fluid-attenuated inversion recovery; MS, multiple sclerosis; PD, proton density.

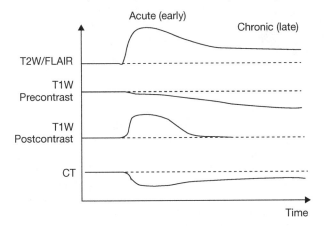

FIGURE 8.2   Time course of MRI change in MS lesion. Note early development of contrast enhancement and T2-weighted change and later development of T1 "black hole" changes.

MS, multiple sclerosis.

damage. For example, given the preferential distribution of MS lesions throughout the corpus callosum and callososeptal junction, chronic MS patients eventually develop striking callosal volume loss. Deep white matter lesions and periventricular lesions lead to marked enlargement of the ventricles (see Figures 8.5, 8.10, and 8.11). The degenerative phase of MS leads to cortical volume loss with apparent widening of the sulci.

Variations in Appearance and Potential Look-Alikes

Like many tissues, when subjected to pathological insult, the brain can only respond macroscopically in several ways. Since MRI typically images a tissue's macroscopic response rather than the pathology itself, many different pathologies or diseases can have a similar appearance. Specifically, MRI exquisitely measures water concentration within tissues, which can be altered in two ways: (a) vasogenic

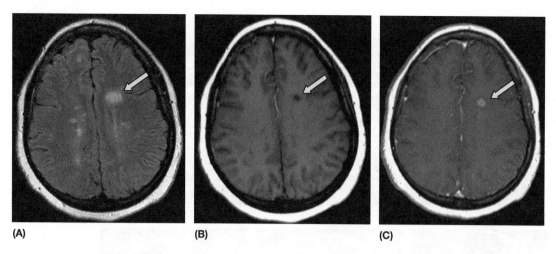

(A) (B) (C)

FIGURE 8.3   A 39-year-old woman with moderate disease burden MS. Axial FLAIR image (A) shows numerous patchy foci of FLAIR bright signal throughout the deep periventricular and pericallosal white matter of both hemispheres. The largest lesion in the left frontal lobe shows relatively fluffy, ill-defined margins on the FLAIR image (arrow, A), corresponding dark signal on precontrast T1 image (arrow, B), and avid enhancement following contrast administration (arrow, C) consistent with a new or acute lesion with active demyelination.

FLAIR, fluid-attenuated inversion recovery; MS, multiple sclerosis.

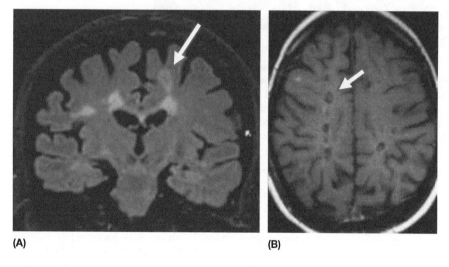

(A) (B)

FIGURE 8.4   Coronal FLAIR (A) and axial T1 (B) images in this patient with known, long-standing MS show bilateral deep white matter lesions with sharp, well-defined margins and corresponding profoundly dark T1 signal consistent with late or chronic lesions. These T1 dark foci are commonly referred to as "black holes."

FLAIR, fluid-attenuated inversion recovery; MS, multiple sclerosis.

edema which allows excess water to enter the brain parenchyma from leaky vessels, or (b) the destruction or alteration of myelin (which is hydrophobic) which allows excess water to enter the now more-hydrophilic lesion. Thus, although extremely sensitive in the detection of white matter pathology, unfortunately many MRI abnormalities common in MS are nonspecific and can be seen in a variety of other disease processes, which are difficult to distinguish by imaging alone (see Figure 8.7). An additional difficulty is that the number, size, and overall burden of brain and spinal cord disease can vary dramatically depending on the stage at which an MS patient is imaged and the severity of their disease.

NONSPECIFIC WHITE MATTER DISEASE

The most common differential diagnostic consideration for multiple nonenhancing foci of bright T2 or FLAIR signal in the supratentorial white matter without associated mass effect is nonspecific white matter disease (NSWMD), which are multiple small foci of white matter injury thought secondary to the sequelae of chronic, clinically silent, microvascular ischemia. These white matter changes are often associated with generalized, diffuse brain parenchymal volume loss frequently noted in patients over 50 years old (16), and can be accentuated in patients with chronic hypertension or diabetes. An example of nonspecific, likely chronic microvascular ischemic changes is included in Figure 8.7.

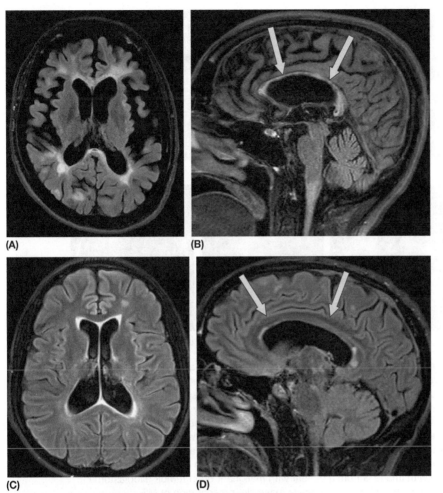

(A)   **(B)**   **(C)**   **(D)**

FIGURE 8.5   Upper row axial FLAIR (A) and sagittal FLAIR (B) images from a middle-aged woman with advanced MS demonstrate severe burden, patchy and near confluent bright signal abnormality throughout the periventricular and subcortical white matter with marked associated thinning of the corpus callosum (arrows, B) and marked generalized brain parenchymal volume loss greater than expected for age. Axial FLAIR (C) and sagittal FLAIR (D) images from a young, newly diagnosed patient with MS demonstrate relatively fewer white matter lesions with volume of the corpus callosum and overall brain parenchymal volume intact.

FLAIR, fluid-attenuated inversion recovery; MS, multiple sclerosis.

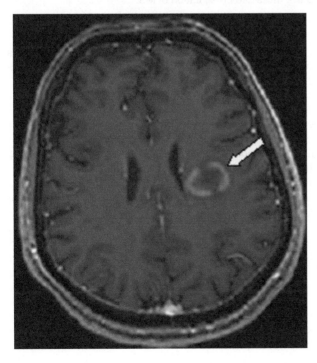

FIGURE 8.6   Lesion (arrow) within the deep white matter of the left cerebral hemisphere of this patient with known MS demonstrates incomplete ring of enhancement characteristic for acute demyelination. In patients not yet diagnosed with MS who present for the first time with neurological symptoms, identifying this "incomplete ring" pattern of enhancement on MRI of the brain can be an important clue to suggest underlying demyelinating disease.

MS, multiple sclerosis.

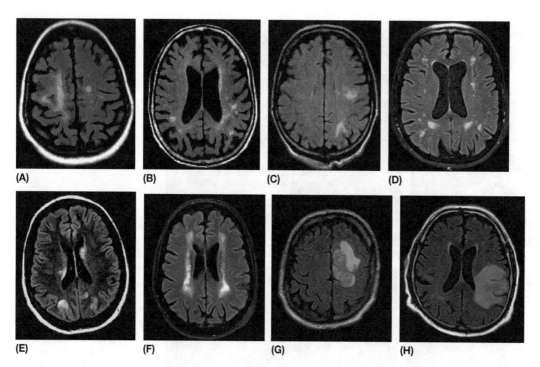

FIGURE 8.7 Examples of mimics and potential look-alikes based on imaging alone: Several axial FLAIR images from patients with entirely different diagnoses. Image A is a patient with lymphoma. Image B is an older patient with hypertension and nonspecific chronic microvascular white matter changes. Image C is a patient with progressive multifocal leukoencephalopathy from reactivation of the JC virus. Image D is a patient with giant cell arteritis demonstrating changes secondary to recurrent inflammation involving the cerebrovascular blood vessels. Image E is a patient with progressive reversible encephalopathy syndrome. Image F is a patient with Fahr's disease, an inherited neurological disorder of abnormal calcium deposition within the brain. Images G and H both demonstrate mass-like areas of signal abnormality with image G from a patient with malignant brain tumor (glioblastoma multiforme) and image H from a patient with the tumefactive mass-like presentation of MS.

FLAIR, fluid-attenuated inversion recovery; MS, multiple sclerosis.

Though the imaging appearance of early or mild MS and mild chronic microvascular ischemic change can be nearly identical, nonimaging factors such as age, gender, other disease, and clinical presentation may help distinguish them. Several imaging features may favor MS over NSWMD. The distribution of lesions can be a distinguishing factor. Lesions involving the corpus callosum and along the callososeptal junction are more common in MS while relatively rare in chronic microvascular disease. The degree of volume loss specifically involving the corpus callosum is also generally greater in MS than in a patient with chronic microvascular ischemic change, which is more often associated with generalized volume loss involving the entirety of the brain and manifested by prominence of the cortical sulci. NSWMD also infrequently affects the anterior temporal lobes and the cerebellum. Since the cortex and subcortical U-fibers are hyperperfused from an abundant capillary network, NSWMD is rarely seen in those locations. White matter lesions of long-standing MS more commonly demonstrate corresponding T1 hypointensity (17) whereas those of chronic microvascular ischemia

are often T1 isointense. Finally, although enhancement is common with acute MS, it is extremely atypical for lesions of chronic microvascular ischemia.

NEUROMYELITIS OPTICA

Neuromyelitis Optica (NMO; formally known as Devic's syndrome) is a relapsing, inflammatory, demyelinating disorder of the CNS with imaging features occasionally similar to those of conventional MS. Unlike MS, however, NMO characteristically preferentially involves the spinal cord and the optic nerves with relative sparing of the brain parenchyma. Moreover, to be able to suggest a diagnosis of NMO, the MRI appearance of the brain must be either normal or not meet diagnostic criteria for MS (18). Up to 60% of NMO patients have T2/FLAIR hyperintense white matter lesions, which are nonspecific and their presence does not exclude NMO as the diagnosis. A number of NMO spectrum disorders (NMOSD) have been described which typically include a longitudinally extensive transverse myelitis extending over three vertebral body segments, and optic neuritis.

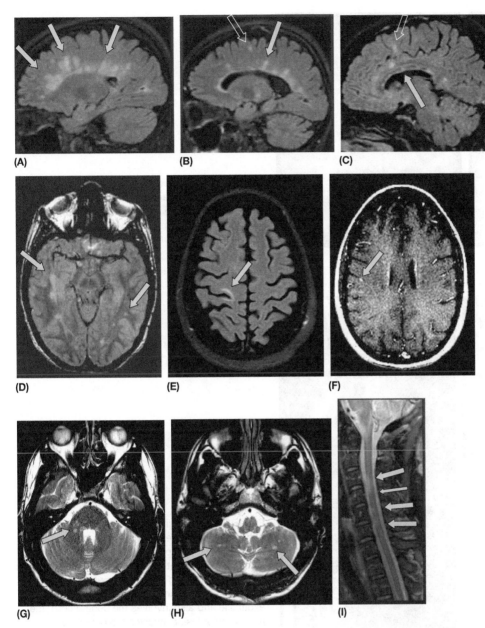

FIGURE 8.8 Examples of MS demyelinating lesions in characteristic locations pertinent to the McDonald Criteria as included in Table 8.2. Sagittal FLAIR images (A–C) demonstrate perpendicularly oriented periventricular lesions along the callososeptal margins and corpus callosum (arrow, C) in a "dot-dash" pattern classic for MS. Additional juxtacortical or subcortical white matter lesions are seen on sagittal FLAIR images (B, C, open arrows) and in the temporal lobes on axial FLAIR image (D). Axial FLAIR image (E) demonstrates juxtacortical lesion spanning the subcortical white matter and portions of the overlying cortex (arrow), with postcontrast T1-weighted axial image (F) demonstrating small enhancing cortical lesion (arrow) consistent with a tiny focus of active demyelination. Axial T2-weighted images (G, H) demonstrate infratentorial lesions within the right brachium pontis (arrow, G) and both cerebellar hemispheres (arrows, H), with several spinal cord lesions designated by the arrows on sagittal PD image (I).

FLAIR, fluid-attenuated inversion recovery; MS, multiple sclerosis.

Current consensus criteria allow diagnosis of NMOSD with involvement of one of six core clinical characteristics implicating specific regions (optic nerve, spinal cord, area postrema of dorsal medulla, brainstem, diencephalon, or cerebrum), along with detection of aquaporin-4 antibody (AQP4-IgG) and exclusion of alternative diagnoses (19).

The classic, imaging appearance of the spine in NMO consists of a prominent cord lesion, often enhancing and expansile, with T2 hyperintensity, at least three vertebral segments in length, and primarily involving the central part of the spinal cord (18) (Figure 8.10). Although as many as 25% of MS cases have been documented to involve only the spinal cord (9,20,21), most MS spinal cord lesions (or foci of T2 hyperintensity) tend to be substantially smaller than those of NMO, measuring less than two vertebral body segments in length, and tend to be located along the periphery of the cord (21) (Figure 8.8). In contrast, the cord lesions of NMO tend to be larger or longer in length, and involve the central cord (Figure 8.10). In the acute phase, the cord lesions of both NMO and MS can be associated with focal cord expansion and enhancement. In both diseases, chronic lesions are eventually associated with volume loss.

In both MS and NMO, optic neuritis is characterized by a swollen optic nerve or chiasm lesion associated with abnormal T2 signal and inflammatory changes of the adjacent retro-orbital fat planes (Figure 8.11a). A relationship between optic neuritis and MS has been well documented, with an overall risk of developing MS

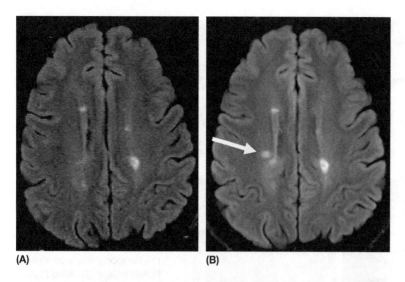

(A) (B)

FIGURE 8.9 Dissemination in Time. Careful side-by-side comparison of two axial FLAIR images acquired 15 months apart demonstrates interval appearance of a new lesion within the deep, right frontoparietal white matter (arrow, B).

FLAIR, fluid-attenuated inversion recovery.

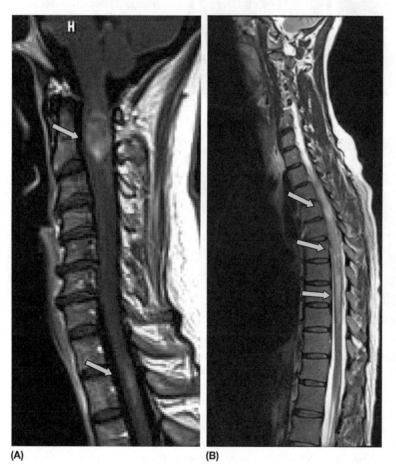

(A) (B)

FIGURE 8.10 Sagittal images from two different patients with demyelinating lesions of the spinal cord. T1-weighted postcontrast image (A) from a known MS patient demonstrates two short segment enhancing lesions (arrows). While the superior most enhancing lesion is somewhat expansile and also involves the central cord, the more inferior lesion involves the periphery of the cord and both are relatively short in length, less than two vertebral segments, and typical of MS. In contrast, sagittal T2-weighted image (B) from a patient with NMO demonstrates expansile abnormal T2 bright signal (arrows) throughout a much larger or longer portion of the central cervical and thoracic cord.

MS, multiple sclerosis; NMO, Neuromyelitis Optica.

approximated at 50% within 15 years following initial presentation with optic neuritis (22). Among patients with a normal brain MRI during documented optic neuritis, the risk of developing MS is nearly three times higher for females, and more than twice as likely to develop when the retrobulbar portion of the optic nerve was involved as opposed to the anterior optic nerve (22). Careful attention to the cisternal optic nerves and chiasm is recommended as lesions in this location may frequently go undetected (Figure 8.11b).

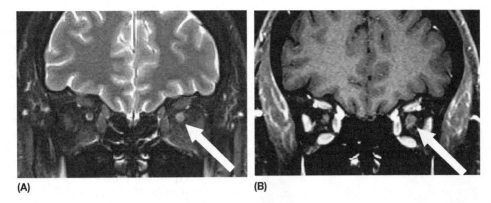

(A)   **(B)**

FIGURE 8.11A   Fat-saturated coronal T2-weighted images (A) and fat-saturated postcontrast coronal T1-weighted MR images from two different patients with optic neuritis. Both patients (A and B) demonstrate asymmetric enlargement and enhancement of the left optic nerve (arrows) consistent with optic neuritis. Patient B also demonstrates somewhat fuzzy, ill-defined T2 bright signal surrounding the left optic nerve consistent with inflammatory fat stranding.

MR, magnetic resonance.

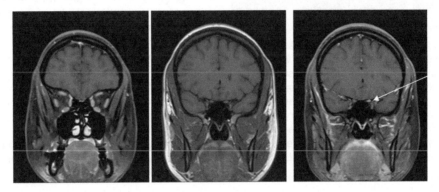

FIGURE 8.11B   A 36-year-old female patient with NMO. Fat-saturated postcontrast coronal T1-weighted MR image (left) demonstrates unremarkable intra-orbital optic nerves. Coronal precontrast T1 image (middle), and corresponding fat-saturated postcontrast T1 image (right) demonstrates enhancement of the cisternal left optic nerve (arrow).

MR, magnetic resonance; NMO, Neuromyelitis Optica.

TECHNICAL CONSIDERATIONS AND PITFALLS

FLAIR images provide excellent contrast between the normal white matter and the bright signal intensity of demyelinating plaques, and are thus fundamental to the evaluation of any patient with suspected MS. Although FLAIR images are very sensitive to white matter injury, they are unfortunately also very prone to artifact, or the presence of signal abnormality not secondary to the actual disease but something extraneous. The most common causes of MRI artifact are patient motion and "pulsation" artifact, or pulsations from an adjacent vascular structure causing the overlay of abnormal signal across the image (see Figure 8.12). For this reason, T2-weighted and PD imaging sequences are often more reliable in assessing for demyelinating plaques or lesions in the brain stem and cerebellum, or for confirming the presence of a lesion that may be suspected on FLAIR.

While the FLAIR imaging sequence is particularly vulnerable to many types of artifacts, all MRI sequences will be degraded by patient motion (Figure 8.13). Thus, for certain patients unable to stay still within the scanner because of claustrophobia, anxiety, or other clinical disability, anesthesia or sedation may be required to obtain an optimally diagnostic MRI exam. The presence of various types of hardware can also limit the diagnostic utility of MRI. For example, dental braces cause loss of signal throughout the anterior-most portions of the brain, and mascara on eyelashes may cause localized loss of signal along the anterior orbits. Problems inherent with the MRI scanner such as inhomogeneity of the magnetic field or magnetic coils can also cause signal abnormalities limiting lesion detection.

The ability to detect lesions depends not only on the pulse sequence and imaging parameters, but also on the field strength of the MRI machine (23,24). In one series studying 15 patients definitively diagnosed with MS, those imaged on a 4 T strength MRI machine had nearly one-third more lesions detected when compared with imaging performed on a 1.5 T strength MRI machine (23). In a similar study comparing known MS patients imaged on a 3 T strength MRI machine versus a 1.5 T strength MRI machine, overall lesion volume was higher by 12% when imaged on

the higher field strength MRI machine (24). Although 3 T strength MRI machines are now more common in the everyday clinical practice setting, the use of ultra-high magnetic field strength MRI at field strengths of 7 T has been historically limited to research (25) but hold promise for continued clinical application, and may see Food and Drug Administration (FDA) approval in the next few years.

A number of novel imaging approaches are currently under investigation. One of these which holds promise in terms of providing quantifiable MRI signal data that could be generalizable across institutions is that of magnetic resonance fingerprinting (MRF). This utilizes a pseudo randomized acquisition that causes signals from different tissue types to have a unique signal evolution, which can then be processed and compared with a pattern recognition algorithm to match the "fingerprints" to a predefined dictionary, and thus provide quantitative maps of the magnetic parameters (26,27). The goal of utilizing such imaging biomarkers is to overcome qualitative limitations and bridge to more quantifiable imaging, for example, increased specificity regarding pathological tissue substrates and better estimate damage outside of a focal lesion (28). This new imaging method has the potential to provide new dimensions of tissue contrast that are simply not combinations or variations of currently available T1W and T2W images. In addition to providing new contrast for focal lesions, MRF maps are quantifiable and can show correlations to disease within normal appearing white matter (28,29).

A close relationship between inflammatory MS plaques and cerebral microvasculature abnormalities has been shown histologically (30). With the advent and refinement of high-field MRI at 7 T and greater (31), the fine anatomy of the

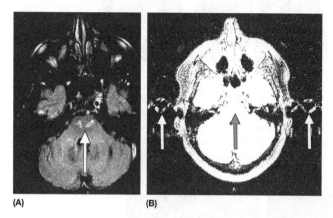

FIGURE 8.12 Axial FLAIR image (A) demonstrates two areas of bright signal within the brain stem of this patient with known MS (arrow). This same image with parameters adjusted to highlight subtle differences (B) reveals that these apparent bright spots are secondary to pulsation artifact extending throughout the image (arrows) rather than secondary to actual new lesions within the brain stem. Though FLAIR sequences are fundamental to any imaging protocol to evaluate for MS, FLAIR sequences are unfortunately prone to artifact.

FLAIR, fluid-attenuated inversion recovery; MS, multiple sclerosis.

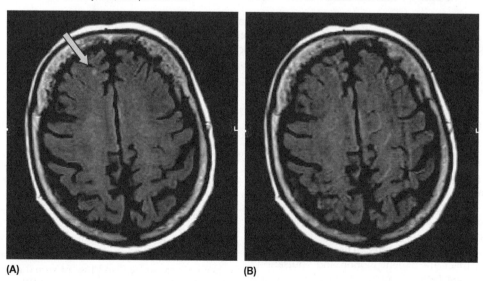

FIGURE 8.13 Axial FLAIR images at the same level from a patient being evaluated for MS demonstrate a FLAIR bright lesion in the subcortical white matter of the right frontal lobe (arrow) seen when the patient is holding still (A), but virtually undetectable when the patient is moving within the MRI scanner (B).

FLAIR, fluid-attenuated inversion recovery; MS, multiple sclerosis.

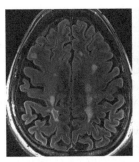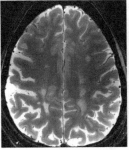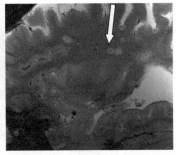

FIGURE 8.14 7 T imaging in a patient with MS. Axial FLAIR (left) image demonstrates white matter demyelinating plaques. Axial T2*-weighted GRE (middle) image at the same level, with a magnified corresponding sagittal T2*-weighted GRE (right) demonstrates the central medullary vein seen en-face as a black dot within the center of the plaque (arrow). 7 T offers exquisite fine vascular detail within the white matter while clearly depicting the white matter lesions.

FLAIR, fluid-attenuated inversion recovery; MS, multiple sclerosis.

periventricular veins is able to be imaged with exquisite detail (Figure 8.14). The presence of a central small vein on 7 T imaging could be a distinctive feature of MS, possibly differentiating from other conditions such as NMO or Susac syndrome (32). Studies have examined the association of MS lesions with veins, with the goal of determining the frequency with which MS lesions are peri-venous, and to examine whether identifying these lesions has predictive value. A prospective study utilizing 7 T T2* imaging examined patients with suspected MS demonstrated a high association with follow-up diagnosis and percentage perivenous lesions greater than 40% (33). However, implementation has some limitations as counting lesions is time consuming, and other diseases may have greater than 40% of the lesions associated with central veins (34). Other classification paradigms have been proposed, for example only assessing 10 white matter lesions provides greater than 90% accuracy (35). Another recent paradigm proposes three simple criteria: Inflammatory demyelination could be diagnosed if there are six or more morphologically characteristic lesions. If there are less than six, but the morphologically characteristic lesions outnumber nonperivenous lesions, inflammatory demyelination could be diagnosed. If neither of these criteria are met, inflammatory demyelination should not be diagnosed (36).

CLINICAL APPLICATIONS IN DISEASE MONITORING

MRI has become instrumental in monitoring patients already diagnosed with definitive MS, and allows for the objective assessment of disease severity, disease activity, and disease progression—specifically important in assessing responsiveness to therapy. Since its introduction into mainstream medicine in the 1980s, MRI has been estimated by some authors to detect MS disease activity 5 to 10 times more frequently than the clinical evaluation alone would suggest (37)—implying that many lesions found on MRI may be clinically silent. For this reason, MRI findings are often correlated with additional patient report measures when making clinical decisions regarding any potential changes in therapy.

Although no standardized guidelines exist, generally an MRI of the brain (with potential additional imaging of the cervical and thoracic spine) is performed at least once during course of disease to obtain further diagnostic confirmation. Follow-up imaging is often obtained if new diagnostic questions should arise or new neurological symptoms develop potentially suggesting comorbid conditions other than MS. Furthermore, most clinical practices will obtain imaging prior to starting new treatment, and then 6 months and 1 year into the treatment to assess response. In general, for those patients who develop three or more active lesions on subsequent MRI scans and demonstrate clinically active disease manifested by relapses and progression of disability, a change in treatment strategy is usually recommended. Note that a new "rebaselining" MRI may be needed once a new treatment is fully effective to exclude the possibility that new lesions actually occurred before full efficacy of the chosen agent.

With the advent of new effective MS therapies, the risk for progressive multifocal leukoencephalopathy (PML) has increased in patients with JC virus antibodies (Figure 8.15). Surveillance MRI can detect PML in the presymptomatic phase, which improves survival and outcomes (38). FLAIR and T2 weighted imaging demonstrates a characteristic involvement of subcortical fibers with a sharp border toward the cortex and ill-defined border toward the white matter. Diffusion imaging is useful to depict the acute demyelination in PML lesions (39). Infrequently (<50%), PML lesions may demonstrate enhancement with gadolinium, which is often ill-defined (40). However, if the therapy is stopped, postcontrast imaging is useful to depict superimposed immune reconstitution syndrome.

The growing development and implementation of "big data" are now involving MS, and will continue to do so. A goal is to make every MS patient effectively a datapoint, rather than those enrolled in research programs, whose disease is carefully measured in all its aspects,

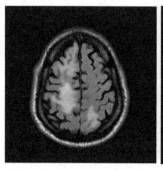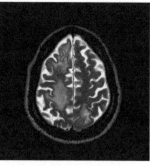

FIGURE 8.15 Axial FLAIR (left) and T2 (right) images at the same level from a patient with MS on natalizumab demonstrates development of patchy white matter signal abnormalities, with involvement of the subcortical U-fibers. The findings are consistent with PML.

FLAIR, fluid-attenuated inversion recovery; MS, multiple sclerosis; PML, progressive multifocal leukencephalopathy.

thereby permitting data-based decision making when compared to real life populations. This goal necessitates standardization of data metrics for clinical and research purposes, and one example of a recent clinical implantation is MS-PATHS (Multiple Sclerosis Partners Advancing Technology and Health Solutions) (41). This encompasses standardized MS history and performance testing at all clinical visits, across multiple institutions (currently numbering 10) and standardized imaging utilizing identical MRI scanning parameters. Central to the MRI protocols are common 3D T1 and FLAIR sequences, which will permit accurate quantitative assessment for volumes of both lesions and brain parenchyma, in particular any interval change. In addition, in cooperation with MS neurologists, the radiology reports for MS studies has now been standardized across insitutitons to highlight MS measures most relevant to MS disease assessment and treatment algorithms.

MRI SAFETY

MRI examination with 1.5 to 3 T strength MRI scanners has now become the standard of care across much of the United States. While MRI is safe for the majority of the population, each patient must be screened prior to undergoing an MRI exam or coming too close to the MRI scanner, and general access to the public is restricted in areas having magnetic fields above 0.5 mT (42).

One of the greatest potential hazards around an MRI machine is the missile effect from ferromagnetic objects such as oxygen cylinders, scissors, pens, or other common metallic objects. When in proximity to the magnetic field created by the MRI scanner, these objects will rapidly accelerate toward the bore of the MRI scanner, potentially damaging those objects or injuring people in their path. For this reason, all patients and healthcare workers are scanned with metal detectors prior to entering the MRI suite, and are required to remove any and all ferromagnetic metallic objects beforehand. Likewise, all metallic objects in and

around the MRI scanner must be constructed from specialized MRI-safe materials. Those patients with bullet fragments, shrapnel, or other forms of metal embedded into their bodies may require additional imaging and clinical evaluation to ascertain whether or not it would be safe for them to undergo an MRI examination.

Patients with implantable devices must also be screened prior to undergoing MRI examination. Certain implantable devices, such as pacemakers, may be deactivated by a magnetic field, and those patients with certain cardiac conditions requiring constant cardiac pacing may require specialized examination in a closely monitored setting with their electrophysiologist or cardiology staff nearby. Certain metallic devices may absorb energy and increase in temperature when exposed to radiofrequency pulses within the magnetic field. Moreover, because of the torque produced by the magnetic field, ferromagnetic devices such as certain aneurysm clips, implanted electrodes, cochlear implants, or internal drug infusion pumps may also move or migrate during the MRI exam, potentially posing significant hazard. It is thus important for all patients to make their MRI technician aware of the make and model of any and all implanted medical devices they may have prior to entering the MRI scanner.

Though the U.S. Food and Drug Administration has not established guidelines with respect to the safety of MRI in pregnant women, according to the Policies, Guidelines, and Recommendations for MR Imaging Safety and Patient Management issued by the Safety Committee of the Society for Magnetic Resonance Imaging in 1991, "MR imaging may be used in pregnant women if other non-ionizing forms of diagnostic imaging are inadequate or if the examination provides important information that would otherwise require exposure to ionizing radiation such as fluoroscopy or computed tomography (CT)." When possible, MRI is commonly delayed until the second or third trimester owing to the theoretical concern over tissue heating caused by the radiofrequency pulses. Intravenous contrast agents are generally not recommended, as they are known to cross the placenta and their long-term effects are not yet well known.

Orders for noncontrast MRI brain and/or cervical spine imaging are increasing in prevalence for MS patients in whom no active disease is suspected. However in the setting of suspected active inflammation, or in patients unable to provide detailed history, gadolinium contrast-enhanced imaging may be indicated. The risk of nephrogenic systemic fibrosis can be significantly mitigated by avoiding contrast in patients with severe renal dysfunction, and by utilizing macrocyclic contrast agents. Evidence has shown some gadolinium retention in the brain (43,44) and other body tissues with all gadolinium-based contrast agents, although this is higher with linear agents as a result of molecular dissociation. However, no current evidence exists to indicate that this gadolinium retention results in patient harm, and the current FDA recommendation is currently to not restrict gadolinium use on this basis.

KEY POINTS FOR PATIENTS AND FAMILIES

- Data have emerged that small amounts of gadolinium are retained in the body including the brain, although no known clinical impact exists.

- Postcontrast imaging holds more utility in the assessment of a specific clinical question, with a trend toward noncontrast imaging for disease monitoring.

REFERENCES

1. Inglese M. Multiple sclerosis: new insights and trends. *AJNR Am J Neuroradiol.* 2006;27:954–957.
2. Rocca MA, Anzalone N, Falini A, et al. Contribution of magnetic resonance imaging to the diagnosis and monitoring of multiple sclerosis. *Radiol Med.* 2013;118:251–264. Epub ahead of print.
3. McDonald WI, Compston A, Edan G, et al. Recommended diagnostic criteria for multiple sclerosis: guidelines from the International Panel on the diagnosis of multiple sclerosis. *Ann Neurol.* 2001;50:121–127.
4. Polman CH, Reingold SC, Edan G, et al. Diagnositc criteria for multiple sclerosis: 2005 revisions to the "McDonald Criteria." *Ann Neurol.* 2005;58:840–846.
5. Polman CH, Reingold SC, Banwell B, et al. Diagnostic criteria for multiple sclerosis: 2010 revisions to the McDonald Criteria. *Ann Neurol.* 2011;69:292–302.
6. Barkhof F, Filippi M, Miller DH, et al. Comparison of MR imaging criteria at first presentation to predict conversion to clinically definite MS. *Brain.* 1997;120:2059–2069.
7. Traboulsee A, Simon JH, Stone L, et al. Revised recommendations of the consortium of MS centers task force for a standardized MRI protocol and clinical guidelines for the diagnosis and follow-up of multiple sclerosis. *AJNR Am J Neuroradiol.* 2016;3:394–401.
8. Strangel M, Penner IK, Kallman B, et al. Towards the implementation of 'no evidence of disease activity' in multiple sclerosis treatment: the multiple sclerosis decision model. *Ther Adv Neurol Discord.* 2015;1:3–13.
9. Ge Y. Multiple sclerosis: the role of MR imaging. *AJNR Am J Neuroradiol.* 2006;27:1165–1176.
10. Truyen L, van Waesberghe JH, van Walderveen MA, et al. Accumulation of hypointense lesions ("black holes") on T1 spin-echo MRI correlates with disease progression in multiple sclerosis. *Neurology.* 1996;47:1469–1476.
11. Adams CW, Abdulla YH, Torres EM, et al. Periventricular lesions in multiple sclerosis: their perivenous origin and relationship to granular ependymitis. *Neuropathol Appl Neurobiol.* 1987;13:141–152.
12. Lisanti CJ, Asbach P, Bradley WG. The ependymal "dot-dash" sign: an MR imaging finding of early multiple sclerosis. *AJNR Am J Neuroradiol.* 2005;26:2033–2036.
13. Gean-Marton AD, Vezina LG, Marton KI, et al. Abnormal corpus callosum: a sensitive and specific indicator of multiple sclerosis. *Radiology.* 1991;180:215–221.
14. Rovira A, Swanton J, Tintore M, et al. A single, early magnetic resonance imaging study in the diagnosis of multiple sclerosis. *Arch Neurol.* 2009;5:287–292.
15. Montalban X, Tintore M, Swanton J, et al. MRI criteria for MS in patients with clinically isolated syndromes. *Neurology.* 2010;74:427–434.
16. Fazekas F, Chawluk JB, Alavi A, et al. MR Signal abnormalities at 1.5T in Alzheimer's dementia and normal aging. *AJNR Am J Neuroradiol.* 1987;8:421–426.
17. Wallace CJ, Seland TP, Fong TC. Multiple sclerosis: the impact of MR imaging. *AJR Am J Roentgenol.* 1992;158:849–857.
18. Wingerchuk DM, Lennon VA, Pittock SJ, et al. Revised diagnostic criteria for Neuromyelitis optica. *Neurology.* 2006;66(10):1485–1489.
19. Wingerchuk DM, Banwell B, Bennett JL, et al. International consensus diagnostic criteria for Neuromyelitis Optica spectrum disorders. *Neurology.* 2016;2:177–189.
20. Ikuta F, Zimmerman HM. Distribution of plaques in seventy autopsy cases of multiple sclerosis in the United States. *Neurology.* 1976;26:26–28.
21. Tartaglino LM, Friedman DP, Flanders AE, et al. Multiple sclerosis in the spinal cord: MR appearance and correlation with clinical parameters. *Radiology.* 1995;195:725–732.
22. Optic Neuritis Study Group. Multiple sclerosis risk after optic neuritis: final optic neuritis treatment trial follow-up. *Arch Neurol.* 2008;65(6):727–732.
23. Keiper MD, Grossman RI, Hirsch JA, et al. MR identification of white matter abnormalities in multiple-sclerosis: a comparison between 1.5T and 4T. *AJNR Am J Neuroradiol.* 1998;19:1489–1493.
24. Sicotte NL, Voskuhl RR, Bouvier S, et al. Comparison of multiple sclerosis lesions at 1.5 and 3.0 Tesla. *Invest Radiol.* 2003;38:423–427.
25. Kolia K, Maderwald S, Putzki N, et al. First clinical study on ultra-high-field MR imaging in patients with multiple sclerosis: comparison of 1.5T and 7T. *AJNR Am J Neuroradiol.* 2009;30:699–702.
26. European Society of Radiology. Magnetic Resonance Fingerprinting—a promising new approach to obtain standardized imaging biomarkers from MRI. *Insights Imaging.* 2015;6:163–165.
27. Ma D, Gulani V, Seiberlich, N, et al. Magnetic resonance fingerprinting. *Nature.* 2013;495:187–192.
28. Filippi M, Absinta M, Rocca MA. Future MRI tools in multiple sclerosis. *J Neurol Sci.* 2013;331:114–18.
29. Nakamura K, Deshmane A, Guruprakash D, et al. A novel method for quantification of normal appearing brain tissue in multiple sclerosis: magnetic resonance fingerprinting. Abstract P4.158. Presented at: 68th Annual Meeting of the American Academy of Neurology; April 19, 2016; Vancouver, Canada.
30. Adams CW, Poston RN, Buk SJ. Pathology, histochemistry and immunocytochemistry of lesions in acute multiple sclerosis. *J Neurol Sci.* 1989;92:291–306.
31. Christoforidis GA, Bourekas EC, Baujan M, et al. High resolution MRI of the deep brain vascular anatomy at 8 Tesla: susceptibility-based enhancement of the venous structures. *J Comput Assist Tomogr.* 1999;23:857–866.
32. Filippi M, Rocca MA, Ciccarelli O, et al. MRI criteria for the diagnosis of multiple sclerosis: MAGNIMS consensus guidelines. *Lancet Neurol.* 2016;3:292–303.
33. Mistry N, Dixon J, Tallantyre E, et al. Central veins in brain lesions visualized with high-field magnetic resonance imaging: a pathologically specific diagnostic biomarker for inflammatory demyelination in the brain. *JAMA Neurol.* 2013;70:623–810.
34. Sati P, Oh J, Constable RT, et al. The central vein sign and its clinical evaluation for the diagnosis of multiple sclerosis: a consensus statement from the North American Imaging in Multiple Sclerosis Cooperative. *Nat Rev Neurol.* 2016;12:714–722.
35. Tallantyre EC, Dixon, JE, Donaldson I, et al. Ultra-high-field imaging distinguishes MS lesions from asymptomatic white matter lesions. *Neurology.* 2011;6:534–539.
36. Mistry N, Abdel-Fahim R, Samaraweera A, et al. Imaging central veins in brain lesions with 3T T2*-weighted magnetic resonance imaging differentiates multiple sclerosis from microangiopathic brain lesions. *Mult Scler.* 2016;22:1289–1296.
37. Barkhof F, Scheltens P, Frequin ST, et al. Relapsing-remitting multiple sclerosis: sequential enhanced MR imaging vs clinical

findings in determining disease activity. *AJR Am J Roentgenol.* 1992;159:1041–1047.

38. Dong-Si T, Richman S, Wattjes MP, et al. Outcome and survival of asymptomatic PML in natalizumab-treated MS patients. *Ann Clin Tranl Neurol.* 2014;1:755–764.

39. Wattles, MP, Barkof F. Diagnosis of natalizumab-associated progressive multifocal leukencephalopathy using MRI. *Curr Opin Neurol.* 2014;27:260–270.

40. Youstry TA, Pelletier D, Cadavid D, et al. Magnetic resonance imaging pattern in natalizumab-associated progressive multifocal leukencephalopathy. *Ann Neurol.* 2012;72:779–787.

41. Bermel R, Mowry E, Krupp L, et al. Multiple sclerosis advancing technology and health solutions (MS PATHS): initial launch experience. *Neurology.* 2017;88(suppl 16):P1.372.

42. Bushberg JT, Seibert SA, Leidholdt EM, Jr., et al. *The Essential Physics of Medical Imaging.* Philadelphia, PA: Lippincott Williams & Wilkins; 2002.

43. Radbruch A, Weberling LD, Kieslich PJ, et al. Gadolinium retention in the dentate nucleus and globus pallidus is dependent on the class of contrast agent. *Radiology.* 2015;275:783–791.

44. Kanal E, Tweedle MF. Residual or retained gadolinium: practical implications for radiologists and our patients. *Radiology.* 2015;275:630–634.

9

Tools and Tests for Multiple Sclerosis

Robert A. Bermel

KEY POINTS FOR CLINICIANS

- Blood tests play an important role in excluding mimics of multiple sclerosis (MS).
- Spinal fluid analysis can help establish an inflammatory basis for abnormal imaging findings and help exclude mimics of MS in atypical situations, but is only occasionally required to make the diagnosis of MS.
- Evoked potentials can help to establish dissemination in space consistent with the diagnosis of MS, but are not specific for MS.
- Biomarker blood tests exist to help establish the diagnosis of neuromyelitis optica and assess individual risk for complications associated with natalizumab.
- Biomarkers are not yet available to predict an individual patient's response to a specific therapy.
- Optical coherence tomography is a newer technology that can track retinal neurodegeneration and monitor for macular edema in patients on fingolimod therapy for MS.

The diagnosis of MS is made clinically on the basis of a synthesis of the history, examination, imaging, and paraclinical testing where necessary (1). No single paraclinical test can confirm or exclude MS with certainty. The brain MRI has emerged as the foremost test suggesting the diagnosis of MS if abnormal with typical features, or excluding the diagnosis of MS if normal. Paraclinical testing can be used to support the diagnosis of MS by fulfilling the criteria for dissemination in space (usually, evoked potentials [EPs] or optical coherence tomography [OCT]) and verifying an inflammatory etiology for the neurological disorder (spinal fluid analysis). The ubiquitous availability of MRI and its utility in diagnosing MS makes it a test that is now commonly performed early in the course of neurological symptoms. When the brain MRI is definitively abnormal but not classic for MS, it raises the possibility of an alternative neurological diagnosis, and blood and spinal fluid tests can be used to exclude "mimics" of MS at the time of diagnosis. When the brain MRI is mildly abnormal and the clinician views the diagnosis of MS as unlikely, testing such as EPs and spinal fluid analysis can be utilized to show a lack of central nervous system (CNS) pathology, in order to more definitively exclude the diagnosis of MS.

BLOOD TESTS

The differential diagnosis of MS (discussed in detail in Chapter 10) is broad, and multiple alternative disease entities can cause similar symptoms and a similar imaging appearance to MS. When atypical clinical features make the exclusion of mimics essential, blood tests play a key role (2). Even when the diagnosis of MS is secure, blood tests are indicated in order to exclude the presence of comorbid conditions, which can occur at high frequency. Finally, there are also blood tests which can be used to help guide therapeutic decision making.

> *When atypical clinical features make the exclusion of mimics essential, blood tests play a key role.*

Testing to exclude mimics of MS is performed if prompted by red flags on the history or exam (see Chapter 10). The specific tests sent are guided by the specific clinical scenario. Some of the most commonly ordered tests are for rheumatological or autoimmune diseases, which can cause CNS demyelination (Table 9.1). Many of these possibilities can be reliably distinguished from MS on the basis of clinical features, imaging findings, or lab results. Other organ-specific autoimmune diseases, such as thyroid autoimmunity and pernicious anemia, occur with higher frequency in patients with MS, have some symptomatic overlap with MS, and therefore justify screening (Table 9.1). Antinuclear antibody (ANA) is commonly positive in MS at low or moderate titres and if present in isolation without clinical signs does not indicate systemic lupus erythematosus and typically needs no further evaluation. Prior to initiating disease-modifying therapy for MS, it is often prudent to send tests of liver and kidney function, given the effect of some MS treatments on these organs. With the growing emphasis on vitamin D supplementation in patients with MS, some clinicians choose to check vitamin D levels to guide the dosage of vitamin D (3). Immunity to varicella zoster virus is required (whether by exposure or vaccination) prior to utilizing some immunosuppressive therapies to treat MS, so this status is also often evaluated.

There are reports that antiglycan antibodies occur with increased frequency in MS, and serological tests for those have been proposed as a tool aiding in the diagnosis of MS at early stages or to help distinguish patients who are more likely to experience disability progression (4). Although these serological tests are commercially available, they have limited specificity and sensitivity and have not been independently replicated. At this point, they are not commonly utilized in clinical practice. MRI and in some cases spinal fluid results are used preferentially to inform diagnosis and prognosis in MS, and it is not clear that antiglycan antibody testing would significantly affect treatment decisions even in cases where the MRI and other testing are equivocal.

The neuromyelitis optica IgG antibody (NMO-IgG) is a blood test that has approximately a 76% sensitivity and 94% specificity for neuromyelitis optica (NMO), and is now a key asset in making the diagnosis of NMO (5). NMO-IgG is an autoantibody directed against the aquaporin-4 water channel on astrocyte foot processes, and is now recognized as the pathogenic autoantibody responsible for the manifestations of NMO (6). The discovery of this autoantibody has solidified NMO as a unique pathological entity distinct from MS and requiring a different treatment regimen. NMO-IgG should be tested if inflammatory demyelination is suspected as a mechanism and clinical or imaging features are suggestive of NMO or atypical for MS. Testing in the blood is sufficiently sensitive in most cases, but on rare occasions this test will be positive in the cerebrospinal fluid (CSF) when it is negative in the blood.

> The neuromyelitis optica IgG antibody is now a key asset in making the diagnosis of NMO.

Although there are not currently any predictive biomarker tests that help to guide choice of therapy on the basis of efficacy in individuals, there are some tests which can guide choice of MS therapy on the basis of risk of a therapeutic complication. A 2-step serological assay for antibodies to the JC virus (JCV) in the blood is currently utilized to help determine risk of progressive multifocal leukoencephalopathy (PML), a complication associated with some MS therapies, particularly natalizumab (7). The pathogenesis of PML is thought to require multiple steps, beginning with acquisition of the JCV and requiring time for the virus harbored in individuals regardless of immune status, to become neurotropic. Only then, in immunocompromised hosts, can the virus cause PML. The prevalence of anti-JCV antibodies is approximately 56% in the MS population (8), and the current recommendation is to check JCV antibody status every 6 months in patients who initially test negative and are being treated with natalizumab. Thus, testing for JCV antibody status allows lower-risk utilization of natalizumab for at least limited and sometimes long periods of time in patients who have not been previously exposed to the virus. Other tests for risk stratification include ECG for cardiac risks and retinal examination for ophthalmological risks related to fingolimod.

TABLE 9.1 Common Blood Tests Sent at the Time of MS Diagnosis

TESTS WHICH MAY HELP TO IDENTIFY MIMICS OF MS OR COMORBID CONDITIONS	TESTS WHICH MAY IMPACT OR HELP TO GUIDE MS TREATMENT
Erythrocyte sedimentation rate	Complete blood count
Antinuclear antibody[a]	Renal and liver function tests
Thyroid stimulating hormone level	JC virus antibody status
Vitamin B$_{12}$ level	Varicella antibody status
	Hepatitis remote exposure panel
	Tuberculosis screen (Quantiferon)
Copper level	Vitamin D level
Antineutrophil cytoplasmic antibodies	
Rheumatoid factor	
SSA/SSB (Sjogren's antibodies)	
Extractable nuclear antigen antibodies	
Antiphospholipid antibodies	
Aquaporin-4 antibody (neuromyelitis optica IgG)	
Lyme titers	

[a]ANA is commonly positive in MS at low or moderate titres and does not typically require further evaluation.
MS, multiple sclerosis.

> Testing for JCV antibody status allows lower-risk utilization of natalizumab in patients who have not been previously exposed to the virus.

Blood tests to either predict the response to therapy (predictive biomarkers) or prognosis in MS (prognostic biomarkers) would be helpful to guide therapeutic decision making, but are not currently available. In their absence, MRI remains the primary means for measuring MS disease burden, degree of disease activity, and assessing response to therapy.

> *Blood tests to either predict the response to therapy or prognosis in MS would be helpful to guide therapeutic decision making, but are not currently available.*

LUMBAR PUNCTURE/SPINAL FLUID ANALYSIS

If the clinical history, examination, and imaging are typical for MS, spinal fluid analysis is not a requirement in order to make the diagnosis of MS. Some situations in which spinal fluid analysis is useful in supporting a diagnosis of MS include the following:

> *If the clinical history, examination, and imaging are typical for MS, spinal fluid analysis is not a requirement in order to make the diagnosis of MS.*

1. Exclusion of other alternative etiologies (infectious, inflammatory, granulomatous disorders) if atypical features are present
2. Diagnosis of some cases of primary progressive MS (PPMS) (especially to distinguish PPMS from neurodegenerative disorders)
3. Diagnosis of MS in older individuals or those with vascular risk factors, where white matter lesions on MRI may have a vascular or other non-MS etiology
4. In patients with pacemakers or other reasons precluding MRI, if the diagnosis of MS is suspected
5. In situations where disease-modifying therapy is being considered (such as after a clinically isolated syndrome) but imaging and EPs alone provide insufficient evidence to support a diagnosis of MS

The brain MRI is the most predictive test for determining the risk of future attacks after a clinically isolated syndrome (9). However, CSF studies do add additional predictive value, with the presence of oligoclonal bands in the CSF conferring almost double the risk of a second attack, independent of brain MRI (10). If CSF analysis is being considered in this situation for risk estimation, it is generally only if the brain MRI is equivocal and the patient or physician would change their decision to start disease-modifying therapy on the basis of the result.

> *The brain MRI is the most predictive test for determining the risk of future attacks after a clinically isolated syndrome.*

In the most recent recommendations of the International Panel on Diagnosis of MS, pertinent to situation no. 5 noted previously, spinal fluid evidence of intrathecal antibody synthesis is again formally supported as a substitute for dissemination in time (DIT) criteria. Specifically, demonstration of CSF oligoclonal bands in the absence of atypical CSF findings allows a diagnosis of MS to be made, even if the MRI findings on the baseline scan do not meet the criteria for DIT and in advance of either a second attack or MRI evidence of a new or active lesion on subsequent imaging (11).

When CSF is sent for analysis, multiple tests on the fluid are generally requested, guided by the clinical scenario (Table 9.2). The core findings from CSF analysis that support a diagnosis of MS are qualitative or quantitative evidence of intrathecal antibody synthesis, in the form of oligoclonal bands or elevated IgG index. Oligoclonal bands are identified by electrophoresis of proteins present in CSF compared to the patient's own serum, and generally defined as present and unique to the CSF if there are two or more bands present in the CSF that are not present in the serum. It is a qualitative test that evaluates for unique immunoglobulins in the CSF that are not present in the serum (12). The IgG index (Figure 9.1) is a quantitative representation of the amount of intrathecal IgG present, controlling for both the amount of albumin present in the CSF and the ratio of IgG to CSF in the blood. The IgG index is compared to a fraction derived from a reference population, and is interpreted as high if it exceeds the level defined as abnormal on the basis of the reference used for

TABLE 9.2 CSF Tests Commonly Sent When Evaluating for MS

ALWAYS SHOULD BE ORDERED IF CONSIDERING MS	SOMETIMES MAY BE ORDERED ON THE BASIS OF CLINICAL SUSPICION AND LABORATORY RELIABILITY
Cell count and differential Total protein quantification Glucose quantification Oligoclonal bands evaluation (CSF and serum electrophoresis) IgG index and IgG synthesis rate	Cytology and/or flow cytometry (if clinical suspicion for lymphoma or other malignancy) Borrelia antibody titers (if clinical suspicion for lyme disease) VDRL (if clinical suspicion for syphilis) Culture and other infectious antigen tests Free kappa light chains

CSF, cerebrospinal fluid; MS, multiple sclerosis; VDRL, venereal disease research laboratory.

$$IgG\,index = \frac{(CSF\,IgG\,/\,CSF\,albumin)}{(Serum\,IgG\,/\,Serum\,albumin)}$$

FIGURE 9.1 CSF IgG index derivation.

CSF, cerebrospinal fluid.

the individual laboratory. The IgG synthesis rate is another quantitative marker of intrathecal antibody synthesis. It is the calculated amount (in milligram per 24 hours) of de novo IgG being produced in the CSF compartment based on measured serum and CSF values of albumin and IgG, plus constants derived from a normal reference population (13). Its value parallels that of the IgG index.

> *The core findings from CSF analysis that support a diagnosis of MS are qualitative (the presence of two or more oligoclonal bands) or quantitative (elevated IgG index) evidence of intrathecal antibody synthesis.*

Though evidence of oligoclonal bands or elevation of IgG index is supportive of the diagnosis, these findings are not specific for MS. Oligoclonal bands and elevated IgG index can be found in many neurological disorders. Other CSF tests commonly associated with MS are even less specific. If CSF protein is high, then the IgG synthesis rate may be falsely elevated. Detection of myelin basic protein in the CSF occurs in many neurological and nonneurological disorders and should not be used in isolation to support a diagnosis of MS.

> *Detection of myelin basic protein in the CSF occurs in many neurological and nonneurological disorders and should not be used in isolation to support a diagnosis of MS.*

The performance characteristics of CSF laboratory measures can vary substantially on the basis of the methodology used. Electrophoresis using isoelectric focusing is increasingly becoming the standard method used to evaluate for oligoclonal bands because of its sensitivity (12). Assays for free kappa light chains may augment the diagnostic specificity for MS in some situations, but currently have low utility because of the wide methodological variability. Knowing the analytical method used and normative values associated with the individual laboratory where CSF testing was performed can help in the proper interpretation of the test results.

> *Knowing the analytical method used and normative values associated with the individual laboratory where CSF testing was performed is helpful for proper interpretation of the test results.*

Neither oligoclonal bands nor IgG index can be utilized as a marker of response to disease-modifying therapy in MS. Even after immunoablation and hematopoetic stem cell transplantation in patients with MS, CSF findings of oligoclonal bands and elevated IgG index remain abnormal (14). Assays for the presence of neuron-specific markers in the CSF have been proposed as a measure of disease activity or neuroaxonal damage in MS, but none are currently utilized in widespread clinical practice. N-acetyl aspartate and CSF neurofilament heavy or light chains have all received recent attention as potential candidates (15), although the clinical utility remains uncertain and certainly feasibility of incorporating CSF testing into the routine monitoring of MS would present a challenge.

EVOKED POTENTIALS

EPs are an electrophysiological test where the delay is measured between the presentation of a sensory stimulus (whether visual, somatosensory, or auditory) and its low voltage evoked cortical potential. By averaging multiple stimulus presentations and responses, the timing of the cortical potential of interest can be measured with high accuracy, and compared to a known reference interval. A delay in the peak occurrence of the EP (i.e., an increased latency in the P100 peak) is evidence for dysfunction in the pathway of interest, with demyelination being a common cause. However, increased latency is nonspecific and can be caused by a number of different conditions.

Visual EPs and somatosensory EPs are the most commonly utilized EPs and are sensitive tests for demyelination in those respective pathways. Brain stem (auditory) EPs are less commonly utilized. EPs are most useful for demonstration of dissemination in space. For example, they may be useful in the situation of a patient with a single lesion if it demonstrates an asymptomatic conduction delay in a different part of the neuraxis consistent with a second lesion (16). In the setting of neurological symptoms of uncertain etiology, EPs can be useful to demonstrate the presence or absence of conduction delay, though a positive result is not specific for a primary demyelinating etiology. The sensitivity of visual EPs at the time of a clinically isolated syndrome for predicting the development of clinically definite MS has been estimated at between 25% and 85%, with specificity between 63% and 78% (17,18). The wide range of values is testament to the variability of yield based on the characteristics of patients put forth for EP testing, variability in methodology and quality control, and the definition of the outcome of interest.

In the setting of neurological symptoms of uncertain etiology, evoked potentials can be useful to demonstrate the presence or absence of conduction delay, though a positive result is not specific for a primary demyelinating etiology.

In general, EPs now play a limited role in making the diagnosis of MS, as they add very little sensitivity to current MRI of the brain and spinal cord which when combined with CSF studies as needed, typically provide sufficient diagnostic certainty.

OPTICAL COHERENCE TOMOGRAPHY

OCT is an office-based imaging method that uses near-infrared light to generate high-resolution cross-sectional images (in this case of the retina), analogous to B-mode ultrasound (19). Two areas of the retina are imaged using OCT: the peripapillary region and the macular region. The peripapillary region is useful for measuring the thickness of the retinal nerve fiber layer (RNFL—measured circumferentially around the optic nerve head), at the point just before these developmentally unmyelinated axons coalesce to form the optic nerve. Volume or thickness of the macula can also be measured, and abnormal pathology including macular edema (a possible complication of fingolimod therapy for MS) can be sensitively detected. Newer OCT analysis techniques focus on segmentation of individual retinal layers, permitted by the high-resolution spectral domain OCT instruments currently in use (Figure 9.2). One such measure of emerging interest is the thickness of the

retinal ganglion cell layer (GCL) (20). Measured at the macula, it is a way to assess the integrity of a layer of first-order sensory neurons. Thus, the three measures most commonly in use to monitor MS using OCT are the peripapillary RNFL thickness, total macular volume, and GCL thickness.

OCT is an office-based imaging method that uses near-infrared light to generate high-resolution cross-sectional images (in this case of the retina), analogus to B-mode ultrasound.

Though OCT has been used for a number of years by ophthalmologists to monitor nerve fiber layer thinning in glaucoma, applications for neurological diseases, especially MS, which commonly affects the optic nerves, are relatively new. From large cross-sectional and smaller longitudinal studies, it is known that the RNFL (and also macular volume and GCL) becomes thinned most dramatically after optic neuritis, but also during the course of MS in the absence of classic optic neuritis (21). OCT has also helped to elucidate the time course of axon loss after optic neuritis. By 3 months after the event, RNFL loss becomes apparent (Figure 9.3), and is largely complete by 6 months (22).

For these reasons, OCT is considered standard in these clinical situations:

1. Evaluating for macular edema prior to starting and while on fingolimod therapy for MS
2. To identify RNFL thinning to demonstrate a history of remote optic neuritis

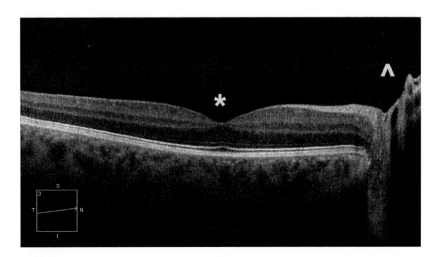

FIGURE 9.2 High resolution OCT image including both the macula (white star) and optic nerve head (caret symbol), demonstrating the ability to resolve individual retinal layers.

OCT, optical coherence tomography.

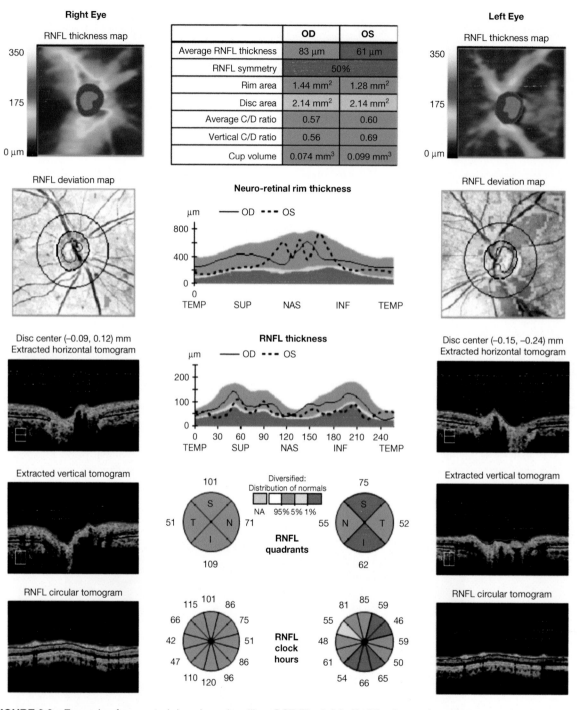

FIGURE 9.3 Example of a spectral domain peripapillary OCT. The left half of the figure shows images and measurements from the right eye (OD) of a patient with MS who previously experienced optic neuritis in the left eye (OS). The average RNFL thickness is normal OD (83 uM), and significantly thinned OS (61 uM). Images from top to bottom of the figure show (a) heat map of RNFL thickness (blue = thinner, red = thicker); (b) fundus photo demarcating the optic nerve head (outlined in black) and peripapillary circle where the RNFL is measured (purple circle); and colorized images of the RNFL show the actual cross-sectional tomograms taken from the (c) mid-horizontal slice, (d) mid-vertical slice, and (e) peripapillary circle. All boxes containing numerical measurements are shaded green, yellow, or red corresponding to the top 95%, top 99%, and bottom 1% compared to a normative database.

MS, multiple sclerosis; OCT, optical coherence tomography; RNFL, retinal nerve fiber layer; OD, oculus dexter; OS, oculus sinister.

Spectral domain (high definition) OCT has emerged as the test of choice to screen for macular edema prior to and after starting fingolimod therapy for MS. OCT can also help identify conduction delay in a patient with nonspecific visual symptoms (i.e., not typical for optic neuritis) or who is visually asymptomatic.

In addition, OCT is being explored in these clinical situations:

1. During recovery from acute optic neuritis, to quantify axon loss relative to visual deficits
2. On a yearly or biyearly basis, for monitoring longitudinal neurodegeneration in MS

In certain circumstances, if a patient with optic neuritis has a persistent severe deficit despite a standard course of intravenous methylprednisolone (IVMP), an OCT showing preserved axonal integrity may prompt additional immunotherapy, whether a second course of IVMP, plasma exchange, or intravenous immunoglobulin G (IVIG) (23).

> *Spectral domain (high definition) OCT has emerged as the test of choice to screen for macular edema prior to and after starting fingolimod therapy for MS.*

Though OCT has the potential to become useful as a tool to monitor longitudinal neurodegeneration or axon loss, neuroprotective therapies do not yet exist to intervene on that process. Some physicians will still request OCT for longitudinal monitoring, to establish a patient's baseline in anticipation of an effective neuroprotective therapy in the future.

SUMMARY

Paraclinical tests are used less frequently owing to the increased reliance on MRI to establish the diagnosis of MS and monitor its treatment; they still play a vital role in some clinical situations. The utility of spinal fluid analysis to support the diagnosis of MS has been reemphasized in the most recent recommendations of the International Panel on Diagnosis of MS. OCT is an emerging technology that is useful for exploring the mechanisms and time course of damage and recovery in MS, while also serving as a tool in the clinic to monitor retinal neurodegeneration and screen for macular edema. Current research efforts are focused on developing biomarker tests to inform prognosis or response to specific therapies in MS.

ACKNOWLEDGMENT

Supported by RG 4449A1/T from the National Multiple Sclerosis Society (USA).

REFERENCES

1. Polman CH, Reingold SC, Banwell B, et al. Diagnostic criteria for multiple sclerosis: 2010 revisions to the McDonald Criteria. *Ann Neurol.* 2011;69:292–302.
2. Miller DH, Weinshenker BG, Filippi M, et al. Differential diagnosis of suspected multiple sclerosis: a consensus approach. *Mult Scler.* 2008;14:1157–1174.
3. Mowry EM. Vitamin D. Evidence for its role as a prognostic factor in multiple sclerosis. *J Neurol Sci.* 2011;311:19–22.

KEY POINTS FOR PATIENTS AND FAMILIES

- Accurately establishing the diagnosis of MS is important, and in most cases that can be done using a combination of the medical history, neurological examination, and MRI. If any of those components expose atypical features or are inconclusive, additional testing may be required to establish the correct diagnosis.

- Even if we are certain that MS is the correct diagnosis, blood tests are often helpful to evaluate for other conditions that are common in patients with MS and may contribute to symptoms, or other tests which guide how we treat MS.

- A "spinal tap" tests for abnormal immune activation around the brain and spinal cord, and in some (but not all) cases is necessary to correctly diagnose or exclude MS. Hearing of the need for a "spinal tap" often provokes anxiety. This is a safe test if done by an experienced practitioner, and is not as uncomfortable as its reputation would suggest.

- OCT is a simple, noninvasive test that measures the thickness of the retina in the back of your eye. This test can be helpful in identifying problems in the visual system to support the diagnosis of MS, evaluating visual symptoms to help understand if they arise from MS, and in safety monitoring related to one of the MS therapies—fingolimod.

4. Schwarz M, Spector L, Gortler M, et al. Serum anti-Glc(α 1,4)Glc(α) antibodies as a biomarker for relapsing-remitting multiple sclerosis. *J Neurol Sci.* 2006;244:59–68.

5. Wingerchuk DM, Lennon VA, Pittock SJ, et al. Revised diagnostic criteria for neuromyelitis optica. *Neurology.* 2006;66:1485–1489.

6. Takahashi T, Fujihara K, Nakashima I, et al. Anti-aquaporin-4 antibody is involved in the pathogenesis of NMO: a study on antibody titre. *Brain.* 2007;130:1235–1243.

7. Gorelik L, Lerner M, Bixler S, et al. Anti-JC virus antibodies: implications for PML risk stratification. *Ann Neurol.* 2010;68:295–303.

8. Bozic C, Richman S, Plavina T, et al. Anti-John Cunnigham virus antibody prevalence in multiple sclerosis patients: baseline results of STRATIFY-1. *Ann Neurol.* 2011;70:742–750.

9. Fisniku LK, Brex PA, Altmann DR, et al. Disability and T2 MRI lesions: a 20-year follow-up of patients with relapse onset of multiple sclerosis. *Brain.* 2008;131:808–817.

10. Tintoré M, Rovira A, Río J, et al. Do oligoclonal bands add information to MRI in first attacks of multiple sclerosis? *Neurology.* 2008;70:1079–1083.

11. Thompson AJ, Banwell BL, Barkhof F, et al. Diagnosis of multiple sclerosis: recommended 2017 revisions of the McDonald criteria. *Lancet Neurol.* 2018;17:162–173.

12. Freedman MS, Thompson EJ, Deisenhammer F, et al. Recommended standard of cerebrospinal fluid analysis in the diagnosis of multiple sclerosis: a consensus statement. *Arch Neurol.* 2005;62:865–870.

13. Tourtellotte WW, Potvin AR, Fleming JO, et al. Multiple sclerosis: measurement and validation of central nervous system IgG synthesis rate. *Neurology.* 1980;30:240–244.

14. Saiz A, Carreras E, Berenguer J, et al. MRI and CSF oligoclonal bands after autologous hematopoietic stem cell transplantation in MS. *Neurology.* 2001;56:1084–1089.

15. Teunissen CE, Iacobaeus E, Khademi M, et al. Combination of CSF N-acetylaspartate and neurofilaments in multiple sclerosis. *Neurology.* 2009;72:1322–1329.

16. Gronseth GS, Ashman EJ. Practice parameter: the usefulness of evoked potentials in identifying clinically silent lesions in patients with suspected multiple sclerosis (an evidence-based review): report of the Quality Standards Subcommittee of the American Academy of Neurology. *Neurology.* 2000;54:1720–1725.

17. Hume AL, Waxman SG. Evoked potentials in suspected multiple sclerosis: diagnostic value and prediction of clinical course. *J Neurol Sci.* 1988;83:191–210.

18. Filippini G, Comi GC, Cosi V, et al. Sensitivities and predictive values of paraclinical tests for diagnosing multiple sclerosis. *J Neurol.* 1994;241:132–137.

19. Frohman EM, Fujimoto JG, Frohman TC, et al. Optical coherence tomography: a window into the mechanisms of multiple sclerosis. *Nat Clin Pract Neurol.* 2008;4:664–675.

20. Petzold A, Balcer LJ, Calabresi PA, et al. Retinal layer segmentation in multiple sclerosis: a systematic review and meta–analysis. *Lancet Neurol.* 2017;16(10):797–812.

21. Pulicken M, Gordon-Lipkin E, Balcer LJ, et al. Optical coherence tomography and disease subtype in multiple sclerosis. *Neurology.* 2007;69:2085–2092.

22. Henderson APD, Altmann DR, Trip AS, et al. A serial study of retinal changes following optic neuritis with sample size estimates for acute neuroprotection trials. *Brain.* 2010;133:2592–2602.

23. Costello F. Evaluating the use of optical coherence tomography in optic neuritis. *Mult Scler Int.* 2011;2011:148394.

10 Differential Diagnosis of Multiple Sclerosis

Megan H. Hyland and Jeffrey A. Cohen

KEY POINTS FOR CLINICIANS

- In patients with a "classic" multiple sclerosis (MS) presentation where MRI is consistent with the diagnosis, consideration of a broad differential diagnosis is unnecessary as the likelihood of an alternative diagnosis is low.
- Nonspecific white matter abnormalities and small vessel ischemic disease are the two most common alternative diagnoses in patients incorrectly labeled with MS.
- While it is important to diagnose MS early on in the disease course so that treatment may be initiated, it is also necessary to prevent mislabeling patients.
- Watch for "red flags," which may point to other diagnoses than MS.
- Be ready to rethink the diagnosis of MS if the course or response to therapy do not fit the usual MS pattern.

Because the differential diagnosis of MS is broad, distinguishing MS from other possible diseases can be challenging at times. The difficulty is illustrated in a survey of MS specialists, which showed that nearly all respondents (over 95%) reported seeing a patient within the past year who had been incorrectly diagnosed with MS (1). Evaluation of potential MS is complicated by the lack of a single, definitive diagnostic test. Attempts to design a blood test for the diagnosis of MS have shown limited success thus far, often demonstrating either suboptimal sensitivity or specificity (2). The role of potential blood tests is still unclear as the results of current tests do not clearly change diagnosis or management in the setting of more well-established clinical and paraclinical information. The currently accepted formal diagnostic criteria are outlined in Chapter 7. In general, MS is diagnosed by weighing data from clinical history, neurological exam, MRI, and, in some cases, evoked potentials or cerebrospinal fluid (CSF) tests. Historically, all of the diagnostic criteria for MS stipulate that the diagnosis cannot be made if an alternative etiology for the symptoms and test results is more plausible (3), making identification of other potential diagnoses crucial.

MULTIPLE SCLEROSIS OR NOT MULTIPLE SCLEROSIS?

The typical MS patient presents with an acute syndrome characterized by focal neurological symptoms indicating a central nervous system (CNS) process, for example, weakness, positive sensory symptoms or sensory loss, monocular vision loss, diplopia, or ataxia. These symptoms typically evolve over several days and usually improve or resolve fully after several weeks or months. Objective findings on neurological examination reflect the site(s) of CNS involvement. The neurological manifestations typically are steroid responsive but also can remit spontaneously. Characteristic MRI findings include ovoid T2 hyperintense lesions in the brain and/or spinal cord, some of which may enhance on post-gadolinium (Gd) T1 images. CSF typically shows normal or mildly elevated protein and mononuclear cell count, and evidence of intrathecal antibody production (oligoclonal bands and/or an elevated IgG index). In such patients, consideration of a broad differential diagnosis is unnecessary as the likelihood of an alternative diagnosis is low. However, a relatively high proportion of patients referred to MS subspecialty clinics for the possibility of MS do not fit this "classic" phenotype and have a higher probability of having a different diagnosis. Important tools for differentiating MS from other diseases include additional focused history taking, laboratory studies, and close examination of MRI lesion patterns, focusing on findings that would be atypical for MS.

In patients with a very typical MS presentation, consideration of a broad differential diagnosis is unnecessary as the likelihood of an alternative diagnosis is low.

Ideally, a uniform diagnostic algorithm could be applied to all patients. Potential diagnostic algorithms have been proposed (4) but are difficult to apply in practice because patients with possible MS come to medical attention for a variety of reasons. Patients may fall into several categories. First, some patients have symptoms and test results consistent with the broad range of potential MS manifestations but with features suggestive of another disease. These are the patients for whom it is most important to keep in mind the full spectrum of potential MS mimics (Table 10.1). Attention to "red flags"—features atypical for MS or indicative of another disease process—is the basis of avoiding misdiagnosis.

A second category of patients with "possible MS" has become common with the increasing use of MRI. These patients often have nonspecific symptoms suggestive of MS or may be asymptomatic but are primarily assessed for MS because of white matter abnormalities on brain MRI. Up to one-third of new diagnostic referrals to an MS center are estimated to be due to an abnormal brain MRI, with one MS center finding that only 11% of those patients ultimately had MS (5). In addition, a survey of MS subspecialists regarding misdiagnosis cited MRI-based diagnoses—nonspecific white matter abnormalities and

small vessel ischemic disease—as the two most common alternative diagnoses in patients incorrectly labeled with MS (1). In this category of patients, particular focus must be placed on patient history and MRI patterns in order to make a correct diagnosis.

A third category of patients includes those with numerous symptoms, often overlapping with those of MS but lacking the classic course and frequently having normal neurological exams and test results. These patients may have underlying medical or psychiatric issues, such as fibromyalgia, depression, sleep disorders, or conversion disorder—and may or may not have superimposed MS. Often, imaging studies show nonspecific T2 hyperintensities, which further raise the question of MS. Although it is important to diagnose MS early on in the disease course so that treatment may be initiated, it is also necessary to prevent mislabeling patients. Ethical concerns that accompany an incorrect MS diagnosis include the difficulty in "undiagnosing" a chronic disease, unnecessary use of long-term, costly medications that carry risk of potential adverse effects, and the risk of other medical conditions being attributed to MS and subsequently not being treated adequately (6).

This chapter attempts to strike a balance between making readers aware of the many red flags and potential alternative diagnoses to MS and highlighting a practical approach to the most commonly seen "possible MS" patient.

TABLE 10.1 Differential Diagnosis of MS by Disease Category

Demyelinating	Acute disseminated encephalomyelitis, NMO spectrum disorder
Infection	Lyme disease, syphilis, PML, AIDS, HTLV-1, Herpes zoster
Autoimmune	SLE, Sjogren's syndrome, vasculitis, neurosarcoidosis, Behçet's disease, Susac's syndrome, celiac disease, thyroid disease, autoimmune encephalitis
Vascular	Multiple embolic infarcts, small vessel ischemia, migraine
Metabolic	Vitamin B_{12} deficiency, copper deficiency
Genetic	Lysosomal disorders, adrenoleukodystrophy, mitochondrial disorders, Fragile X-associated tremor/ataxia syndrome, other genetic disorders, CADASIL, hereditary spastic paraparesis, hereditary ataxias
Neoplastic	Central nervous system lymphoma, primary or metastatic tumor, paraneoplastic syndrome
Neurodegenerative	Motor neuron disease
Spine disease	Vascular malformations, degenerative spine disease

CADASIL, cerebral autosomal dominant arteriopathy with subcortical infarcts and leukoencephalopathy; HTLV-1, human T-lymphotropic virus, type 1; MS, multiple sclerosis; NMO, neuromyelitis optica; PML, progressive multifocal leukoencephalopathy; SLE, systemic lupus erythematosus.

DIAGNOSTIC RED FLAGS

Clinical Red Flags

Certain symptom characteristics—either the type of symptom or time course over which it develops—may support or argue against an MS diagnosis. For example, although pain is common in MS, it would be unlikely for MS to cause certain types of pain directly. Joint pain typically points toward rheumatological autoimmune mimics of MS such as systemic lupus erythematosus (SLE). Similarly, although headaches are common among people with MS, as in the general population, headaches in the setting of MRI white matter changes raise suspicion for cerebral autosomal dominant arteriopathy with subcortical infarcts and leukoencephalopathy (CADASIL) or CNS vasculitis but more often may reflect common headache syndromes such as migraine. Although neck pain can occur with acute MS lesions in the cervical cord, chronic cervicalgia suggests a structural cause such as disc herniation or spinal stenosis. Fever warrants consideration of an infectious or rheumatological etiology. Although cognitive changes are seen in MS, they generally develop gradually later in the disease process, and usually affect processing speed, memory, and executive function. Language is rarely impacted. Acute mental status changes would be more typical for acute disseminated encephalomyelitis (ADEM) or other autoimmune etiology such as CNS SLE or antibody-mediated encephalitis symptoms and exam findings consistent with multiple cranial neuropathies raise suspicion for Lyme disease, neurosarcoidosis, or malignancy. Marked fatigue is a common but relatively nonspecific MS symptom, which usually warrants evaluation of other possible causes, such as sleep apnea, thyroid disease, or vitamin deficiencies. Migrating numbness and/or weakness are common symptoms prompting referral to an MS clinic, but the fluctuating nature typically prompts further investigation for other etiologies. A thorough review of systems for other organ system involvement (e.g., pulmonary disease which may point to neurosarcoidosis) is recommended during the process of diagnosing MS.

The symptoms of MS are varied, making symptom evolution a critical consideration in the diagnostic process. An important red flag is a history of symptoms that do not follow a pattern of the typical MS relapse (evolution over hours to days, persistence over days to weeks, and resolution over weeks to months). Symptoms that only last hours at a time, frequently change location or severity, develop abruptly, or become rapidly cumulative, point away from MS. Other symptom patterns atypical for MS are summarized in Table 10.2. Of note is that primary progressive MS has a disease course that differs from the more common relapsing forms, typically characterized by weakness and spasticity that develop insidiously and worsen slowly over years. Painless progressive difficulty walking often is initially attributed by the patient to knee or back problems, causing the diagnosis of progressive MS to be delayed. Conversely, symptoms of progressive myelopathy should include consideration of mechanical etiologies (i.e., disc herniation) or, more rarely, diseases such as human T-lymphotropic virus, type 1 (HTLV-1) or hereditary spastic paraparesis.

> *Marked fatigue is a common but relatively nonspecific MS symptom.*

Other aspects of patient history that may identify red flags include age of onset and family history. MS is most commonly diagnosed in patients ages 20 to 50 years; younger patients may be more likely to have ADEM or a leukodystrophy while older patients are more likely to have arthritic spine changes or vascular etiologies such as small vessel ischemia, particularly with a history of vascular risk factors. MS has only a relatively minor hereditary component, so a strong family history, particularly of stereotypical manifestations, would be more concerning for a leukodystrophy, mitochondrial disease, hereditary ataxia, or other genetic disorder.

An atypical response to therapy is another red flag suggesting other potential diagnoses. Improvement in symptoms in response to steroid treatment is not specific for MS; it may occur, for example, in other inflammatory

TABLE 10.2 Clinical Red Flags for the Potential Misdiagnosis of MS

Onset of symptoms before age 20 y or after 50 y

Very prominent family history of stereotyped manifestations

Atypical course
- Gradually progressive course from onset—unless considering primary progressive MS—particularly in a young patient or with manifestations other than a myelopathy
- Abrupt development of symptoms

Unifocal manifestations (even if relapsing)

Neurological manifestations unusual for MS

Associated systemic manifestations

Missing features, particularly in long-standing or severe disease
- Lack of oculomotor, optic nerve, sensory, or bladder involvement

Atypical response to treatment
- Lack of any response to corticosteroids
- Exceptionally rapid or dramatic response to corticosteroids or disease-modifying treatments
- Lack of any response to potent disease therapies such as natalizumab

MS, multiple sclerosis.

disorders, malignancy, and spinal vascular malformations or mechanical compression. However, MS symptoms typically do not respond immediately when steroids are initiated or worsen acutely after cessation of steroid treatment; this pattern would be suggestive of a steroid-responsive mimic such as neurosarcoidosis. Additionally, lack of any response to potent MS disease-modifying therapy, such as natalizumab, particularly in the absence of anti-natalizumab neutralizing antibodies, should lead to reconsideration of the MS diagnosis.

> *Lack of any response to a potent MS disease-modifying therapy should lead to reconsideration of the MS diagnosis.*

Imaging Red Flags

MRI is an increasingly important diagnostic tool in MS, and as noted earlier, an "abnormal brain MRI" is a common reason for referral to neurologists, in particular MS subspecialists. White matter hyperintensities on T2-weighted images (i.e., fluid-attenuated inversion recovery [FLAIR]) MRI are a typical finding in MS, but the size, shape, and location of the lesions are vital in differentiating MS from other etiologies. A summary of MRI findings that may help differentiate MS from other diseases is shown in Table 10.3.

MS lesions may be punctate (less than 3 mm), making them harder to distinguish from lesions due to small vessel ischemic disease including migraine, but in MS, patients often have a combination of larger (>6 mm) and

TABLE 10.3   Distinguishing MRI Features of Selected MS Mimics

PML	Confluent posterior cerebral T2 lesions with decreased signal on T1-weighted images, gradual enlargement, absent Gd-enhancement or faint enhancement of the leading edge
NMO spectrum disorder	Longitudinally extensive lesions in the spinal cord, corpus callosum or optic nerve; brain lesions in the diencephalon or dorsal medulla (area postrema)
HTLV-1 associated myelopathy	Thoracic spinal cord atrophy, sparse cerebral lesions
SLE and Sjogren's syndrome	Lesions predominantly in the subcortical white matter, gray matter involvement
Vasculitis	Ischemic lesions or cerebral infarcts, gray matter involvement, vascular or meningeal Gd-enhancement
Neurosarcoidosis	Parenchymal mass lesions with persistent Gd-enhancement, vascular or meningeal Gd-enhancement
Behçet's disease	Predominantly brain stem involvement
Susac's syndrome	Gray matter involvement or atypical callosal lesions
Vitamin B_{12} deficiency	Abnormal signal limited to the dorsal cervical spinal cord
Leukodystrophies	Diffuse white matter abnormality
Adrenomyeloneuropathy	Symmetric lesions in posterior cerebral white matter
Mitochondrial disorders	Multifocal gray or white matter lesions, basal ganglia calcifications
Spinocerebellar degenerations	Brain stem or cerebellar atrophy without signal abnormality
Motor neuron disease	Typically normal MRI, or symmetrical atrophy, or abnormal T2 hyperintensity in the pyramidaltracts
CADASIL	Lack of involvement of corpus callosum, cerebellum, optic nerves, or spinal cord; temporal lobe predominance; involvement of deep gray structures Presence of lacunar infarcts
CNS lymphoma	Unifocal or multifocal lesions with gradual enlargement or mass effect, gray matter involvement, persistent Gd-enhancement, vascular enhancement
Spinal vascular malformation	Patchy increased T2 signal in the spinal cord with faint Gd-enhancement or cord enlargement, possibly visible draining veins, absent or nonspecific cerebral lesions
Fragile X syndrome	Confluent white matter involvement; basal ganglia, brain stem, and cerebellar lesions; symmetric middle cerebellar peduncle involvement

CADASIL, cerebral autosomal dominant arteriopathy with subcortical infarcts and leukoencephalopathy; CNS, central nervous system; Gd, gadolinium; HTLV-1, human T-lymphotropic virus, type 1; MS, multiple sclerosis; NMO, neuromyelitis optica; PML, progressive multifocal leukoencephalopathy; SLE, systemic lupus erythematosus.

smaller lesions. MS lesions can be a variety of shapes, but typical lesions are ovoid or "flame-shaped." Although lack of classically shaped lesions is not necessarily a red flag, the expectation of such lesions increases in patients with a larger lesion burden. The location of lesions is also important in the differential diagnosis. MS lesions are characteristically seen in periventricular, juxtacortical, and cortical locations when located supratentorially, while small vessel ischemic lesions typically spare the immediate periventricular and callosal regions. Sagittal images are helpful when an MS diagnosis is being considered because they best demonstrate callosal lesions. One location red flag to consider is a predominance of temporal lesions—although MS lesions often occur around the temporal horn, a high proportion of temporal lobe lesions is potentially suggestive of CADASIL. In contrast, complete sparing of the temporal lobe is common with small vessel ischemic disease. MS lesions frequently involve the cerebellum and brain stem, but a predominance of brain stem lesions suggests a possibility of neurosarcoidosis or Behçet's disease.

> *Sagittal images are helpful when a MS diagnosis is being considered because they best demonstrate callosal lesions.*

Other imaging sequences are often helpful in distinguishing MS from other etiologies. In MS, T2 hyperintense lesions may be hypointense on T1-weighted images, representing areas of increased axonal loss following prior inflammation. Diffusion weighted imaging may occasionally present a "reverse" red-flag: the presence of restricted diffusion is a common finding in acute stroke but is also possible in acute MS lesions and should be considered with an appropriately corresponding history.

The pattern of Gd-enhancement often is useful in distinguishing MS lesions from another pathology. MS lesions often show either uniform Gd-enhancement or an open-ring pattern, with the presence of additional nonenhancing lesions. The Gd-enhancement typically resolves within 1 to 2 months. Closed ring lesions, enhancement of all lesions, or enhancement lasting more than 2 months raise the possibility of malignancy, infection, or other inflammatory conditions, such as neurosarcoidosis. PML may look similar to MS lesions on T2-weighted imaging initially, but classically is distinguished by gradual enlargement without enhancement or with only mild enhancement limited, often limited to the leading edge. Of note, natalizumab-associated PML may have an increased incidence of enhancement and has been seen in up to one-third of patients. Meningeal or vascular enhancement raises concern for neurosarcoidosis or CNS vasculitis.

Typically, in early MS, some but not all MRI lesions show Gd-enhancement that persists in an individual lesion for 4 to 8 weeks and exhibits a diffuse or open-ring pattern.

Gd-enhancement with other characteristics should prompt consideration of other diagnoses.

Spinal cord MRI is a useful but frequently underutilized diagnostic tool. Intramedullary T2 hyperintensities in the cervical or thoracic spinal cord are much more specific for MS than brain lesions and help to point toward the diagnosis of MS if the brain lesions appear nonspecific. MS lesions typically involve one to two spinal levels, are more frequent in the cervical spine, and often have a patchy distribution. Longitudinally extensive (more than three cord segment) lesions are atypical for MS and are more likely to indicate neuromyelitis optica (NMO) spectrum disorder or a metabolic etiology such as B_{12} or copper deficiency. Lesions that are predominantly in the posterior columns are generally seen in tertiary syphilis or B_{12} deficiency. Another red flag on spine imaging is persistent Gd-enhancement which is generally more concerning for neurosarcoidosis, malignancy, or vascular malformations.

CSF Red Flags

"Classic" CSF findings are outlined earlier in the chapter and include signs of intrathecal antibody production. These can be absent in patients with otherwise typical MS, but in the setting of a marked pleocytosis, particularly if there is a significant proportion of cells other than lymphocytes and macrophages, or markedly elevated protein levels, other diagnoses should be considered, particularly infection, other inflammatory disorders, or malignancy. Conversely, while CSF oligoclonal bands may facilitate an MS diagnosis, both oligoclonal band and IgG index elevation may be present in other inflammatory or infectious conditions.

CSF oligoclonal bands and IgG index elevation may be present in other inflammatory or infectious conditions.

MIMICS BY DISEASE CATEGORY

A comprehensive description of all potential MS mimics is outside the scope of this text, but selected key points are outlined here. Other demyelinating etiologies are addressed in detail in separate chapters. The importance of distinguishing NMO spectrum disorder from MS is noteworthy because it is often overlooked and the therapeutic approach is different than that for MS.

Infectious etiologies are frequently considered when red flags arise. For example, PML is more likely to cause visual field abnormalities than typical MS vision changes, which most often are due to optic neuropathy. Additional history or exam findings may also point toward an infectious cause, for example, classic erythema migrans raises the possibility of CNS manifestations of Lyme disease. However, it is important to note that evidence of systemic Lyme disease does not prove it as the cause of the MS-like illness; in endemic areas, the infection and MS may be coincident and not causally linked. A broader scope of infectious possibilities should be considered in immunocompromised patients, those with risk factors for HIV infection, or with a history of travel to areas with higher incidences of certain infectious diseases.

Inflammatory and autoimmune diseases can be most difficult to distinguish from MS because the MRI and CSF findings can be similar. In these cases, clinical symptoms may be very helpful in guiding additional diagnostic testing. Classic sicca symptoms are suggestive of Sjögren's syndrome, while a malar rash may suggest SLE. Dry skin and brittle hair/nails suggest thyroid disease (another frequently concomitant rather than causal disease process). Prominent gastrointestinal symptoms warrant additional evaluation for celiac disease. Oral or genital ulcers are concerning for Behçet's disease. Hearing loss warrants consideration of Susac's syndrome. Although cranial nerve nuclei can be affected in MS, extensive cranial nerve involvement is more typical of neurosarcoidosis. Bloodwork may be helpful in confirming inflammatory etiologies, but certain tests—antinuclear antibody (ANA) and angiotensin converting enzyme (ACE) levels—may be modestly elevated in MS. In the absence of other indications of SLE or sarcoidosis, mildly elevated ANA and ACE levels do not require further investigation. Conversely, if clinical suspicion for neurosarcoidosis is high in spite of negative ACE levels, further assessment with chest imaging or PET scan may be warranted as serum and CSF ACE levels are not highly sensitive. High ANA titers and the presence of other autoantibodies are more specific for SLE.

Metabolic etiologies should be considered in patients with gastrointestinal malabsorption (e.g., history of gastric bypass surgery). In patients with borderline B_{12} (cobalamin) deficiency, blood tests for methylmalonic acid and homocysteine levels should also be checked. Nitrous oxide abuse also leads to functional B_{12} deficiency as it irreversibly binds to the cobalt ion of methylcobalamin and prevents further metabolism. Concurrent myelopathy and sensory neuropathy is characteristic of both B_{12} and copper deficiency. The latter is uncommon but should be considered in patients taking zinc supplements as zinc inhibits the absorption of copper.

The most common malignancy mistaken for MS is primary CNS lymphoma. CSF examination may demonstrate cytologically abnormal lymphocytes but usually is normal or demonstrates only nonspecific abnormalities of protein or pleocytosis. However, spinal tap may still be useful because a finding of oligoclonal bands and an elevated IgG index would argue more strongly in favor of a demyelinating etiology. CNS lymphoma often is steroid responsive, but the response usually is self-limited. Persistent Gd-enhancement or gradual enlargement of MRI lesions should raise the question of malignancy. Ultimately, brain biopsy may be needed for diagnostic confirmation.

CNS lymphoma often is steroid responsive, but the response usually is self-limited.

DIAGNOSTIC ALGORITHM

If the history, exam, and MRI findings are characteristic of MS, CSF studies and evoked potentials usually are not necessary. Limited additional bloodwork is suggested to look for more common MS mimics as they can often occur concomitantly and may be easily treated (e.g., thyroid disease, B_{12} deficiency). Thus, the evaluation of such patients may be limited to

- Comprehensive medical and neurological history and examination
- Cranial MRI including axial and sagittal FLAIR images, axial proton density or T2-weighted images (better visualization of posterior fossa), and T1-weighted images pre- and post-Gd administration
- Limited blood studies, potentially including complete blood count, thyroid stimulating hormone, ANA, syphilis screen, (FTA-ABS), vitamin B_{12} level, Lyme titer (in endemic areas)

The utility of more extensive bloodwork is often debated. In patients with manifestations characteristic of MS, the yield is low and false positive results can be misleading.

Additional testing, such as CSF studies, spinal imaging, and/or VEPs should be considered in less typical cases.

Additional testing, such as CSF studies, spinal imaging, and/or visual evoked potentials (VEPs) should be considered in less typical cases. The specific testing should be guided by the features of the patient, including the presence of red flags.

Patients with abnormal brain MRI in the absence of characteristic clinical manifestations of MS require careful consideration. In patients with atypical histories and nonspecific symptoms, MRI of the brain and spinal cord may be sufficient to rule out MS, but additional tests should be considered as needed. It is important, however, not to assign the diagnosis of MS merely on the basis of exclusion of other diagnoses.

CONCLUSIONS

MS often presents in a typical or straightforward fashion. In such patients, the additional work-up can be limited to MRI studies and modest bloodwork. Clinicians must remain vigilant to ensure that the evolution of manifestations and response to therapy continue to indicate MS. However, many patients referred to MS clinics may not actually have MS. A high proportion of these patients have abnormal brain MRIs and/or nonspecific symptoms and should only be diagnosed with MS with caution. It is reasonable to monitor patients periodically in whom testing is equivocal rather than prematurely assigning an MS diagnosis. Careful attention must also be given to identification of red flags because they can indicate the need to search for a potentially uncommon but treatable alternative diagnosis.

KEY POINTS FOR PATIENTS AND FAMILIES

- MS may sometimes be easy to diagnose but there are also times where the diagnosis is unclear and may take time to make.
- MS diagnosis is not based on the number of symptoms, but on the pattern of symptoms, neurological findings on exam, MRI features, and sometimes other diagnostic test results (i.e., CSF studies). It requires expertise to make a firm diagnosis of MS.
- Many other conditions may at times look like MS and should be considered when the history, exam, imaging, or other results suggest other diagnoses.
- Many people with nonspecific white matter lesions are evaluated for the diagnosis of MS, but often they do not actually have this disease.

REFERENCES

1. Solomon AJ, Klein EP, Bourdette D. "Undiagnosing" multiple sclerosis: the challenge of misdiagnosis in MS. *Neurology.* 2012;78:1986–1991.
2. Brettschneider J, Jaskowski TD, Tumani H, et al. Serum anti-GAGA4 IgM antibodies differentiate relapsing remitting and secondary progressive multiple sclerosis from primary progressive multiple sclerosis and other neurological diseases. *J Neuroimmunol.* 2009;217:95–101.
3. Polman CH, Reingold SC, Banwell B, et al. Diagnostic criteria for multiple sclerosis: 2010 revisions to the McDonald Criteria. *Ann Neurol.* 2011;69(2):292–302.
4. Miller DH, Weinshenker BG, Filippi M, et al. Differential diagnosis of suspected multiple sclerosis: a consensus approach. *Mult Scler.* 2008;14:1157–1174.
5. Carminoso MJ, Brousseau KM, Arciniegas DB, et al. Initial evaluations for multiple sclerosis in a university multiple sclerosis center: outcomes and role of magnetic resonance imaging in referral. *Arch Neurol.* 2005;62:585–590.
6. Boissy AR, Ford, PJ. A touch of MS: therapeutic mislabeling. *Neurology.* 2012;78:1981–1985.

SUGGESTED READING

Barned S, Goodman AD, Mattson DH. Frequency of anti-nuclear antibodies in multiple sclerosis. *Neurology.* 1995;45:384–385.

Greco CM, Tassone F, Garcia-Aroncena D, et al. Clinical and neuropathologic findings in a woman with the *FMR1* premutation and multiple sclerosis. *Arch Neurol.* 2008;65(8):1114–1116.

Halperin JJ, Logigian EL, Finkel MF, et al. Practice parameters for the diagnosis of patients with nervous system Lyme borreliosis (Lyme disease). *Neurology.* 1996;46:619–627.

Kumar N, Gross JB, Jr, Ahlskog JE. Copper deficiency myelopathy presents a clinical picture like subacute combined degeneration. *Neurology.* 2004;63(1):33–39.

LaMantia L, Erbetta A. Headache and inflammatory disorders of the central nervous system. *Neurol Sci.* 2004;25(suppl 3):148–153.

Logigian EL, Kaplan RF, Steere AC. Chronic neurologic manifestations of Lyme disease. *N Engl J Med.* 1990;323:1438–1444.

McDermott C, White K, Bushby K, et al. Hereditary spastic paraparesis: a review of new developments. *J Neurol Neurosurg Psychiatry.* 2000;69(2):150–160.

Natowicz MR, Benjjani B. Genetic disorders that masquerade as multiple sclerosis. *Am J Med Genet.* 1994;49(2):149–169.

O'Riordan JI. Central nervous system white matter diseases other than multiple sclerosis. *Curr Opin Neurol.* 1997;10:211–214.

Rudick RA, Miller AE. Multiple sclerosis or multiple possibilities: the continuing problem of misdiagnosis. *Neurology.* 2012;78:1904–1906.

Singhal S, Rich P, Markus HS. The spatial distribution of MR imaging abnormalities in cerebral autosomal dominant arteriopathy with subcortical infarcts and leukoencephalopathy and their relationship to age and clinical features. *AJNR Am J Neuroradiol.* 2005;26(10):2481–2487.

Solomon AJ, Bourdette DN, Cross AH, et al. The contemporary spectrum of multiple sclerosis misdiagnosis: a multicenter study. *Neurology.* 2016;87(13):1393–1399.

Stern BJ. Neurological complications of sarcoidosis. *Curr Opin Neurol.* 2004;17(3):311–316.

Theodoridou A, Settas L. Demyelination in rheumatic diseases. *J Neurol Neurosurg Psychiatry.* 2006;77(3):290–295.

Thompson AJ, Polman CH, Miller DH, et al. Primary progressive multiple sclerosis. *Brain.* 1997;210:1085–1096.

Wingerchuk DM, Banwell B, Bennett JL, et al. International consensus diagnostic criteria for neuromyelitis optica spectrum disorders. *Neurology.* 2015;85:1–13.

Younger DS. Vasculitis of the nervous system. *Curr Opin Neurol.* 2004;17(3):317–336.

PART III. TREATMENT

2018 American Academy of Neurology Guidelines for Multiple Sclerosis Disease-Modifying Therapy

Alexander D. Rae-Grant

In April 2018, the American Academy of Neurology (AAN) published a systematic review and guidelines for disease-modifying therapy (DMT) for multiple sclerosis (MS) (1,2). The systematic review analyzed seven clinical questions related to DMT in patients with relapsing remitting, secondary and primary progressive MS, as well as those with clinically isolated syndromes. Twenty-three different medications were included in this systematic review, including Food and Drug Administration (FDA)- and European Medicines Agency (EMA)-approved medicines and off label use of medicines with moderate-to-high-quality evidence. Recommendations were developed by an expert panel using an electronic modified Delphi process. Thirty recommendations were developed for starting, switching, and stopping MS DMT. The systematic review and recommendation process followed Institute of Medicine recommendations for guideline development (3).

Some key points to take away from these recommendations include the following:

1. Proper diagnosis of MS is the gateway to treatment with DMT; avoiding misdiagnosis is as important as early diagnosis in MS care.
2. Engaging the patient actively in a dialogue about the role of DMT, their readiness to initiate therapy, specific patient characteristics that may affect choice of medicine, and ongoing monitoring for adherence is key to success in the use of DMT.
3. Clinicians should be ready to recommend switching DMTs when patients have ongoing disease activity as measured by relapses and/or new MRI lesions.
4. Counselling about DMTs before pregnancy is important and consists of evaluating risks of medication in pregnancy, risks of certain medications for teratogenicity and infertility, and evaluating the ongoing risk of MS relapses in an individual patient.
5. The decision of which medicine to use should include an evaluation of the disease activity in the patient; higher disease activity should prompt a higher efficacy medication earlier in the disease course.
6. There may be a subgroup of patients with MS where disease activity is low enough, risk is high enough, and disability is large enough that further DMT treatment is not helpful. However, the committee was not able to come to consensus on a specific indicator for stopping DMT.

7. The committee did not have enough evidence to decide whether a high-efficacy initial strategy was better or worse than a standard escalation (or stepped) approach, although studies are underway to evaluate this question. In addition, there was limited data to compare medications in most cases; further pragmatic clinical trials will be helpful in evaluating comparative efficacy in the clinic population.

AAN GUIDELINE COMMITTEE RECOMMENDATIONS

Starting Recommendations

1. **Level B:** Clinicians should counsel people with newly diagnosed MS about specific treatment options with DMT at a dedicated treatment visit.
2. **Level A:** Clinicians must ascertain and incorporate/review preferences in terms of safety, route of administration, lifestyle, cost, efficacy, common adverse effects (AEs), and tolerability in the choice of DMT in people with MS being considered for DMT.
   Level A: Clinicians must engage in an ongoing dialogue regarding treatment decisions throughout the disease course with people with MS.
3. **Level B:** Clinicians should counsel people with MS that DMTs are prescribed to reduce relapses and new MRI lesion activity. DMTs are not prescribed for symptom improvement in people with MS.
   Level A: Clinicians must counsel people with MS on DMTs to notify the clinicians of new or worsening symptoms.
4. **Level B:** Clinicians should evaluate readiness or reluctance to initiate DMT and counsel on its importance in people with MS who are candidates to initiate DMT.
5. **Level B:** Clinicians should counsel about comorbid disease, adverse health behaviors, and potential interactions of the DMT with concomitant medications when people with MS initiate DMTs.
6. **Level B:** Clinicians should evaluate barriers to adherence to DMT in people with MS.
   Level B: Clinicians should counsel on the importance of adherence to DMT when people with MS initiate DMTs.

7. **Level B:** Clinicians should discuss the benefits and risks of DMTs for people with a single clinical demyelinating event with two or more brain lesions that have imaging characteristics consistent with MS.

   Level B: After discussing the risks and benefits, clinicians should prescribe DMT to people with a single clinical demyelinating event and two or more brain lesions characteristic of MS who decide they want this therapy.

8. **Level C:** Clinicians may recommend serial imaging at least annually for the first 5 years and close follow-up rather than initiating DMT in people with clinically isolated syndrome (CIS) or relapsing forms of MS who are not on DMT, have not had relapses in the preceding 2 years, and do not have active new MRI lesion activity on recent imaging.

9. **Level B:** Clinicians should offer DMTs to people with relapsing forms of MS with recent clinical relapses or MRI activity.

10. **Level B:** Clinicians should monitor for medication adherence, AEs, tolerability, safety, and effectiveness of the therapy in people with MS on DMTs.

    Level B: Clinicians should follow up either annually or according to medication-specific risk evaluation and mitigation strategies (REMS) in people with MS on DMTs.

11. **Level B:** Clinicians should monitor the reproductive plans of women with MS and counsel regarding reproductive risks and use of birth control during DMT use in women of childbearing potential who have MS.

12. **Level B:** Clinicians should counsel men with MS on their reproductive plans regarding treatment implications before initiating treatment with teriflunomide or cyclophosphamide.

13. **Level B:** Because of the high frequency of severe AEs, clinicians should not prescribe mitoxantrone to people with MS unless the potential therapeutic benefits greatly outweigh the risks.

14. **Level B:** Clinicians should prescribe alemtuzumab, fingolimod, or natalizumab for people with MS with highly active MS.

    Level C: Clinicians may direct people with MS who are candidates for DMTs to support programs.

15. **Level C:** Clinicians may recommend azathioprine or cladribine for people with relapsing forms of MS who do not have access to approved DMTs.

16. **Level C:** Clinicians may initiate natalizumab treatment in people with MS with positive anti-JCV antibody indexes above 0.9 only when there is a reasonable chance of benefit compared with the low but serious risk of progressive multifocal leukoencephalopathy (PML).

17. **Level B:** Clinicians should offer ocrelizumab to people with primary progressive multiple sclerosis (PPMS) who are likely to benefit from this therapy unless there are risks of treatment that outweigh the benefits.

Switching Recommendations

1. **Level B:** Clinicians should monitor MRI disease activity from the clinical onset of disease to detect the accumulation of new lesions in order to inform treatment decisions in people with MS using DMTs.

   Level B: Clinicians should recognize that relapses or new MRI-detected lesions may develop after initiation of a DMT and before the treatment becomes effective in people with MS who are using DMTs.

   Level B: Clinicians should discuss switching from one DMT to another in people with MS who have been using a DMT long enough for the treatment to take full effect and are adherent to their therapy when they experience one or more relapses, two or more unequivocally new MRI-detected lesions, or increased disability on examination, over a 1-year period of using a DMT.

2. **Level B:** Clinicians should evaluate the degree of disease activity, adherence, AE profiles, and mechanism of action of DMTs when switching DMTs in people with MS with breakthrough disease activity during DMT use.

3. **Level B:** Clinicians should discuss a change to noninjectable or less frequently injectable DMTs in people with MS who report intolerable discomfort with the injections or in those who report "injection fatigue" on injectable DMTs.

4. **Level B:** Clinicians should inquire about medication AEs with people with MS who are taking a DMT and attempt to manage these AEs, as appropriate.

   Level B: Clinicians should discuss a medication switch with people with MS for whom these AEs negatively influence adherence.

5. **Level B:** Clinicians should monitor laboratory abnormalities found on requisite laboratory surveillance (as outlined in the medication's package insert) in people with MS who are using a DMT.

   Level B: Clinicians should discuss switching DMT or reducing dosage or frequency (where there are data on different doses [e.g., interferons, teriflunomide, azathioprine]) when there are persistent laboratory abnormalities.

6. **Level B:** Clinicians should counsel people with MS considering natalizumab, fingolimod, rituximab, ocrelizumab, and dimethyl fumarate about the PML risk associated with these agents.

   Level B: Clinicians should discuss switching to a DMT with a lower PML risk with people with MS taking natalizumab who are or become JCV antibody positive, especially with an index of above 0.9 while on therapy.

7. **Level B:** Clinicians should counsel that new DMTs without long-term safety data have an undefined risk of malignancy and infection for people with MS starting or using new DMTs.

   Level B: If a patient with MS develops a malignancy while using a DMT, clinicians should promptly discuss switching to an alternate DMT, especially for people with MS using azathioprine, methotrexate, mycophenolate, cyclophosphamide, fingolimod, teriflunomide, alemtuzumab, or dimethyl fumarate.

Level B: People with MS with serious infections potentially linked to their DMT should switch DMTs (does not pertain to PML management in people with MS using DMT).

8. **Level B:** Clinicians should check for natalizumab antibodies in people with MS who have infusion reactions before subsequent infusions, or in people with MS who experience breakthrough disease activity with natalizumab use.

   Level B: Clinicians should switch DMTs in people with MS who have persistent natalizumab antibodies.

9. **Level A:** Physicians must counsel people with MS considering natalizumab discontinuation that there is an increased risk of MS relapse or MRI detected disease activity within 6 months of discontinuation.

   Level B: Physicians and people with MS choosing to switch from natalizumab to fingolimod should initiate treatment within 8 to 12 weeks after natalizumab discontinuation (for reasons other than pregnancy or pregnancy planning) to diminish the return of disease activity.

10. **Level B:** Clinicians should counsel women to stop their DMT before conception for planned pregnancies unless the risk of MS activity during pregnancy outweighs the risk associated with the specific DMT during pregnancy.

    Level B: Clinicians should discontinue DMTs during pregnancy if accidental exposure occurs, unless the risk of MS activity during pregnancy outweighs the risk associated with the specific DMT during pregnancy.

    Level B: Clinicians should not initiate DMTs during pregnancy unless the risk of MS activity during pregnancy outweighs the risk associated with the specific DMT during pregnancy.

Stopping Recommendations

1. **Level B:** In people with relapsing remitting multiple sclerosis (RRMS) who are stable on DMT and want to discontinue therapy, clinicians should counsel people regarding the need for ongoing follow-up and periodic reevaluation of the decision to discontinue DMT.

   Level B: Clinicians should advocate that people with MS who are stable (i.e., no relapses, no disability progression, stable imaging) on DMT should continue their current DMT unless the patient and physician decide a trial off therapy is warranted.

2. **Level B:** Clinicians should assess the likelihood of future relapse in individuals with secondary progressive multiple sclerosis (SPMS) by assessing patient age, disease duration, relapse history, and MRI-detected activity (e.g., frequency, severity, time since most recent relapse or gadolinium-enhanced lesion).

   Level C: Clinicians may advise discontinuation of DMT in people with SPMS who do not have ongoing relapses (or gadolinium-enhanced lesions on MRI activity) and have not been ambulatory (EDSS 7 or greater) for at least 2 years.

3. **Level B:** Clinicians should review the associated risks of continuing DMTs versus those of stopping DMTs in people with CIS using DMTs who have not been diagnosed with MS.

Level A recommendation denotes a practice recommendation that must be done. *Must* recommendations are rare, as they are based on high confidence in the evidence and require both a high magnitude of benefit and low risk.

Level B recommendation denotes a practice recommendation that should be done. *Should* recommendations tend to be more common, as the requirements are less stringent but still based on the evidence and benefit–risk profile.

Level C recommendation denotes a practice recommendation that may be done. *May* recommendations represent the lowest allowable recommendation level the AAN considers useful within the scope of clinical practice and can accommodate the highest degree of practice variation.

REFERENCES

1. Rae-Grant ADG, Marrie RA, Rabinstein A, et al. Practice guideline recommendations summary: disease-modifying therapies for adults with multiple sclerosis. *Neurology* 2018;90:777–88.
2. Rae-Grant A DG, Marrie RA, Rabinstein A, et al. Comprehensive systematic review summary: disease-modifying therapies for adults with multiple sclerosis. *Neurology* 2018;90:789–800.
3. Institute of Medicine. *Clinical Practice Guidelines We Can Trust.* Washington, DC: National Academies Press; 2011.

11

Approach to Disease-Modifying Therapy

Laura E. Baldassari and Jeffrey A. Cohen

KEY POINTS FOR CLINICIANS

- Management of relapsing multiple sclerosis (MS) involves treatment of relapses, disease-modifying therapy (DMT), and symptomatic management.
- The short-term goal of DMT is to prevent relapses and MRI lesion activity.
- The long-term goal of DMT is to prevent disability worsening and transition to secondary progressive disease.
- There are over a dozen DMTs with regulatory approval and they have diverse mechanisms of action for treatment of relapsing forms of MS.
- Current treatment strategies include escalation, starting with high-efficacy DMT, and treating to target.
- Selection of DMT and treatment strategy is dependent on the patient's preferences, their disease course, comorbidities, response to therapy, and safety/tolerability of the medication.
- Recommended monitoring while on DMT includes clinical follow-up every 3 to 6 months and MRI 6 to 12 months after starting therapy.
- More research is needed to help establish guidelines for appropriately stopping DMT.

INTRODUCTION

Relapsing remitting multiple sclerosis (RRMS) comprises approximately 85% to 90% of MS cases at diagnosis (1). It is a chronic disease characterized by periodic relapses (also called attacks or exacerbations) that represent new focal inflammatory disease activity. The rate of relapse varies among patients, as does the degree of recovery. As a result, patients can accumulate neurologic disability over time from incomplete recovery from relapses or transition to secondary progressive MS (SPMS). Therefore, the current approach to RRMS treatment involves management of relapses, prevention of relapses via disease-modifying therapy (DMT), and symptomatic management.

Over the past several years, there have been significant advances in DMT development and treatment strategies. Over a dozen approved MS DMTs have diverse mechanisms of action, potency, safety profiles, and usage considerations that must be taken into account with DMT selection and ongoing management. This chapter presents an overview of these medications, highlighting important differences among them that affect the settings in

which they should be used. Refer to Chapters 13 and 14 for discussion of mechanism of action, efficacy, safety, and practical aspects of use in more detail.

CONCEPTS OF MS DISEASE MANAGEMENT

Goals of DMT

Institution of MS DMTs has both short- and long-term therapeutic goals. The short-term goals include prevention of relapses and MRI lesion activity. The long-term goals include prevention of disability worsening and transition to secondary progressive disease. The anticipated benefits must be weighed against potential side effects and safety concerns. Individual patients have different priorities.

Early Treatment Initiation

It is increasingly accepted that early treatment of RRMS is important to prevent ongoing inflammation and relapses (2,3). In the early stages, MS inflammation and tissue damage tends to be subclinical with relatively preserved compensatory and recovery mechanisms (4–6). Longitudinal studies suggest that the development of new MRI lesions exceeds the incidence of clinical relapses by up to 10 times (2,7). Additionally, studies have demonstrated that patients in the early stages of disease can have brain atrophy and cortical lesions (though the latter are not detected on traditional MRI) (8). This early destruction often portends worse prognosis, as the patient's clinical disease course begins with an already lowered neurological reserve and decreased ability to compensate or recover from subsequent relapses.

As a result, there is increased risk of evolution to a secondary progressive course with ongoing, untreated inflammatory disease. The concept of a "therapeutic window" has been proposed, where inflammatory activity predominantly occurs early in the disease course and is, therefore, most amenable to DMT. Studies have suggested that this therapeutic window closes when degenerative activity becomes an important driver of disability, namely when patients reach an Expanded Disability Status Scale (EDSS) of 3.0 (moderate disability) (6,9). The inflammatory activity of MS tends to decrease as neurodegeneration increases over time, making the DMTs less effective later in the disease course (10–12).

Prognosis in MS

Disease severity in MS varies significantly from patient to patient and can range from fulminant to what is referred to as "benign MS." Patients can present with fulminant or aggressive disease, requiring high-potency medications to rapidly control the inflammatory disease activity. Alternatively, patients can have relatively infrequent relapses and slow or no disability accrual. It is nearly impossible to predict an individual patient's prognosis early in the disease. However, patients who present with certain prognostic indicators may have a worse long-term course and therefore should have more aggressive initial treatment. Poor prognostic indicators include high posterior fossa or spinal cord lesion burden on MRI, overall high either T2 or gadolinium-enhancing lesion burden on MRI, or frequent relapses with incomplete recovery (13).

Most patients with MS accumulate disability and evolve to a SPMS course, but multiple studies demonstrate that patients treated with DMT have substantially decreased risk of conversion to SPMS compared to patients in the pre-DMT era (14,15). Based on this information, early DMT initiation should be the default approach in most patients with relapsing forms of MS and those with active inflammation, but it may be reasonable to postpone DMT in some patients with very mild disease or based on patient preference. However, the clinician needs to continue monitoring such patients and remain vigilant for indications of ongoing disease activity. There are few patients who ultimately prove to have benign MS, but they cannot be reliably identified early. Moreover, patients who have a mild course in terms of physical disability can experience cognitive impairment, which can be extremely disabling in some cases (2,16,17).

Current Treatment Strategies

The concept of treat to target was recently introduced as a treatment approach in MS, but is often utilized for the management of rheumatologic diseases (9,18). Treat to target refers to establishment of a predefined goal, or target, for treatment, along with a monitoring plan and criteria for changing or stopping DMT. We recommend utilizing this approach for all patients.

Two potential strategies employed in the treat-to-target approach include escalation and early treatment with high-potency medication. Escalation is the classic treatment paradigm in MS. It refers to initiating a safe, but generally less efficacious, DMT in order to reduce long-term safety concerns. In this strategy, patients transition over time to more potent and potentially less safe medications as needed for breakthrough disease activity, also called inadequate treatment response. Although this approach is appealing from a safety perspective, the strategy can delay the time to achieve optimal control of inflammatory disease activity, therefore subjecting patients to risk of ongoing relapses, tissue injury, and disability worsening.

Early treatment with high-efficacy medications involves utilizing more potent medication, which previously were considered second- or even third-line, early in the DMT sequence. Although safety concerns may arise with the use of high-potency medications, this strategy is gaining popularity due to increasing focus of early, effective control of inflammatory disease. Some clinicians utilize this approach for patients with highly active disease at presentation to rapidly achieve control of inflammation. It is important to note that this strategy of starting with high-efficacy medications is often erroneously referred to as "induction"; induction generally refers to use of DMTs with prolonged effects (such as alemtuzumab and mitoxantrone), which are then followed by a safer and less potent maintenance therapy.

Several criteria have been proposed as targets in a treat to target approach: no evidence of disease activity (NEDA), the Rio Score, and the modified Rio Score (9). The concept of NEDA emerged following a post hoc analysis of the AFFIRM trial of natalizumab and was originally referred to as "disease activity free status" (19). This term evolved over time to NEDA3, indicating the absence of: (a) relapses, (b) confirmed disability worsening on EDSS, and (c) MRI lesion activity. Due to its focus on inflammatory components of MS, NEDA3 does not include brain atrophy, an important correlate of cognitive disability and neurodegeneration which also contribute to disease progression (20,21). Recent work suggests addition of brain atrophy as a fourth dimension to NEDA, thus creating

NEDA4 (22). NEDA4's added focus of neurodegeneration may better capture this element of disease progression, but may be difficult to achieve since MS DMTs are primarily focused on reducing inflammatory activity. NEDA3 is an attractive candidate for a treatment target, but is considered stringent and somewhat difficult to achieve in clinical practice, potentially leading to excessive rates of "treatment failures" and DMT switching.

The Rio and modified Rio Scores were developed in 2008 and 2012, respectively, in a cohort of patients receiving interferon-beta (23–26). These scores integrate clinical and MRI data, with the intention of predicting suboptimal response to interferon-beta. The modified Rio Score differed from the original Rio Score in terms of MRI lesion and relapse scoring. Based on these scores, patients are categorized as responders or nonresponders. Patients can receive an indeterminate modified Rio Score, prompting repeat evaluation at 6 months. If within those 6 months the patient experienced a relapse or had more than one new MRI lesion, they were considered nonresponders (25).

Although the original and modified Rio Scores can provide a useful framework for determining suboptimal response to DMT, NEDA is a more popular treat to target goal. The Rio Scores are less stringent than NEDA, were only validated in patients receiving interferon-beta, and do not adequately reflect the degree to which MS experts are aiming to control disease activity in MS. In terms of the NEDA construct, NEDA3 does not entirely capture ongoing neurodegenerative pathology, making NEDA4 more attractive conceptually. However, NEDA4 may be difficult to implement in clinical practice because DMTs are primarily designed to prevent inflammatory activity, and brain atrophy determination is not available in most clinical centers. NEDA4 may therefore be more applicable in the research setting.

Other Factors in DMT Selection

When selecting an initial DMT for an individual patient, there are several additional factors to consider in addition to safety and potency.

COMORBIDITIES

If a patient has a history of malignancy, it is generally advisable to avoid immunosuppression. Patients with gastrointestinal disorders or chronic gastrointestinal complaints should generally avoid dimethyl fumarate given the relatively high rate of diarrhea and abdominal pain. As diabetes is a known independent risk factor for macular edema, fingolimod should be used with caution in diabetics (27). Patients with cardiac disease should avoid fingolimod given its propensity to affect cardiac rate and conduction. Interferon-beta is associated with incident or worsening depression, and should not be prescribed to patients with preexisting, treatment-resistant mood disorders. Patients with preexisting liver disease should avoid DMTs that can cause hepatotoxicity, including interferon-beta, natalizumab, fingolimod, and teriflunomide. Specifically,

patients at risk of hepatitis B reactivation should not receive ocrelizumab.

Other practical considerations regarding comorbidities involve route of DMT administration. If a patient is significantly underweight, he or she may have difficulty with injections so other routes of administration should be considered. Intramuscular injections are contraindicated in patients requiring therapeutic anticoagulation. Patients who have undergone bariatric surgery may have inadequate absorption of oral medications, though additional research is needed to better characterize absorption of oral DMTs (28).

AGE

A patient's age is also a major consideration in DMT selection. Older patients have higher potential for decreased overall DMT tolerability, so the benefits of treatment should outweigh the risks of DMT use in this setting (29). For example, older patients are at higher risk of lymphopenia associated with dimethyl fumarate use (30). Regarding pediatric MS, data from controlled clinical trials are limited but a recent Phase III randomized controlled trial reported significant relapse rate reduction associated with fingolimod use in a pediatric population; the observed safety profile was similar to that seen in adults as well (31,32). However, the general approach to treatment is based on extrapolation from clinical trials in adults, as well as expert consensus (33). Generally, interferon-beta and glatiramer acetate are considered first-line therapies, and natalizumab is considered for highly active disease. Ongoing studies of fingolimod, dimethyl fumarate, and teriflunomide in the pediatric MS population will help guide their use in this patient population (33).

JC VIRUS ANTIBODY STATUS

Progressive multifocal leukoencephalopathy (PML) is a potentially fatal infection of the central nervous system caused by the John Cunningham (JC) virus. As a result of the potential PML risk, natalizumab is administered in the United States via a Risk Evaluation and Mitigation Strategies (REMS) program called MS TOUCH. Additionally, recommended clinical monitoring for PML while on natalizumab includes brain MRI and JC virus antibody testing every 6 months. The JC virus antibody test is commonly positive, as a high proportion of the general population has been exposed to the virus. Reports of seropositivity prevalence range from 31% to 91%, with a recent multinational study of MS patients reporting a prevalence of 57.1% (34). Based on the accumulating experience, the MS TOUCH program provides risk estimates for PML taking into account a patient's JC virus antibody titer, duration of exposure to natalizumab, and prior exposure to immunosuppression (35). Clinicians should test a patient's JC virus status when considering natalizumab and discuss with the patient the risks of PML versus the benefits of this highly potent medication. When a patient is seropositive for JC virus and other DMT options are available, natalizumab is generally avoided. Patients who seroconvert to become JC seropositive are usually switched to another therapy.

PML is a particular concern with natalizumab but is also rarely associated with dimethyl fumarate and fingolimod use. There is also a potential risk of PML with ocrelizumab, as there are reports of PML in rheumatologic and oncologic patients receiving rituximab, another anti-CD20 monoclonal antibody (36,37). It is, therefore, important for clinicians to remain vigilant for signs of PML while on these agents. Prolonged lymphopenia in the setting of dimethyl fumarate may be associated with higher PML risk, though some patients who developed PML while on dimethyl fumarate did not have severe lymphopenia (38). Additionally, rare cases of PML have been reported in patients taking fingolimod, although severe lymphopenia is not a risk factor for PML with fingolimod. The PML risk stratification via JC virus antibody titer is not established for these medications, so it is difficult to provide a patient with a precise PML risk estimate in the setting of a positive JC virus titer when starting fingolimod or dimethyl fumarate. Currently, the estimated risk of PML with dimethyl fumarate is about 1/50,000, and with fingolimod is 1/18,000 (39).

Monitoring While on DMT

Appropriate assessment of DMT effectiveness and safety involves evaluation of both clinical and radiographic parameters, in addition to medication-specific laboratory monitoring (Table 11.1). Monitoring is important to evaluate for inadequate treatment response, which may indicate need to change DMT. Inadequate treatment response is often defined clinically as relapses or disability worsening, and radiographically as new lesions (either T2 hyperintensities or gadolinium enhancing) on MRI.

No generally accepted guidelines for monitoring exist. Clinical monitoring is usually indicated every 3 to 6 months initially after starting a new DMT, which should include evaluation for effectiveness, as well as safety and

TABLE 11.1 Suggested Monitoring Guidelines for Patients With RRMS

MEASURE	TIMING
MRI brain +/- cervical spine	Baseline 6 months after starting DMT Every 12 months thereafter
Interval history	Every 3 to 6 months
Neurological assessment Targeted neurological examination Quantitative measures (EDSS, MSFC)	Every 6 months, or when feasible
DMT-specific laboratory evaluation	As recommended for each DMT

DMT, disease-modifying therapy; EDSS, Expanded Disability Status Scale; MSFC, Multiple Sclerosis Functional Composite; RRMS, relapsing remitting multiple sclerosis.

tolerability. Regarding DMT effectiveness, a clinician should evaluate for the presence of new symptoms, relapse, or disability worsening. Quantitative measures of neurological performance are also integral to ongoing assessment of DMT effectiveness in the clinical setting. Such quantitative measures include the EDSS (40) and the Multiple Sclerosis Functional Composite (MSFC). The MSFC originally included the 9-Hole Peg Test, Timed 25-Foot Walk, and Paced Auditory Serial Addition Test (PASAT) (41). Recent expert consensus proposed substituting the PASAT with the symbol digit modalities test improves evaluation of information processing speed (42). The same group also recommended adding the Sloan low contrast letter acuity test to assess vision.

Assessment of medication safety and tolerability includes querying a patient for medication side effects and compliance. Another important element of this safety monitoring includes DMT-specific laboratory testing, which often includes routine bloodwork (i.e., complete blood count and hepatic function panel).

Disease activity on MRI tends to exceed that of clinical relapses, so regular MRI monitoring is important particularly in the early stages of disease (43). MRI should be performed as a baseline at the time of starting a new DMT, followed by an MRI approximately 6 months later then annually. More or less frequent MRIs may be appropriate depending on the patient's prior level of disease activity. Ocular Coherence Tomography (OCT) is another modality that is gaining popularity as an imaging biomarker for usage in MS, although its place in the routine monitoring of patients and their response to DMT is not yet established (44).

Another consideration in management of some DMTs is that of neutralizing antibodies. Interferon-beta and the monoclonal antibodies, specifically natalizumab, can stimulate formation of neutralizing antibodies, potentially affecting the pharmacokinetics and effectiveness of the DMT. Neutralizing antibodies to interferon-beta are often checked routinely after 1 year, and natalizumab after 6 months of treatment. If neutralizing antibodies are present, switching DMT is warranted. If a patient has a relapse or another indication of disease activity while on interferon-beta or natalizumab, neutralizing antibodies should be checked as well. The clinical relevance of neutralizing antibodies to alemtuzumab, rituximab, and ocrelizumab is less clear.

Changing DMT

Formal guidelines for changing DMTs are not yet established. The decision to change from one DMT to another involves multiple considerations and should be based on the treatment strategy or paradigm that is decided upon by the patient and clinician. Changing DMT is a highly individualized decision that will vary from patient to patient, and as a result it is important to discuss both objective evidence and patient preferences in this setting.

Additionally, a clinician should integrate information regarding clinical and radiographic effectiveness and tolerability of a medication.

If a patient reports experiencing side effects despite well-controlled disease activity, a clinician should first consider available side effect mitigation strategies (e.g., NSAIDs for constitutional side effects of interferon-beta, aspirin for flushing from dimethyl fumarate) if possible. There are situations where DMT side effects significantly reduce tolerability and medication compliance, resulting in treatment discontinuation and subsequent change in DMT. A change in DMT due to side effects does not necessarily need to be to a more potent medication. However, the new DMT should have a different route, mechanism of action, and safety profile than the first DMT in order to avoid ongoing tolerability issues.

Inadequate treatment response is the other major reason why patients change DMT. If clinical or radiographic disease activity is observed, a clinician should first confirm compliance with the medication. If a patient reports compliance, DMT typically should be changed to either a more potent agent or one with a different mechanism of action.

Another issue that arises with changing DMT is the trade-off between preserving efficacy and avoiding combined toxicity during the transition from one DMT to another. Generally, changing to and from the injectable therapies (interferon-beta and glatiramer acetate) is safe and does not require a washout period. When considering increasingly potent therapies, more complicated situations arise for which there is no currently available evidence to guide management. The duration of a washout period is a compromise between balancing safety concerns, specifically infection in the setting of immunosuppression, and the risk of disease activity. In general, 2 to 3 months is considered as an adequate washout period, but should be shorter (1–2 months) in patients with highly active disease. If a patient is changing DMT due to inadequate treatment response, a prolonged washout period will increase that breakthrough disease activity risk even more so. The suggested washout period length is also affected by the presence and severity of lymphopenia, but this is considered on an individual patient basis. This balance between safety and preventing disease activity should be thoughtfully considered.

Stopping DMT

Generally, there are two scenarios in which stopping DMT is considered. The first is older patients, generally over the age of 55 years, with clinical and radiographic stability for over 3 to 5 years. The other scenario where a clinician could consider stopping DMT is in an older patient with secondary progressive disease, specifically continued disability progression despite stable disease on MRI. The impetus for DMT discontinuation is even higher in either of these scenarios if a patient is experiencing side effects from the DMT or having financial difficulty paying for the DMT. No widely accepted guidelines have been established, but research to address this question is ongoing.

DISEASE MODIFYING THERAPIES FOR RRMS

Mechanisms of Action

DMTs have diverse mechanisms of action and resultant effects on the immune system. The major categories of DMT mechanisms of action include immunomodulation, alteration of cell trafficking, and cell depletion (Table 11.2). However, it is important to note that the precise therapeutic mechanism of action is not fully understood for any MS DMT. Although the category does not necessarily correlate with potency, it is important that clinicians be familiar with mechanisms of action of these highly specialized immunotherapies in order to make informed decisions regarding DMT transitions. For example, one should carefully consider the timing of transitioning to a cell-depleting therapy following fingolimod, as the lymphocytes targeted by cell depletion are sequestered within lymph nodes and may not be effectively depleted. When changing a patient's DMT due to inadequate treatment response, a clinician should consider a DMT with a different mechanism of action.

Immunomodulation refers to a drug that has effects on immune function, but does not cause general immunosuppression. Immunomodulatory therapies for MS include interferon-beta (interferon-beta-1b subcutaneous injection [Betaseron and Extavia], interferon-beta-1a intramuscular injection [Avonex], interferon-beta-1a subcutaneous injection [Rebif], and pegylated interferon-beta-1a subcutaneous injection [Plegridy]), glatiramer acetate (Copaxone and Glatopa), and dimethyl fumarate (Tecfidera).

Interferon-beta is thought to cause a shift in cytokine expression from a pro-inflammatory to an anti-inflammatory profile, among other mechanisms described in Table 11.2 (45). Glatiramer acetate was originally developed as an immunologic mimic of myelin basic protein, but now is thought to function as an altered ligand for major histocompatibility complex (MHC) Class II molecules, therefore inhibiting T-lymphocyte activation and inducing T-regulatory lymphocytes (46). Dimethyl fumarate activates the nuclear factor (erythroid-derived 2)-like 2 pathway, which is involved in oxidative stress responses and immune function (47).

DMTs in the second category interfere with trafficking of lymphocytes. Natalizumab (Tysabri) is a monoclonal antibody targeting alpha-4 integrin, a molecule expressed on lymphocytes. Binding of natalizumab prevents interaction between alpha-4 integrin and vascular cell adhesion molecule-1 expressed on vascular

TABLE 11.2 DMT Mechanisms of Action

CATEGORY	MEDICATION	SPECIFIC MECHANISM OF ACTION
Immunomodulation	Dimethyl fumarate (Tecfidera)	Activates nuclear factor (erythroid-derived 2)-like 2 pathway, which is involved in response to oxidative stress
	Glatiramer acetate (Copaxone, Glatopa)	Random synthetic polypeptides, originally intended to be immunologic mimic of myelin basic protein Altered ligand for MHC II molecules Inhibits T-lymphocyte activation and induces regulatory cells when presented to T lymphocytes (46)
	Interferon-beta (Avonex, Rebif, Betaseron, Extavia, Plegridy)	Shifts profile of cytokine expression from Th1 (pro-inflammatory) to Th2 (anti-inflammatory) Modulates B- and T-lymphocyte function Decreases matrix metalloproteinases, reducing blood–brain barrier disruption (45,62)
Interference with cell trafficking	Fingolimod (Gilenya)	Sphingosine-1-phosphate receptor modulator Prevents lymphocyte egress from lymph nodes (49)
	Natalizumab (Tysabri)	Binds alpha-4-integrin, blocking interaction with vascular cell-adhesion molecule-1 Inhibits lymphocyte migration into the central nervous system (48)
Cell depletion	Alemtuzumab (Lemtrada)	Anti-CD52 monoclonal antibody Antibody-dependent lysis of B and T lymphocytes
	Mitoxantrone (Novantrone)	Anthracenedione-based chemotherapeutic agent Intercalates into DNA, interferes with DNA repair, RNA synthesis resulting in cell cycle arrest Impairs B lymphocyte, T lymphocyte, and macrophage proliferation
	Ocrelizumab (Ocrevus)	Anti-CD20 monoclonal antibody Depletes B lymphocytes
	Teriflunomide (Aubagio)	Inhibits mitochondrial dihydroorotate dehydrogenase and therefore interferes with pyrimidine synthesis Results in reduced proliferation of activated T and B lymphocytes (50)

DMT, disease-modifying therapy.

endothelial cells. As a result, lymphocytes are not able to traverse the blood–brain barrier (48). Fingolimod (Gilenya) down-modulates sphingosine-1-phosphate receptors, inhibiting lymphocyte egress from lymph nodes (49).

Finally, several DMTs function via depleting certain cell populations, including mitoxantrone (Novantrone), teriflunomide (Aubagio), alemtuzumab (Lemtrada), and ocrelizumab (Ocrevus). Mitoxantrone interferes with RNA synthesis and subsequent proliferation of B lymphocytes, T lymphocytes, and macrophages. Teriflunomide inhibits mitochondrial dihydroorotate dehydrogenase and subsequently interferes with pyrimidine synthesis, resulting in reduced proliferation of activated T and B lymphocytes (50). Alemtuzumab is a monoclonal antibody that binds to CD52, a cell surface molecule found on lymphocytes and several other cells of the immune system, resulting in their destruction via antibody- and complement-mediated cytolysis (51). In addition to its cell-depleting effects, the prolonged benefit observed with use of alemtuzumab is likely due to immune reconstitution with a more regulatory, rather than inflammatory, profile (52). Ocrelizumab is an anti-CD20 monoclonal antibody that depletes B lymphocytes (53).

Administration

DMTs for MS are administered via injectable (subcutaneous or intramuscular), oral, or intravenous (IV) routes. Injectable medications include interferon-beta (subcutaneous or intramuscular) and glatiramer acetate (subcutaneous). Oral medications include dimethyl fumarate, fingolimod, and teriflunomide. The IV DMTs include ocrelizumab, natalizumab, mitoxantrone, and alemtuzumab. Mode of administration is an important issue for some patients. Clinicians should incorporate the different routes of administration into their discussions with patients about DMT selection, as patients may have preferences in this regard.

Potency

The approved DMTs have a broad range of potency and, therefore, vary in their role in the management of MS (54). It may be misleading to compare efficacy of DMTs across clinical trials, and few formal head to head comparisons exist. Therefore, clinicians must be cautious in interpretation of the literature and extrapolating relative effectiveness from clinical trial data. With this important caveat,

DMTs considered to be high potency include natalizumab, alemtuzumab, mitoxantrone, and ocrelizumab. Interferon-beta, glatiramer acetate, and teriflunomide are considered lower potency (29). Fingolimod and dimethyl fumarate, are thought to have intermediate potency.

Potency is an important consideration in selecting a DMT, as increased potency tends to be accompanied by increased safety issues. Depending upon the approach to treatment, discussed earlier in this chapter, clinicians should take potency into account with a patient's disease severity and preferences. It is important to determine whether a higher potency drug is warranted given the increased risk sometimes associated with its use.

Onset of Action

Overall, the kinetics of onset of action and reaching full potency are not known precisely for any agent. Biologic effects can be seen very early for all DMTs, particularly high-potency agents, but it generally takes several months or more for their therapeutic benefit to fully manifest. Patients presenting with aggressive disease warrant prompt control of inflammatory disease activity. In such cases, a clinician should consider a high-potency DMT, temporary benefit from a course of corticosteroids, and early MRI to confirm disease control.

Safety

Safety is another important consideration when selecting a DMT, for both patients and clinicians. Safety concerns that occur with certain DMTs include laboratory abnormalities (i.e., cytopenias or liver enzyme elevation), infections, and other conditions specific for certain DMTs. For example, lymphopenia can be a side effect of interferon-beta and dimethyl fumarate. Fingolimod results in lymphopenia as well, but this is an expected effect due to its mechanism of lymphocyte sequestration. Liver enzyme elevation can be observed with use of interferon-beta, dimethyl fumarate, fingolimod, teriflunomide, and natalizumab. Appropriate, medication-specific laboratory monitoring while on DMTs is extremely important for many DMTs and should be discussed at the time of DMT initiation.

In general, increased drug potency is accompanied by increased safety issues. Examples of major safety concerns that have arisen in the setting of potent DMT use include PML with several agents but particularly natalizumab, secondary autoimmune phenomena with alemtuzumab, and infections with various DMTs.

Tolerability

The major characteristics of DMTs that contribute to tolerability are route of administration and side effects. Some patients may be averse to self-injection and therefore oral or IV options should be considered. DMTs have specific anticipated side effects, which should be discussed prior to initiation. For example, interferon-beta can cause flu-like symptoms, which can be quite problematic for some patients but can be mitigated with nonsteroidal anti-inflammatory drug administration prior to injection. Dimethyl fumarate can cause flushing, abdominal pain, or diarrhea that can adversely affect its tolerability as well. Other specific DMT side effects are discussed in detail in Chapters 13 and 14. Tolerability is an important factor in patient compliance with DMTs, another major element of MS management.

Convenience

The DMTs have various degrees of convenience to patients. Oral medications are often considered the most convenient from the patient perspective. For some patients, infrequent infusion also is attractive, particularly given the essentially ensured compliance with such regimens. However, patients who live in rural areas may have limited accessibility to a specialized infusion center. Patients with full-time employment may also have difficulty regularly taking time off from work for an infusion. Other considerations include the need to refrigerate many of the injectable medications, which can impair a patient's ability to travel or participate in other activities.

Cost and Access

The cost of each MS DMT is very high, and has risen over time out of proportion to inflation (55). The average annual cost for an MS DMT was over $54,000 in 2013, and continues to increase (56). The MS DMTs do not have a significant cost differential that affects utilization in the clinical setting. However, a patient's insurance status often affects the choice of DMT. Based upon contractual arrangements (and not necessarily clinical reasons), many insurers have preferred algorithms for the order of DMT prescribed. Providers often must submit an appeal to prescribe medications that do not align with the sequence. Importantly, many of the pharmaceutical companies offer co-pay assistance or free drug programs, which can be very helpful in patients who are under-insured or completely uninsured.

Long-Term Experience

Generally, interferon-beta and glatiramer acetate are perceived as the safest medications, which in part arises from long-term experience with them. They were first approved in the 1990s, allowing an almost 30-year longitudinal experience with both short- and long-term safety issues. As a result, clinicians can generally assure patients that these medications are safe long-term and do not result in significant adverse health effects, although almost all of them still require clinical and laboratory monitoring.

Conversely, the newer medications do not have as much information available regarding long-term safety. In general, the potential long-term concerns with immunosuppression include malignancy and infection. The recently approved DMTs will require longer term postmarketing surveillance to better establish a long-term safety record. This unknown long-term safety may influence a patient's decision to go on a newer DMT, and such patients may opt for interferon-beta or glatiramer acetate instead.

Reproductive Attributes

MS is a chronic disease that often affects women of childbearing age. Therefore, clinicians and patients should discuss reproductive plans and potential implications on choice of DMT. In general, no currently available DMT is advisable in the setting of pregnancy or breastfeeding. However, glatiramer acetate is considered the safest DMT in pregnancy, with a pregnancy category B rating in the prior Food and Drug Administration (FDA) system. Interferon-beta, dimethyl fumarate, fingolimod, alemtuzumab, and natalizumab are all category C. Mitoxantrone is category D, and teriflunomide is pregnancy category X (57). Ocrelizumab has not been assigned a pregnancy category.

Given the potential for teratogenicity and other reproductive effects, effective contraceptive strategies and family planning should be discussed with patients prior to starting a DMT and readdressed during treatment with DMT.

Additional consideration should be given when selecting a DMT for women of childbearing potential. For example, prescription of teriflunomide in this patient population is complicated given its high risk of teratogenicity and extremely long half-life. It is advisable for men taking teriflunomide also to practice contraception, as the drug is present in semen (57).

CONCLUSIONS

Over the past 20 years, over a dozen medications have received regulatory approval for MS. These immunotherapies have diverse mechanisms of action and properties that affect the settings in which they should be used. Given the advancements made thus far, we anticipate ongoing success with more stringent control of MS disease activity over time.

Treatment for relapsing forms of MS should begin as early as possible to prevent ongoing inflammation and resultant accumulation of tissue damage and disability. Several paradigms for treatment exist, with the goal to prevent clinical relapses, new lesions on MRI, and progressive disability. It is unclear whether this goal is best accomplished via gradual escalation in therapy intensity or starting with highly effective therapy. Clinicians should discuss the goals of therapy and DMT initiation decisions with patients to set clear expectations and elicit ongoing feedback regarding patient preferences. Regular laboratory, clinical, and radiographic monitoring are extremely important for patients on DMT. Guidelines for changing and stopping DMT are not yet clearly established, and these decisions are complicated and need to be tailored to the individual clinical situation.

PATIENT CASE An otherwise healthy 28-year-old woman with recently diagnosed relapsing remitting MS comes to clinic to establish care and discuss DMT initiation. She originally presented with left optic neuritis, and MRI revealed four gadolinium-enhancing lesions, as well as a mild to moderate burden of T2 hyperintense lesions in her brain and cervical spine. Lumbar puncture was notable for the presence of nine unique cerebrospinal fluid oligoclonal bands, and blood tests for potential MS mimics were negative.

What initial DMT do you recommend? What elements of a treatment strategy are important to discuss with the patient?

Given her presentation with high inflammatory activity, indicated by her gadolinium enhancing lesion burden on MRI, early and highly efficacious DMT initiation is warranted. It is important to discuss appropriate targets for treatment with the patient, as well as the need to control the inflammatory component of her disease. The clinician also should ask about her preferences regarding an acceptable drug safety profile and route of administration. We would elect to start her on a higher potency agent given her relatively high MRI lesion burden and lesion activity at presentation.

The clinician has a conversation with her regarding treatment strategy, and she is concerned about the number of lesions already on her brain MRI. After a discussion of potential targets, she and her neurologist

(continued)

(continued)

decide on NEDA3 as her treatment goal. The options of natalizumab, ocrelizumab, dimethyl fumarate, and fingolimod were discussed. She opted to initiate therapy with fingolimod due to safety and convenience preferences, as well as a history of intermittent diarrhea that may reduce tolerability of dimethyl fumarate. She is scheduled for a 3-month follow-up clinic visit and 6-month follow-up MRI.

She completes the necessary screening and starts fingolimod. At the 3-month visit, the medication is well tolerated. She reports compliance with fingolimod, and her laboratory monitoring demonstrates expected lymphopenia. A hepatic function panel and OCT are normal. At the 6-month visit, she again is tolerating fingolimod without side effects and denies any clinical changes or symptoms of relapse. Brain MRI, however, demonstrates three new gadolinium-enhancing lesions.

What do you do at this point?

Given her ongoing lesion activity on MRI despite 6 months of consistent fingolimod therapy, changing DMT is recommended based on the NEDA3 goal. A clinician should then discuss the options of natalizumab and ocrelizumab, and obtain a JC virus antibody titer to help guide this decision.

She is JC virus antibody negative, and opts to start natalizumab. How should the transition from fingolimod to natalizumab be conducted?

Unfortunately, no guidelines exist to assist in this decision regarding the optimal washout period. A longer washout period length increases theoretical safety concerns from an immunosuppression and infection standpoint, but the patient will be at risk for further disease activity and/or rebound. Given the fact that she is JC virus negative, as well as the respective mechanisms of action of fingolimod and natalizumab, there is not a clear indication for a washout period in this transition.

She tolerates the monthly natalizumab infusions well, and follow-up brain MRI after 6 months does not show any gadolinium-enhancing lesions or new T2 hyperintense lesions. She is again JC virus seronegative. Following 1 year of therapy with natalizumab, monitoring brain MRI again appears stable. However, JC virus antibody has become positive, with an index value of 1.8, and this is confirmed 1 month later.

What do you do now?

At this point, her persistently positive JC virus antibody in the setting of less than 24 months of natalizumab exposure and no prior immunosuppression, her risk of PML is estimated to be less than 1/1,000; this risk increases to 3/1,000 after 2 years of therapy (35). With her high JC virus antibody index (>1.5), her risk of PML is closer to 1/1,000, and if the index remains high, her risk will increase to 8.1/1,000 after 24 months of therapy (58). A change in therapy is therefore indicated at this point, and a reasonable option would be ocrelizumab, another highly potent medication with lower PML risk. However, if needed, she could remain on natalizumab for up to 2 years with minimal increase in her PML risk. It is currently unclear whether prior use of intermediate- to high-potency MS DMTs, such as dimethyl fumarate and fingolimod, increases the risk of natalizumab-associated PML. Due to concern regarding PML, the patient opted to change to ocrelizumab.

She transitioned to ocrelizumab after appropriate screening. Again, discussion regarding the appropriate washout period is warranted. Based upon studies of natalizumab discontinuation, the highest risk for recurrence or rebound of disease activity occurs after 8 weeks post-treatment discontinuation (59–61). Therefore, a 1- to 2-month washout period following her last infusion of natalizumab is recommended before starting ocrelizumab. Given her JC virus seropositivity and previous highly active disease, close MRI monitoring at the time of changing therapy and at 3 months is warranted as well.

Follow-up brain MRIs at 3 and 6 months remained stable, without any new or gadolinium-enhancing lesions, or findings concerning for PML. She denied any symptoms suggestive of relapse. Therefore, she continued on ocrelizumab.

KEY POINTS FOR PATIENTS AND FAMILIES

- There are three major parts to the management of MS;
  - Treatment of relapses
  - Prevention of disease activity (relapses or new MRI lesions)
  - Management of symptoms (via wellness, other medications, and other allied health services [rehabilitation, psychology, etc.])
- DMTs for MS are designed to prevent further disease activity, and do not directly restore function or improve symptoms;
- DMTs should be started early to prevent future relapses, disease activity, and disability worsening over time;
- It is important to discuss dosing, route of administration, and potential side effects with your provider when selecting a DMT;
- Several strategies for MS DMT management exist, including whether to start on a stronger medication initially or to escalate as needed over time in response to disease activity. You should discuss these strategies with your provider when starting a DMT;
- After starting a DMT, monitoring for its effectiveness involves both regular clinical (office visits) and imaging (MRI) evaluations. Most DMTs also require regular bloodwork for safety monitoring;
- If disease activity continues while on a DMT, you and your provider should discuss whether changing to a different DMT is indicated and which medications are appropriate options

REFERENCES

1. Lublin FD, Reingold SC, Cohen JA, et al. Defining the clinical course of multiple sclerosis: the 2013 revisions. *Neurology.* 2014;83(3):278–286.
2. MS Coalition. *The Use of Disease-Modifying Therapies in Multiple Sclerosis: Principles and Current Evidence.* 2017. Available at: http://www.nationalmssociety.org/getmedia/5ca284d3-fc7c-4ba5-b005-ab537d495c3c/DMT_Consensus_MS_Coalition_color
3. Merkel B, Butzkueven H, Traboulsee AL, et al. Timing of high-efficacy therapy in relapsing-remitting multiple sclerosis: a systematic review. *Autoimmun Rev.* 2017;16(6):658–665.
4. Gallo A, Rovaris M, Riva R, et al. Diffusion-tensor magnetic resonance imaging detects normal-appearing white matter damage unrelated to short-term disease activity in patients at the earliest clinical stage of multiple sclerosis. *Arch Neurol.* 2005;62(5):803–808.
5. Rovaris M, Gambini A, Gallo A, et al. Axonal injury in early multiple sclerosis is irreversible and independent of the short-term disease evolution. *Neurology.* 2005;65(10):1626–1630.
6. Confavreux C, Vukusic S, Adeleine P. Early clinical predictors and progression of irreversible disability in multiple sclerosis: an amnesic process. *Brain.* 2003;126(pt 4):770–782.
7. McFarland HF, Frank JA, Albert PS, et al. Using gadolinium-enhanced magnetic resonance imaging lesions to monitor disease activity in multiple sclerosis. *Ann Neurol.* 1992;32(6):758–766.
8. Dalton CM, Chard DT, Davies GR, et al. Early development of multiple sclerosis is associated with progressive grey matter atrophy in patients presenting with clinically isolated syndromes. *Brain.* 2004;127(pt 5):1101–1107.
9. Smith AL, Cohen JA, Hua LH. Therapeutic targets for multiple sclerosis: current treatment goals and future directions. *Neurotherapeutics.* 2017;14(4):952–960.
10. Frischer JM, Bramow S, Dal-Bianco A, et al. The relation between inflammation and neurodegeneration in multiple sclerosis brains. *Brain.* 2009;132(pt 5):1175–1189.
11. Bruck W, Stadelmann C. Inflammation and degeneration in multiple sclerosis. *Neurol Sci.* 2003;24(suppl 5):S265–267.
12. Leray E, Yaouanq J, Le Page E, et al. Evidence for a two-stage disability progression in multiple sclerosis. *Brain.* 2010;133(pt 7):1900–1913.
13. Rush CA, MacLean HJ, Freedman MS. Aggressive multiple sclerosis: proposed definition and treatment algorithm. *Nat Rev Neurol.* 2015;11(7):379–389.
14. Bergamaschi R, Quaglini S, Tavazzi E, et al. Immunomodulatory therapies delay disease progression in multiple sclerosis. *Mult Scler.* 2016;22(13):1732–1740.
15. Tedeholm H, Lycke J, Skoog B, et al. Time to secondary progression in patients with multiple sclerosis who were treated with first generation immunomodulating drugs. *Mult Scler.* 2013;19(6):765–774.
16. Ramsaransing GS, De Keyser J. Predictive value of clinical characteristics for 'benign' multiple sclerosis. *Eur J Neurol.* 2007;14(8):885–889.
17. Sayao AL, Devonshire V, Tremlett H. Longitudinal follow-up of "benign" multiple sclerosis at 20 years. *Neurology.* 2007;68(7):496–500.
18. Smolen JS. Treat-to-target as an approach in inflammatory arthritis. *Curr Opin Rheumatol.* 2016;28(3):297–302.
19. Havrdova E, Galetta S, Hutchinson M, et al. Effect of natalizumab on clinical and radiological disease activity in multiple sclerosis: a retrospective analysis of the Natalizumab Safety and Efficacy in Relapsing-Remitting Multiple Sclerosis (AFFIRM) study. *Lancet Neurol.* 2009;8(3):254–260.
20. Damasceno A, Damasceno BP, Cendes F. No evidence of disease activity in multiple sclerosis: implications on cognition and brain atrophy. *Mult Scler.* 2016;22(1):64–72.
21. De Stefano N, Airas L, Grigoriadis N, et al. Clinical relevance of brain volume measures in multiple sclerosis. *CNS Drugs.* 2014;28(2):147–156.
22. Kappos L, De Stefano N, Freedman MS, et al. Inclusion of brain volume loss in a revised measure of 'no evidence of disease activity' (NEDA-4) in relapsing-remitting multiple sclerosis. *Mult Scler.* 2016;22(10):1297–1305.

23. Rio J, Castillo J, Rovira A, et al. Measures in the first year of therapy predict the response to interferon beta in MS. *Mult Scler.* 2009;15(7):848–853.

24. Sormani M, Signori A, Stromillo M, et al. Refining response to treatment as defined by the Modified Rio Score. *Mult Scler.* 2013;19:1246–1247.

25. Sormani MP, De Stefano N. Defining and scoring response to IFN-beta in multiple sclerosis. *Nat Rev Neurol.* 2013;9:504–512.

26. Sormani MP, Rio J, Tintore M, et al. Scoring treatment response in patients with relapsing multiple sclerosis. *Mult Scler.* 2013;19(5):605–612.

27. Jain N, Bhatti MT. Fingolimod-associated macular edema: incidence, detection, and management. *Neurology.* 2012;78(9):672–680.

28. Geraldo Mde SP, Fonseca FLA, Gouveia MFV, et al. The use of drugs in patients who have undergone bariatric surgery. *Int J Gen Med.* 2014;7:219–224.

29. Comi G, Radaelli M, Soelberg Sorensen P. Evolving concepts in the treatment of relapsing multiple sclerosis. *Lancet.* 2017;389(10076):1347–1356.

30. Longbrake EE, Naismith RT, Parks BJ, et al. Dimethyl fumarate-associated lymphopenia: risk factors and clinical significance. *Mult Scler J Exp Transl Clin.* January-December 2015;1. pii: 2055217315596994. Epub July 31, 2015.

31. Chitnis T, Arnold DL, Banwell B, et al. PARADIGMS: a randomised double-blind study of fingolimod versus interferon β-1a in paediatric multiple sclerosis [abstract 276]. In: *7th Joint ECTRIMS-ACTRIMS Meeting.* 2017.

32. Novartis landmark Phase III trial shows fingolimod significantly reduces relapses in children and adolescents with MS | Novartis [press release]. September 5, 2017.

33. Narula S, Banwell B. Pediatric demyelination. *Continuum (Minneapolis, Minn).* 2016;22(3):897–915.

34. Bozic C, Subramanyam M, Richman S, et al. Anti-JC virus (JCV) antibody prevalence in the JCV Epidemiology in MS (JEMS) trial. *Eur J Neurol.* 2014;21(2):299–304.

35. Biogen Idec. Tysabri (R) [package insert]. Cambridge, MA: Biogen Idec;2016.

36. Molloy ES, Calabrese LH. Progressive multifocal leukoencephalopathy: a national estimate of frequency in systemic lupus erythematosus and other rheumatic diseases. *Arthritis Rheu.* 2009;60(12):3761–3765.

37. Paues J, Vrethem M. Fatal progressive multifocal leukoencephalopathy in a patient with non-Hodgkin lymphoma treated with rituximab. *J Clin Virol.* 2010;48(4):291–293.

38. Lehmann-Horn K, Penkert H, Grein P, et al. PML during dimethyl fumarate treatment of multiple sclerosis: how does lymphopenia matter? *Neurology.* 2016;87(4):440–441.

39. Berger JR. Classifying PML risk with disease modifying therapies. *Mult Scler Relat Disord.* 2017;12:59–63.

40. Kurtzke JF. Rating neurologic impairment in multiple sclerosis: an expanded disability status scale (EDSS). *Neurology.* 1983;33(11):1444–1452.

41. Fischer JS, Rudick RA, Cutter GR, et al. The Multiple Sclerosis Functional Composite Measure (MSFC): an integrated approach to MS clinical outcome assessment. National MS Society Clinical Outcomes Assessment Task Force. *Mult Scler.* 1999;5(4):244–250.

42. Cohen JA, Reingold SC, Polman CH, et al. Disability outcome measures in multiple sclerosis clinical trials: current status and future prospects. *Lancet Neurol.* 2012;11(5):467–476.

43. Paty DW, Li DK. Interferon beta-lb is effective in relapsing-remitting multiple sclerosis. II. MRI analysis results of a multicenter, randomized, double-blind, placebo-controlled trial. 1993 [classical article]. *Neurology.* 2001;57(12)(suppl 5):S10-15.

44. Brandt AU, Martinez-Lapiscina EH, Nolan R, et al. Monitoring the course of MS with optical coherence tomography. *Curr Treat Options Neurol.* 2017;19(4):15.

45. Dhib-Jalbut S, Marks S. Interferon-beta mechanisms of action in multiple sclerosis. *Neurology.* 2010;74(suppl 1):S17-24.

46. Schrempf W, Ziemssen T. Glatiramer acetate: mechanisms of action in multiple sclerosis. *Autoimmun Rev.* 2007;6(7):469–475.

47. Biogen Idec. Tecfidera (R) [package insert]. Cambridge, MA:Biogen Idec;2017.

48. Ransohoff RM. Natalizumab for multiple sclerosis. *N Engl J Med.* 2007;356(25):2622–2629.

49. Brinkmann V. FTY720 (fingolimod) in multiple sclerosis: therapeutic effects in the immune and the central nervous system. *Br J Pharmacol.* 2009;158(5):1173–1182.

50. Bar-Or A, Pachner A, Menguy-Vacheron F, et al. Teriflunomide and its mechanism of action in multiple sclerosis. *Drugs.* 2014;74(6):659–674.

51. Ruck T, Afzali AM, Lukat KF, et al. ALAIN01--Alemtuzumab in autoimmune inflammatory neurodegeneration: mechanisms of action and neuroprotective potential. *BMC Neurol.* 2016;16:34.

52. Zhang X, Tao Y, Chopra M, et al. Differential reconstitution of T cell subsets following immunodepleting treatment with alemtuzumab (anti-CD52 monoclonal antibody) in patients with relapsing-remitting multiple sclerosis. *J Immunol.* 2013;191(12):5867–5874.

53. Longbrake EE, Cross AH. Effect of multiple sclerosis disease-modifying therapies on B cells and humoral immunity. *JAMA Neurol.* 2016;73(2):219–225.

54. Cross AH, Naismith RT. Established and novel disease-modifying treatments in multiple sclerosis. *J Intern Med.* 2014;275(4):350–363.

55. Hartung DM, Bourdette DN, Ahmed SM, et al. The cost of multiple sclerosis drugs in the US and the pharmaceutical industry: too big to fail? *Neurology.* 2015;84(21):2185–2192.

56. Adelman G, Rane SG, Villa KF. The cost burden of multiple sclerosis in the United States: a systematic review of the literature. *J Med Econ.* 2013;16(5):639–647.

57. Cree BA. Update on reproductive safety of current and emerging disease-modifying therapies for multiple sclerosis. *Mult Scler.* 2013;19(7):835–843.

58. Plavina T, Subramanyam M, Bloomgren G, et al. Anti-JC virus antibody levels in serum or plasma further define risk of natalizumab-associated progressive multifocal leukoencephalopathy. *Ann Neurol.* 2014;76(6):802–812.

59. Jokubaitis VG, Li V, Kalincik T, et al. Fingolimod after natalizumab and the risk of short-term relapse. *Neurology.* 2014;82(14):1204–1211.

60. Kappos L, Radue EW, Comi G, et al. Switching from natalizumab to fingolimod: a randomized, placebo-controlled study in RRMS. *Neurology.* 2015;85:29–39.

61. Sangalli F, Moiola L, Ferre L, et al. Long-term management of natalizumab discontinuation in a large monocentric cohort of multiple sclerosis patients. *Mult Scler Relat Disord.* 2014;3(4):520–526.

62. Dhib-Jalbut S. Mechanisms of action of interferons and glatiramer acetate in multiple sclerosis. *Neurology.* 2002;58(8)(suppl 4):S3-9.

12 Relapse Management in Multiple Sclerosis

Andrew L. Smith and Robert J. Fox

KEY POINTS FOR CLINICIANS

- A hallmark of multiple sclerosis (MS) is the clinical relapse, an episode of new or worsening MS symptoms not due to fever or infection lasting more than 1 day.
- In a patient with an established diagnosis of MS, a typical clinical relapse needs little further evaluation besides consideration of infection and alternative diagnoses.
- Relapse management commonly involves high-dose corticosteroids—typically 1,000 mg daily for 3 to 5 days, followed by short oral prednisone taper.
- Management of MS symptoms is sometimes helpful.
- Clinical recovery takes several weeks or months, although residual symptoms can persist indefinitely.

In approximately 85% of patients, MS begins with a relapsing–remitting phase, in which neurological manifestations develop in the context of acute relapses (1). An MS relapse is defined as new or worsening neurological symptoms which persist for more than 24 hours in the absence of fever or infection (2). In clinical trials, the definition of a relapse usually requires objective neurological findings on examination; however, in clinical practice, the overall clinical picture is more important than objective findings. Typical symptoms of an MS relapse include blurred vision, diplopia, numbness, motor weakness, vertigo, or ataxia, but vary from case to case. Symptoms typically come on and worsen over several days or weeks, although occasionally symptoms can be sudden and maximal at onset, mimicking a stroke. Sensory symptoms in the extremity will often start in the toes or fingers and gradually progress proximally up the limb and sometimes into the trunk. Sensory symptoms involving the trunk can be described as a tightness sensation, informally called the "MS hug." Weakness can be seen, but usually numbness is more prominent than weakness. Urinary and bowel symptoms can include urgency and frequency, although incontinence is rare during an acute MS relapse.

Neurological findings on examination depend on the affected system. Optic neuritis can present with reduced visual acuity, color desaturation, visual field cut, visual distortion (i.e., "looking through glass soda block"), papillitis on fundoscopy, rapid afferent pupillary defect, and mild retro-orbital pain with eye movement. Diplopia from internuclear ophthalmoplegia is common in MS and manifests with adduction weakness in one or both eyes with a dissociated abductor nystagmus. Sensory symptoms can include numbness, paraesthesia, and less commonly pain. Objective sensory loss is often absent despite the patient reporting sensory changes, though a sensory level on the trunk may at times occur.

Most MS relapses will recover spontaneously over several weeks or months and leave only minor residual symptoms, regardless of treatment. However, not all relapses recover completely. Early in the disease, most disability accrual is the result of incomplete relapse recovery (3). Several arguments suggest benefit from active relapse treatment with corticosteroids. First, clinical trials found corticosteroids to accelerate clinical recovery from a relapse. Second, pathological studies have found greater than 10,000 transected axons/mm^3 in MS lesions with active inflammation (4). This irreversible axonal injury argues for aggressive reduction of inflammation to minimize permanent tissue damage.

Most MS relapses improve regardless of treatment.

EVALUATION

In a patient without the diagnosis of MS, evaluation of an MS relapse focuses on making an accurate diagnosis of MS and excluding other potential diagnoses (see Chapters 7 and 10). In the patient with an established diagnosis of MS, evaluation is more limited, mainly ruling out "pseudorelapses." Pseudorelapse is defined as a worsening of previous MS symptoms during a period of illness, particularly a febrile illness or metabolic derangement. Bladder infections, respiratory infections, and skin infections (e.g., decubitus ulcers) are common culprits. Becoming overheated may precipitate a worsening of symptoms. Emotional distress and sleep deprivation can also worsen previous neurological symptoms and mimic an MS relapse through worsened fatigue, sensory symptoms, gait, and overall reduced level of function. Clinical relapses need to be differentiated from transient day-to-day fluctuations in neurological symptoms, which are common in MS patients.

Once the causes of pseudorelapse have been explored, little further workup needs to be done for a typical relapse. Importantly, an MS relapse is a clinical diagnosis; therefore, imaging studies are generally considered neither necessary nor indicated during the initial evaluation and management of an MS relapse. Assuming no red flags that are listed in Table 12.1 are discovered, then most uncomplicated relapses in a patient with known MS can often be evaluated by telephone.

TABLE 12.1   Red Flags in "MS Relapse"

- Fever: suggests possible infection
- Urinary symptoms: suggests possible urinary infection
- Relapses more than once every 2–3 mo: suggests pseudorelapses or alternative diagnosis
- Patients receiving highly active anti-inflammatory therapy such as natalizumab: consider opportunistic infection such as PML
- Incomplete response to corticosteroids: although incomplete response to corticosteroids is not rare, it should raise the consideration of alternative diagnosis, including NMOSD or infection

MS, multiple sclerosis; NMOSD, neuromyelitis optica spectrum disorder; PML, progressive multifocal leukoencephalopathy.

In patients taking highly active anti-inflammatory therapy like natalizumab, alemtuzumab, rituximab, or ocrelizumab, clinical relapses are uncommon, but come with new concerns. Out of all of the highly efficacious treatments, natalizumab represents a special case. Relapse symptoms early in the course of treatment with natalizumab (i.e., <6 months) may suggest the presence of neutralizing antibodies against the therapy. Relapse symptoms later in the course of treatment with natalizumab (i.e., >6 months of therapy) should raise concerns of treatment-related complications like progressive multifocal leukoencephalopathy (PML). While all moderately and highly efficacious therapies carry a risk of PML, the risk is higher with natalizumab. Therefore, any evidence of disease activity on natalizumab after 6 months of treatment should be considered PML until proven otherwise.

> *PML should be considered with relapse symptoms more than 6 months after starting any highly efficacious therapy, with the concern being highest with natalizumab.*

Superimposed medical conditions need to be differentiated from an MS relapse, particularly when the presentation is atypical for an MS relapse. For example, sudden onset symptoms should raise a concern for stroke, particularly in patients with vascular risk factors. Cardiac ischemia should be considered in a patient with left arm sensory symptoms, such as pain and heaviness. Paroxysmal events may suggest seizures or tonic spasms. Some patients with MS describe their tonic spasms as "relapses," stating they have multiple "relapses" in a given day. Patients rarely have more than a few true relapses in a year, so it is sometimes helpful for a clinician to clarify with patients on their concept of relapses.

> *Relapse = Exacerbation = Attack = Bout of MS*

Most relapses respond to a single course of corticosteroids. When symptoms do not improve within 1 to 2 weeks, alternative or contributing diagnoses should be considered. Potential conditions include infection (particularly urinary tract infections, which can be asymptomatic), emotional distress, depression, and anxiety. Gradually, progressive neurological symptoms from progressive MS can sometimes be confused with an MS relapse. MRI studies of the affected area (e.g., spinal cord for partial transverse myelitis relapse) can help evaluate for persistent inflammation, which manifests as gadolinium enhancement and edema, as well as a mechanical etiology such as disc disease. On the other hand, imaging at the time of relapse is not usually helpful with either diagnosing the relapse, treating the relapse, or planning changes in therapy. Waiting for an MRI to be performed may unnecessarily slow the beginning of relapse therapy.

MANAGEMENT

The overall goal of relapse management is to stop active inflammation, limit damage secondary to active inflammation, accelerate and improve clinical recovery, and (ideally) delay the next clinical relapse. Table 12.2 outlines the typical management for MS relapse.

TABLE 12.2 Typical Management for an MS Relapse

- In a patient with known MS, confirm typical symptoms of MS relapse
- Screen for infection—bladder, respiratory, skin
- Treat with a 3-d course of 1 g/d IVMP or 1,250 mg/d prednisone, followed by 9-d prednisone taper: 60 mg daily for 3 d, 40 mg daily for 3 d, 20 mg daily for 3 d
- Clinical follow-up in about 6–8 wk to confirm good recovery of symptoms and consider need to change long-term MS therapy
- In a patient with incomplete recovery, consider alternative/contributing conditions, then re-treat with 3–5 d of IVMP and prednisone taper
- If still incomplete recovery, consider imaging affected area to help differentiate active inflammation from established injury and consider treatment with plasma exchange.

IVMP, intravenous methylprednisolone; MS, multiple sclerosis.

Corticosteroids

The mainstay of MS relapse management is corticosteroids. First reported in 1951 (5), it was not until 1970 that an influential controlled trial showed that adrenocorticotropic hormone (ACTH) improves recovery from a clinical relapse (6). Reports of benefit from high-dose intravenous methylprednisolone (IVMP) in several autoimmune disorders led to single-arm studies of IVMP in MS (7,8). Three randomized trials compared the efficacy of ACTH and IVMP (9–11). The most influential of these trials was a randomized, placebo-controlled, double-blind comparison of IVMP for 3 days versus intramuscular ACTH for 14 days (11). Both treatment groups improved significantly but there were no significant differences between the groups up to 90 days after treatment. The investigators concluded that IVMP was an effective alternative to ACTH, required shorter treatment durations, and was better tolerated. Based upon those studies, most clinicians then abandoned ACTH for treatment of clinical relapses and instead utilized IVMP.

Corticosteroids are the mainstay of MS relapse treatment.

Additional placebo-controlled studies of IVMP provided consistent evidence that high-dose corticosteroids were beneficial compared to placebo (Table 12.3). A meta-analysis and a *Cochrane Review* found convincing evidence to support the use of IVMP to treat acute relapses (12,13). Several small studies have followed patients over 1 year after a course of IVMP and reported improved outcomes in the patients treated with IVMP compared to either placebo or low-dose corticosteroids (14–16).

The optimal dose and route of administration for corticosteroids are not clearly defined. Doses ranging from 500 to 2,000 mg/d (IV [intravenous] or oral) for 3 to 5 days have been found to hasten recovery from MS relapses, whereas a single infusion of high-dose corticosteroid was found to be minimally effective (Table 12.4). Doses of 500 to 2,000 mg/d (IV or oral) for 3 to 5 days are appropriate for the treatment of MS relapses. Low or moderate doses of oral corticosteroids are used by some clinicians, particularly for mild relapses. The Optic Neuritis Treatment Trial suggested that low-dose corticosteroids were associated with an increased rate of recurrent optic neuritis, compared with placebo (16). However, this was not a primary end point for the study and has not been confirmed in other trials and thus should not guide therapy. Several trials—including a recent trial—have suggested that high-dose oral therapy are similarly effective as the IVMP (17,19). High-dose oral therapies have an advantage of not requiring nursing administration and can be taken on the patient's schedule. However, high-dose oral prednisone treatment bioequivalent dose is 1,250 mg. This requires taking up to twenty-five 50 mg pills per day, which may be difficult for patients and raise concerns by pharmacists.

Corticosteroids accelerate the recovery from MS relapses.

Side effects from corticosteroids are common, but typically mild (Table 12.5). Many of the common side effects of corticosteroids can be managed with proper education and over-the-counter medications, when

TABLE 12.3 Placebo-Controlled Trials of High-Dose Corticosteroids for MS Relapses

STUDY	YEAR	TREATMENT REGIMENS	N	RESULT
Durelli et al. (17)	1986	15 d of IVMP, tapering from 15 mg/kg/d down to 1 mg/kg/d vs. placebo	20	MP better than placebo
Milligan et al. (18)	1987	IVMP 500 mg/d for 5 d vs. placebo	22	MP better than placebo
Sellebjerg et al. (14)	1998	Oral MP 500 mg/d for 5 d vs. placebo	51	Higher proportion of patients with improvement in oral MP group

IV, intravenous; MP, methylprednisolone; MS, multiple sclerosis; N, total number of subjects.

TABLE 12.4   Clinical Trials Comparing Different Types or Doses of Corticosteroids for MS Relapses

STUDY	YEAR	TREATMENT REGIMENS	N	OUTCOME
Bindoff et al. (22)	1988	IVMP 1,000 mg/d for 1 d IVMP 1,000 mg/d for 5 d	32	Improved disability in the 5-d-treated group
Alam et al. (23)	1993	IVMP 500 mg/d for 5 d Oral MP 500 mg/d for 5 d	35	No difference between groups over 1 mo
La Mantia et al. (15)	1994	IVMP 100 mg/d, tapering off over 14 d vs. IVMP 40 mg/d, tapering over 14 d vs. IV dexamethasone 8 mg/d, tapering over 14 d	31	High rate of worsening in low-dose MP group after treatment
Barnes et al. (24)	1997	IVMP 1,000 mg/d for 3 d, vs. Oral MP 48 mg/d, tapering over 21 d	80	No significant difference in disability over 24 wk
Oliveri et al. (25)	1998	IVMP 2,000 mg/d for 5 d, vs. IVMP 500 mg/d for 5 d	29	No significant difference in disability over 2 mo, but lower MRI activity in high-dose group
Martinelli et al. (26)	2009	IVMP 1,000 mg/d for 5 d, vs. Oral MP 1,000 mg/d for 5 d	40	No significant difference in reduction in gadolinium-enhancing lesions
Le Page et al. (19)	2015	IVMP 1,000 mg/d for 3 d vs. Oral MP 1,000mg/d for 3 d	200	No significant difference in improvement (decrease of at least one point in most affected Kurtzke Functional System Scale), without need for retreatment with corticosteroids by 28 d

IV, intravenous; MP, methylprednisolone; MS, multiple sclerosis; N, total number of subjects.

TABLE 12.5   Side Effects of Corticosteroids

Common side effects associated with a course of corticosteroids
Metallic taste
Insomnia
Dysphoria
Anxiety
Increased appetite
Edema
Headache
Myalgia
Easy bruising
Acne
Gastrointestinal distress/heartburn
Flushing
Palpitations
Uncommon but important adverse effects associated with a course of corticosteroids include:
Anaphylaxis
Osteonecrosis/aseptic necrosis
Psychosis
Euphoria or depression
Exacerbation of preexisting peptic ulcer disease, diabetes mellitus, hypertension, affective disorders
Cataract formation

TABLE 12.6   Key Information for Patients and Families for Clinical Relapse Management

– Clinical relapses are new or worsening neurological symptoms that persist for more than a day or two, and that are not due to infection or fever.
– It is not always easy to differentiate symptoms of an MS relapse from other symptoms. Communicating with your care provider can help recognize what is an MS relapse and what is not.
– Clinical relapses usually are treated with corticosteroids to shorten symptom duration and help improve recovery of inflamed tissue.
– Corticosteroids are typically well tolerated, but can cause some side effects, including:
  – metallic taste
  – irritability
  – insomnia
  – weight gain
– Rarely, corticosteroids can cause more significant psychiatric symptoms.
– Repeated or long-term corticosteroid use can cause thinning of the bones (osteoporosis), but a short-term course like that used for an MS relapse is not thought to have significant impact on bone health. Rarely, corticosteroids will cause permanent injury to the hip or shoulder joint (aseptic necrosis).
– Most relapse symptoms recover over several weeks to months, but some symptoms can persist long term. Long-term symptoms can often be managed with targeted treatments.

needed (Table 12.6). A common side effect is a feeling of well-being or mild euphoria, which typically is welcomed by patients. Anxiety and irritability, especially in newly diagnosed MS patients, are common and should be treated with reassurance and a short-acting anxiolytic medication, if needed. Insomnia is frequent and can be managed with a short-acting sedative–hypnotic. Patients should be warned about increased appetite. It is often useful for patients to receive their first dose of IV corticosteroids under outpatient

medical supervision. This supervision helps with medication education, as well as monitoring and management of side effects. Mania and psychosis are rare and, when seen, can be managed with phenothiazines, antipsychotics, or lithium carbonate (20). Allergic reactions are typically against the preservative, and using preservative-free IVMP preparations can reduce this reaction. Anaphylactoid reactions are rare and thought to be related to immunoglobulin E (IgE) response to the succinate portion of methylprednisolone (21). Sensitization protocols are available for those with severe allergic reactions to preservative-free IVMP but require admission to an intensive care monitoring unit for each treatment.

Adrenocorticotropic Hormone

In late 1980s ACTH had largely fallen out of favor as the treatment for acute relapse of MS. However, there has been a resurgence in use of ACTH in the past 5 to 10 years. Several lines of research argue that ACTH may be superior to exogenously administered corticosteroids. ACTH is the principal agonist for the melanocortin receptor (MCR) system and binds to five subreceptors (MC1R–MC5R). In addition to its role stimulating the natural production of cortisol through its interaction with MC2R in the adrenal gland, ACTH binds to the other receptors, which leads to further down-regulation of several pro-inflammatory cytokines and may confer additional neuroprotection (27,28). While ACTH has similar side effects to steroids, some patients report tolerating ACTH better. Moreover, ACTH may have a reduced risk for osteoporosis and avascular necrosis of the hip (29).

Despite the purported advantages of ACTH, there is little evidence-based data to support its use over methylprednisolone or other exogenous corticosteroids. Some have suggested that ACTH is an alternative to high-dose corticosteroids for patients who do not respond to or tolerate corticosteroids (30), but the evidence to support this claim is currently limited to anecdotal clinical experience. While ACTH may have some theoretical benefits, its prohibitive cost (approximately US$29,000 per vial), similar efficacy to IVMP, easy availability of oral MP and other corticosteroid preparations (for patients without IV access), and absence of evidence-based studies in support of its superiority make the use of ACTH as a first line therapy in MS relapses problematic (27). Its role as a second-line treatment for MS relapse also has not been demonstrated. ACTH has a comparable cost of plasma exchange and does not require central access. However, for severe relapse, plasma exchange is generally preferred due to its demonstrated effectivess (31–35). Based on the current evidence, the use of ACTH is limited to those who have moderately severe relapses, who are unable to tolerate or fail to respond to high-dose glucocorticoid steroids and have contraindications for plasma exchange.

Intravenous Immunoglobulins

Intravenous immunoglobulins (IVIGs) have been used as a second line therapy to treat acute relapses of MS. While anecdotal evidence and small nonblinded case series supports the use of IVIG in relapses (36), clinical trials demonstrate that IVIG was neither superior to placebo nor was there an added benefit when used in combination with steroids (37) (Table 12.7). Furthermore, IVIG carries the risk of infusion reactions, thrombosis, renal dysfunction, and aseptic meningitis. Therefore, the use of IVIG is limited to those who cannot tolerate steroids or ACTH and those who either have contraindications to plasma exchange (PLEX) or cannot receive PLEX due to logistical reasons.

Plasmapheresis

Plasmapheresis (also called plasma exchange, PLEX, or apheresis) is often used to treat severe MS relapses that have failed to respond to standard therapy. Clinical trials support the use of PLEX as a highly effective treatment for acute MS relapses (33,41). The main reasons for the second line status of PLEX is its requirement of a central line dialysis catheter, risks of complications, prolonged treatment course, and high cost. With every other day dosing schedule, a full course of PLEX can take 10 to 14 days (Table 12.8). Many patients require hospitalization throughout the course of plasmapheresis treatment. Beside the risk of infection due to central access, PLEX can also cause electrolyte abnormalities, depletion of coagulation factors, infusion reactions, and a temporary immunodeficient state. Due to these drawbacks, PLEX is usually only considered in patients who have failed to improve after one or two courses of IVMP or for those with a severe relapse.

Symptomatic Therapy

Targeted management of relapse symptoms is sometimes needed (Table 12.9). This management can include physical or occupational therapy for gait or arm dysfunction, urinary catheter for acute urinary retention, short-term analgesics for pain, antiemetics and phenothiazines for vertigo, antiepileptics for tonic spasms, and an eye patch for diplopia. Patient education is an important component of MS relapse management, both regarding MS relapses in general (Table 12.6) as well as management of corticosteroid side effects (Table 12.5). Admission for relapses is usually limited to those patients unable to recover at home because of mobility or other functional issues.

Recovery from a clinical relapse usually starts within a couple days of corticosteroid initiation and continues for many months. When relapses do not respond sufficiently to corticosteroid treatment, plasma exchange or immune globulin can be considered, although neither of these are Food and Drug Administration (FDA)-approved for treatment of an MS relapse.

A clinical relapse indicates ongoing MS inflammation, which in turn indicates that the current long-term disease-modifying therapy may be insufficient to control the disease. Early in the treatment course of a disease-modifying therapy (i.e., <6 months), a clinical relapse may be tolerated as the therapy is becoming effective. If a clinical relapse occurs after about 6 months on a long-term

TABLE 12.7 Clinical Trials Comparing Different Types or Doses of IVIG for MS Relapses

STUDY	YEAR	TREATMENT REGIMENS	N	OUTCOME
Sorensen et al., TARIMS Study Group (38)	2004	IVMP 1,000 mg/d for 3 d IVIG 1g/kg 24 hr before treatment IVMP 1,000 mg/d for 3 d	76	Mean change in Z-Scores of the individual Targets neurological deficit at 12 wk.
Visser et al. (39)	2004	IVMP 500 mg/d for 5 d IV methyl-prednisolone 0.5 g directly followed by 0.4 g/kg for 5 d	35	EDSS at 4 wk
Roed et al. (40)	2005	IVMP 100 mg/d, tapering off over 14 d vs. IVMP 40 mg/d, tapering over 14 d vs. IV dexamethasone 8 mg/d, tapering over 14 d	31	Contrast Sensitivity

IVIG, intravenous immunoglobulin; MS, multiple sclerosis; N, total number of subjects.

TABLE 12.8 Clinical Trials Comparing Different Types or Doses of PLEX for MS Relapses

STUDY	YEAR	TREATMENT REGIMENS	N	OUTCOME
Weiner HL, Dau PC, Khatri BO, et al. (31)	1989	IM ACTH and oral cyclophosphamide + 11 PLEX IM ACTH and oral cyclophosphamide + 11 sham PLEX	116	Rate of sustain clinical improvement
Weinshenker BG, O'Brien PC, Petterson TM, et al. (33)	1999	Sham PLEX PLEX	22	standardized clinical scales for the targeted neurologic deficits

ACTH, adrenocorticotropic hormone; IM, intramuscular; MS, multiple sclerosis; N, total number of subjects; PLEX, plasma exchange.

disease-modifying therapy (and perhaps earlier with a highly effective therapy, such as natalizumab), it may be appropriate to consider changing long-term disease-modifying therapy.

SPECIAL CONSIDERATIONS

Neuromyelitis Optica Spectrum Disorder

Neuromyelitis optica spectrum disorder (NMOSD) is a related neuroinflammatory disorder secondary to a specific autoantibody with the same name, NMOSD. Initial treatment for an NMOSD relapse is similar to that of MS;

TABLE 12.9 Symptomatic Therapy to Consider as Adjunctive Treatment With Corticosteroids

SYMPTOM	TREATMENT
Gait or arm dysfunction	Physical and/or occupational therapy
Urinary retention	Urinary catheter, urology evaluation
Pain	Short-term analgesic
Vertigo	Antiemetic, phenothiazine
Tonic spasm	Antiepileptic medications
Diplopia	Eye patch

however, patients with NMOSD often have an incomplete response to corticosteroids and recurrent relapse as early as several weeks or months later. Therefore, NMOSD, patients generally receive a longer corticosteroid taper (typically several months) and different long-term treatments (see Chapter 37). When corticosteroids are not sufficiently effective, plasmapheresis is often used to improve recovery. In contrast to MS, NMOSD pathology from relapses are associated marked tissue injury and necrosis associated with NMOSD relapses. Due to the severity of the pathological changes, starting treatment for all NMO relapses as soon as possible after relapse onset is critical. Aggressive evaluation of seemingly mild new symptoms is required to detect potential new relapses in NMOSD. Relapses can rapidly progress in severity over hours to days. Disability accumulation in NMOSD is driven by relapses, because incomplete recovery from an NMOSD relapse is common. Therefore, a higher urgency is required to begin treatments for relapses in NMOSD than in MS.

> *NMOSD relapses are managed similarly as MS relapses, but are treated more urgently and more aggressively than MS relapses.*

MRI Relapse

By definition, clinical relapses are clinical manifestations of acute MS inflammation. However, active inflammation is sometimes observed as gadolinium-enhancing lesions on MRI in patients without any symptoms. The severe tissue injury observed in pathological studies of active inflammation suggest that this disease activity as seen on MRI may benefit from a course of corticosteroids, although no studies have formally evaluated this potential benefit.

PATIENT CASE   A 36-year-old woman with a 3-year history of known multiple sclerosis (MS) calls reporting 5 days of gradually progressive paraesthesia in her left leg—starting first in her toes, and now up to her waist. She has never had these symptoms before.

Question: What evaluation is needed? What management do you recommend?

Answer: The clinical picture is most consistent with a partial myelitis secondary to an MS relapse. After asking her about potential infections, no further evaluation is typically needed. It is reasonable to treat her at this point with a course of high-dose corticosteroids (e.g., 3 days of 1 g/d intravenous methylprednisolone [IVMP] or 1.25 g/d of prednisone, followed by a 12-day prednisone taper). Information about the side effects of corticosteroids and expectation of treatment response should be reviewed with her.

She calls during the last few days of the prednisone taper and reports that although sensory symptoms improved for a few days immediately after high-dose steroids corticosteroids, they now have returned and have progressed to involve her left hand and arm to the shoulder.

Question: What do you do now?

Answer: This still appears most consistent with an MS relapse, despite not responding to a course of high-dose corticosteroids. At this point, it is important to exclude infection, so a urinalysis would be appropriate, even without urinary symptoms. A repeat course of high-dose corticosteroids is indicated (e.g., 5 days of 1 g/d IVMP, followed by a 12-day prednisone taper). Generally during re-treatment, IV steroids are preferred over oral steroids. It would also be appropriate to schedule a follow-up in about 2 to 3 weeks with MRI of the cervical spine (likely location of the symptomatic lesion), and imaging here will evaluate both for active inflammation and alternative etiologies, such as compressive disc disease. Brain MRI would also be helpful as a broad-based assessment of ongoing inflammation. At the follow-up visit, consideration should include whether her current disease-modifying therapy is sufficiently effective in controlling active inflammation.

KEY POINTS FOR PATIENTS AND FAMILIES

- Limit concentrated sugars (to lessen the risk of hyperglycemia), limit salt (to decrease fluid retention), and encourage foods rich in potassium (to avoid hypokalemia).
- To help prevent gastritis, an acid blocker (e.g., ranitidine) may be helpful.
- Insomnia typically responds to short-acting hypnotic at bedtime.
- In patients with known hypertension, blood pressure should be monitored by the infusion nurse.
- In patients with known diabetes mellitus or past history of corticosteroid-associated hyperglycemia, blood sugar should be monitored closely. Involvement of the patient's primary care provider can be helpful.
- Irritability is common, although typically only needs patient counseling.
- Severe affective side effects (e.g., psychosis) are rare, but may respond to antipsychotic medication such as lithium.

REFERENCES

1. Markowitz CE. Multiple sclerosis update. *Am J Manag Care.* 2013;19:s294–300.
2. Berkovich R. Treatment of acute relapses in multiple sclerosis. *Neurotherapeutics.* 2013;10:97–105. doi:10.1007/s13311-012-0160-7.
3. Lublin FD, Baier M, Cutter G. Effect of relapses on development of residual deficit in multiple sclerosis. *Neurology.* 2003;61:1528–1532.
4. Trapp BD, Peterson J, Ransohoff RM, et al. Axonal transection in the lesions of multiple sclerosis. *N Engl J Med.* 1998;338:278–285. doi:10.1056/NEJM199801293380502.
5. Glaser GH, Merritt HH. Effects of ACTH and cortisone in multiple sclerosis. *Trans Am Neurol Assoc.* 1951;56:130–133.
6. Rose AS, Kuzma JW, Kurtzke JF, et al. Cooperative study in the evaluation of therapy in multiple sclerosis. ACTH vs. placebo—final report. *Neurology.* 1970;20:1–59.
7. Buckley C, Kennard C, Swash M. Treatment of acute exacerbations of multiple sclerosis with intravenous methyl-prednisolone. *J Neurol Neurosurg Psychiatry.* 1982;45:179–180.
8. Dowling PC, Bosch VV, Cook SD. Possible beneficial effect of high-dose intravenous steroid therapy in acute demyelinating disease and transverse myelitis. *Neurology.* 1980;30:33–36.
9. Abbruzzese G, Gandolfo C, Loeb C. "Bolus" methylprednisolone versus ACTH in the treatment of multiple sclerosis. *Ital J Neurol Sci.* 1983;4:169–172.
10. Barnes MP, Bateman DE, Cleland PG, et al. Intravenous methylprednisolone for multiple sclerosis in relapse. *J Neurol Neurosurg Psychiatry.* 1985;48:157–159.
11. Thompson AJ, Kennard C, Swash M, et al. Relative efficacy of intravenous methylprednisolone and ACTH in the treatment of acute relapse in MS. *Neurology.* 1989;39:969–971.
12. Miller DM, Weinstock-Guttman B, Bethoux F, et al. A meta-analysis of methylprednisolone in recovery from multiple sclerosis exacerbations. *Mult Scler.* 2000;6: 267–273. doi:10.1177/135245850000600408.
13. Filippini G, Brusaferri F, Sibley WA, et al. Corticosteroids or ACTH for acute exacerbations in multiple sclerosis. *Cochrane Database Syst Rev.* 2000:CD001331. doi:10.1002/14651858.CD001331.
14. Sellebjerg F, Frederiksen JL, Nielsen PM, et al. Double-blind, randomized, placebo-controlled study of oral, high-dose methylprednisolone in attacks of MS. *Neurology.* 1998;51:529–534.
15. La Mantia L, Eoli M, Milanese C, et al. Double-blind trial of dexamethasone versus methylprednisolone in multiple sclerosis acute relapses. *Eur Neurol.* 1994;34:199–203.
16. Beck RW, Cleary PA, Anderson MM, Jr., et al. A randomized, controlled trial of corticosteroids in the treatment of acute optic neuritis. The Optic Neuritis Study Group. *N Engl J Med.* 1992;326:581–588. doi:10.1056/NEJM199202273260901.
17. Durelli L, Cocito D, Riccio A, et al. High-dose intravenous methylprednisolone in the treatment of multiple sclerosis: clinical-immunologic correlations. *Neurology.* 1986;36:238–243.
18. Milligan NM, Newcombe R, Compston DA. A double-blind controlled trial of high dose methylprednisolone in patients with multiple sclerosis: 1. Clinical effects. *J Neurol Neurosurg Psychiatry.* 1987;50:511–516.
19. Le Page E, Veillard D, Laplaud DA, et al. Oral versus intravenous high-dose methylprednisolone for treatment of relapses in patients with multiple sclerosis (COPOUSEP): a randomised, controlled, double-blind, non-inferiority trial. *Lancet.* 2015;386:974–981. doi:10.1016/S0140-6736(15)61137-0.
20. Falk WE, Mahnke MW, Poskanzer DC. Lithium prophylaxis of corticotropin-induced psychosis. *JAMA.* 1979;241:1011–1012.
21. Burgdorff T, Venemalm L, Vogt T, et al. IgE-mediated anaphylactic reaction induced by succinate ester of methylprednisolone. *Ann Allergy Asthma Immunol.* 2002;89:425–428. doi:10.1016/S1081-1206(10)62046-7.
22. Bindoff L, Lyons PR, Newman PK, et al. Methylprednisolone in multiple sclerosis: a comparative dose study. *J Neurol Neurosurg Psychiatry.* 1988;51:1108–1109.
23. Alam SM, Kyriakides T, Lawden M, et al. Methylprednisolone in multiple sclerosis: a comparison of oral with intravenous therapy at equivalent high dose. *J Neurol Neurosurg Psychiatry.* 1993;56:1219–1220.
24. Barnes D, Hughes RA, Morris RW, et al. Randomised trial of oral and intravenous methylprednisolone in acute relapses of multiple sclerosis. *Lancet.* 1997;349:902–906.
25. Oliveri RL, Valentino P, Russo C, et al. Randomized trial comparing two different high doses of methylprednisolone in MS: a clinical and MRI study. *Neurology.* 1998;50:1833–1836.
26. Martinelli V, Rocca MA, Annovazzi P, et al. A short-term randomized MRI study of high-dose oral vs intravenous methylprednisolone in MS. *Neurology.* 2009;73:1842–1848. doi:10.1212/WNL.0b013e3181c3fd5b.
27. Gettig J, Cummings JP, Matuszewski K. H.p. Acthar gel and cosyntropin review: clinical and financial implications. *P T.* 2009;34:250–257.
28. Catania A, Gatti S, Colombo G, et al. Targeting melanocortin receptors as a novel strategy to control inflammation. *Pharmacol Rev.* 2004;56:1–29. doi:10.1124/pr.56.1.1.
29. Arnason BG, Berkovich R, Catania A, et al. Mechanisms of action of adrenocorticotropic hormone and other melanocortins relevant to the clinical management of patients with multiple sclerosis. *Mult Scler.* 2013;19:130–136. doi:10.1177/1352458512458844.
30. Ross AP, Ben-Zacharia A, Harris C, et al. Multiple sclerosis, relapses, and the mechanism of action of adrenocorticotropic hormone. *Front Neurol.* 2013;4:21. doi:p10.3389/fneur.2013.00021.
31. Weiner HL, Dau PC, Khatri BO, et al. Double-blind study of true vs. sham plasma exchange in patients treated with immunosuppression for acute attacks of multiple sclerosis. *Neurology.* 1989;39:1143–1149.
32. Rodriguez M, Karnes WE, Bartleson JD, et al. Plasmapheresis in acute episodes of fulminant CNS inflammatory demyelination. *Neurology.* 1993;43:1100–1104.
33. Weinshenker BG, O'Brien PC, Petterson TM, et al. A randomized trial of plasma exchange in acute central nervous system inflammatory demyelinating disease. *Ann Neurol.* 1999;46:878–886.
34. Bennetto L, Totham A, Healy P, et al. Plasma exchange in episodes of severe inflammatory demyelination of the central nervous system. A report of six cases. *J Neurol.* 2004;251:1515–1521. doi:10.1007/s00415-004-0588-8.
35. Meca-Lallana JE, Rodriguez-Hilario H, Martinez-Vidal S, et al. [Plasmapheresis: its use in multiple sclerosis and other demyelinating processes of the central nervous system. An observation study]. *Rev Neurol.* 2003;37:917–926.
36. Elovaara I, Kuusisto H, Wu X, et al. Intravenous immunoglobulins are a therapeutic option in the treatment of multiple sclerosis relapse. *Clin Neuropharmacol.* 2011;34:84–89. doi:10.1097/WNF.0b013e31820a17f3.
37. Dudesek A, Zettl UK. Intravenous immunoglobulins as therapeutic option in the treatment of multiple sclerosis. *J Neurol.* 2006;253(suppl 5):V50–58. doi:10.1007/s00415-006-5007-x.
38. Sorensen PS, Haas J, Sellebjerg F, et al. IV immunoglobulins as add-on treatment to methylprednisolone for acute relapses in MS. *Neurology.* 2004;63:2028–2033.
39. Visser LH, Beekman R, Tijssen CC, et al. A randomized, double-blind, placebo-controlled pilot study of i.v. immune globulins in combination with i.v. methylprednisolone in the treatment of relapses in patients with MS. *Mult Scler.* 2004;10:89–91. doi:10.1191 /1352458504ms978sr.
40. Roed HG, Langkilde A, Sellebjerg F, et al. A double-blind, randomized trial of IV immunoglobulin treatment in acute optic neuritis. *Neurology.* 2005;64:804–810. doi:10.1212/01.WNL.0000152873.82631.B3.
41. Cortese I, Chaudhry V, So YT, et al. Evidence-based guideline update: plasmapheresis in neurologic disorders: report of the Therapeutics and Technology Assessment Subcommittee of the American Academy of Neurology. *Neurology.* 2011;76:294–300. doi:10.1212/WNL.0b013e318207b1f6.

13 Treating Relapsing Forms of Multiple Sclerosis: Injection and Oral Therapies

Le H. Hua

KEY POINTS FOR CLINICIANS

- There are currently 15 approved disease-modifying therapies for multiple sclerosis (MS).
- The injectable therapies are interferon-beta, glatiramer acetate, and daclizumab (daclizumab was withdrawn from market in March 2018).
- The oral therapies are fingolimod, teriflunomide, and dimethyl fumarate.
- These can be considered first-line therapies, except for daclizumab, which should be reserved for second- or third-line therapies due to severe adverse safety concerns.
- Interferons, glatiramer acetate, and teriflunomide have established favorable long-term safety profiles.
- The risks with fingolimod and dimethyl fumarate continue to evolve, as during the postmarketing period, a small number of progressive multifocal encephalopathy cases have been discovered. It remains too early to determine risk mitigation strategies currently.
- The risks of daclizumab will also likely continue to evolve in the postmarketing surveillance period.

INTRODUCTION

There has been an overwhelming increase in available therapies for relapsing forms of MS since the first disease-modifying therapy (DMT) was approved in 1993. The DMTs have varying mechanisms, routes of administration, efficacy, and safety profiles. The decision of which therapy to use can be challenging, but also allows for improved tailoring of therapy specific to individuals based on disease characteristics and patient preferences. At present, there are more than 15 approved DMTs for MS, and this chapter focuses on the injectable and oral treatment options. Chapter 14 will focus on infusion therapies. Mechanism of action, trial results, start-up and monitoring, risk stratification, and typical patients will be covered, respectively, for interferons, glatiramer acetate (GA), daclizumab (DAC), fingolimod, teriflunomide, and dimethyl fumarate (DMF). Tables covering trial results and safety considerations for reference are provided, but are not intended for cross-trial comparisons (Tables 13.1 and 13.2).

INTERFERON BETA

Mechanism of Action

There are several formulations of interferon (IFN) beta which vary in dosing frequency: IFN beta-1b administered subcutaneously every other day (Betaseron and Extavia), IFN beta-1a administered intramuscularly once a week (Avonex) or subcutaneously three times per week (Rebif), and peginterferon beta-1a administered subcutaneously every 2 weeks (Plegridy). IFN beta-1b is developed in *Escheria coli* and not glycosylated, whereas IFN beta-1a is produced in the Chinese hamster ovarian cell lines and is glycosylated (16). The clinical importance of these differences is unknown in MS. Brand names will be subsequently used for IFN beta therapy when clarification of the specific formulation is necessary.

IFN beta was developed for use in MS, based on the recognition that there was lower endogenous IFN beta production in patients with MS. IFN beta is thought to have anti-inflammatory and immunodulatory effects

TABLE 13.1   Summary of Pivotal Clinical Trial Results Leading to Drug Approval for MS

DISEASE-MODIFYING THERAPY	RELATIVE REDUCTION IN ANNUALIZED RELAPSE RATE (%)	MRI OUTCOMES: RELATIVE REDUCTION IN NEW T2 LESIONS (%)/Gd-ENHANCING LESIONS (%)	RELATIVE DISABILITY REDUCTION (%)
IFNβ-1b 0.25 mg SC QOD (1,2)	34	83/—	29 (NS)
IFNβ-1a 30 mcg IM weekly (3)	18	34.3/32.3	36
IFNβ-1a 22 mcg SC TIW and 44 mcg SC TIW (4,5)	29 (22 mcg) 32 (44 mcg)	67/22 (22 mcg) 78/67 (44 mcg)	32 (22 mcg) 28 (44 mcg)
Pegylated IFNβ-1a 125 mcg SC every 2 wk (6)	27	67/86	38
GA 20 mg SC daily (7,8)	29	30/29	12 (NS)
GA 40 mg SC TIW (9)	34	34.7/44.8	—
Daclizumab 150 mg SC monthly (10)*	45[a]	54/60[a]	27[a]
Fingolimod 0.5 mg PO daily (11,12)	54	75/82	27–34
Teriflunomide 7 mg PO and 14 mg PO daily (13)	31.2 (7 mg) 31.5 (14 mg)	44/57.1 (7 mg) 76.7/80.4 (14 mg)	20 (NS) (7 mg) 26 (14 mg)
Dimethyl fumarate 240 mg PO BID (14,15)	44–53	71–85/74–90	38

*Withdrawn from market in March 2018.
[a]Daclizumab is compared to IFNβ-1a. All other relative rate reductions are compared to placebo.
BID, twice daily; GA, glatiramer acetate; Gd, gadolinium; IFNβ, interferon β; IM, intramuscular; MS, multiple sclerosis; PO, oral; QOD, every other day; NS, not significant; SC, subcutaneous; TIW, three times weekly.

TABLE 13.2   Side Effects and Safety Considerations for Disease Modifying Therapies in MS

DISEASE-MODIFYING THERAPY	ROUTE AND DOSE	COMMON SIDE EFFECTS	SAFETY CONSIDERATIONS	MONITORING RECOMMENDATIONS
IFNβ therapies	IFNβ-1b 0.25 mg SC QOD IFNβ-1a 30 mcg IM weekly IFNβ-1a 22mcg SC TIW IFNβ-1a 44 mcg SC TIW Pegylated IFNβ-1a 125 mcg SC every 2 wk	Flu-like symptoms, depression, injection site reactions, headaches	Transaminitis, leukopenia	CBC, LFT at 1, 3, 6 mo and every 6–12 mo thereafter. Thyroid function as clinically indicated
Glatiramer acetate	20 mg SC daily 40 mg SC TIW	Injection site reactions, lipoatrophy, postinjection systemic reactions	None	None
Daclizumab*	150 mg SC monthly	Injection site reactions, rash, infections, depression	Transaminitis, liver failure, cutaneous reactions, autoimmunity	Baseline LFT, screening for tuberculosis, and hepatitis exposure. Monthly LFTs while on medication and for 6 mo after discontinuation

(continued)

TABLE 13.2   Side Effects and Safety Considerations for Disease Modifying Therapies in Multiple Sclerosis (*continued*)

DISEASE-MODIFYING THERAPY	ROUTE AND DOSE	COMMON SIDE EFFECTS	SAFETY CONSIDERATIONS	MONITORING RECOMMENDATIONS
Fingolimod	0.5 mg PO daily	Bradycardia, headache, diarrhea, cough, infections	Macular edema, symptomatic bradycardia, and heart block, cryptococcus meningitis, PRES, PML	Baseline: CBC, LFT, VZV IgG, ECG, eye exam, and first-dose observation Monitoring: eye exam for macular edema at 3–4 mo, and periodically. CBC and LFT every 3–6 mo
Teriflunomide	7 mg PO 14 mg PO daily	Gastrointestinal side effects, hair thinning, headaches	Liver failure, teratogenicity	Baseline and monthly LFT for 6 mo at start-up. Screen for tuberculosis exposure. CBC and LFT periodically while on medication
Dimethyl fumarate	240 mg PO BID	Flushing, gastrointestinal side effects	PML, liver injury, lymphopenia	CBC and LFT at baseline and every 3–6 mo while on medication

*Withdrawn from market in March 2018.

BID, twice daily; CBC, complete blood count; IM, intramuscular; LFT, liver function test; MS, multiple sclerosis; PML, progressive multifocal leukoencephalopathy; PO, oral; PRES, posterior reversible encephalopathy syndrome; QOD, every other day; SC, subcutaneous; TIW, three times weekly; VZV, varicella zoster virus.

by inhibiting T-cell activation and proliferation, inducing apoptosis of autoreactive T cells, cytokine modulation and enhancing anti-inflammatory responses, and inhibition of leukocyte migration across the blood–brain barrier (17).

Trial Results

The pivotal trials leading to approval of IFN beta therapies demonstrated annualized relapse rate (ARR) reductions of 18% to 34%, when compared to placebo. Secondary MRI endpoints of relative reduction in new T2 lesions and gadolinium (Gd) enhancing lesions ranged from 34% to 83% and 22% to 67%, respectively (1–5). Disability endpoints were not significant for Betaseron (1). Disability outcomes were the primary endpoint for the Avonex trial, which demonstrated a 36% reduction in 6-month confirmed disability progression compared to placebo (3). Compared to placebo, Rebif showed 32% to 38% relative reduction in disability (4). Dose comparison trials of IFN beta treatments suggest higher efficacy with higher dose formulations (18,19).

A pegylated IFN beta-1a formulation was approved in 2014 based on the results of the ADVANCE trial (6). Compared to placebo, pegylated IFN beta-1a demonstrated an ARR reduction of 27%, relative reduction in T2 lesions of 67%, and Gd enhancing lesions by 86%. There was also a 38% relative reduction in 3-month confirmed disability progression. These results are comparable to the pivotal IFN beta trials.

Safety and adverse events were similar across all IFN beta trials. Common adverse events were influenza-like symptoms (fevers, chills, myalgias, malaise), depression, neutropenia, lymphopenia, elevated transaminases, and thyroid dysfunction. Some patients also report worsening of headaches with IFN beta use.

Start-Up, Monitoring, and Risk Stratification

Each IFN beta formulation has a dose titration schedule which allows for improved tolerability. The target dose of Avonex is 30 mcg intramuscular weekly. Titration starts with 7.5 mcg for the first week and increases by 7.5 mcg weekly to reach the full 30 mcg dose (20). Rebif is available at 22 and 44 mcg doses subcutaneous three times per week. Titrations schedule begins with 20% of the total dose for the first 2 weeks, then half the dose for 2 weeks, and reaching full dose at week 5 (21). The target dose of Betaseron and Extavia is 0.25 mg subcutaneous every other day. Titration starts at 0.625 mg every other day for 2 weeks, and increases by 0.625 mg every 2 weeks to reach the full 0.25 mg dose starting week 7 (22). Finally, Plegridy is dosed at 125 mcg subcutaneous every 2 weeks. Titrations start at 63 mcg on day 1, 94 mcg on day 15, and the full dose of 125 mcg on day 29 (23).

> *Each IFN beta formulation has a dose titration schedule which allows for improved tolerability.*

Patients need to have baseline complete blood counts (CBCs), liver function testing (LFT), and thyroid function testing. CBC and LFT should be monitored while on medication at intervals of 1, 3, and 6 months after treatment start, and then periodically thereafter, for example, every 6 to 12 months. Thyroid function should be monitored as clinically indicated. In the past, the development of neutralizing antibodies (NAbs) to IFN beta led to concern regarding potential decreased efficacy. Higher doses were associated with higher rates of NAb formation (24). The necessity of measuring NAbs to IFN beta have decreased, particularly as there are many alternative DMTs available for patients who demonstrate disease activity while on IFN beta therapy. In Europe, however, the guidelines suggest checking for presence of NAbs at 12 and 24 months. Patients who are positive for NAbs should be retested 3 to 6 months later, and treatment discontinued with high titers of NAbs.

Typical Patients

The IFN beta have established efficacy, favorable safety profiles, and are generally well tolerated. They are approved as first-line therapy for relapsing MS. Avonex, Betaseron, and Extavia are also approved for use in patients with a clinically isolated syndrome (CIS). Avonex and Plegridy offer less frequent dosing intervals than the other IFN beta. Overall, IFN beta is ideal for use in patients with mild disease, who are risk adverse, and are able to manage injections.

> *Overall, IFN beta is ideal for use in patients with mild disease, who are risk adverse, and are able to manage injections.*

GLATIRAMER ACETATE

Mechanism of Action

GA is a complex polypeptide mixture of L-glutamic acid, L-lysine, L-alanine, and L-tyrosine, initially developed to induce demyelination in the experimental autoimmune encephalomyelitis (EAE) mouse. Surprisingly, this mixture was found to be protective, and thus further developed as a treatment for MS. The mechanism of action of GA accounting for its clinical benefit in MS is incompletely understood but is hypothesized to involve competition with myelin autoantigens at the major histocompatibility complex class II binding site on antigen presenting cells, induction of antigen-specific Th2 T cells leading to bystander suppression of inflammation, and stimulation of neurotrophic factor secretion by immune cells (25).

Trial Results

The phase 3 trial that lead to approval of GA showed relative reduction in ARR of 29% compared to placebo (7). There was a reduction in confirmed one-point disability progression of 12%; however, this was not significant. A separate, shorter, placebo-controlled trial was completed to evaluate MRI outcomes, and showed relative reduction in T2 lesions by 30% and Gd lesions by 29% (8). Years later, the Glatiramer Acetate Low-frequency Administration (GALA) study demonstrated that a 40 mg three times per week formulation was similarly efficacious, with a relative reducing in ARR by 34% compared to placebo, a 34.7% relative reduction in T2 lesions, and 44.8% relative reduction in Gd lesions (9). Disability outcomes were not evaluated. Safety and tolerability were comparable to GA 20 mg daily dosing.

Recently several generic formulations of GA 20 mg daily have been submitted for approval (Momenta/Sandoz, Mylan/NATCO, and Synthon/Pfizer). The U.S. Federal Drug Agency approved generic GA (Glatopa-Momenta/Sandoz) based on equivalent biophysiochemical properties and effects in the EAE model. Contrastingly, the European Medicines Agency advised Synthon to perform an equivalency trial for their generic GA product (26). This led to the GATE trial, a multicenter, randomized, double blind, active- and placebo-controlled phase 3 trial, using MRI as a primary outcome to compare generic versus brand formulations. Results from the GATE trial revealed equivalent efficacy, tolerability, and safety for the generic GA (Synthon) compared to brand GA (Teva) (27).

Common side effects for GA are injection site tenderness, induration, pruritis, and erythema. Immediate postinjection reactions can also infrequently occur consisting of flushing, palpitations, dyspnea, and anxiety occurring within minutes of injection and resolving up to 30 minutes later. With prolonged use, patients can develop lipoatrophy, with resultant scarring at site of injections.

Start-Up, Monitoring, and Risk Stratification

GA is administered subcutaneously and available as either 20 mg daily or 40 mg three times per week (28). There are no dose titration or laboratory monitoring requirements for GA. Unique among the MS DMTs, there were no adverse effects on embryo-fetal development, delivery or offspring growth, and development when GA was administered in animal studies and is generally considered safe in pregnancy.

> *Unique among the MS DMTs, there were no adverse effects on embryo-fetal development, delivery or offspring growth, and development when GA was administered in animal studies and is generally considered safe in pregnancy.*

Typical Patients

Similar to IFN beta, GA also has established efficacy, favorable safety profiles, and is generally well tolerated. GA is approved for relapsing MS as well as CIS. It is also ideal for use in patients with mild disease, who are risk adverse, and are able to manage injections. As mentioned earlier, GA is considered safe in pregnancy and pregnant patients can remain on GA during the first trimester (29). As there are no effects on blood counts and liver function, GA can also be useful in patients where recurrent lymphopenia or transaminitis are concerns.

DACLIZUMAB (Withdrawn From Market in March 2018)

Mechanism of Action

DAC is a humanized anti-CD25 monoclonal antibody, which modulates interleukin-2 signaling, and leads to expansion of CD56bright natural killer cells, inhibition of T-cell activation, and reduces development of lymphoid tissue inducer cells (30). It was initially developed to prevent rejection in renal transplant patients. Based on its immune effects, DAC was explored for use in MS. A high-yield process (HYP) was developed for long-term subcutaneous administration and less antibody-dependent cytotoxicity compared to the intravenous formulation.

Trial Results

The DECIDE study was the phase 3 trial that lead to the approval of DAC in MS (10). This was a double-blind, multicenter randomized controlled trial comparing DAC to intramuscular IFN beta-1a. Results from trial showed that DAC had a 45% relative risk reduction in ARR when compared to IFN beta-1a. There were no statistically significant differences in 3-month confirmed disability progression; however, 6-month confirmed disability progression was reduced by 27% compared to IFN beta-1a. For MRI endpoints, DAC had 54% relative reduction in T2 lesions and 60% relative reduction in Gd-enhancing lesions when compared to IFN beta-1a.

DAC was relatively well tolerated with 14% discontinuing treatment due to adverse events during the trial. Side effects include skin reactions (rash, dermatitis, eczema), transaminitis, infections, and depression. Severe risks include other immune-mediated disorders (skin reactions, lymphadenopathy, noninfectious colitis) and liver toxicity including autoimmune hepatitis.

Start-Up, Monitoring, and Risk Stratification

DAC-HYP is a 150 mg subcutaneous injection given monthly (31). Patients who receive treatment with DAC are required to enroll in a Risk Evaluation and Mitigation Strategy (REMS) program due to autoimmunity and liver failure risks. Baseline testing for liver function, tuberculosis exposure, and hepatitis B and C virus are required. Monthly LFT is required while on treatment and for an additional 6 months after discontinuing therapy.

> *Patients who receive treatment with DAC are required to enroll in a REMS program due to autoimmunity and liver failure risks.*

Typical Patients

DAC is a high-efficacy treatment, with significant reductions in ARR and MRI endpoints against an active comparator. However, due to its safety profile, would be reserved as a second- or third-line agent. Its subcutaneous mechanism may be favorable compared to intravenous options for those with limited access to an infusion center or poor venous access. Patients would need to be able to comply with REMS requirement of monthly liver testing. DAC has not been associated with progressive multifocal leukoencephalopathy (PML) in renal transplant usage or trials with MS; however, longer follow-up is needed to further assess risk of PML.

FINGOLIMOD

Mechanism of Action

Fingolimod was developed during the search for novel drug compounds from analysis of fungal metabolites believed to have medicinal effects in folk medicine. This novel compound, originally named FTY720, appeared to have benefits in organ transplantation through nonimmunosuppressant mechanisms. Further studies led to the discovery that fingolimod binds to and modulates the sphingosine 1 phosphate (S1P) receptor (32). By binding to the S1P receptors, fingolimod is thought to sequester lymphocytes in lymph nodes, thus decreasing the inflammatory response in MS, although other mechanisms may underlie fingolimod's potential for neuroprotection, as fingolimod crosses the blood–brain barrier, and S1P and S1P receptors are found in the central nervous system (CNS). S1P receptor interaction also accounts for the cardiovascular (bradycardia, slowed atrioventricular conduction, increased blood pressure), pulmonary, and macular edema side effects for fingolimod (33).

Trial Results

Fingolimod was the first oral therapy to be approved for relapsing MS. The two pivotal phase 3 studies were the FREEDOMS trial (24-month double blind, randomized trial of oral fingolimod compared to placebo) and the TRANSFORMS trial (12-month double blind, double dummy randomized trial of oral fingolimod compared to intramuscular IFN beta-1a) (11,12). Two doses of fingolimod, 0.5 and 1.25 mg, were studied in the trials; however, only the 0.5 mg dose was approved as there was comparable efficacy to the higher dose, with a more favorable safety profile. In FREEDOMS, fingolimod 0.5 mg showed a relative reduction in ARR by 54%, and a 27% relative risk reduction in 3-month confirmed disability progression at 24 months compared to placebo. There was also a significant relative reduction in 6-month confirmed disability progression of 34%. New T2 lesions and Gd-enhancing lesions showed relative reductions of 75% and 82%, respectively. In TRANSFORMS, ARR was relatively reduced by 52% compared to IFN beta-1a. MRI endpoints of new T2 lesions and Gd-enhancing lesions were relatively reduced by 35% and 55%, respectively. Disability progression was similar among treatment groups during the 1-year study.

Fingolimod is very well tolerated, with only 5% to 7.5% discontinuing the 0.5 mg dose formulation due to adverse events. Common side effects include bradycardia, headache, transaminitis, diarrhea, cough, influenza, sinusitis, back pain, abdominal pain, and extremity pain. Rare safety concerns include atrioventricular block, macular edema, PML, posterior reversible encephalopathy syndrome, herpes viral infections and cryptococcal infections, and basal cell carcinoma. A handful of PML cases have been reported in the postmarketing surveillance period.

Start-Up, Monitoring, and Risk Stratification

Fingolimod is a once daily pill. Prior to starting this medication, baseline testing requirements include CBC, LFT, varicella zoster virus (VZV) immunity, baseline electrocardiogram, and testing for macular edema. Patients in whom testing for VZV antibody is negative should undergo vaccination and treatment delayed for 1 month to allow for full vaccination effects. Testing for macular edema should occur after 3 to 4 months on treatment and periodically thereafter on treatment as indicated. A first-dose observation period of 6 hours, in which heart rate and blood pressure are monitored hourly, is required at initiation and again if drug is discontinued for more than 14 days. Heart rate should start to recover by the end of the 6 hours; otherwise, observation needs to continue until resolved. High-risk patients (those at risk of symptomatic bradycardia, heart block, prolonged QTc interval, and/or those taking other drugs with risk of torsades de pointes), should be monitored overnight. Recent myocardial infarction, unstable angina, stroke, transient ischemic attack, and heart failure are contraindications. Fingolimod should also be avoided in patients with Mobitz type II second-degree or third-degree atrioventricular (AV) block, sick sinus syndrome, or baseline QTc interval ≥ 500 milliseconds (34).

High-risk patients (those at risk of symptomatic bradycardia, heart block, prolonged QTc interval, and/or those taking other drugs with risk of torsades de pointes), should be monitored overnight. Recent myocardial infarction, unstable angina, stroke, transient ischemic attack, and heart failure are contraindications.

John Cunningham (JC) virus antibody positivity can also be obtained, although it is uncertain how this should change management. PML risk stratification strategies have not been developed for fingolimod as the very small number of cases thus far does not indicate trends suggestive of increased risk. Fingolimod leads to lymphopenia due to the drug mechanism of lymphocyte sequestration in lymph nodes, and thus makes monitoring peripheral lymphocyte subsets difficult to interpret. In the clinical trials fingolimod was discontinued with absolute lymphocyte counts less than 0.2×10^9/L; however, there does not appear to be an increased risk of infections related to lower lymphocyte counts in the postmarketing period. Risk of lymphopenia needs to be weighed against benefits of ongoing treatment in these individuals. Lymphocyte counts can take months to recover after stopping therapy.

Lymphocyte counts can take months to recover after stopping therapy.

Typical Patients

Fingolimod has a favorable efficacy and tolerability profiles and can be considered in patients who are treatment naïve or second line after failure of initial treatment. Once daily dosing is an attractive option for many patients. Due to safety concerns, more start-up monitoring is required compared to other DMTs, but after treatment initiation, most patients do well and are able to remain on fingolimod.

TERIFLUNOMIDE
Mechanism of Action

Teriflunomide is an active metabolite of leflunomide, which is approved for use in rheumatoid arthritis. Based on its safety and efficacy in rheumatoid arthritis, drug developers sought to extend leflunomide to other autoimmune conditions, but focused the development of its active metabolite teriflunomide in MS. Teriflunomide reversibly inhibits dihydroorotate dehydrogenase, which is involved in new pyrimidine synthesis for rapidly dividing cells, while preserving the salvage pathway for resting lymphocytes (35).

This is thought to reduce T- and B-cell proliferation and have anti-inflammatory effects. Teriflunomide also targets cytokine signaling pathways and has direct modulatory effects on T and B cells and innate immune cells; however, the clinical significance of these effects is unknown.

Trial Results

The TEMSO trial was a randomized trial evaluating teriflunomide at 7 and 14 mg doses compared to placebo (13). Results showed relative risk reductions in ARR of 31.2% and 31.5% for 7 and 14 mg doses, respectively, compared to placebo, and relative reductions in 3-month confirmed disability progression of 20% and 26%, respectively, for the 7 and 14 mg doses; however, the 7 mg dose was not significant. MRI endpoints demonstrated relative reductions in T2 lesions of 44% and 76.7% for 7 and 14 mg doses, respectively, and reduction in Gd-enhancing lesions of 57.1% and 80.4% for 7 and 14 mg doses, respectively.

In the TENERE trial, teriflunomide 7 and 14 mg doses were compared to IFN beta-1a 44 mcg three times weekly formulation in a rater-blinded randomized trial (36). Primary outcome of time to treatment failure was not significantly different between groups. ARR was similar between teriflunomide 14 mg and IFN beta-1a; however, ARR rate was higher on teriflunomide 7 mg.

Common side effects are hair thinning, gastrointestinal disturbance (diarrhea, nausea), headaches, and transaminitis. Hepatotoxicity is a potential risk based on reports of liver failure on leflunomide. This medication is considered teratogenic even if the patient is male, and therefore counselling regarding contraception is imperative. Only 9% to 11% discontinued teriflunimode in the clinical trial due to adverse events.

> This medication is considered teratogenic even if the patient is male, and therefore counselling regarding contraception is imperative.

Start-Up, Monitoring, and Risk Stratification

Teriflunomide is available in 7 and 14 mg doses (37). Prior to starting treatment, baseline CBC and LFT should be obtained. Additional screening for latent tuberculosis also needs to be completed. Liver enzymes should be monitored monthly for first 6 months. Blood counts and liver enzymes should be checked periodically while on treatment. Teriflunomide needs to be avoided in pregnant patients, and should also be avoided in patients who are planning pregnancy. This medication may still be detected years after use and therefore elimination methods with activated charcoal or cholestyramine are required for rapid wash out, particularly for accidental pregnancy or severe adverse effects.

> This medication may still be detected years after use and therefore elimination methods with activated charcoal or cholestyramine are required for rapid wash out, particularly for accidental pregnancy or severe adverse effects.

Typical Patients

Teriflunimode can be considered first-line therapy for patients with MS, or second-line therapy for those patients who need to switch treatment for tolerability issues. It can also be considered in sequencing after using higher efficacy agents. Its efficacy is comparable to IFNs, and oral route may be better for patients who are unable to self-inject or needle averse. It has good long-term safety data based on its parent drug, leflunimode. It should be avoided in those with severe liver disease.

DIMETHYL FUMARATE
Mechanism of Action

Dimethyl fumarate (DMF) was developed under the name BG-12, and was based on the success of fumaric acid esters in psoriasis in Germany. Fumaric acid and its esters are found naturally in some plants and mushrooms and were first studied in dermatology for use in psoriasis based on the hypothesis that a metabolic defect in the Krebs cycle was the cause of the disease. The chemist, Walter Schweckendiek, tested this on himself and published the positive results in 1959. It was mainly used off label until 30 years later, when formal clinical trials took place, leading to approval of fumaric acid esters (Fumaderm) in 1994. DMF is the dimethyl ester of fumaric acid and is metabolized to monomethyl fumarate in the intestine and has improved gastrointestinal tolerability compared to mixed fumaric acid esters. Monomethyl fumarate is considered the active metabolite exerting immune effects. Its exact immunomodulatory effects are unknown, but studies have demonstrated reduction in peripheral blood mononuclear cells and cytokine shifts from Th1 pro-inflammatory cytokines to Th2 anti-inflammatory cytokines. DMF also activates transcription of the nuclear (erythroid-derived 2) related factor (Nrf2) pathways, and thus has antioxidant and possible neuroprotective effects (38).

Trial Results

The DEFINE study was a randomized, double-blind, placebo-controlled study assessing DMF 240 mg twice daily and 240 mg three times daily doses (14). Relative reduction in ARR for the 240 mg twice daily dose was 53% and three times daily dosing was 48% compared to placebo. There was a 38% and a 34% relative risk reduction in confirmed disability progression for the twice daily and three times daily doses. MRI endpoints for relative reduction in new T2 lesions was 85% and 74%, and for Gd lesions was 90% and 73% for twice daily and thrice daily, respectively. The CONFIRM study was also a randomized, placebo-controlled study evaluating 240 mg twice daily and 240 mg three times daily dosing, but also included GA as a reference comparator at the request of regulatory agencies (15). It was not powered for superiority or non-inferiority to GA. Relative reductions in ARR were 44%, 51%, and 29% for DMF twice daily, DMF thrice daily, and GA versus placebo, respectively. Differences in disability progression were not significant for the three treatment groups versus placebo (21% for DMF twice daily, 24% for DMF thrice daily, 7% for GA). Relative reductions in MRI endpoints for new T2 lesions were 71%, 73%, and 54%, and for Gd lesions were 74%, 65%, and 61% for DMF twice daily, DMT thrice daily, and GA, respectively. Based on the results of the two studies, approval was only pursued with the twice daily dosing.

The discontinuation rate for DMF due to adverse events during the trial was 12% to 16%. Side effects with DMF include flushing and gastrointestinal symptoms (diarrhea, abdominal cramping, nausea), which decreases after the first 2 months of use. Other side effects include transaminitis, lymphopenia, and increased risk of infections.

Start-Up, Monitoring, and Risk Stratification

DMF is an oral pill taken twice daily (39). The typical titration schedule is 120 mg twice daily for 7 days, then 240 mg twice daily. For those with intolerable side effects, an alternate titration schedule can be attempted, such as starting with 25% of the dose for 1 week, and increasing by 25% weekly until goal dose is attained at week 4. Flushing side effects can be reduced by taking DMF with food and/or taking aspirin 30 minutes before taking DMF.

Flushing side effects can be reduced by taking DMF with food and/or taking aspirin 30 minutes before taking DMF.

Prior to starting, baseline lab testing for CBC and LFT should be obtained, and repeated every 3 to 6 months while on treatment.

In the postmarketing period, several cases of PML have been associated with DMF. There appears to be an association with prolonged lymphopenia with all but one case of PML, with prolonged lymphopenia less than 0.5×10^9/L. This association is consistent with the reports of PML on patients exposed to fumaric acid esters with lymphopenia. The Food and Drug Administration (FDA) has updated the prescribing information to include recommendations to discontinue treatment if lymphocyte counts remain less than 0.5×10^9/L for greater than 6 months (39). JC virus antibody positivity can also be obtained, although it is uncertain how this should change management as PML risk stratification strategies have also not been developed for DMF. The FDA also updated the label to include risk of liver injury, with postmarketing cases of serum aminotransferases greater than 5-fold the upper limit of normal and total bilirubin greater than 2-fold the upper limit of normal. Liver abnormalities resolved with treatment discontinuation, but some patients required hospitalization.

The FDA has updated the prescribing information to include recommendations to discontinue treatment if lymphocyte counts remain less than 0.5×10^9/L for greater than 6 months.

Typical Patients

DMF also has a favorable efficacy and safety profile. It can be considered first- or second-line treatment in relapsing MS. Treatment start-up is simple with minimal laboratory monitoring requirements. Twice daily dosing may be difficult for some patients. For patients who prefer oral treatment, DMF has less concerns for patients with comorbid cardiovascular conditions compared to other oral options.

PATIENT CASE 1 A previously healthy 22-year-old woman awoke with blurred vision in her right eye that worsened over 2 days. She went to see her optometrist who performed an eye exam. They did not see any acute pathology. An MRI scan of her brain and orbits showed retro-orbital right optic nerve enhancement. There were also three periventricular lesions, one of which was considered an asymptomatic enhancing lesion. She was diagnosed with multiple sclerosis and treated with intravenous high-dose steroids for 3 days for her acute optic neuritis and her vision recovered after 2 weeks. Her neurologist advised her to start disease-modifying therapy. The patient was given information regarding the first-line therapies: IFN beta, glatiramer acetate (GA), fingolimod, teriflunomide, and dimethyl fumarate (DMF). She informed her neurologist that she was recently married and interested in becoming pregnant in the next few years but did not have any immediate plans. Based on her pregnancy plans, GA was determined to be the best choice for her, and she preferred less frequent injection. She was started on GA 40 mg subcutaneous three times per week.

> **PATIENT CASE 2** A 38-year-old woman with multiple sclerosis is currently on IFN beta-1b for the past 4 years, started immediately after her diagnosis. She was doing well until 3 weeks ago when she developed numbness from the waist down. MRI studies revealed one enhancing lesion in her thoracic spine, and one new T2 lesion in her brain compared to the previous year. Her neurologist treated her current relapse with high-dose oral steroids, as she had difficulty getting to an infusion center. Her neurologist also recommended changing disease-modifying therapy (DMT) as she had both clinical and radiological progression on IFN beta. The patient no longer wanted to perform injections and asked about oral options. She was given information regarding fingolimod, teriflunomide, and dimethyl fumarate (DMF). Her spinal cord lesion was concerning for higher risk of disability, and she did not feel she was able to take a medication twice daily. She was interested in fingolimod. She has no other medical conditions, no prior cardiac issues, and is not on any additional medications. She underwent baseline laboratory testing, which were normal and had previously received varicella zoster virus vaccination. Baseline electrocardiogram was normal, and she successfully completed the 6-hour first-dose observation period without difficulty. One year later, she continues to tolerate fingolimod, remains clinically stable, and MRIs do not show new disease activity.

KEY POINTS FOR PATIENTS AND FAMILIES

- Disease-modifying therapies for multiple sclerosis have been shown to reduced relapses, MRI disease activity, and disability progression.

- Interferon beta and glatiramer acetate were the first therapies to be approved for multiple sclerosis in the 1990s.

- New oral therapies, fingolimod, teriflunomide, and dimethyl fumarate were approved in 2010, 2012, and 2013, respectively.

- Daclizumab is a highly efficacious injection approved in 2016, but has a strict laboratory monitoring program to monitor for liver dysfunction.

- Treatment choice should be made with patient input on preferred routes of administration, risk aversion, and ability to comply with monitoring requirements.

- Patients also need to share other medical conditions, prescribed and nonprescribed medications, and pregnancy plans to guide treatment decisions.

REFERENCES

1. IFNB Multiple Sclerosis Study Group. Interferon beta-1b is effective in relapsing-remitting multiple sclerosis. I. Clinical results of a multicenter, randomized, double-blind, placebo-controlled trial. *Neurology.* 1993;43(4):655–655. doi:10.1212/WNL.43.4.655.
2. Paty DW, Li DKB, The UBC MS/MRI Study Group, et al. Interferon beta-1b is effective in relapsing-remitting multiple sclerosis. II. MRI analysis results of a multicenter, randomized, double-blind, placebo-controlled trial. *Neurology.* 1993;43(4):662–667. doi:10.1212/WNL.43.4.662.
3. Jacobs LD, Cookfair DL, Rudick RA, et al. Intramuscular interferon beta-1a for disease progression in relapsing multiple sclerosis. *Ann Neurol.* 1996;39(3):285–294.
4. PRISMS (Prevention of Relapses and Disability by Interferon beta-1a Subcutaneously in Multiple Sclerosis) Study Group. Randomised double-blind placebo-controlled study of interferon beta-1a in relapsing/remitting multiple sclerosis. *Lancet.* 1998;352(9139):1498-1504.
5. Li DK, Paty DW. Magnetic resonance imaging results of the PRISMS trial: a randomized, double-blind, placebo-controlled study of interferon-beta1a in relapsing-remitting multiple sclerosis. Prevention of Relapses and Disability by Interferon-beta1a Subcutaneously in Multiple Sclerosis. *Ann Neurol.* 1999;46(2):197–206.
6. Calabresi PA, Kieseier BC, Arnold DL, et al. Pegylated interferon beta-1a for relapsing-remitting multiple sclerosis (ADVANCE): a randomised, phase 3, double-blind study. *Lancet Neurol.* April 2014. doi:10.1016/S1474-4422(14)70068-7.
7. Johnson KP, Brooks BR, Cohen JA, et al. Copolymer 1 reduces relapse rate and improves disability in relapsing-remitting multiple sclerosis: results of a phase III multicenter, double-blind, placebo-controlled trial. *Neurology.* 1995;45(7):1268–1276. doi:10.1212/WNL.45.7.1268.
8. Comi G, Filippi M, Wolinsky JS. European/Canadian multicenter, double-blind, randomized, placebo-controlled study of the effects of glatiramer acetate on magnetic resonance imaging–measured disease activity and burden in patients with relapsing multiple sclerosis. *Ann Neurol.* 2001;49(3):290–297.
9. Khan O, Rieckmann P, Boyko A, et al. Three times weekly glatiramer acetate in relapsing-remitting multiple sclerosis. *Ann Neurol.* 2013;73(6):705–713. doi:10.1002/ana.23938.
10. Kappos L, Wiendl H, Selmaj K, et al. Daclizumab HYP versus interferon beta-1a in relapsing multiple sclerosis. *N Engl J Med.* 2015;373(15):1418–1428. doi:10.1056/NEJMoa1501481.

11. Kappos L, Radue E-W, O'Connor P, et al. A placebo-controlled trial of oral fingolimod in relapsing multiple sclerosis. *N Engl J Med.* 2010;362(5):387–401. doi:10.1056/NEJMoa0909494.

12. Cohen JA, Barkhof F, Comi G, et al. Oral fingolimod or intramuscular interferon for relapsing multiple sclerosis. *N Engl J Med.* 2010;362(5):402–415. doi:10.1056/NEJMoa0907839.

13. O'Connor P, Wolinsky JS, Confavreux C, et al. Randomized trial of oral teriflunomide for relapsing multiple sclerosis. *N Engl J Med.* 2011;365(14):1293–1303.

14. Gold R, Kappos L, Arnold DL, et al. Placebo-controlled phase 3 study of oral BG-12 for relapsing multiple sclerosis. *N Engl J Med.* 2012;367(12):1098–1107. doi:10.1056/NEJMoa1114287.

15. Fox RJ, Miller DH, Phillips JT, et al. Placebo-controlled phase 3 study of oral BG-12 or glatiramer in multiple sclerosis. *N Engl J Med.* 2012;367(12):1087–1097. doi:10.1056/NEJMoa1206328.

16. Annibali V, Mechelli R, Romano S, et al. IFN-β and multiple sclerosis: from etiology to therapy and back. *Cytokine Growth Factor Rev.* 2014;26(2):221–228. doi:10.1016/j.cytogfr.2014.10.010.

17. Dhib-Jalbut S, Marks S. Interferon-beta mechanisms of action in multiple sclerosis. *Neurology.* 2010;74(suppl 1):S17–S24. doi:10.1212/WNL.0b013e3181c97d99.

18. Durelli L, Verdun E, Barbero P, et al. Every-other-day interferon beta-1b versus once-weekly interferon beta-1a for multiple sclerosis: results of a 2-year prospective randomised multicentre study (INCOMIN). *Lancet.* 2002;359(9316):1453–1460.

19. Schwid SR, Panitch HS. Full results of the Evidence of Interferon Dose-Response-European North American Comparative Efficacy (EVIDENCE) study: a multicenter, randomized, assessor-blinded comparison of low-dose weekly versus high-dose, high-frequency interferon beta-1a for relapsing multiple sclerosis. *Clin Ther.* 2007;29(9):2031–2048. doi:10.1016/j.clinthera.2007.09.025.

20. *Avonex(R) [package insert].* Cambridge, MA: Biogen Inc.; 1996. Available at: https://www.avonex.com/content/dam/commercial/multiple-sclerosis/avonex/pat/en_us/pdf/Avonex_Prescribing_Information.pdf. Accessed July 30, 2017.

21. *Rebif(R) [package insert].* Rockland, MA: EMD Serono, Inc.; 1996. Available at: http://www.emdserono.com/ms.country.us/en/images/Rebif_PI_tcm115_140051.pdf?Version=.

22. *Betaseron(R) [package insert].* Whippany, NJ: Bayer HealthCare Pharmaceuticals Inc.; 1993. Available at: https://labeling.bayerhealthcare.com/html/products/pi/Betaseron_PI.pdf. Accessed July 30, 2017.

23. *Plegridy(R) [package insert].* Cambridge, MA: Biogen Inc.; 2014. Available at: https://www.plegridy.com/content/dam/commercial/multiple-sclerosis/plegridy/pat/en_us/pdf/november/plegridy-prescribing-information.pdf. Accessed July 30, 2017.

24. Govindappa K, Sathish J, Park K, et al. Development of interferon beta-neutralising antibodies in multiple sclerosis—a systematic review and meta-analysis. *Eur J Clin Pharmacol.* 2015;71(11):1287–1298. doi:10.1007/s00228-015-1921-0.

25. Varkony H, Weinstein V, Klinger E, et al. The glatiramoid class of immunomodulator drugs. *Expert Opin Pharmacother.* 2009;10(4):657–668. doi:10.1517/14656560902802877.

26. Hua LH, Cohen JA. Considerations in the development of generic disease therapies for multiple sclerosis. *Neurol Clin Pract.* 2016;6(4):369–376. doi:10.1212/CPJ.0000000000000267.

27. Cohen J, Belova A, Selmaj K, et al. Equivalence of generic glatiramer acetate in multiple sclerosis: a randomized clinical trial. *JAMA Neurol.* 2015 Dec;72(12):1433-1441. doi: 10.1001/jamaneurol.2015.2154.

28. *Copaxone(R) [package insert].* Overland Park, KS: Teva Neuroscience, Inc.; 1996. Available at: https://www.copaxone.com/Resources/pdfs/PrescribingInformation.pdf. Accessed July 30, 2017.

29. Herbstritt S, Langer-Gould A, Rockhoff M, et al. Glatiramer acetate during early pregnancy: a prospective cohort study. *Mult Scler.* 2016;22(6):810–816. doi:10.1177/1352458515623366.

30. Bielekova B. Daclizumab therapy for multiple sclerosis. *Neurotherapeutics.* 2013;10(1):55–67. doi:10.1007/s13311-012-0147-4.

31. *Zinbryta® [package insert].* Cambridge, MA: Biogen Inc.; 2016. Available at: https://www.zinbryta.com/content/dam/commercial/multiple-sclerosis/zinbryta/na/en_us/pdfs/zinbryta-prescribing-information.pdf. Accessed July 30, 2017.

32. Chun J, Brinkmann V. A Mechanistically novel, first oral therapy for multiple sclerosis: the development of fingolimod (FTY720, Gilenya). *Discov Med.* 2011;12(64):213–228.

33. Cohen JA, Chun J. Mechanisms of fingolimod's efficacy and adverse effects in multiple sclerosis. *Ann Neurol.* 2011;69(5):759–777. doi:10.1002/ana.22426.

34. *Gilenya(R) [package insert].* Stein, Switzerland: Novartis Pharma Stein AG; 2010. Available at: https://www.pharma.us.novartis.com/sites/www.pharma.us.novartis.com/files/gilenya.pdf. Accessed July 30, 2017.

35. Claussen MC, Korn T. Immune mechanisms of new therapeutic strategies in MS: teriflunomide. *Clin Immunol.* 2012;142(1):49–56. doi:10.1016/j.clim.2011.02.011.

36. Vermersch P, Czlonkowska A, Grimaldi LM, et al. Teriflunomide versus subcutaneous interferon beta-1a in patients with relapsing multiple sclerosis: a randomised, controlled phase 3 trial. *Mult Scler J.* October 2013. doi:10.1177/1352458513507821.

37. *Aubagio(R) [package insert].* Cambridge, MA: Genzyme Corporation; 2012. Available at: http://products.sanofi.us/aubagio/aubagio.pdf. Accessed July 30, 2017.

38. Linker RA, Gold R. Dimethyl fumarate for treatment of multiple sclerosis: mechanism of action, effectiveness, and side effects. *Curr Neurol Neurosci Rep.* 2013;13(11):394. doi:10.1007/s11910-013-0394-8.

39. *Tecfidera(R) [package insert].* Cambridge, MA: Biogen Inc.; 2013. Available at: https://www.tecfiderahcp.com/content/dam/commercial/multiple-sclerosis/tecfidera/hcp/en_us/pdf/Tecfidera_PI.pdf. Accessed July 30, 2017.

14 | Treating Relapsing Forms of Multiple Sclerosis: Infusion Therapies

Jenny J. Feng and Daniel Ontaneda

KEY POINTS FOR CLINICIANS

- There are six infusion therapies for the treatment of relapsing forms of multiple sclerosis (MS)—including DNA-disrupting agents (mitoxantrone and cyclophosphamide) and monoclonal antibodies (natalizumab, alemtuzumab, rituximab, and ocrelizumab).

- Mitoxantrone use is limited by risk of dose-dependent cardiotoxicity and therapy-related acute leukemia.

- Cyclophosphamide has mixed and limited clinical trial results but may have more anti-inflammatory effects in younger patients with active disease.

- Natalizumab is a highly effective agent that has been associated with progressive multifocal leukoencephalopathy (PML), a rare but serious adverse event. Therefore, patients should be appropriately risk stratified prior to initiating therapy using John Cunningham virus (JCV) serology. Subjects who are JCV negative carry a low risk of PML. Positive JCV serology, history of prior immunosuppression use, and a longer duration of natalizumab use increase the risk of PML.

- Alemtuzumab is a highly effective disease modifying agent and is approved in treatment of refractory relapsing MS patients. Alemtuzumab use is associated with serious risk of autoimmune disorders and requires stringent monitoring.

- Despite lack of phase three trials in relapsing MS, rituximab is frequently used off-label in cases with disease activity where contraindications or failures of previous therapies exist.

- Ocrelizumab is the only approved medication for the treatment of both relapsing–remitting MS (RRMS) and primary progressive MS (PPMS). In clinical trials it was well tolerated with favorable risk and side effect profile and may be considered in treatment naïve and nontreatment naïve patients.

INTRODUCTION

Infusion therapies represent a category of MS disease-modifying agents (DMTs) administered by scheduled intravenous infusion (IV). Infusion therapies include both older chemotherapeutic medications (cyclophosphamide and mitoxantrone) and more recently developed monoclonal antibodies (natalizumab, ocrelizumab, rituximab, alemtuzumab). The group of infusion therapies as a whole tends to be more potent and have the advantage of being administered less frequently than oral or injectable therapies.

Greater efficacy, however, may come at the price of higher risks. In prescribing infusion therapies, clinicians must take each drug's risk and benefit profiles into consideration as well as patient demographics and preferences in order to develop personalized treatment plans. Infusion therapies are most commonly used in relapsing active disease that has not responded to first-line therapies and/or patients who are demonstrating signs of rapidly progressive disabling disease. However, improvement in safety profiles of more recently approved monoclonal infusion agents make first-line use increasingly common. In this review, we will highlight the mechanism of action, efficacy, and risks of the different infusion DMTs for relapsing forms of MS. We will review the available infusion medications for MS, starting with DNA-disrupting agents followed by monoclonal antibodies. Table 14.1 presents a summary of the infusion therapies reviewed.

MITOXANTRONE (NOVANTRONE)

Mitoxantrone, an anthracenedione compound that intercalates into DNA, causing disruptions in DNA synthesis, also acts as a type II topoisomerase inhibitor and interferes with DNA repair mechanisms. It was found to have immunomodulatory effects by suppressing T cells, B cells, macrophages, and reduces the level of inflammatory cytokines (1).

Mitoxantrone was originally developed as a chemotherapy agent and is Food and Drug Administration (FDA) approved for treatment of acute nonlymphocytic leukemia and drug-resistant prostate cancer. In 2000, it was approved for the treatment of relapsing MS based on evidence from several randomized controlled trials. In a randomized, placebo-controlled trial involving secondary progressive MS (SPMS) or worsening relapsing–remitting MS (RRMS) patients, mitoxantrone was shown to reduce disability progression and relapse rate (2). In another trial involving SPMS and RRMS patients, fewer patients who had received mitoxantrone combined with intravenous methylprednisolone (IVMP) had enhancing lesions at 6 months when compared to patients who received IVMP alone (3). Mitoxantrone monotherapy in SPMS reduced the relapse rate and number of enhancing lesions when compared to IVMP (4).

Although common side effects of mitoxantrone include nausea, alopecia, hypotension, rashes, urinary tract infection (UTI), and menstrual disorders, its most serious side effects—cardiotoxicity and leukemia, limit its clinical use. Cardiac function must be evaluated prior to starting each mitoxantrone dose, and in patients with left ventricular ejection fraction (LVEF) less than 50%, mitoxantrone is contraindicated. Similarly, in patients whose LVEF decreases by greater than 10%, mitoxantrone should be discontinued. Rapid infusion also carries a higher risk; thus, a slow infusion over 30 minutes is preferred. The cumulative lifetime dose of mitoxantrone is a primary risk factor for cardiotoxicity. Because of this, the lowest effective dose should be used and maximum total lifetime dose is limited at 140 mg/m^2 (5). Higher cumulative doses are also correlated with higher incidence of leukemia.

Postmarketing surveillance has indicated that the incidence of ventricular dysfunction, congestive heart failure, and therapy-related acute leukemia (TRAL) are 12%, 0.8%, and 0.3%, respectively (6).

Mitoxantrone is typically recommended to be administered for no longer than 2 years at the dosing of 12mg/m^2 intravenously every 3 months. It also has been studied as a short-term induction therapy given as 12mg/m^2 monthly for 6 months in patients with aggressive form of relapsing MS (7).

Given that leukopenia, thrombocytopenia, and lymphopenia will be observed approximately 3 months after induction, complete blood count (CBC) with platelets should be checked prior to each treatment and the dosing of mitoxantrone should be adjusted depending on the degree of hematological suppression.

Despite its efficacy in reducing disability progression and relapse rate, mitoxantrone is now seldom used in North America. The concerns for cumulative dose-dependent side effects, and the availability of alternative DMTs with fewer treatment-related risks, has reduced its use over the past few years in the United States (8). It remains an option in patients with aggressive relapsing disease that is refractory to other treatments when other highly effective therapies are not available, and is still used in other regions such as Latin America.

CYCLOPHOSPHAMIDE (CYTOXAN)

Cyclophosphamide is an antineoplastic agent that was developed in the 1950s. It is metabolized in the liver into phosphoramide mustard, which acts as a DNA intercalating agent disrupting mitosis and leading to cell death. Rapidly dividing cells are especially affected. For this reason, it was FDA approved for the treatment of hematologic malignancies such as lymphomas, leukemia, and a variety of solid tumors. Cyclophosphamide was later found to have immunomodulatory and immunosuppressive effects via suppression of T and B cells, and alteration of pro- and anti-inflammatory cytokines secretion in favor of an anti-inflammatory state (9).

Cyclophosphamide was initially tested for use in MS in 1966 (10); however, there has been a paucity of large-scale randomized clinical trials that investigate the effects of cyclophosphamide in relapsing forms of MS. The first clinical trial included relapsing MS and progressive MS patients demonstrated that IV infusion of cyclophosphamide did not produce significant effects compared to adrenocorticotropic hormone (ACTH) or cortisol (11). Subsequently, an open-label, uncontrolled trial demonstrated that IV cyclophosphamide stabilized neurological decline as well as relapse rate in relapsing MS (12). In another trial including RRMS patients with refractory disease and rapidly deteriorating neurological function, cyclophosphamide infusions led to improvement in radiologic measures of disease (13). In recent years, a randomized, double blind trial involving SPMS patients failed to reach significance in its primary end point on time to disability progression; however, it did demonstrate some effects in reducing risk of progression on secondary analysis. The group that received cyclophosphamide had low tolerability to the drug and experienced higher dropout rates. This may have affected statistical analysis of the outcome measure (14).

Cyclophosphamide is generally well tolerated, despite significant safety concerns. Common and transient side effects include nausea, vomiting, and alopecia. Urinary

TABLE 14.1 Summary of Infusion Therapies Characteristics, Administration, and Monitoring Parameters

	DOSING	MECHANISM OF ACTION	ADVERSE EFFECTS	PREGNANCY CATEGORY	PRIOR TO INITIATING	MONITORING
Mitoxantrone	12 mg/m^2 IV every 3 mo for 24 mo per MIMS protocol 12–20 mg IV with 1 g IV methylprednisolone every mo for 6 mo per French British protocol Lifetime maximum 140 mg/m^2	Anthracenedione, topoisomerase inhibitor	Gonadal failure Amenorrhea Liver toxicity Cardiotoxicity (arrhythmia, congestive heart failure) Leukemia Alopecia IRR	D	Echocardiogram CBC with differential and platelets Pregnancy test in reproductive age females	CBC with differential and platelets prior to each dose, and every 6 mo for 5 y posttreatment Echocardiogram prior to each infusion, and annually for 5 y after discontinuation LFTs
Cyclophosphamide	No established treatment protocol 600 mg/m^2 IV every other day and daily IVMP × 8 d followed by 600–1,000 mg/m^2 IV every 4–8 wk with or without IVMP	Metabolite phosphoramide mustard is a DNA intercalating agent	Transient nausea/vomiting Reversible alopecia Urinary dysfunction, bladder cancer, hemorrhagic cystitis Infertility Liver toxicity	D, can be excreted in breast milk	LFT UA Pregnancy test in reproductive age females	UA and LFT when indicated
Natalizumab	300 mg IV monthly	Anti-α4-integrin monoclonal Ab	IRR Fatigue GI side effects Mild infections (URI/UTI) PML	C	JCV Ab MRI Brain Pregnancy test in reproductive age females	Annual MRI brain JVC Ab every 6–12 mo CBC every 6–12 mo LFT every 6–12 mo Anti-natalizumab Ab
Alemtuzumab	First course: 12 mg IV daily × 5 d Second course: 12 mg IV daily × 3 d 12 mo from first course Third course (as needed): 12 mg IV daily × 3 d when appropriate per disease course	Anti-CD52 monoclonal Ab	Autoimmune diseases (thyroid, renal, hematologic) Malignancy Lymphopenia IRR	C, and may be excreted in human milk	CBC with differential and platelets sCr TSH UA Skin exam HPV testing Also recommend: LFTs, VZV IgG, HIV, hepatitis serology, TB screening, pregnancy test in reproductive age females	TSH, free T4 every 3 months × 48 mo after final infusion CBC with differential and platelets monthly sCr monthly UA with microscopy monthly Annual skin exam Annual HPV screening and gynecological exam

(continued)

TABLE 14.1 Summary of Infusion Therapies Characteristics, Administration, and Monitoring Parameters (*continued*)

	DOSING	MECHANISM OF ACTION	ADVERSE EFFECTS	PREGNANCY CATEGORY	PRIOR TO INITIATING	MONITORING
Rituximab	No established guidelines -500 or 1,000 mg IV every 6–12 mo. (Swedish registry) Or 1,000–2,000 mg IV subdivided into two infusions given within 1 mo followed by 375 mg/m² IV weekly × 4 doses. (Naismith) Or 1,000 mg IV day 1 and day 15. (Hauser)	Anti-CD 20 monoclonal Ab	IRR Mild infections	C	CBC with differential and platelets Hepatitis B screening	CBC with differential and platelets to monitor for neutropenia when indicated
Ocrelizumab	Initial dose: 300 mg IV followed by 300 mg IV 2 wk after initial dose Then: 600 mg IV every 6 mo	Anti-CD 20 monoclonal Ab	IRR Mild infections (URI/UTI) Malignancy	No current category, but contraception advised prior to initiating infusion and for 6 mo post last infusion	Hepatitis B screening Pregnancy test in reproductive age females	Routine breast cancer screening

Ab, antibody; CBC, complete blood count; GI, gastrointestinal; HPV, human papilloma virus; IgG, immunoglobulin; IRR, infusion-related reactions; IV, intravenous; IVMP, intravenous methylprednisolone; JCV, John Cunningham virus; LFT, liver function tests; MIMS, Mitoxantrone in Multiple Sclerosis Study Group; PML, progressive multifocal leukoencephalopathy; sCr, serum creatine; TB, tuberculosis; TSH, thyroid stimulating hormone; UA, urinalysis; URI, upper respiratory infection; UTI, urinary tract infection; VZV, varicella zoster virus.

dysfunction can occur in many patients, and can be associated with a risk of bladder cancer and hemorrhagic cystitis. Since cyclophosphamide is metabolized through the hepatic system, in less than 10% of patients there can be elevation of hepatic enzymes and liver toxicity. It can also interfere with fertility in both males and females and menstruation in females. It is a pregnancy category D drug that can cause serious birth defects, and women who are breastfeeding should avoid cyclophosphamide since it can be excreted in breast milk (15).

There is no established treatment protocol for cyclophosphamide in MS. Commonly used IV regimen usually involves induction with every other day IV cyclophosphamide 600 mg/m² along with daily IVMP during the course of induction for 8 days and a 600 to 1,000 mg/m² dose given IV every 4 to 8 weeks with or without IVMP. In some cases cyclophosphamide can be combined with interferon beta or glatiramer acetate (16).

Despite mixed results in RRMS, cyclophosphamide does appear to exhibit some positive effects in disease activity due to its anti-inflammatory effects, especially in subgroup analysis involving patients with more active disease. Significant safety concerns limit the use of cyclophosphamide in clinical practice and for these reasons, in MS it remains a seldom-used medication.

NATALIZUMAB (TYSABRI)

Natalizumab is a selective humanized monoclonal antibody (Ab) that targets alpha 4 integrin, an adhesive molecule found on lymphocytic cell surfaces that mediates endothelial adhesion. Natalizumab blocks the adhesion of lymphocytes to central nervous system (CNS) endothelial cells, thus inhibiting the migration of lymphocytes into CNS space across the blood–brain barrier (BBB).

In placebo-controlled trials, natalizumab has been shown to have robust effects against relapses and radiographic evidence of disease activity. It significantly reduced the risk of confirmed disability progression (CDP) by 42%, relapse rate by 68%, and new or enlarging T2 lesions by 83% in a randomized placebo-controlled phase 3 trial involving RRMS patients (17). In patients who relapsed despite being on interferon beta therapy, the addition of natalizumab significantly reduced probability of progression, reduced annualized relapse rate (ARR), and improved radiographic disease burden (18).

Natalizumab has a half-life of approximately 16 days and its biological effects persist for 12 weeks. It is typically administered as 300 mg IV every 4 weeks. Baseline brain MRI with and without contrast should be obtained prior to initiating natalizumab as well as John Cunningham virus (JCV) Ab.

Natalizumab is a generally well-tolerated agent. Common side effects include infusion-related reactions, which can occur in up to a quarter of patients, as well as headache, fatigue, gastrointestinal side effects, and infections such as UTI and upper respiratory infection (URI). Ab to natalizumab can develop in up to 6% of patients, which

can block the biologic effects of natalizumab and render it ineffective, and can increase risk for hypersensitivity reactions. Timing to onset of hypersensitivity can be immediate or delayed, and is most common during the second dose; up to 1% of patients can potentially develop anaphylaxis. The hypersensitivity effects can be ameliorated with administration of antihistamines and corticosteroids in pretreatment.

The FDA approved natalizumab for treatment of relapsing MS in 2004. However, after three cases of progressive multifocal encephalopathy (PML) were associated with natalizumab, it was taken off the market in February 2005 until further investigations were made with regard to its relationship to PML. In July 2006, it was made commercially available once again for the treatment of RRMS.

PML is a progressive brain infection caused by the reactivation of JCV. The risk of PML in patients on natalizumab was initially reported to be 1/1,000 in 2006 (19). Since then, the total number of natalizumab-associated PML cases, as of June 2017, is 731 out of 170,900 patients, with 728 being MS patients. Total doses of natalizumab prior to PML diagnosis ranges from 8 to 134 doses, with an average duration of 49 months on natalizumab (Biogen data on-file).

Natalizumab-treated patients can be risk stratified based on history and clinical data (Table 14.2). JCV Ab should be checked prior to initiating natalizumab as JCV infections is a prerequisite for development of PML. Patients without anti-JCV antibodies are at lower risk of developing PML, approximately less than 0.09/1,000. It is important to note whether a patient has been on immunosuppressive treatment prior to natalizumab, as prior immunosuppression (IS) use confers a 2- to 4-fold increase in PML risk. The duration of natalizumab also positively correlates with risk of developing PML, with a time-responsive risk increase in approximately 14% of PML cases developed within the first 24 months and the majority developed in patients who received greater than 24 months of therapy (19).

In addition to the three factors mentioned earlier, JCV Ab index is another marker that may be able to assist in risk stratification—patients diagnosed with PML had higher titers than patients without PML (20). Currently in clinical practice,

TABLE 14.2 Risk-Stratification for PML in Natalizumab-Treated Patients

ANTI-JCV NEGATIVE		
<1/1,000		
ANTI-JCV POSITIVE		
NATALIZUMAB EXPOSURE DURATION	NO PRIOR IS USE	PRIOR IS USE
1–24 mo	<1/1,000	1/1,000
25–48 mo	3/1,000	12/1,000
49–72 mo	6/1,000	13/1,000

JCV, John Cunningham virus; PML, progressive multifocal leukoencephalopathy IS, immunosuppression.

it is generally accepted that in natalizumab-treated patients with JCV index of greater than 1.5, the risk of PML is higher (21). For patients with JCV index less than 0.9, along with no prior IS, the risk of PML is considerably lower than those with JVC index greater than 1.5. Table 14.2 presents estimated risk of PML based on factors described earlier.

MRI is deemed the most critical tool in detecting PML, as early lesions may be subclinical and early detection makes early intervention possible. For these reasons, patients on natalizumab should have MRI conducted at least every 6 months and JCV Ab and index should be checked every 6-12 months. Cerebrospinal fluid (CSF) screening for PML, specifically for the JCV polymerase chain reaction (PCR), is specific, but is not 100% sensitive as low DNA titers may be hard to detect. Multiple cases of JCV PCR-negative PML have been reported (22), likely due to titers below laboratory detection threshold.

If a clinical suspicion for PML exists, natalizumab should be discontinued immediately. MRI brain with and without contrast, CSF testing, and JCV PCR should be obtained. Plasma exchange can be initiated to accelerate removal of natalizumab, at the recommended frequency of every other day for a total of five sessions. In rare cases of diagnostic uncertainty, brain biopsy may be required.

Given its potency, natalizumab is a good choice in cases of patients with active disease. In JCV-negative patients, the use of natalizumab as a first-line agent has been increasingly popular. In JCV-positive patients, risk and benefit have to be weighed carefully and alternative options should be considered. Its use in progressive disease is limited given the negative results from a recent large study of SPMS with natalizumab (23).

ALEMTUZUMAB (LEMTRADA)

Alemtuzumab is a humanized monoclonal Ab directed against cell surface protein CD52. CD52 is found on both B and T cells, with the highest concentrations found on memory B cells and myeloid dendritic cells. Infusion of alemtuzumab depletes cells in the adaptive immune system while leaving cells of the innate immune system intact. It also modulates the cytological profile of reconstituted lymphocytes after depletion (24,25).

Prior to its utilization in treatment of MS, alemtuzumab, also known as Campath, MabCampath, and Campath-1H, was developed as a chemotherapy agent to treat malignancies including lymphoma. The FDA-approved alemtuzumab in 2014 for the treatment of RRMS in patients who have failed two or more DMTs on the basis of two registration studies. In the CARE MS I study alemtuzumab was compared to interferon beta 1a as a first-line treatment for RRMS patients and reduced ARR by 55%. There was also a greater proportion of patients on alemtuzumab who remained relapse-free compared to interferon beta (26). Similar efficacy was reported in a phase 3 randomized trial of alemtuzumab compared to interferon beta as a second-line treatment for RRMS (Care-MS II) in patients who experienced one or more relapses while on interferon or glatiramer acetate. This trial demonstrated that alemtuzumab produced significant reduction in relapses and also in disability progression (27). In another open label study of patients who experienced two or more relapses despite being on interferon, alemtuzumab was shown to be effective in reducing relapse rate and improving expanded disability status (EDSS) (28).

The half-life of alemtuzumab is approximately 21 days, its clearance mechanism is not currently understood; thus, no dosing adjustments for renal or hepatic impairments have been advised. A single course can result in lymphopenia with recovery at various rates.

Alemtuzumab is administered in two separate infusion courses. The first treatment course consists of a 12 mg daily infusion over 5 consecutive days, followed by second treatment course of a 12 mg daily infusion for 3 consecutive days 12 months following the first course. Premedication with corticosteroids or corticosteroids with antihistamine agents is recommended prior to infusion and during the first 3 days of treatment course. Acyclovir 200 mg given twice daily initiated on the day of first infusion and continued for 2 years is also recommended.

The most common side effects after receiving alemtuzumab are infusion-related reactions (~90%) and mild to moderate infections (~70%). However, its most severe side effects are secondary autoimmunity including immune thrombocytopenic purpura (2%), autoimmune thyroiditis (10%–34%), and nephropathies (0.3%) such as glomerulonephritis and anti-glomerular basement membrane disease. In another multicenter prospective cohort, cumulative risk for developing autoimmune diseases following alemtuzumab infusion is reported to be 23%, timing of onset is most commonly seen between months 12 to 18 and 30 to 36 following treatment (29). Rare incidences of malignancies were also reported following alemtuzumab infusion—including thyroid cancer, melanoma, and lymphoma. There is a currently approved Risk Evaluation and Mitigation Strategies (REMS) for alemtuzumab by FDA, last updated in April 2016.

CBC with platelets, serum creatinine, thyroid stimulating hormone (TSH), and urinalysis should be obtained prior to drug administration. In addition, when clinically indicated, it is recommended to obtain liver function enzymes (LFTs), varicella zoster virus (VZV) immunoglobulin G (IgG), HIV testing, hepatitis serology, tuberculosis screening, and pregnancy test prior to initiation of alemtuzumab. After initial infusion, CBC with platelets and serum creatinine should be checked monthly until 48 months after the second infusion. TSH should be checked every 3 months following initial infusion and until 48 months after last infusion. Urinalysis should be checked monthly following the initial infusion. Other monitoring parameters include annual HPV screening, annual gynecological exams, and baseline and annual skin exams (for melanoma). Prophylaxis with oral antivirals is also recommended for prevention of herpetic infections.

Alemtuzumab exhibits significant effects in reducing relapses and MRI disease activity and sustaining relapse-free periods. Sustained effects of alemtuzumab not requiring further infusions or additional treatments have been reported. Furthermore, its unique infusion schedule of two courses 1 year apart can be utilized to tailor treatment, for example, in female patients who wish to become pregnant in between infusions. However, due to alemtuzumab's side effect profile of autoimmune disorders and some risk of malignancy, it is generally reserved as a second-line agent for actively relapsing patients who have failed other DMTs, and in whom other infusion DMTs with better safety profiles are contraindicated.

RITUXIMAB (RITUXAN)

Rituximab is a chimeric monoclonal Ab that targets CD20, which is primarily expressed on B-cell surfaces and a minority of T cells. It functions via depletion of peripheral and CNS B and to a lesser extent T cells. Initially FDA approved in 1997 for treatment of refractory B-cell non-Hodgkin's lymphoma, now it is approved to treat a variety of autoimmune and paraneoplastic conditions across several fields of medicine. In MS, rituximab has been used anecdotally to treat patients with disease refractory to other DMTs. Despite its widespread use in MS, no large phase 3 trial has examined its effect in relapsing forms of MS. Larger, long-term phase 3 trials are less likely to be pursued in the setting of multiple newer anti-CD20 antibodies being developed and investigated; however, several observational studies are being conducted. Of the completed trials in RRMS, rituximab did demonstrate encouraging results—an open label study of RRMS patients who received rituximab infusions at weeks 0, 2, 24, and 26 reported reduction in clinical relapses and radiographic burden of disease when compared to pretreatment baseline (30). A phase 2 study of 104 RRMS patients who received rituximab had fewer contrast-enhancing lesions (CELs) and relapses compared to patients who received placebo (31). B-cell suppression was maintained for at least 24 weeks beyond the initial infusion period. Reduction in enhancing lesions and improved clinical scores were seen with rituximab infusions weekly over 4 weeks as an add-on therapy for a small cohort of patients with refractory MS who relapsed at least once despite being on injectable therapy (32). In a large retrospective observational study comparing rituximab to interferon beta and glatiramer, rituximab demonstrated significant relapse rate reduction and drug tolerability, however, improvements in EDSS were not found to be significant (33).

For primary progressive disease, a large trial involving rituximab failed to show delay in disease progression or brain atrophy; however, it did reduce T2 lesion volume accruement and subgroup analysis demonstrated an effect in disease progression in younger patients (age <51 years) with more severe active disease and CELs at baseline (34).

Rituximab is well tolerated, with a majority of patients reporting mild infectious events such as URI, UTI, and nasopharyngitis (>10%), and infusion-related reactions such as headache and chills (69.6%). B-cell depletion is usually achieved by week 2 of infusion and persists for at least 24 to 48 weeks (31). Decreased immunoglobulin levels can result in an increase in infections and there are reports of neutropenia associated with rituximab as well (35,36).

Despite the lack of adequate large randomized phase 3 controlled trials in RRMS, rituximab has been frequently used off-label as an alternative to currently FDA-approved DMT for MS in the United States. Rituximab remains as an option for patients with active relapsing disease who are intolerant of other DMTs or if other DMTs are unavailable. Several international healthcare systems have approved its use in MS as well as large private healthcare systems in the United States.

OCRELIZUMAB (OCREVUS)

Ocrelizumab is a humanized recombinant monoclonal anti-CD20 Ab that binds to a different but overlapping epitope compared to rituximab. Developed after observation that rituximab was effective in B-cell depletion in MS, ocrelizumab has demonstrated effects in RRMS and PPMS. In a phase 3 double blind, interferon-controlled trials in RRMS, ocrelizumab was compared with interferon beta 1a and significantly reduced ARR by 45%, reduced risk to CDP by 34% at 6 months, and significantly reduced the number of CELs as well as new/enlarging T2 lesions (37). In PPMS, ocrelizumab was shown to delay 3 months disability progression by 24% when compared to placebo. Secondary outcomes including brain atrophy, T2 lesion accumulation, and total T2 lesion volume were also positive (38). It was approved by FDA in March 2017 as the first DMT indicated for the treatment of both relapsing and primary progressive forms MS.

The approved dose for ocrelizumab consists of an initial dose of 300 mg followed by a second 300 mg dose 2 weeks later. Thereafter, ocrelizumab is infused every 6 months at a single dose of 600 mg.

Ocrelizumab is generally well tolerated based on existing data for both MS and non-MS population. The most common side effects include infusion-related reactions (34%–40%), which can be treated by pretreating with appropriate antihistamine agents and methylprednisolone prior to each infusion. Mild infections, which include URI, UTI, and nasopharyngitis respond well to antibiotics. There is also an increased risk of developing mild–moderate herpes-related infections (5%) after receiving ocrelizumab; thus, it is contraindicated in patients with active herpes. Hepatitis B reactivation can occur as also described with other anti-CD20 therapies; thus, hepatitis B virus screening should be performed in patients prior to initial infusion. Ocrelizumab is contraindicated in patients with acute hepatitis B. There is also an increased risk of malignancy (<1%), specifically breast cancer in females; thus, routine cancer screening should also be performed in patients who receive ocrelizumab.

Anti-ocrelizumab antibodies occurred in only 0.4% of patients and there are currently insufficient data to determine the effect of neutralizing antibodies in regard to safety and efficacy.

The half-life of ocrelizumab is 26 days. B-cell depletion is achieved around week 2 following initial infusion and remains at negligible levels until recovery at approximately week 72. Effect on CELs appears to be prompt with most of the effect occurring in the first 4 weeks after medication initiation. Previously when ocrelizumab was investigated in rheumatologic diseases, trials were halted early due to opportunistic infections, and this may be related to the underlying disease and use of concomitant medications. However, in MS populations studied, there have been no increases in opportunistic infections when compared to interferon. There has been a single case of PML reported with ocrelizumab use; however, it was felt to be related to recent natalizumab administration. There are no reported PML cases that have been solely attributed to ocrelizumab to date.

Ocrelizumab is a treatment option for non-treatment-naïve patients with RRMS in the setting of ongoing disease activity, especially in the presence of JCV-positive serology, where other highly effective treatments are likely to carry higher risk. Given its overall favorable safety profile to date it also is a reasonable consideration in treatment-naïve patients, especially in those with high levels of disease activity at baseline. As more real world data are collected with this medication, its use as a first-line agent will likely increase over time. In primary-progressive MS it is the only medication approved. Of note, the medication was studied in a group of patients under age 55, in which approximately one quarter of patients had enhancing lesions at baseline. Its utility in patients older than 55 years and those without evidence of inflammatory lesions over sustained periods of time remains unclear (Table 14.3).

TABLE 14.3   Pivotal Phase 3 Trials for FDA-Approved Infusion Therapies for RRMS

DRUG	TRIAL	EFFECT ON DISABILITY	EFFECT ON RELAPSE RATE	EFFECT ON RADIOGRAPHIC DISEASE MEASURES
Mitoxantrone	MIMS (randomized, double blind, placebo controlled) (2)	−0.13 improvement in EDSS (compared to 0.24 in placebo group)	68% reduction in ARR	74% decrease in number of CELs 85% decrease in number of new/enlarging T2 lesions
Natalizumab	AFFIRM (randomized, double-blind, placebo controlled) (18)	42% risk reduction to CDP	68% reduction ARR	92% reduction in number of CELs 82% reduction in number of new/enlarging T2 lesions
Alemtuzumab	CARE-MS I (randomized, double-blind, IFNβ-1a controlled, treatment-naïve patients) (26)	27% risk reduction to CDP (nonsignificant)	54.9% reduction in ARR	63% reduction in number of CELs 17% reduction in number of new/enlarging T2 lesions
	CARE-MS II (randomized, double-blind, IFNβ-1a controlled, refractory patients) (27)	42% risk reduction to CDP	49.4% reduction in ARR	61% reduction in CELs 32% reduction in new/enlarging T2 lesions
Ocrelizumab	Opera I/II (randomized, double-blind, IFNβ-1a controlled) (37)	37% risk reduction to CDP	47% reduction in ARR	94% and 95% reduction in number of CELs. 77% and 83% reduction in number of new/enlarging T2 lesions

ARR, annualized relapse rate; CDP, confirmed disability progression; CEL, contrast-enhancing lesion; EDSS, expanded disability status scale; FDA, Food and Drug Administration; IFN, interferon; RRMS, relapsing–remitting MS

CONCLUSION

In the advent of an increasing number of disease-modifying therapies to treat relapsing form of MS, the currently available infusion monoclonal antibodies are notable as high-efficacy options. They are currently used for patients with breakthrough disease activity and in treatment-naïve patients with highly active disease. Their use in treatment-naïve patients will likely become more common as the question of escalation versus early highly effective treatment is now being considered by both patients and clinicians. It is important to note that each therapy has its own unique profile of side effects and monitoring parameters; thus, careful screening of risk factors, stringent post-administration monitoring and symptom-based management are needed. As data from postmarketing surveillance expand for the newer infusion monoclonal medications, clinicians will have a better understanding of risk and will be able to tailor treatment to individual patient needs.

KEY POINTS FOR PATIENTS AND FAMILIES

- There are currently six infusion therapies that can be used intravenously for the treatment of relapsing MS, four of which are FDA approved.
- Infusion therapies are more potent in reducing inflammation and delaying disability, and require less frequent dosing compared to oral and injectable therapies.
- Given the unique efficacy and side effect profile of each agent, choice of infusion therapy is guided by patient preference, disease status and disability progression, dosing frequency, and tolerability of side effects.
- Stringent monitoring is recommended due to incidence of some rare but serious adverse effects.
- All infusion therapies should be avoided in pregnant patients.

REFERENCES

1. Fidler JM, DeJoy SQ, Gibbons JJ. Selective immunomodulation by the antineoplastic agent mitoxantrone. I. Suppression of B lymphocyte function. *J Immunol.* 1986;137(2): 727–732. Available at: http://www.jimmunol.org/content/137/2/727? ijkey=87589caa02173468ac503af904cf17b34ce267ba&keytype2=tf_ipsecsha. Accessed July 22, 2017.

2. Hartung H-P, Gonsette R, König N, et al. Mitoxantrone in progressive multiple sclerosis: a placebo-controlled, double-blind, randomised, multicentre trial. *Lancet.* 2000;360(9350):2018–2025.

3. Edan G, Miller D, Clanet M, et al. Therapeutic effect of mitoxantrone combined with methylprednisolone in multiple sclerosis: a randomised multicentre study of active disease using MRI and clinical criteria. *J Neurol Neurosurg Psychiatry.* 1997;62(2):112–118. doi:10.1136/JNNP.62.2.112.

4. van de Wyngaert FA, Beguin C, D'Hooghe MB, et al. A double-blind clinical trial of mitoxantrone versus methylprednisolone in relapsing, secondary progressive multiple sclerosis. *Acta Neurol Belg.* 2001;101(4):210–216. Available at: http://www.ncbi.nlm.nih.gov/pubmed/11851027. Accessed July 22, 2017.

5. Rivera VM, Jeffery DR, Weinstock-Guttman B, et al. Results from the 5-year, phase IV RENEW (Registry to Evaluate Novantrone Effects in Worsening Multiple Sclerosis) study. *BMC Neurol.* 2013;13:80. doi:10.1186/1471-2377-13-80.

6. Marriott JJ, Miyasaki JM, Gronseth G, et al. Evidence report: The efficacy and safety of mitoxantrone (Novantrone) in the treatment of multiple sclerosis: report of the Therapeutics and Technology Assessment Subcommittee of the American Academy of Neurology. *Neurology.* 2010;74(18):1463–1470. doi:10.1212/WNL.0b013e3181dc1ae0.

7. Edan G, Comi G, Le Page E, et al. Mitoxantrone prior to interferon beta-1b in aggressive relapsing multiple sclerosis: a 3-year randomised trial. *J Neurol Neurosurg Psychiatry.* 2011;82(12):1344–1350. doi:10.1136/jnnp.2010.229724.

8. Martinelli Boneschi F, Vacchi L, Rovaris M, et al. Mitoxantrone for multiple sclerosis. In: Martinelli Boneschi F, ed. *Cochrane Database of Systematic Reviews.* Chichester, UK: John Wiley & Sons, Ltd; 2013. doi:10.1002/14651858.CD002127.pub3.

9. Smith DR, Balashov KE, Hafler DA, et al. Immune deviation following pulse cyclophosphamide/methylprednisolone treatment of multiple sclerosis: increased interleukin-4 production and associated eosinophilia. *Ann Neurol.* 1997;42(3):313–318. doi:10.1002/ana.410420307.

10. Aimard G, Girard PF, Raveau J. Multiple sclerosis and the auto-immunization process. Treatment by antimitotics. *Lyon Med.* 1966;15(6):345–352.

11. Cendrowski W. Treatment of multiple sclerosis with intravenous hydrocortisone hemisuccinate in combination with cyclophosphamide or cytosine arabinoside. *Neurol Neurochir Pol.* 1974;8(1):47–52. Available at: http://www.ncbi.nlm.nih.gov/pubmed/4407711. Accessed July 31, 2017.

12. Gonsette RE, Demonty L, Delmotte P. Intensive immunosuppression with cyclophosphamide in multiple sclerosis. *J Neurol.* 1977;214(3):173–181. doi:10.1007/BF00316148.

13. Gobbini MI, Smith ME, Richert ND, et al. Effect of open label pulse cyclophosphamide therapy on MRI measures of disease activity in five patients with refractory relapsing–remitting multiple sclerosis. *J Neuroimmunol.* 1999;99(1):142–149. doi:10.1016/S0165-5728(99)00039-9.

14. Brochet B, Deloire MSA, Perez P, et al. Double-blind controlled randomized trial of cyclophosphamide versus methylprednisolone in secondary progressive multiple sclerosis. *PLOS ONE.* 2017;12(1):e0168834. doi:10.1371/journal.pone.0168834.

15. Portaccio E, Zipoli V, Siracusa G, et al. Safety and tolerability of cyclophosphamide "pulses" in multiple sclerosis: a prospective study in a clinical cohort. *Mult Scler J.* 2003;9(5):446–450. doi:10.1191/1352458503ms926oa.

16. Weiner HL, Cohen JA. Treatment of multiple sclerosis with cyclophosphamide: critical review of clinical and immunologic effects. *Mult Scler J*. 2002;8(2):142–154. doi:10.1191/1352458502ms790oa.

17. Polman CH, O'Connor PW, Havrdova E, et al. A Randomized, placebo-controlled trial of natalizumab for relapsing multiple sclerosis. *N Engl J Med*. 2006;354(9):899–910.

18. Rudick RA, Stuart WH, Calabresi PA, et al. Natalizumab plus interferon beta-1a for relapsing multiple sclerosis. *N Engl J Med*. 2006;354(9):911–923.

19. Bloomgren G, Richman S, Hotermans C, et al. Risk of natalizumab-associated progressive multifocal leukoencephalopathy. *N Engl J Med*. 2012;366(20):1870–1880. doi:10.1056/NEJMoa1107829.

20. Plavina T, Subramanyam M, Bloomgren G, et al. Anti-JC virus antibody levels in serum or plasma further define risk of natalizumab-associated progressive multifocal leukoencephalopathy. *Ann Neurol*. 2014;76(6):802–812. doi:10.1002/ana.24286.

21. Warnke C, von Geldern G, Markwerth P, et al. Cerebrospinal fluid JC virus antibody index for diagnosis of natalizumab-associated progressive multifocal leukoencephalopathy. *Ann Neurol*. 2014; 76(6):792–801. doi:10.1002/ana.24153.

22. Kuhle J, Gosert R, Buhler R, et al. Management and outcome of CSF-JC virus PCR-negative PML in a natalizumab-treated patient with MS. *Neurology*. 2011;77(23):2010–2016. doi:10.1212/WNL.0b013e31823b9b27.

23. Steiner D, Arnold DL, Freedman MS, et al. Natalizumab versus placebo in patients with secondary progressive multiple sclerosis (SPMS): results from ASCEND, a multicenter, double-blind, placebo-controlled, randomized phase 3 clinical trial. *Poster presented at: 68th Annual Meeting of the American Academy of Neurology*; April 14; 2016; Vancouver, BC.

24. Rao SP, Sancho J, Campos-Rivera J, et al. Human peripheral blood mononuclear cells exhibit heterogeneous CD52 expression levels and show differential sensitivity to alemtuzumab mediated cytolysis. *PLOS ONE*. 2012;7(6):e39416. doi:10.1371/journal.pone.0039416.

25. Hill-Cawthorne GA, Button T, Tuohy O, et al. Long term lymphocyte reconstitution after alemtuzumab treatment of multiple sclerosis. *J Neurol Neurosurg Psychiatry*. 2012;83(3):298–304.

26. Cohen JA, Coles AJ, Arnold DL, et al. Alemtuzumab versus interferon beta 1a as first-line treatment for patients with relapsing-remitting multiple sclerosis: a randomised controlled phase 3 trial. *Lancet*. 2012;380(9856):1819–1828.

27. Coles AJ, Twyman CL, Arnold DL, et al. Alemtuzumab for patients with relapsing multiple sclerosis after disease-modifying therapy: a randomised controlled phase 3 trial. *Lancet*. 2012;380(9856):1829–1839.

28. Fox EJ, Sullivan HC, Gazda SK, et al. A single-arm, open-label study of alemtuzumab in treatment-refractory patients with multiple sclerosis. *Eur J Neurol*. 2012;19(2):307–311. doi:10.1111/j.1468-1331.2011.03507.x.

29. Cossburn M, Pace AA, Jones J, et al. Autoimmune disease after alemtuzumab treatment for multiple sclerosis in a multicenter cohort. *Neurology*. 2011;77(6):573–579. doi:10.1212/WNL.0b013e318228bec5.

30. Bar-Or A, Calabresi PAJ, Arnold D, et al. Rituximab in relapsing-remitting multiple sclerosis: a 72-week, open-label, phase I trial. *Ann Neurol*. 2008;63(3):395–400.

31. Hauser SL, Waubant E, Arnold DL, et al. B-cell depletion with rituximab in relapsing-remitting multiple sclerosis. *N Engl J Med*. 2008;358(7):676–688.

32. Naismith RT, Piccio L, Lyons JA, et al. Rituximab add-on therapy for breakthrough relapsing multiple sclerosis: a 52-week phase II trial. *Neurology*. 2010;74(23):1860–1867.

33. Spelman T, Frisell T, Piehl F, et al. Comparative effectiveness of rituximab relative to IFN-β or glatiramer acetate in relapsing-remitting MS from the Swedish MS registry. *Mult Scler J*. June 2017:135245851771366. doi:10.1177/1352458517713668.

34. Hawker K, O'Connor P, Freedman MS, et al. Rituximab in patients with primary progressive multiple sclerosis: results of a randomized double-blind placebo-controlled multicenter trial. *Ann Neurol*. 2009;66(4):460–471.

35. Wolach O, Bairey O, Lahav M. Late-onset neutropenia after rituximab treatment. *Medicine (Baltimore)*. 2010;89(5):308–318. doi:10.1097/MD.0b013e3181f2caef.

36. Dunleavy K, Tay K, Wilson WH. Rituximab-associated neutropenia. *Semin Hematol*. 2010;47:180–186. doi:10.1053/j.seminhematol.2010.01.009.

37. Hauser SL, Bar-Or A, Comi G, et al. Ocrelizumab versus Interferon beta-1a in relapsing multiple sclerosis. *N Engl J Med*. 2017;376(3):221–234. doi:10.1056/NEJMoa1601277.

38. Montalban X, Hauser SL, Kappos L, et al. Ocrelizumab versus placebo in primary progressive multiple sclerosis. *N Engl J Med*. 2017;376(3):209–220. doi:10.1056/NEJMoa1606468.

15

Treating Progressive Multiple Sclerosis

Carrie M. Hersh

KEY POINTS FOR CLINICIANS

- Primary progressive multiple sclerosis (PPMS) is defined by progressive accrual of disability in the absence of relapses.
- Secondary progressive multiple sclerosis (SPMS) is defined as an initial relapsing–remitting disease course followed by gradual clinical progression with or without relapses.
- Recent changes have been proposed to the classification of progressive MS that focus on presence (or absence) of disease activity and continued disability progression. These proposals will help identify patients for PPMS and SPMS clinical trials and treatment.
- Ocrelizumab is the first disease-modifying therapy approved for PPMS and suggests a role for B-cell therapy for both the inflammatory and perhaps neurodegenerative phases of progressive multiple sclerosis (MS).
- Numerous therapeutics for the treatment of PPMS and SPMS with unique mechanisms of action are currently in the investigatory phase, including siponimod, high-dose biotin, and ibudilast.
- Concerted efforts are currently in progress via the Progressive MS Alliance, Multiple Sclerosis Outcome Assessments Consortium, and the International Collaborative on Progressive MS to identify robust metrics for measuring MS-related disability in progressive MS and, as an extension, developing novel neurotherapeutics.
- Symptomatic therapies and neurorehabilitation are important management strategies to improve quality of life and function in progressive MS.

DEFINITION OF PROGRESSIVE MULTIPLE SCLEROSIS

MS is a chronic, inflammatory, demyelinating, and neurodegenerative disease of the central nervous system (CNS) that affects the white and gray matter of the brain and spinal cord. Approximately, 85% of patients present with a relapsing–remitting MS (RRMS) disease course at onset, defined as alternating episodes of new or worsening symptoms (relapses), followed by complete or partial recovery of symptoms (remission). About two-thirds of RRMS patients will transition to SPMS, a clinical form of MS that is characterized by gradual accumulation of disability independent of relapses over time. PPMS occurs in about 10% of patients, characterized as gradual worsening of neurologic disability from disease onset with absence of distinct relapses or remissions (1). The term "progressive MS" is a collective term for both SPMS and PPMS.

CLINICAL FEATURES, DISEASE COURSE, AND IMPLICATIONS FOR TARGETED DISEASE THERAPY

There are two important limitations in clinical practice for managing progressive MS, which can reflexively pose a challenge in developing an effective individualized therapeutic strategy:

1. Identification of the distinct time of transition from a RRMS to SPMS disease course, typically defined as a period of 6 to 12 months of gradual disability progression proceeding the relapsing phase.
2. Identification of PPMS at symptom onset as distinct from a relapsing–remitting disease course with slower or delayed onset of subsequent relapses.

The recognition of progressive MS can therefore be delayed past a point where irreversible or "fixed" disability has already incurred. There are no MRI or laboratory biomarkers yet available that effectively identify patients with progressive MS. Thus, practitioners are tasked with recognizing a progressive disease course based on careful clinical observation and scrutiny.

In SPMS there are several risk factors that shorten the transition time to clinical progression from a relapsing–remitting disease course: advanced age at the time of onset; initial presentation of posterior fossa or spinal cord syndromes; incomplete recovery of function following the initial relapse; higher number of relapses within the first 5 years of disease onset; and higher disability early in the disease course (2). A feature that distinguishes PPMS from the more common presentation of RRMS, besides a slower, insidious onset of symptoms, is an older age at presentation (40–50 years old). Most studies show that PPMS patients are typically about 10 years older than those presenting with RRMS (3,4). It should also be noted that relapses may still occur in patients with SPMS, and occasionally even in individuals with PPMS (5). Although the term "progressive relapsing" MS was previously generally accepted to define the latter phenotype, new criteria have since been proposed to simplify the classification.

An international panel of MS experts recently proposed changes to the classification of MS to more effectively characterize the clinical course of progressive MS (6). One of the changes included the categorization of progressive disease as either phenotypically manifesting active inflammation ("active") or no active inflammation ("nonactive") via new clinical relapses and/or new T2 and/or gadolinium-enhancing (GdE) MRI lesions within the past year. Another proposed change was the categorization of progressive disease on the presence or absence of continued gradual clinical decline ("with progression" or "without progression") (see Figure 15.1). These proposed recommendations were built to allow clearer conceptualization of progressive MS and more efficient recruitment of progressive MS patients into clinical trials.

Since the inauguration of disease-modifying therapies (DMTs) in 1993, there have been dramatic advances in the MS field. These breakthroughs have primarily centered on the development of agents targeting inflammation to modify the overall disease course in relapsing MS. However, up until recently, there has been a significant unmet need in developing effective neurotherapeutics for PPMS and SPMS, specifically for progressive disease that is inactive but progressive. This dearth of treatment for

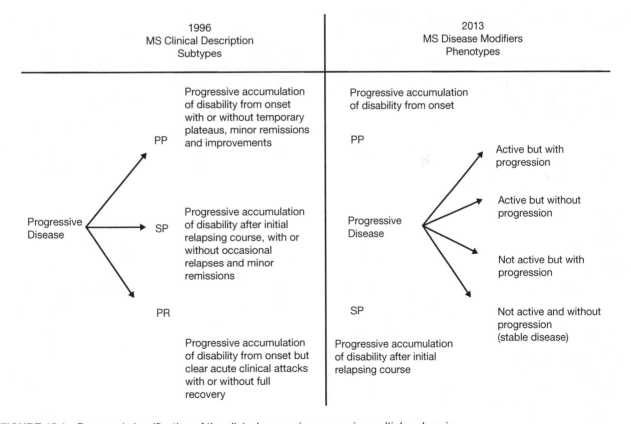

FIGURE 15.1 Proposed classification of the clinical course in progressive multiple sclerosis.

Source: Lublin FD, Reingold SC, Cohen JA, et al, Defining the clinical course of multiple sclerosis: the 2013 revisions. *Neurology*. 2014; 83:278-286 and http://n.neurology.org/content/83/3/278.long.

progressive MS stems from an incomplete understanding of the disease pathogenesis, lack of validated outcome measures, and mostly negative clinical trial experiences to date.

PATHOGENESIS AND NEUROTHERAPEUTIC IMPLICATIONS

In RRMS, a predominant pathological feature is the breakdown of the blood–brain barrier with subsequent focal inflammatory demyelination. In progressive MS, inflammation is a less defining pathological hallmark. Instead, progressive MS is characterized by neurodegeneration of the white and gray matter resulting in brain and spinal cord atrophy on a background of mild–moderate inflammation (7). Predominant factors driving neurodegeneration include mitochondrial dysfunction due to defective oxidative phosphorylation and nitric oxide production, resulting in a chronic state of virtual hypoxia due to unmet energy demands (8), and age-dependent iron accumulation in myelin and oligodendrocytes leading to oxidative tissue damage (9).

Growing evidence supports a strong pathogenic role of B lymphocytes on MS disease activity and implicates a unique neurotherapeutic target, as suggested by the OLYMPUS trial (10). This notion is further substantiated by postmortem brain tissue from patients with SPMS that showed meningeal lymphoid follicles containing proliferating B cells (11). Diffuse T lymphocyte- and B lymphocyte-driven meningeal inflammation has also been demonstrated in PPMS, resulting in extensive demyelination and neurite loss in the cortical gray matter, leading to a more severe clinical disease course (12).

A fundamental question that remains is whether or not there are innate differences in the inflammatory response of relapsing versus progressive forms of MS, given the failure of most anti-inflammatory DMTs in progressive MS to date (8), including interferon beta (13–16), cladribine (17), glatiramer acetate (18), rituximab (10), and fingolimod (19) (see Table 15.1). Although mitoxantrone showed reduced progression of disability and clinical relapses in a population of patients with RRMS and SPMS (20), significant safety concerns restrict its use in clinical practice. In either case, the key neurodegenerative pathophysiologic mechanisms that underlie progressive MS, namely PPMS and SPMS that is inactive yet still progressive, warrant further understanding to identify targets beyond the inflammatory aspects of disease that will more effectively uncover robust neurotherapeutics.

TABLE 15.1 Placebo-Controlled Clinical Trials in PMS

AGENT/STUDY	YEAR	DISEASE COURSE	STUDY DURATION (MONTHS)	SAMPLE SIZE	SUMMARY OF OUTCOMES
Interferon beta-1b SC qod Dose: 4 million IU SC × 2 wk, then 8 million IU SC qod (EUSPMS) (13)	1998	SPMS	36	718	Significant benefit: delay in progression of disability, defined as sustained increase in EDSS for at least 3 mo
Cladribine Dose: 0.07 mg/kg/d SC for 5 consecutive days every 4 wk for either two or six cycles (total dose, 0.7 mg/kg or 2.1 mg/kg, respectively) (17)	2000	SPMS	12	159	No significant benefit: mean change in disability (EDSS)
Interferon beta-1a SC tiw Dose: 22 or 44 mcg SC tiw (SPECTRIMS) (14)	2001	SPMS	36	618	No significant benefit: time to confirmed progression of disability
Mitoxantrone Dose: (5 mg/m² [exploratory group] or 12 mg/m² IV) every 3 mo (MIMS) (20)	2002	RRMS, SPMS	24	194	Significant benefit: reduced progression of disability and clinical exacerbations
Interferon beta-1a weekly Dose: 60 mcg IM weekly (IMPACT) (15)	2002	SPMS	24	436	No significant benefit: EDSS
Interferon beta-1b SC qod Dose: 8 million IU (or adjusted for body weight/size, 5 million IU/mL) SC qod (NASPMS) (16)	2004	SPMS	36[a]	939	No significant benefit

(continued)

TABLE 15.1 Placebo-Controlled Clinical Trials in PMS (*continued*)

AGENT/STUDY	YEAR	DISEASE COURSE	STUDY DURATION (MONTHS)	SAMPLE SIZE	SUMMARY OF OUTCOMES
Glatiramer acetate Dose: 20 mg SC daily (PROMISE) (18)	2007	PPMS	36	943	No significant benefit: sustained accumulation of disability
Rituximab Dose: two 1,000 mg IV infusions every 24 wk (OLYMPUS) (10)	2009	PPMS	24	439	No significant benefit: time to confirmed disease progression
Fingolimod Dose: 0.5 mg PO daily (INFORMS) (19)	2016	PPMS	36	823	No significant benefit: 3-mo confirmed disability progression

aTrial was stopped early due to lack of clinical benefit.

EDSS, Expanded Disability Status Scale; IM, intramuscular; IU, international units; IV, intravenous; PMS, progressive multiple sclerosis; PO, oral; PPMS, primary progressive multiple sclerosis; qod, every other day; RRMS, relapsing–remitting MS; SC, subcutaneous; SPMS, secondary progressive multiple sclerosis; tiw, three times per week.

Overall, an incomplete understanding of progressive MS pathogenesis has slowed the development of effective therapies and requires further inquiry. Nevertheless, the field recently made a substantial advancement in neurotherapeutics with the approval of the first DMT indicated for PPMS, ocrelizumab. This exciting breakthrough is encouraging for the future development of neuroprotective and neurorestorative agents, providing more complete control of a highly heterogeneous and complex disease.

APPROVED DMT FOR PPMS

Ocrelizumab

Ocrelizumab is a humanized monoclonal antibody that targets CD20 on B lymphocytes. Ocrelizumab depletes B lymphocytes through various mechanisms including complement-dependent cytolysis, direct antibody–dependent cytolysis, and apoptosis (21). Driven by positive results in the subgroup analysis of the OLYMPUS trial investigating rituximab in PPMS, a phase III trial of ocrelizumab with similar study design was conducted in patients with PPMS against a placebo-controlled group (ORATORIO) (22). Key eligibility criteria included patients who were between 18 and 55 years of age, carried a diagnosis of PPMS (per 2005 revised McDonald Criteria), scored between 3.0 and 6.5 on the Expanded Disability Status Scale (EDSS), had duration of MS symptoms of less than 15 years if EDSS was > 5.0 at screening or less than 10 years if EDSS ≤5.0 at screening, and had a documented history of elevated immunoglobulin G (IgG) index or at least one IgG oligoclonal band on cerebrospinal fluid testing. Patients were randomly assigned in a 2:1 ratio to receive ocrelizumab 600 mg intravenous (IV) (initially divided into two 300 mg IV infusions 14 days apart) or matching placebo every 6 months. About 488 patients were assigned to receive ocrelizumab, and 244 patients were assigned to placebo. Among the total enrollees, 402 patients (82%) assigned to ocrelizumab and 174 (71%) assigned to placebo completed 120 weeks of the trial.

The primary end point was the percentage of patients with disability progression confirmed at 12 weeks in a time-to-event analysis. Disability progression was defined as an increase in the EDSS of at least 1.0 point from baseline that was sustained for at least 12 weeks if the baseline score was ≤5.5 or an increase of at least 0.5 points sustained over at least 12 weeks if the baseline score was ≤5.5. The investigation met its primary endpoint with 12-week confirmed disability progression of 32.9% in ocrelizumab versus 39.3% in the placebo group (hazard ratio: 0.76; 95% confidence interval [CI]: 0.59–0.98, $p = 0.03$) with a relative risk reduction of 24.0% and number needed to treat of 16 patients. In a secondary end point analysis, the percentage of patients with 24-week confirmed disability progression was 29.6% with ocrelizumab versus 35.7% with placebo (hazard ratio: 0.75; 95% CI: 0.58–0.98, $p = 0.04$) with a relative risk reduction of 25%. The results also favored ocrelizumab with respect to ambulation speed as measured by the Timed 25-Foot Walk (T25FW, $p = 0.04$), change in the total volume of T2-weighted brain MRI lesions ($p < 0.001$), and change in brain volume ($p = 0.02$). Details on the results of these secondary endpoints are highlighted in Table 15.2.

The results of a subgroup analysis of efficacy endpoints in patients with and without GdE lesions at baseline were directionally consistent with the findings in the overall trial population. The trial was not powered to detect between-group differences among these subgroups, but the results suggest that active inflammation at baseline might represent a possible treatment-effect-modifying factor. In other words, patients with earlier, more active disease (e.g., clinical relapses and/or new MRI disease activity) might have increased benefit from ocrelizumab compared to those who have more advanced, "purely" progressive MS. The ORATORIO trial enrollment criteria excluded PPMS patients older than 55 years of age. Therefore, experience from clinical practice and extension phase data are warranted to further clarify treatment effects in an older MS population.

In a safety analysis, infusion-related reactions, upper respiratory tract infections, and oral herpes infections were more frequent with ocrelizumab than with placebo. Neoplasms occurred in 2.3% of patients who received ocrelizumab and in 0.8% of patients who received placebo. The imbalance in observed neoplasms in ocrelizumab warrants continued evaluation in the context of what is expected in an aging MS population and other anti-CD20 therapies (23,24). In the postmarketing experience, one case of progressive multifocal leukoencephalopathy (PML) was reported in a German patient with relapsing MS who transitioned from natalizumab to ocrelizumab through a compassionate use program (26). These results affirm that long-term clinical experience is warranted to better identify future safety signals and thereby stratify potential risks.

EMERGING THERAPEUTICS IN THE PIPELINE

Siponimod

Siponimod (BAF312) is an oral selective sphingosine-1 phosphate (S1P) modulator, specifically targeting S1P-1 and S1P-5 receptors, and demonstrating greater selectivity than fingolimod (31). Siponimod therefore results in fewer organ-specific side effects based on the narrower distribution of S1P receptors throughout the body. Siponimod reduces circulation and infiltration of autoreactive lymphocytes into the CNS. It might exert its CNS effects by modulating neurobiological processes via S1P-1 and S1P-5 receptors on astrocytes and oligodendrocytes. A recent phase II trial demonstrated a reduction in brain MRI lesions and relapses by up to 80% of patients treated with siponimod versus placebo (32).

EXPAND, the largest phase III, randomized, double-blind, placebo-controlled study in SPMS to date, included over 1,600 patients from 31 different countries. SPMS patients with or without relapses and aged 18–60 years with an EDSS score from 3.0 to 6.5 were enrolled. Siponimod (2 mg once daily oral pill) reduced the risk of 3-month confirmed disability progression by 21% compared with placebo ($p = 0.013$) (33). Other results from the EXPAND study showed improvements compared with placebo in 12- and 24-month annualized relapse rate, the percentage change in brain volume, and change from baseline in T2 lesion volume. Based on the results in the given population, the optimal patient for siponimod would presumably be younger with earlier, more active disease. However, even patients with secondary progressive disease for over 3 years and EDSS scores of 6.5 seemed to gain some benefit in the clinical trial. These data suggest a potential therapeutic role for patients with SPMS, possibly

even impacting those with a less inflammatory disease course. Overall, siponimod was well tolerated with a relatively benign safety profile.

High-Dose Biotin

Biotin (Vitamin H) is a ubiquitous water-soluble vitamin that acts as a coenzyme for various carboxylases involved in key steps of energy metabolism and fatty acid synthesis (26). A small case series recently described the treatment of "biotin responsive basal ganglia disease," an orphan neurometabolic disease caused by mutations in the SLC19A3 gene coding for a thiamine transporter, with high doses of biotin (5–10 mg/kg/d) (27). Five patients with optic neuropathy and leukoencephalopathy also clinically responded to high-dose biotin, one of which was later found to have SPMS (28).

These findings prompted the development of a small pilot study investigating the effectiveness of high-dose biotin (100–300 mg/d) in both SPMS and PPMS (29). Evaluation criteria were variable across the 23 consecutive patients who were studied, including both quantitative and qualitative measurements. The preliminary data suggested that high doses of biotin might have a positive benefit in disability progression in progressive MS across visual and spinal cord pathways. The proposed mechanism of benefit likely stems from biotin's role in targeting metabolic processes that provides energy production in a mismatched system of increased energy demand and a decreasing available reserve.

A French multicenter phase III double-blind, placebo-controlled trial investigating high-dose biotin (MD1003, 100 mg biotin tid) was conducted in progressive MS patients (either primary progressive or secondary progressive without recent relapses). The primary outcome of this study was the proportion of patients with disability reversal at 9 months, confirmed at 12 months, defined as a decrease in the EDSS score of ≥ 1 point (≥ 0.5 for EDSS 6.0–7.0) or a $\geq 20\%$ decrease in the T25FW. 12.6% of the MD1003 group versus 0% of the placebo group met the primary endpoint ($p < 0.005$) (30). This trial showed that high-dose biotin reversed MS-related disability in some progressive MS patients, and importantly, demonstrated that this effect was sustained over 1 year.

THERAPEUTICS UNDER INVESTIGATION

Ibudilast

Ibudilast (MN-166) is a nonselective phosphodiesterase (PDE-4 and PDE-10) inhibitor that also blocks the macrophage migration inhibitory factor. Earlier studies have shown that, together, these effects suppress the formation of pro-inflammatory cytokines and promote the production of brain growth factors (34). A phase II trial of ibudilast in patients with RRMS demonstrated no beneficial effect on the rate of newly active lesions and relapses but did show reduction in brain atrophy rates, suggesting a potential neuroprotective effect (35).

A phase IIb study (SPRINT-MS) comparing ibudilast (50 mg twice daily oral pill) to placebo in either PPMS or SPMS is in progress in over 28 different centers across the United States. As of July 2016, half of the 255 enrolled patients completed the 96-week-long treatment schedule (NCT01982942) (36). For the primary endpoint of whole brain atrophy, ibudilast demonstrated a statistically significant 48% reduction in the rate of progression of whole brain atrophy compared to placebo ($p = 0.04$) in the modified ITT (intent-to-treat) population as measured by MRI analysis using brain parenchymal fraction (BPF). There were no significant outliers driving the results, and a modified sensitivity analysis was consistent with the primary analysis. Ibudilast also demonstrated a reduction in the progression of cortical atrophy compared to placebo as a secondary endpoint. Ibudilast had no effect on the progression of retinal nerve fiber layer thinning on optical coherence tomography.

Simvastatin

Statins, hydroxymethylglutaryl-CoA reductase inhibitors, demonstrate immunomodulatory and neuroprotective effects in cerebrovascular disease (37). In this context, statins are potentially an attractive neurotherapeutic agent for progressive MS. Previous experimental allergic encephalomyelitis (EAE) models and open label trials showed decreased disease activity in patients with MS (38). A recent phase II trial (MS-STAT) showed a statistically significant reduction in the annualized rate of whole brain atrophy in patients treated with simvastatin 80 mg daily compared to placebo (−0.25% per year adjusted difference between the two groups; $p = 0.003$). In summary, patients treated with high-dose simvastatin showed a 43% reduction in the annualized rate of whole-brain atrophy versus placebo (39). It is important to note, however, that this metric has not been strongly linked to outcomes important to MS patients (e.g., cognition, symptoms, and overall function) and should be considered when designing future phase III clinical trials.

Amiloride, Riluzole, and Fluoxetine

The MS-SMART study is a four-arm phase II clinical trial investigating amiloride, riluzole, and fluoxetine compared with placebo (NCT01910259). Amiloride, a potassium-sparing diuretic, has been found to reduce functional neurologic deficits in previous EAE studies (40). Riluzole, an established disease therapy for amyotrophic lateral sclerosis, is an inhibitor of tetradotoxin-sensitive voltage-gated sodium channels with antiglutamatergic effects (41). Fluoxetine, a selective serotonin reuptake inhibitor, presumably has neuroprotective properties through suppression of microglia activation and enhancement of brain-derived neurotrophic factor in animal models (42,43). The mechanism of studying multiple therapeutics simultaneously is to minimize exposure to placebo while hastening the identification of an effective treatment strategy.

Restorative Therapies

Several potential restorative therapies are currently in the early phases of investigation in progressive MS.

ANTI-LINGO-1

Leucine-rich repeat and immunoglobulin-like domain containing neurite outgrowth inhibitor receptor-interacting protein-1 (LINGO-1) is a cell surface protein expressed in neural cells. It is a negative modulator of axonal myelination via inhibition of the differentiation of oligodendrocyte precursor cells to mature oligodendrocytes (44). In this context, blockage of LINGO-1 may represent a potential strategy for remyelination and preservation of axonal integrity in MS. A randomized, double-blind phase II trial (SYNERGY) of a novel anti-LINGO-1 monoclonal antibody (opicinumab, BIIB033) investigated the impact on disease progression in patients with RRMS and SPMS (45). Patients with either RRMS or relapsing SPMS were randomized either to one of four doses of IV opicinumab (3, 10, 30, or 100 mg/kg) in addition to IM interferon beta-1a or placebo. Out of 418 patients, 334 completed the 72-week study.

The primary endpoint of the study was the percentage of participants with 3-month confirmed improvement of neurophysical and/or cognitive function, using a multicomponent endpoint comprising the EDSS, T25FW, 9-Hole Peg Test, and 3-Second Paced Auditory Serial Addition Test. In summary, the investigators did not appreciate a linear dose response. Participants receiving the middle doses (10 and 30 mg/kg) achieved the strongest benefit with no detectable effects in the lowest and highest doses. Analyses also showed that opicinumab was more effective in younger patients and those with shorter disease duration and less severe whole brain volume loss at baseline. Although this U-shaped dose relationship failed to meet its primary endpoint, investigators plan to utilize what has been learned in the phase IIb trial by further investigating the middle dose that appears to have the strongest benefit (10 mg/kg) and recruiting patients most likely to be responders (younger individuals with early active disease) into future clinical trials.

STEM CELL THERAPY

Stem cell transplantation has been proposed as a second-line treatment strategy for refractory MS. The mechanism behind its role in MS is presumably through the eradication of autoreactive cells, thereby resetting the aberrant immune response to self-antigens, possibly promoting CNS regeneration (46). In an open label proof-of-concept clinical trial in patients with SPMS with clinical evidence of optic nerve involvement, infusion of autologous bone marrow–derived mesenchymal stem cells improved visual acuity and visual evoked response latency (47). A phase II trial of autologous bone marrow infusion in patients with SPMS or PPMS is in progress (NCT01815632).

Table 15.2 summarizes various clinical trials to date in progressive MS.

TABLE 15.2 Emerging Therapeutics for Progressive Multiple Sclerosis: Select Phase II and Phase III Clinical Trials

AGENT/STUDY	CLINICAL TRIAL PHASE	PLACEBO-CONTROLLED	STUDY DURATION (MONTHS)	DISEASE COURSE	SAMPLE SIZE	SUMMARY OF OUTCOMES
Ocrelizumab[a] Dose: 300 mg IV Day 1/Day 15 600 mg IV q6 months (ORATORIO) (14)	III	Yes	24	PPMS	732	Significant benefit • 12-wk confirmed disability progression in 32.9% of ocrelizumab patients vs. 39.3% of placebo (HR: 0.76, $p = 0.03$) • 24-week confirmed disability progression in 29.6% of ocrelizumab patients vs. 35.7% of placebo (HR: 0.75, $p = 0.04$) • Worsening of T25FW by 38.9% with ocrelizumab vs. 55.1% with placebo ($p = 0.04$) • 3.4% decrease in total T2 lesion volume with ocrelizumab vs. 1.09% with placebo ($p < 0.001$) • 0.90% decrease in brain volume loss with ocrelizumab vs. 1.09% with placebo ($p = 0.02$) No significant benefit • Physical Component Summary score of the 26-Item Short-Form Health Survey ($p = 0.60$)
High-dose biotin Dose: 100 mg PO tid (MD1003) (24)	III	Yes	12 (12-mo extension)	PPMS, SPMS	154	Significant benefit • 12.6% of MD1003 patients vs. 0% placebo met primary endpoint of sustained reversal of MS-related disability, defined as an EDSS decrease of ≥1 point (≥0.5 for EDSS 6–7) or a ≥20% decrease in T25FW ($p = 0.005$) • 9.9% of patients on MD1003 during core/extension vs. 31.7% in placebo/MD1003 in core/extension phase had EDSS progression at month 18, confirmed at month 24 ($p = 0.005$) No significant benefit • 4.2% of MD1003 patients and 13.6% placebo had EDSS progression at month 9, confirmed at month 12, in the core phase ($p = 0.07$) Caution in interpretation • 50% of patients received fampridine during the trial • 40% of patients were treated with a concomitant DMT

(continued)

TABLE 15.2 Emerging Therapeutics for Progressive Multiple Sclerosis: Select Phase II and Phase III Clinical Trials (*continued*)

AGENT/STUDY	CLINICAL TRIAL PHASE	PLACEBO-CONTROLLED	STUDY DURATION (MONTHS)	DISEASE COURSE	SAMPLE SIZE	SUMMARY OF OUTCOMES
Siponimod Dose: 2 mg PO daily (BAF312; EXPAND) (27)	III	Yes	40	SPMS	1530	Significant benefit • 21% reduction in confirmed 3-mo disability progression with siponimod compared to placebo ($p = 0.013$) Caution in interpretation • Patients with relapsing SPMS were included[b]
Ibudilast Dose: 50 mg PO bid (SPRINT) (30)	II	Yes	24	PPMS, SPMS	255	Significant benefit • 48% reduction in the rate of progression of whole brain atrophy compared to placebo ($p = 0.04$) • Reduction in the progression of cortical atrophy compared to placebo No significant benefit • No effect on the progression of retinal nerve fiber layer thinning on optical coherence tomography
Simvastatin Dose: 80 mg PO daily (MS-STAT) (33)	II	Yes	24	SPMS	140	Significant benefit • 43% reduction in annualized rate of whole brain atrophy in simvastatin group compared to placebo • −0.254 mean difference in EDSS, favoring simvastatin over placebo ($p < 0.01$) • −4.78 mean difference in total MSIS-29, favoring simvastatin over placebo ($p < 0.05$) No significant benefit • MSFC ($p > 0.10$), new/enlarging T2 lesions ($p = 0.176$), or rate of relapse ($p = 0.473$) Caution in interpretation • Patients with relapsing SPMS were included • Expected effects of simvastatin on inflammation were not shown • Disability outcome (brain atrophy) was a surrogate measure and not the current standard metric in phase III trials (EDSS)

(*continued*)

TABLE 15.2 Emerging Therapeutics for Progressive Multiple Sclerosis: Select Phase II and Phase III Clinical Trials (*continued*)

AGENT/STUDY	CLINICAL TRIAL PHASE	PLACEBO-CONTROLLED	STUDY DURATION (MONTHS)	DISEASE COURSE	SAMPLE SIZE	SUMMARY OF OUTCOMES
Amiloride, Riluzole, Fluoxetine Dose Amiloride: 5 mg PO daily × 4 wk 5 mg PO bid Dose Riluzole 50 mg PO daily × 4 wk 50 mg PO bid Dose Fluoxetine 20 mg PO daily × 4 wk 20 mg PO bid (MS-SMART)	II	Yes	24	SPMS	440	——
Opicinumab Dose ranges: 3, 10, 30, or 100 IV q4 weeks (anti-LINGO-1; SYNERGY) (39)	IIb	Yes	18	RRMS, SPMS	418	Significant benefit • Patients receiving middle doses (10 and 30 mg/kg) met primary endpoint, defined as the percentage of participants with 3-mo confirmed improvement of neurophysical and/or cognitive function[c] No significant benefit • Patients receiving lowest (3 mg/kg) and highest (100 mg/kg) doses did not show significant benefit Caution in interpretation • Difficult to interpret nonlinear dose relationship • Patients were treated concomitantly with interferon beta-1a • Study population included patients with RRMS and relapsing SPMS

[a]Only approved disease-modifying therapy to date for PPMS.

[b]Inclusion of SPMS patients with relapses potentially confounds the interpretation of beneficial effects in neurodegeneration versus effects on inflammation.

[c]Investigators used a multicomponent endpoint comprising the EDSS, Timed 25-Foot Walk, 9-Hole Peg Test, and 3-Second Paced Auditory Serial Addition Test.

bid, twice daily; EDSS, Expanded Disability Status Scale; HR, hazard ratio; IV, intravenous; MSFC, Multiple Sclerosis Functional Composite; MSIS, Multiple Sclerosis Impact Scale; PO, oral; PPMS, primary progressive multiple sclerosis; RRMS, relapsing–remitting MS; SPMS, secondary progressive multiple sclerosis; T25FW, Timed 25 Foot Walk; tid, three times daily.

SYMPTOM AND DISABILITY MANAGEMENT

Progressive MS, like RRMS, is associated with a heterogeneous array of symptoms and functional deficits that result in a wide range of disability. Symptoms that contribute to the loss of independence and restriction in social activities critically impose upon quality of life and raise healthcare costs and utilization of resources. Individualized treatment of physical symptoms such as motor weakness, pain, mobility dysfunction, spasticity, and bladder and bowel disturbances; in addition to "invisible" symptoms such as fatigue, depression/anxiety, and cognitive and affective disorders is paramount.

Although pharmacotherapy can be beneficial and recommended when appropriate, nonpharmacological approaches can be equally, if not more, effective in progressive MS. An integral aspect of symptomatic treatment is physical and occupational therapy to help patients compensate for existing limitations and prevent disability-related injury. A regular strengthening, stretching, balance training, and fall prevention regimen instructed by an experienced therapist can be highly effective. Utilization of health psychology/counseling and social work resources to help patients manage life complications and stress that accompany progressive disability are key. Some institutions have access to a comprehensive rehabilitation team, which is particularly resourceful in managing MS-related spasticity, including Botox therapy and in some cases baclofen pump management for severe and/or intractable spasticity. In summary, a multidisciplinary approach is a highly effective strategy for treating the chronic symptoms of progressive MS.

Specifics on symptomatic therapy fall outside the scope of this chapter and are further discussed in Chapters 17–32 of this book.

CURRENT LANDSCAPE OF TREATING PROGRESSIVE MS: CHALLENGES AND FUTURE DIRECTIONS

The landscape for the development of effective treatment strategies for progressive MS is one of substantial need and significant promise. Currently, progressive MS lends many challenges to different disciplines: the *scientist* in understanding the pathogenesis of the disorder, the *clinical researcher* in identifying robust markers for measuring effective therapeutics in clinical trials, the *healthcare provider* in managing a chronic condition in clinical practice with few available, robust treatment strategies, and the *patient* for living day to day with a chronic, disabling illness.

Consider the concept of *failed trials* as opposed to *failed therapeutics*, whereby limitations in study design, specifically the absence of an effective therapeutic target, has led to delays in robust treatment strategies for progressive MS (48), notably PPMS and SPMS without active disease and continued progression. An example is the failure of fingolimod to show beneficial effects in PPMS in the INFORMS trial, in which greater than 40% of patients were greater than 50 years of age and greater than 85% of patients had no GdE lesions on baseline brain MRI (19). In summary, the trial population included an older, more advanced and predominantly neurodegenerative PPMS group, thereby selecting out patients with more inflammatory disease who would likely be better responders.

The incomplete understanding of the pathogenesis of progressive MS has made the identification of potential therapeutic targets difficult. Although targeting acute inflammation is a viable metric for relapsing MS, predicting clinical efficacy in phase II and phase III trials for progressive MS requires a more refined and focused assessment tool. One consideration for the failure of prior clinical trials investigating existing DMTs in progressive MS is lack of a sensitive, robust metric. Currently used clinical markers of disability such as the EDSS (49) and Multiple Sclerosis Functional Composite (MSFC) (50) have their own inherent limitations. EDSS is subject to high inter-rater variability (51), relies heavily on lower extremity function (52), does

not include a meaningful cognitive component (53), and is overall insensitive to longitudinal change (54). The MSFC is limited in that it only assesses a restricted amount of neurologic function including arm, leg, visual, and cognitive features; and is not routinely measured in clinical practice. The challenge remains in identifying a metric that is easy to capture, sensitive to longitudinal change, quantitative, and strongly correlates with patient-reported function.

Concerted efforts are currently in progress to better identify new clinical outcome assessment tools that will enhance the development of effective therapeutics in progressive MS. The International Progressive MS Alliance is an expanding global coalition of MS organizations that aims to expedite the development of therapies for effective modification and symptom management of progressive MS (55). The Multiple Sclerosis Outcome Assessments Consortium (MSOAC), a conglomerate of industry, academic, regulatory, and patient representatives, strives to develop and support the adoption of new clinical outcome assessment tools for use in future MS clinical trials. The International Collaborative on Progressive MS has identified key priority areas for research that will leverage resources across disciplines and accelerate development of effective therapies in PMS (56) (see Table 15.3).

Clinical trials are now adopting unique metrics to more efficiently measure clinical efficacy outcomes in progressive MS (57) that capture the predominantly neurodegenerative aspect of the disease. Although this continues to remain a priority area of research, brain atrophy overall is the preferred method of monitoring the neurodegenerative process in progressive MS (58) and is a plausible surrogate measure of disability. This is a promising outcome metric, for sensitive and reproducible methods enable small amounts of brain atrophy to be detected over 1 year or less. Further, sample sizes for proof-of-concept trials that use brain atrophy as a primary outcome measure may be less

---

TABLE 15.3 International Collaborative on Progressive MS Key Priority Areas

1) Discovery of experimental models that reproduce key clinical and pathologic features of PPMS and SPMS.

2) Identification and validation of biologic targets and opportunities to repurpose existing MS medications for use in treating progressive MS.

3) Recognition and validation of proof-of-concept clinical trial outcomes.

4) Development of precise, reproducible, and broad-based clinical outcome measures that are both sensitive to change and predictive over time.

5) Optimization of symptom management and rehabilitation strategies that can help reduce the impact of disability and improve the quality of life in patients with PMS.

MS, multiple sclerosis; PMS, progressive multiple sclerosis; PPMS, primary progressive multiple sclerosis; SPMS, secondary progressive multiple sclerosis.
Source: Fox R, Thompson A, Baker D, et al. Setting a research agenda for progressive multiple sclerosis: the International Collaborative on Progressive MS. *Mult Scler.* 2012;18:1534–1540.

than those required for clinical disability endpoints (59). However, whole-brain atrophy alone may not sufficiently correlate with patient-related function and should be considered when designing clinical trials and interpreting what this means from a phenotypic perspective. Other possible metrics include cerebrospinal fluid (CSF) biomarkers such as neurofilament chains, glial fibrillary acidic protein, tau, and S100b protein (60,61). Metabolomics profiling methods

---

PATIENT CASE A 53-year-old African American woman presents to the office with a diagnosis of multiple sclerosis (MS) since 2008 (44 years old), after having neurologic symptoms since 2005 (41 years old). She initially developed insidious onset of weakness in her left leg. Over the years, she noticed gradual progression of weakness in the left leg that slowly started to involve the right leg. She did not have any relapses over the next 20 years, but she admitted to a slow clinical decline, specifically worsening of weakness in her legs, poor mobility, painful bilateral leg spasticity, and urinary retention with frequent urinary tract infections (UTIs). She started walking with a cane in 2009 and then progressed to use of a rollator in 2012. She stopped working in 2010, mainly due to her mobility impairment.

Brain MRI showed multiple nonenhancing periventricular and juxtacortical lesions. She had one lesion in the left cerebellar hemisphere. Multiple lesions appeared dark on T1-weighted sequences, consistent with chronic demyelination. Spinal cord MRI showed extensive patchy lesion burden throughout the cervical and thoracic spine, mostly involving the dorsolateral aspect of the spinal cord. Neurologic exam showed a spastic paraparetic and ataxic gait with left upper extremity dysdiadochokinesia.

She was treated with glatiramer acetate and interferon beta-1a for several months each in 2008 and 2009, but discontinued therapy due to injection-site reactions and lack of clinical benefit. Symptomatic therapies were not started. The patient was subsequently lost to neurologic follow-up for over 10 years. During this time, she continued to slowly worsen and started losing hope.

Discussion: This patient has a classic presentation of primary progressive multiple sclerosis (PPMS) that had been suboptimally controlled over the years, leading to significant disability with an Expanded Disability Status Scale (EDSS) score of 6.5. After presenting to a tertiary referral MS center, emphasis was immediately placed on a multidisciplinary symptom–management strategy to optimize function and quality of life. She was started on baclofen and tizanidine for MS-related spasticity, but she had poor tolerability and discontinued the medications immediately. Subsequently, she started Botox therapy with improvement in her spasticity to the point where her pain levels were manageable and had an easier time of performing hygienic maneuvers. She also enrolled in physical and occupational therapy with MS-certified specialists, after which time she developed improvement in her mobility, balance, and upper extremity dexterity with a significant reduction in fall frequency. She was also evaluated by a urology team, at which point she was started on tamsulosin with good benefit. Patient then transitioned to intermittent self-catheterization with excellent clinical efficacy. She no longer has recurrent UTIs.

Given the primary progressive disease course, relatively young age (<55 years old), continued clinical decline, and no other significant comorbidities, patient will be starting ocrelizumab for targeted disease therapy. Patient is now hopeful about her future.

KEY POINTS FOR PATIENTS AND FAMILIES

- PPMS is a form of MS where patients develop slow clinical decline from the onset of symptom development.
- SPMS is a form of MS that follows RRMS. Patients may still experience relapses, but gradually worsen over time in between relapses.
- A new classification has been proposed for progressive MS that categorizes the disease state as active and/or progressive. This revised nomenclature will help healthcare providers recognize whether or not DMTs might be beneficial.
- Ocrelizumab is the first DMT approved for PPMS. Multiple novel therapeutics for progressive MS are currently in the investigative stages.
- Symptomatic therapy and rehabilitation are key in managing progressive MS to improve function and quality of life.

have also gained attention (62). Optimistically, the adoption of new study designs with novel outcome measures will pave the way for innovative, emerging therapeutics for progressive MS.

SUMMARY

Although the field of MS has grown rapidly since the inception of DMTs in 1993 for relapsing MS, there are still limitations that have hindered our ability to identify effective treatments for progressive MS: (a) incomplete understanding of the pathogenesis of progressive MS and (b) lack of robust outcome metrics to best identify clinical efficacy in a primarily neurodegenerative disease state. Based on what we have learned from multiple clinical trials investigating both existing and novel therapeutics for progressive MS, responders tend to be younger patients with continued inflammatory disease activity. Individuals with purely progressive MS without active disease continue to be underserved by our present therapeutics, but symptomatic therapies and rehabilitation remain key management strategies in improving quality of life and function for these individuals. Multiple initiatives including the International Progressive MS Alliance and MSOAC are actively working toward filling these knowledge and treatment gaps. The approval of the first DMT indicated for PPMS, ocrelizumab, in addition to positive clinical trial findings for high-dose biotin and siponimod in progressive MS, are encouraging to the MS field and further substantiates the need for robust outcome metrics in testing novel neurotherapeutics. Future strategies hold great promise in managing this disabling, neurodegenerative disease state.

REFERENCES

 1. Compston A, Coles A. Multiple sclerosis. *Lancet*. 2008;372:1502–1517.
 2. Confavreux C, Compston DAS. The natural history of multiple sclerosis. In: Compston DAS, ed. *McAlpine's Multiple Sclerosis*. 4th ed. London, UK: Churchill-Livingstone; 2005.233–243.
 3. Miller DH, Leary SM. Primary-progressive multiple sclerosis. *Lancet Neurol*. 2007;6(10):903–912.
 4. Leary S, Thompson A. Primary progressive multiple sclerosis. *CNS Drugs*. 2005;19(6): 369–376.
 5. Sand IK, Krieger S, Farrell C, et al. Diagnostic uncertainty during the transition to secondary progressive multiple sclerosis. *Mult Scler*. 2014;20:1654–1657.
 6. Lublin FD, Reingold SC, Cohen JA, et al. Defining the clinical course of multiple sclerosis: the 2013 revisions. *Neurology*. 2014;83:278–286.
 7. Lucchinetti CF, Brueck W, Rodriguez M, et al. Multiple sclerosis: lessons from neuropathology. *Semin Neurol*. 1998;18:337–349.
 8. Mahad DH, Trapp BD, Lassmann H. Pathological mechanisms in progressive multiple sclerosis. *Lancet Neurol*. 2015;14:183–193.
 9. Hametner S, Wimmer I, Haider L, et al. Iron and neurodegeneration in the multiple sclerosis brain. *Ann Neurol*. 2013;74:848–861.
10. Hawker K, O'Connor P, Freedman MS, et al. Rituximab in patients with primary progressive multiple sclerosis: results of a randomized double-blind placebo-controlled multicenter trial. *Ann Neurol*. 2009;66:460–471.

11. Magliozzi R, Howell O, Vora A, et al. Meningeal B-cell follicles in secondary progressive multiple sclerosis associate with early onset of disease and severe cortical pathology. *Brain*. 2007;130:1089–1104.
12. Rommer PS, Dudesek A, Stuve O, et al. Monoclonal antibodies in treatment of multiple sclerosis. *Clin Exp Immunol*. 2014;175:373–384.
13. Placebo-controlled multicentre randomised trial of interferon beta-1b in treatment of secondary progressive multiple sclerosis. European Study Group on interferon beta-1b in secondary progressive MS. *Lancet*. 1998;352:1491–1497.
14. Secondary Progressive Efficacy Clinical Trial of Recombinant Interferon beta-1a in MS (SPECTRIMS) Study Group. Randomized controlled trial of interferon beta-1a in secondary progressive MS: clinical results. *Neurology*. 2001;56:1496–1504.
15. Cohen JA, Cutter GR, Fisher JS, et al. Benefit of interferon beta-1a on MSFC progression in secondary progressive MS. *Neurology*. 2002;59:679–687.
16. Panitch H, Miller A, Paty D, et al. Interferon beta-1b in secondary progressive MS: results from a 3-year controlled study. *Neurology*. 2004;63:1788–1795.
17. Rice G, Filippi M, Comi G, et al. The Cladribine Clinical Study Group and for the Cladribine MRI Study Group. Cladribine and progressive MS: clinical and MRI outcomes of a multi-center controlled trial. *Neurology*. 2000;54:1145–1155.
18. Wolinsky JS, Narayana PA, O'Connor P, et al. Glatiramer acetate in primary progressive multiple sclerosis: results of a multinational, multicenter, double-blind, placebo-controlled trial. *Ann Neurol*. 2007;61(1):14–24.
19. Lublin FD, Miller D, Freedman M, et al. Oral fingolimod in primary progressive multiple sclerosis (INFORMS): a phase 3, randomized, double-blind, placebo-controlled trial. *Lancet*. 2016;387(10023):1075–1084.
20. Hartung HP, Gonsette R, Konig N, et al. Mitoxantrone in progressive multiple sclerosis: a placebo-controlled, double-blind, randomised, multicentre trial. *Lancet*. 2002;360(9350):2018–2025.
21. Hauser S, Bar-O A, Comi G, et al. Ocrelizumab versus interferon beta-1a in relapsing multiple sclerosis. *N Engl J Med*. 2017;376:221–234.
22. Montalban X, Hauser S, Kappos L, et al. Ocrelizumab versus placebo in primary progressive multiple sclerosis. *N Engl J Med*. 2017;376:209–220.
23. Nielsen NM, Rostgaard K, Rasmussen S, et al. Cancer risk among patients with multiple sclerosis: a population-based register study. *Int J Cancer*. 2006;118:979–84.
24. Kingwell E, Bajdik C, Phillips N, et al. Cancer risk in multiple sclerosis: findings from British Columbia, Canada. *Brain*. 2012;135:2973–2979.
25. Medscape. July 6, 2017. Available at: http://www.medscape.com/viewarticle/880654. Accessed 1/26/2018.
26. Said HM. Biotin: the forgotten vitamin. *Am J Clin Nutr*. 2002;75:179–180.
27. Tabarki B, Al-Shafi S, Al-Shahwan S, et al. Biotin-responsive basal ganglia disease revisited: clinical, radiographic, and genetic findings. *Neurology*. 2013;80:261–267.
28. Sedel F, Challe G, Vignal C, et al. A novel biotin sensitive leukodystrophy. *J Inherit Metab Dis*. 2011;34:S267.
29. Sedel F, Papeix C, Bellanger A, et al. High doses of biotin in progressive multiple sclerosis: a pilot study. *Mult Scler Relat Disord*. 2015;4:159–169.
30. Tourbah A, Frenay CL, Edan G, et al. MD1003 (high-dose biotin) for the treatment of progressive multiple sclerosis: a randomized double-blind, placebo-controlled study. *Mult Scler*. 2016;22(13):1719–1731.
31. Gonzalez-Cabrera PJ, Brown S, Studer SM, et al. S1P signaling: new therapies and opportunities. *F1000Prime Rep*. 2014;6:109.
32. Selmaj K, Li DK, Hartung HP, et al. Siponimod for patients with relapsing-remitting multiple sclerosis (BOLD): an adaptive, dose-ranging, randomised, phase 2 study. *Lancet Neurol*. 2013;12:756–767.

33. Kappos L, Bar-Or A, Cree B, et al. Efficacy and safety of siponimod in secondary progressive multiple sclerosis - results of the placebo controlled, double-blind, phase III EXPAND study. The 32nd Congress of the European Committee for Treatment and Research in Multiple Sclerosis, London, UK, September 14-17, 2016.

34. Gibson LC, Hastings SF, McPhee I, et al. The inhibitory profile of ibudilast against the human phosphodiesterase enzyme family. *Eur J Pharmacol.* 2006;538:39–42.

35. Barkhof F, Hulst HE, Drulovic J, et al. Ibudilast in relapsing-remitting multiple sclerosis: a neuroprotectant? *Neurology.* 2010;74:1033–1040.

36. Medicinova. SPRINT-MS: safety, tolerability and activity study of ibudilast in subjects with progressive multiple sclerosis. ClinicalTrials. gov. Available at: http://clinicaltrials.gov/ct2/show/NCT01982942. National Institutes of Health sponsored multicentre phase II trial of ibudilast in progressive forms of MS. Accessed 1/06/2018.

37. van der Most PJ, Dolga AM, Nijholt IM, et al. Statins: mechanisms of neuroprotection. *Prog Neurobiol.* 2009;88:64–75.

38. Pihl-Jensen G, Tsakiri A, Frederiksen JL. Statin treatment in multiple sclerosis: a systematic review and meta-analysis. *CNS Drugs.* 2015;29:277–291.

39. Chataway J, Schuerer N, Alsanousi A, et al. Effect of high-dose simvastatin on brain atrophy and disability in secondary progressive multiple sclerosis (MS-STAT): a randomized, placebo-controlled, phase 2 trial. *Lancet.* 2014;383:2213–2221.

40. Vergo S, Craner MJ, Etzensperger R, et al. Acid-sensing ion channel 1 is involved in both axonal injury and demyelination in multiple sclerosis and its animal model. *Brain.* 2011;134:571–584.

41. Cheah BC, Vucic S, Krishnan AV, et al. Riluzole, neuroprotection and amyotrophic lateral sclerosis. *Curr Med Chem.* 2010;17:1942–1999.

42. Zhang F, Zhou H, Wilson BC, et al. Fluoxetine protects neurons against microglial activation-mediated neurotoxicity. *Parkinsoinism Relat Disord.* 2012;18(suppl 1):S213–S217.

43. Alme MN, Wibrand K, Dagestad G, et al. Chronic fluoxetine treatment induces brain region-specific upregulation of genes associated with BDNF-induced long-term potentiation. *Neural Plast.* 2007;2007:26496.

44. Rudick RA, Mi S, Sandrock AW Jr. LINGO-1 antagonists as therapy for multiple sclerosis: in vitro and in vivo evidence. *Expert Opin Biol Ther.* 2008;8(10):1561–1570.

45. Calabresi P, Mellion M, Edwards KR, et al. Efficacy results from the phase 2b SYNERGY Study: treatment of disabling multiple sclerosis with the anti-LINGO-1 monoclonal antibody opicinumab. The 69th Annual Meeting at the American Academy of Neurology, Boston, MA, April 22-28, 2017.

46. Radaelli M, Merlini A, Greco R, et al. Autologous bone marrow transplantation for the treatment of multiple sclerosis. *Curr Neurol Neurosci Rep.* 2014;14:478.

47. Connick P, Kolappan M, Crawley C, et al. Autologous mesenchymal stem cells for the treatment of secondary progressive multiple sclerosis: an open-label phase 2a proof-of-concept study. *Lancet Neurol.* 2012;11:150–156.

48. Shirani A, Okuda D, Stuve O. Therapeutic advances and future prospects in progressive forms of multiple sclerosis. *Neurotherapeutics.* 2016;13:58–69.

49. Kurtzke JF. Rating neurologic impairment in multiple sclerosis: an expanded disability status scale (EDSS). *Neurology.* 1983;33:1444–1452.

50. Fischer JS, Rudick R, Cutter GR. The multiple sclerosis functional composite measure (MSFC): an integrated approach to MS clinical outcome assessment. *Mult Scler.* 1999;5(4):244–250.

51. Palace J, Robertson N. Modifying disability in progressive multiple sclerosis. *Lancet.* 2014;383(9936):2189–2191.

52. Lamers I, Feys P. Assessing upper limb function in multiple sclerosis. *Mult Scler.* 2014 Jun;20(7):775–784.

53. Brissart H, Sauvee M, Latarche C, et al. Integration of cognitive impairment in the expanded disability status scale of 215 patients with multiple sclerosis. *Eur Neurol.* 2010;64:345–350.

54. Kragt JJ, Thompson AJ, Montalban X, et al. Responsiveness and predictive value of EDSS and MSFC in primary progressive MS. *Neurology.* 2008;70(13 pt 2):1084–1091.

55. International progressive MS alliance. Available at: http://www.progressivemsalliance.org/.

56. Fox R, Thompson A, Baker D, et al. Setting a research agenda for progressive multiple sclerosis: the International Collaborative on Progressive MS. *Mult Scler.* 2012;18:1534–1540.

57. Chataway J, Nicholas R, Todd S, et al. A novel adaptive design strategy increases the efficiency of clinical trials in secondary progressive multiple sclerosis. *Mult Scler.* 2011;17:81–88.

58. Miller DH. Biomarkers and surrogate outcomes in neurodegenerative disease: lessons from multiple sclerosis. *NeuroRx.* 2004;1:284–294.

59. Anderson V, Bartlett JW, Fox NC, et al. Detecting treatment effects on brain atrophy in relapsing remitting multiple sclerosis: sample size estimates. *J Neurol.* 2007;254(11):1588–1594.

60. Kuhle J, Plattner K, Bestwick JP, et al. A comparative study of CSF neurofilament light and heavy chain protein in MS. *Mult Scler.* 2013;19:1597–1603.

61. Petzold A, Eikelenboom MJ, Gveric D, et al. Markers for different glial cell responses in multiple sclerosis: clinical and pathological correlations. *Brain.* 2002;125:1462–1473.

62. Botas A, Campbell HM, Han X, et al. Metabolomics of neurodegenerative diseases. *Int Rev Neurobiol.* 2015;122:53–80.

16

Emerging Therapies

Michael D. Kornberg and Peter A. Calabresi

KEY POINTS FOR CLINICIANS

- Current disease-modifying therapies target the peripheral immune system with a primary goal of preventing relapses.
- The next generation of therapies will target intrinsic central nervous system (CNS) mechanisms relevant to progressive multiple sclerosis (MS), such as compartmentalized CNS inflammation, neuro-axonal injury, and remyelination failure.
- Although strategies specifically targeting progressive MS remain far removed from clinical practice, several therapies aiming to improve upon the efficacy/safety of existing drugs are in advanced clinical development.
- Several neuroprotective agents, such as biotin, sodium channel blockers, and statins, have shown positive results in phase 2 trials, with larger studies ongoing or planned.
- Remyelinating/reparative therapies remain in an early developmental stage, with a lead agent (opicinumab) showing mixed results in phase 2 studies, but preclinical work has identified several pipeline strategies undergoing active investigation.
- Therapeutics development for progressive MS will require an improved understanding of the pathogenesis of progression and better clinical outcome measures.

INTRODUCTION

The pace of therapeutics discovery in MS over the past several decades has been remarkable, producing 15 Food and Drug Administration (FDA)-approved disease-modifying therapies. As a whole, these agents substantially impact the disease, not only reducing relapses and short-term disability but also, as increasing evidence indicates, delaying or preventing long-term disability (1–4). Nonetheless, currently available therapies target the peripheral immune system and, with the exceptions of ocrelizumab and mitoxantrone, carry exclusive indications for relapsing forms of MS. These traditional immunologic therapies have largely failed in progressive MS, with the rare successes likely related to patient selection (i.e., younger patients with radiologically active disease) rather than specific targeting of the mechanisms underlying progression.

Although improvements may still be made in the traditional immunologic approach (e.g., development of targeted therapies with more favorable efficacy/ risk profiles than present drugs), the next generation of therapeutics will focus largely on mechanisms relevant to progressive MS, with a goal of arresting progression and restoring function. This includes targeting the compartmentalized inflammation that characterizes progressive MS (consisting of diffuse macrophage/microglial activation and leptomeningeal inflammation), as well as strategies to prevent neurodegeneration and induce remyelination. Although more work is needed to elucidate the pathogenesis of progression and to improve the outcome measures used to assess efficacy, many promising agents already exist within the therapeutic pipeline. This chapter reviews some of the most promising therapies and strategies in development, organized as follows: immunologic, neuroprotective, and remyelinating/ reparative therapies.

EMERGING IMMUNOLOGIC THERAPIES

Immunologic therapies in the most advanced stages of development are still largely targeted at relapsing–remitting MS (RRMS), with a goal either of providing additional high-efficacy options for aggressive disease or eliminating off-target effects to increase safety/tolerability (see Table 16.1). Agents selectively targeting compartmentalized inflammation (either adaptive immune cells that have migrated to the CNS or innate immune resident CNS cells) remain farther from the clinic.

TABLE 16.1 Select Emerging Immunologic Therapies in Advanced Stages of Development

THERAPY	MECHANISM OF ACTION	ROUTE OF ADMINISTRATION/ DOSE	CLINICAL EVIDENCE	SAFETY CONCERNS
aHSCT	Immunoablation followed by reconstitution with autologous stem cells	Varied conditioning and transplant protocols	Primarily small, open-label studies (5,6) Phase 2 (7): 69.6% with no disease activity or progression at 3 y Phase 2 (HALT-MS) (8): 91.3% progression free 86.3% MRI activity free after median 62 months	Complications from immunoablation, primarily infection Overall transplant-related mortality 2.1%–2.8% (5,6), but rates have decreased over time with better patient selection and experience
Cladribine	Purine analog that disrupts DNA synthesis/repair, preferentially depletes lymphocytes	Oral Two to four short courses (daily for 4–5 consecutive days) in year 1, followed by two short courses in year 2	Phase 3: CLARITY (vs. placebo) ARR reduction: 57.6% (3.5 mg/kg) 54.5% (5.25 mg/kg) Decreased risk of disability progression: 20.6% (placebo) vs. 14.3% (3.5 mg/kg) and 15.1% (5.25 mg/kg) Phase 3: ORACLE MS (vs. placebo in CIS) Reduced risk of conversion to MS: 67% (3.5 mg/kg) 62% (5.25 mg/kg)	Lymphopenia Grade 3 or 4 (10): 25.8% (3.5 mg/kg) 45% (5.25 mg/kg) Persistent (96 wk): 21.6% (3.5 mg/kg) 31.5% (5.25 mg/kg) Herpes zoster Neutropenia/ thrombocytopenia (rare)
S1P receptor modulators	Prevent egress of lymphocytes from lymph nodes via S1P$_1$ receptor Improved selectivity for S1P$_1$ receptor vs. fingolimod	Oral	*Ponesimod* Phase 2 (18): Reduced GdE lesions and ARR *Siponimod* Phase 2: BOLD (vs. placebo) Reduced GdE and new/enlarging lesions and ARR Phase 3: EXPAND in SPMS (vs. placebo): 21% decreased risk of disability progression *Ozanimod* Phase 3: SUNBEAM and RADIANCE (vs. weekly IFN β-1a) Reduced ARR	Shorter half-lives than fingolimod Variable degrees of cardiac effects, macular edema, dyspnea
Laquinimod	Oral quinolone 3-carboxamide derivative with broad immune effects	Oral 0.6 mg daily	Phase 3: ALLEGRO (vs. placebo) 23% reduction in ARR 36% decrease in disability progression 33% decrease in brain atrophy Phase 3: BRAVO (vs. placebo) 18% reduction in ARR (nonsignificant) 28% decrease in brain atrophy Phase 3: CONCERTO (time to disease progression vs. placebo in RRMS) No benefit Phase 2: ARPEGGIO (vs. placebo in PPMS) Ongoing	Cardiac side effects at high doses Dose-dependent increase in LFTs (asymptomatic and reversible)

aHSCT, autologous hematopoietic stem cell transplant; ARR, annualized relapse rate; CIS, clinically isolated syndrome; GdE, gadolinium-enhancing; IFN, interferon; MS, multiple sclerosis; PPMS, primary progressive multiple sclerosis; RRMS, relapsing–remitting multiple sclerosis; S1P, selective sphingosine 1-phosphate.

Autologous Hematopoietic Stem Cell Transplant

The rationale underlying autologous hematopoietic stem cell transplant (aHSCT) is to "reset" the immune system and remove autoreactive immune cells by first treating with high-potency immunosuppression to produce chemical immunoablation. The immune system is then repopulated using hematopoietic stem cells derived from the patient, avoiding the complications of allogeneic transplant. Given the serious risks associated with immunoablation, this approach has primarily been studied in patients with very aggressive MS that have failed multiple other therapies. Most of the trials to date have been small, open-label, single-arm studies that differ both in the immunoablative regimen used and the transplant protocol. Nonetheless, several analyses and two phase 2 studies have likely set the stage for a larger, randomized trial comparing aHSCT to other aggressive treatments.

A meta-analysis evaluated 15 studies of aHSCT in MS patients published between 1995 and 2016, including 764 transplanted patients (5). The pooled rate of progression (defined as a sustained increase in Expanded Disability Status Scale [EDSS] score) was 23.3% at 5 years posttransplant, in the absence of ongoing disease modifying therapy. One lesson from this analysis was that younger patients with RRMS see greater benefit, with a pooled 2-year progression rate of 24.8% versus 7.8% in studies including a low versus high proportion of RRMS patients, respectively. Concurrently, a large, retrospective cohort study examined outcomes from 281 patients who underwent aHSCT at 25 different centers from 1995 to 2006 (6). Overall progression-free survival at 5 years was 46%, but again this was greater for patients with relapsing (73%) versus progressive (33%) MS. Building on these lessons, a phase 2 trial of high-intensity immunoablation and aHSCT in 24 MS patients with highly active disease found 69.6% of patients without disease activity or progression after 3 years (7). The effect on new disease activity was profound, as none of the patients experienced clinical or MRI relapse after a median of 6.7 and maximum of 13 years follow-up. Another phase 2 trial, the HALT-MS study, evaluated 24 highly active RRMS patients undergoing aHSCT (8). Progression-free, clinical relapse-free, and MRI activity-free survival were 91.3%, 86.9%, and 86.3%, respectively, after median follow-up of 62 months. Although promising, it must be emphasized that these were open-label studies with careful patient selection, generally excluding patients with significant comorbid conditions.

As mentioned, safety has been a major concern with aHSCT, as immunoablation necessarily leads to cytopenias and therefore a risk of serious infections and other complications. In the meta-analysis and retrospective cohort study described earlier, pooled treatment-related mortality was 2.1% and 2.8%, respectively (5,6). Factors associated with higher mortality have been identified, including progressive disease and higher EDSS score, suggesting that younger patients with RRMS fare better. Notably, mortality with aHSCT appears to have decreased over time, likely driven by greater experience and better patient selection.

In fact, only one treatment-related death has been reported among the 349 patients undergoing aHSCT since 2005 (5). As such, further phase 3 studies may reveal aHSCT as a viable strategy in aggressive MS.

Cladribine

Cladribine (2-chlorodeoxyadenosine), currently FDA approved to treat hairy cell leukemia, has been under development as an oral agent for MS. A purine analog that disrupts DNA metabolism and causes apoptosis, cladribine preferentially depletes T and B lymphocytes because of their high levels of the enzyme necessary for its incorporation into DNA (9). It has a unique dosing regimen among oral agents: two to four short courses (daily treatment for 4–5 consecutive days) in the first year, followed by two short courses during the second year.

Cladribine has been tested in two placebo-controlled phase 3 trials. In the CLARITY study, cumulative doses of 3.5 and 5.25 mg/kg were tested in relapsing MS patients, producing 57.6% and 54.5% reductions in annualized relapse rate (ARR) versus placebo, respectively (10). The risk of 3-month disability progression decreased from 20.6% in the placebo group to 14.3% (33% relative reduction) and 15.1% (31% relative reduction) in the 3.5 and 5.25 mg/kg groups, respectively, with concomitant reductions in brain atrophy rate. Intriguingly, results from a 2-year extension study showed that the effect on ARR is durable even after discontinuation of the drug (11). In the ORACLE MS trial, cladribine was compared to placebo in patients with clinically isolated syndrome (CIS) (12). The risk reduction in time to conversion to clinically definite MS was 67% for the 3.5 mg/kg dose and 62% for the 5.25 mg/kg dose.

The primary safety concern with cladribine is lymphopenia, predictably from its mechanism of action. Lymphocyte counts nadir shortly after each course of treatment, with slow recovery over weeks to months. In CLARITY, 25.8% and 45% of patients experienced grade 3 or 4 lymphopenia at nadir in the 3.5 and 5.25 mg/kg groups, respectively, with persistent lymphopenia at 96 weeks in 21.6% and 31.5% of patients (10). Neutropenia and thrombocytopenia occurred rarely. In CLARITY, there was also concern for increased cancer risk, with 1.1% of cladribine-treated patients developing a malignancy versus none on placebo. This risk was not observed in ORACLE MS; however, a subsequent meta-analysis of cladribine studies found no increased risk of cancer (13).

Although cladribine was approved for use in RRMS in Russia and Australia in 2010, such approval was denied by the European Union in 2010 and by the FDA in 2011. However, with additional safety data from extension studies and a changing landscape of risk/benefit calculations in MS therapeutics, efforts to seek approval have been renewed. The dosing regimen has advantages over some other high-potency treatments, and head-to-head comparisons and longer term safety data may still demonstrate a role for this therapy in aggressive MS.

Selective Sphingosine 1-Phosphate Receptor Modulators

Sphingosine 1-phosphate (S1P) receptors are G protein–coupled receptors comprised of five subtypes (S1P$_{1-5}$), with S1P$_1$ expressed on lymphocytes and controlling egress from peripheral lymph nodes (14). S1P receptor modulators act by causing degradation of S1P$_1$ and "trapping" lymphocytes in the periphery. Fingolimod, a nonselective S1P receptor modulator, was FDA approved for RRMS in 2010. Despite good efficacy, it has a long half-life (6–9 days) and broad side effect profile owing to off-target effects, including potentially dangerous cardiac risks (14,15). As a result, selective S1P receptor modulators are being developed in hopes of limiting side effects while maintaining efficacy.

Furthest along in development are siponimod (targeting S1P$_1$ and S1P$_5$) and the S1P$_1$-selective agents ponesimod and ozanimod. Siponimod and ponesimod have both shown efficacy in clinical and MRI measures of RRMS in phase 2 studies (16–18), and results released from two phase 3 studies of ozanimod in RRMS describe reduced ARR and brain atrophy progression rates compared with intramuscular interferon beta-1a (19,20). The phase 3 EXPAND trial evaluated siponimod 2 mg daily in secondary progressive MS (SPMS) and showed a 21% decreased risk of 3-month confirmed disability versus placebo (21). Although S1P$_5$ expressed by CNS cells, including oligodendrocytes, has been cited as a potential target in progressive MS, the benefit in EXPAND was greatest for younger patients with active disease—suggesting prevention of inflammatory disease activity as the most relevant mechanism.

Although the selective S1P receptor modulators all have shorter half-lives (and therefore a quicker washout period) than fingolimod, it remains to be seen whether their side effect profiles are truly superior. These agents caused variable degrees of bradycardia and cardiac conduction block in phase 2 trials (unsurprisingly given that S1P$_1$ is expressed on atrial myocytes), as well as other side effects seen with fingolimod, such as macular edema and dyspnea (14).

Laquinimod

Laquinimod is an oral quinoline 3-carboxamide derivative with broad immune effects on multiple cell types, including CNS-resident astrocytes and microglia (22). Although studies to date have shown only a modest effect on ARR in RRMS, recent interest in laquinimod stems from a disproportionate impact on measures of disease progression, with animal data suggesting it may target the compartmentalized inflammation that drives neurodegeneration in progressive MS.

In the MS animal model experimental autoimmune encephalomyelitis (EAE), laquinimod prevents formation of meningeal B-cell aggregates (23). In humans, similar leptomeningeal clusters become more frequent in progressive MS and are closely associated with cortical atrophy. In the phase 3 ALLEGRO trial, 0.6 mg/d laquinimod produced a modest 23% reduction in ARR versus placebo, but disability progression and brain atrophy were disproportionately reduced by 36% and 33%, respectively (24). In a second placebo-controlled phase 3 trial, the BRAVO study, 0.6 mg/d laquinimod produced a nonsignificant 18% reduction in ARR but again showed a significant reduction (28%) in brain volume loss (25). An additional placebo-controlled phase 3 trial, CONCERTO, is examining time to disease progression as a primary outcome in RRMS, although initial results released by the sponsors showed no significant effect on this measure (26). A phase 2 trial (ARPEGGIO, NCT02284568) is currently underway in primary progressive MS (PPMS).

Although an increased incidence of cardiovascular events led to discontinuation of the high-dose arms in CONCERTO and ARPEGGIO (1.2 and 1.5 mg/d, respectively), no such events have been reported at the 0.6 mg/d dose in any of the trials (27). Otherwise, the overall safety profile of laquinimod appears favorable, with no increased risk of infection or neoplasm. Dose-dependent increases in liver enzymes were observed but typically were asymptomatic and reversible without withdrawing therapy (22).

Future Directions

Compartmentalized inflammation—chronic activation of innate immune cells and leptomeningeal inflammation—persists in progressive MS and correlates with measures of neurodegeneration, providing a potential immunologic target in this stage of disease. Nonetheless, more work is needed to determine its causality in neuro-axonal injury, as well as how to modulate it pharmacologically and reliably measure it in vivo. Truly "smart" therapies that selectively deplete autoreactive lymphocytes or induce tolerance to myelin-derived antigens likewise remain far from the clinic, although promising approaches are in development. For instance, immunization with autologous Epstein–Barr virus (EBV)-specific T cells (given the postulated role of chronic EBV infection in MS) has produced encouraging phase 1 results (28), as have strategies to induce tolerance via transdermal or peripheral blood mononuclear cell-coupled application of myelin peptides (29,30). Finally, as part of the move toward more precise "personalized" medicine, ongoing research seeks to identify immunologic biomarkers that can predict which therapies are most likely to work for individual patients—such that treatment choices can be tailored for each patient.

EMERGING NEUROPROTECTIVE THERAPIES

Although classically considered a demyelinating disease, neurodegeneration is nearly universal in MS (particularly in progressive MS) and correlates more closely with disability than other pathological and clinical features (31). Neuroprotective therapies thus represent a major goal of current research efforts. Neuro-axonal loss likely results from a combination of inflammation-induced injury and the consequences of chronic demyelination. A number of early-stage therapies are being developed based on the current understanding of mechanisms driving neurodegeneration, the most advanced of which are discussed in the following sections and Table 16.2.

Biotin

The rationale for evaluating high-dose biotin, otherwise known as vitamin B_7, in MS is based on its role as a cofactor for four essential carboxylase enzymes. One of these enzymes is critical for fatty acid synthesis in oligodendrocytes, and the other three produce intermediates of the Krebs cycle—part of the energy-producing pathway in

mitochondria. Accumulating evidence points to energy failure, and mitochondrial dysfunction in particular, as a driver of axonal degeneration in MS. By augmenting mitochondrial function and stimulating fatty acid synthesis, biotin might protect axons and stimulate myelin repair, respectively.

Based on encouraging data from an initial pilot study (32), a small, phase 3 trial of high-dose, pharmaceutical-grade biotin (called MD1003) was conducted in 154 patients with primary or secondary progressive MS with an EDSS score of 4.5 to 7 (the MS-SPI study) (33). MD1003 100 mg three times daily was evaluated versus placebo, with a daring primary endpoint of the proportion of patients experiencing improved disability at month 9, confirmed at month 12. This endpoint was met by 12.6% of the 103 MD1003-treated patients and none of the 51 placebo-treated patients. As a secondary endpoint, the proportion of patients

TABLE 16.2 Select Emerging Neuroprotective Therapies in Clinical Development

THERAPY	MECHANISM OF ACTION	ROUTE OF ADMINISTRATION/ DOSE	CLINICAL EVIDENCE	ADDITIONAL CONSIDERATIONS
Biotin (MD1003)	Cofactor for carboxylase enzymes involved in the Krebs cycle (mitochondrial energy pathway) and fatty acid synthesis Theoretically protects axons from energy depletion and promotes myelin synthesis	Oral 100 mg TID	Phase 3: MS-SPI (vs. placebo) Small size (n = 154) PPMS or SPMS 12.6% experienced improved disability at 9 months vs. none with placebo Larger phase 3: SPI2 Ongoing	Generally safe Can interfere with biotin-based laboratory tests and should be stopped 72 hours before planned testing.
Sodium channel blockers	Protect axons from energy failure and influx of cytotoxic calcium ions Inhibits microglia/macrophage activation	Oral	Phenytoin Phase 2 in acute ON (36): 30% reduction in RNFL loss Amiloride Pilot study in PPMS (37): 14 patients Reduction in brain atrophy rate compared to pretreatment period Phase 2 in ON: ACTION Ongoing Phase 2 in SPMS: MS-SMART Ongoing Oxcarbazepine Phase 2: PROXIMUS Ongoing CSF NfL as measure of neuronal injury	Drugs with long clinical history and well-established safety profiles
Simvastatin	Pleiotropic anti-inflammatory and neuroprotective properties Effects may be both dependent and independent of HMG-CoA reductase inhibition	Oral	Phase 2 in SPMS: MS-STAT Simvastatin 80 mg daily 43% reduction in atrophy rate Improvements in EDSS progression and MSIS-29 Phase 3 in SPMS: MS-STAT2 Ongoing	Simvastatin 80 mg dose has high rate of myopathy/rhabdomyolysis Other HMG-CoA reductase inhibitors may have similar clinical effects

CSF, cerebrospinal fluid; EDSS, Expanded Disability Status Score; MS, multiple sclerosis; MSIS-29, Multiple Sclerosis Impact Scale-29; NfL, neurofilament light; ON, optic neuritis; PPMS, primary progressive MS; RNFL, retinal nerve fiber layer; SPMS, secondary progressive multiple sclerosis; TID, three times daily.

experiencing EDSS progression at month 9 was 4.2% in the MD1003 arm versus 13.6% in the placebo arm, which did not reach statistical significance. Aside from its small size, there were several other methodological weaknesses of the study, such as imbalance in baseline EDSS scores between the two groups and the absence of distinct treating and evaluating physicians. Nonetheless, the data are positive, and a larger phase 3 trial (SPI2, NCT02936037) is currently underway.

Overall, treatment with MD1003 was safe and well tolerated. A concern that arose is the interference of high-dose biotin with biotin-based clinical laboratory tests. These include standard thyroid function tests, and some patients in MS-SPI had false-positive results indicating hyperthyroidism (33). Because many clinical laboratory tests (including emergent tests such as cardiac enzyme levels) employ a biotin-streptavidin system, the potential for interference extends beyond thyroid testing. Practitioners must be aware of this problem, and patients should be counseled to stop biotin supplementation 72 hours before planned blood testing.

Sodium Channel Blockers

Demyelinated axons must redistribute sodium channels to previously myelinated segments in order to maintain the ability to propagate action potentials. This requires increased energy levels to maintain the electrochemical gradient across axonal membranes, ultimately contributing to energy failure and the influx of cytotoxic calcium ions. As such, sodium channel blockers have stirred interest as a potential strategy for neuroprotection in MS, particularly because many are already in clinical use for other conditions such as epilepsy. After initial success in preclinical animal models (34,35), there has been encouraging preliminary data in humans, with several trials ongoing.

A phase 2 study evaluated whether the voltage-gated sodium channel blocker and antiepileptic phenytoin can produce neuroprotection in acute optic neuritis (ON) (36). Patients presenting within 2 weeks of onset were randomized to phenytoin versus placebo and treated for 3 months, with a primary outcome of retinal nerve fiber layer (RNFL) thickness (a measure of optic nerve degeneration) in the affected eye at 6 months, adjusted for RNFL thickness of the unaffected eye at baseline. Treatment with phenytoin produced a 30% reduction in the extent of RNFL loss versus placebo. No significant effect was observed on visual acuity or visual evoked potential (VEP) latency, although the study was not powered to observe such an effect. Another antiepileptic sodium channel blocker with encouraging preclinical data, oxcarbazepine, is currently being tested in a phase 2 trial (PROXIMUS, NCT02104661) in which the primary outcome is levels of neurofilament light (a marker of neuronal damage) in cerebrospinal fluid (CSF). Finally, the acid-sensing ion channel blocker amiloride, currently used in hypertension and congestive heart failure, decreased the rate of brain volume loss and other MRI markers of neurodegeneration in a pilot study of 14 patients with PPMS (37).

Phase 2 studies of amiloride as a neuroprotectant in acute ON (38) (ACTION, NCT01802489) and SPMS (MS-SMART, NCT01910259) have been planned or are underway.

It is worth mentioning that, in addition to providing neuroprotection, sodium channel blockers may also have anti-inflammatory actions on macrophages/microglia, confounding their mechanism of action to some degree (39,40).

Statins

Cholesterol-lowering HMG-CoA reductase inhibitors, commonly referred to as statins, are among the most widely used drugs in medicine. Beyond their specific impact on serum cholesterol levels, however, they exhibit wide-ranging anti-inflammatory and neuroprotective properties and thus have been investigated in progressive MS (41). Supported by preclinical data and a small study showing improved outcomes in ON (42), the phase 2 MS-STAT study evaluated high-dose simvastatin (80 mg daily) in SPMS, with a primary outcome of annualized whole-brain atrophy rate (43). In this 24-month study, simvastatin reduced the annualized atrophy rate by 43%. Although not a primary outcome measure, statistically significant benefits were also shown for EDSS progression and the patient-reported Multiple Sclerosis Impact Scale (MSIS)-29. Based on these encouraging results, a large, phase 3 study of simvastatin 80 mg daily is being planned in patients with SPMS (44) (MS-STAT2).

Future Directions

In addition to the therapies described earlier, a number of other candidates are currently being investigated in clinical trials as neuroprotective agents in MS. Included among these are erythropoietin (45) (NCT01962571), ibudilast (NCT01982942), and idebenone (NCT01854359). Although this work is promising, successful identification and evaluation of potential neuroprotective therapies in the future will require advances in two domains.

First, a better understanding of the mechanisms underlying neuro-axonal injury is needed to identify rational targets for drug design. In this regard, progress in basic/preclinical research has identified mechanisms of injury with potential relevance in MS. For instance, in models of MS, defects in axonal transport and autophagy (the cellular mechanism for clearing damaged cell components) lead to accumulation of damaged axonal mitochondria (46,47). Recent advances in understanding the mechanisms of autophagy in axons and why it fails in disease therefore hold promise in MS (48). Similarly, preclinical research has demonstrated that injured axons execute an active program of self-destruction culminating in depletion of the critical metabolite NAD^+ (49,50). Supplementation with NAD^+ precursors or mutations that increase NAD^+ levels lead to axonal preservation in EAE (51), suggesting the components of this pathway as therapeutic targets. Finally, preclinical studies have identified the complement components C1q and C3 as potential neuroprotective targets in MS. Increased expression of these proteins at synapses leads to microglia-mediated synaptic loss (52), and secretion of C1q by aberrantly activated microglia generates neurotoxic astrocytes that actively kill neurons and oligodendrocytes (53).

A second domain requiring progress is the methods available to measure both neurodegeneration and clinical progression in MS, in order to effectively evaluate therapies in clinical trials. Especially important is the development of validated biomarkers with high predictive value that can be used to screen therapies in small, phase 2 trials before committing to larger studies. Thus far, the acute ON paradigm shows potential, as do measures derived from optical coherence tomography, which not only reflect neurodegeneration from prior optic nerve injury but also correlate with brain atrophy and clinical progression (54).

EMERGING REMYELINATING/REPARATIVE THERAPIES

Finally, a third major goal of therapeutics development in MS is to develop strategies for repairing damage and restoring function. Much effort has focused on inducing remyelination of existing lesions, both to restore function and to prevent further degeneration of demyelinated axons. *De novo* myelination (and remyelination) is mediated by oligodendrocyte precursor cells (OPCs), which are widely distributed, self-renewing cells that are rapidly recruited to areas of myelin injury, where they differentiate into myelinating oligodendrocytes (55). Although OPCs are abundant in adult human brains and present in the majority of chronic MS lesions, remyelination in MS frequently fails, particularly in late-stage and progressive MS patients (56). This failure likely results from a combination of factors, such as inhibitory/toxic components of the lesion environment and the lack of receptive axons. Exciting progress has been made over the last decades to understand and overcome these obstacles. Although remyelinating therapies remain far removed from the clinic, several promising strategies have been identified (see Table 16.3).

Opicinumab

LINGO-1 is a protein expressed by CNS oligodendrocytes and neurons that acts as a negative regulator of oligodendrocyte differentiation and remyelination (57). Opicinumab (also known as BIIB033) is a human monoclonal antibody that antagonizes LINGO-1 and enhances remyelination in preclinical models (58). Much excitement has surrounded the therapeutic potential of opicinumab in MS, and phase 2 trials have been completed in patients with ON and active MS. Although the results of these trials have been mixed, thereby tempering some of this enthusiasm, enough suggestion of benefit exists to pursue larger phase 3 studies.

The RENEW study evaluated opicinumab 100 mg/kg, dosed every 4 weeks for a total of six doses, versus placebo in patients experiencing a first episode of ON, with a primary endpoint of VEP latency at 24 weeks but followed up to 32 weeks (59). In a possibly under-powered study, nonsignificant trends toward improved VEP latency were seen at 24 and 32 weeks in an intention-to-treat analysis, with statistically significant improvement in VEP latency (but not visual acuity) at 32 weeks in a prespecified per-protocol analysis. The SYNERGY trial evaluated four doses of opicinumab (3, 10, 30, and 100 mg/kg), given every 4 weeks for 19 doses, in patients with active RRMS or SPMS, with a primary endpoint of improvement on composite disability scores (60,61). Although the reported results failed to show a linear dose response, the two intermediate doses (10 and 30 mg/kg) led to an increased percentage of improvement responders (65.6% and 68.8%, respectively vs. 51.6% for placebo). These doses may be pursued further in phase 3 trials.

Agents Identified From Cell-Based Screens

One strategy for identifying remyelinating therapies has been to screen existing drugs for their ability to induce OPC differentiation into myelinating oligodendrocytes in vitro, followed by subsequent validation in in vivo models. Using such methods, several promising agents have been identified, including miconazole, clobetasol, and the anti-muscarinics clemastine and benzatropine (62,63). Results released from a phase 2 study of clemastine in MS patients with chronic optic neuropathy demonstrated an improvement in VEP latency with drug treatment, providing proof of principle for the approach and impetus for further clinical trials (64).

Cell-Based Therapies

Another strategy under investigation involves infusion of nonhematopoietic cells to induce remyelination and tissue repair, with two particular cell-based therapies garnering the most interest thus far. The first involves direct injection of neural stem cells or OPCs into the CNS, with a phase 1 safety trial of this approach planned in SPMS patients (65). Although this strategy induces myelination in genetically hypomyelinating animal models, its potential in MS is less clear, since OPCs are abundant in adult human brains but fail to migrate into lesions or differentiate into mature oligodendrocytes when present. A second therapy under investigation involves injection (either intravenous or intrathecal) of mesenchymal stem cells (MSCs), which are pluripotent cells derived from a variety of sources with immunomodulatory and repair-promoting properties in animal models (66). Phase 1 safety trials have been completed in MS patients (67,68) with a phase 2 study currently underway (MESEMS, NCT01854957). Although not designed to evaluate for a treatment effect, a phase 1 study showed no evidence of change in disease activity or neurologic function after MSC infusion (68).

TABLE 16.3   Select Emerging Remyelinating/Reparative Therapies in Clinical Development

THERAPY	MECHANISM OF ACTION	ROUTE OF ADMINISTRATION/DOSE	CLINICAL EVIDENCE	ADDITIONAL CONSIDERATIONS
Opicinumab (BIIB033)	Humanized monoclonal antibody against LINGO-1	Intravenous infusions Given every 4 wk	Phase 2 in acute ON: RENEW 9.1 msec (41%) improvement in VEP latency in PP analysis Nonsignificant improvement in ITT analysis Phase 2 in active RRMS/SPMS: SYNERGY Dose-finding trial 3, 10, 30, and 100 mg/kg doses Improvement in composite disability (vs. placebo) at 10 and 30 mg/kg doses	
Drugs from OPC differentiation screens Includes: Clemastine Benzatropine Miconzaole Clobetasol	Existing drugs found to enhance OPC differentiation in vitro and in animal models		Clemastine Phase 2 study in MS patients with optic neuropathy 1.9 msec improvement in VEP latency after 150 d of treatment	Clemastine has provided proof of principle for this screening method as a means to identify clinically active drugs
Direct injection of NSCs/OPCs	Theoretically provides cellular substrates for remyelination/repair in existing lesions	Intraprenchymal injection into the CNS	Phase 1 trials planned (65)	
Mesenchymal stem cells	Pluripotent cells with immunomodulatory and repair-promoting properties	Intravenous or intrathecal infusion	Phase 1 trials of intrathecal (67) and intravenous (68) administration Phase 2: MESEMS Ongoing	Protocol for preparation and infusion remains nonstandardized

CNS, central nervous system; ITT, intention-to-treat; NSC, neural stem cell; ON, optic neuritis; OPC, oligodendrocyte precursor cell; PP, per-protocol; VEP, visual evoked potential.

Future Directions

Analogous to neuroprotective therapies, further development of remyelinating/reparative therapies will require addressing two main challenges: (a) an incomplete understanding of the mechanisms of remyelination failure and (b) better clinical trial paradigms. With regard to the latter, the most sensitive approach for evaluating efficacy in phase 2 trials remains uncertain, as does the length of treatment necessary to observe an effect.

Regarding the mechanisms of remyelination failure, future research will identify additional factors that either impede or promote OPC migration and differentiation. Some potential therapeutic targets have already been identified but have yet to advance beyond the preclinical stage. For instance, the inflammatory cytokine interferon gamma and astrocyte-derived hyaluronans have both been shown to inhibit OPC differentiation and myelination within inflammatory lesions (69,70). Conversely, immunoregulatory "M2" macrophages/microglia have been demonstrated to promote remyelination both by phagocytosing myelin debris and by secreting pro-regenerative factors (71), and regulatory T lymphocytes directly induce oligodendrocyte differentiation (72). Therapeutic strategies based on these findings hold promise for the future.

CONCLUSIONS

In addition to producing more targeted immunologic therapies with improved safety and efficacy, the future of MS therapeutics lies in halting progression and restoring function. Although obstacles remain, the pace of progress has been rapid and many promising approaches are already in development—giving hope that the next several decades will continue to see great strides in the fight against this debilitating disease.

REFERENCES

1. Wingerchuk DM, Weinshenker BG. Disease modifying therapies for relapsing multiple sclerosis. *BMJ.* 2016;354:i3518.
2. Kavaliunas A, Manouchehrinia A, Stawiarz L, et al. Importance of early treatment initiation in the clinical course of multiple sclerosis. *Mult Scler.* 2017;23:1233–1240.
3. Bergamaschi R, Quaglini S, Tavazzi E, et al. Immunomodulatory therapies delay disease progression in multiple sclerosis. *Mult Scler.* 2016;22:1732–1740.
4. Signori A, Gallo F, Bovis F, et al. Long-term impact of interferon or Glatiramer acetate in multiple sclerosis: a systematic review and meta-analysis. *Mult Scler Relat Disord.* 2016;6:57–63.
5. Sormani MP, Muraro PA, Schiavetti I, et al. Autologous hematopoietic stem cell transplantation in multiple sclerosis: a meta-analysis. *Neurology.* 2017;88:2115–2122.
6. Muraro PA, Pasquini M, Atkins HL, et al. Long-term outcomes after autologous hematopoietic stem cell transplantation for multiple sclerosis. *JAMA Neurol.* 2017;74:459–469.
7. Atkins HL, Bowman M, Allan D, et al. Immunoablation and autologous haemopoietic stem-cell transplantation for aggressive multiple sclerosis: a multicentre single-group phase 2 trial. *Lancet.* 2016;388:576–585.
8. Nash RA, Hutton GJ, Racke MK, et al. High-dose immunosuppressive therapy and autologous HCT for relapsing-remitting MS. *Neurology.* 2017;88:842–852.
9. Beutler E. Cladribine (2-chlorodeoxyadenosine). *Lancet.* 1992;340:952–956.
10. Giovannoni G, Comi G, Cook S, et al. A placebo-controlled trial of oral cladribine for relapsing multiple sclerosis. *N Engl J Med.* 2010;362:416–426.
11. Giovannoni G, Soelberg Sorensen P, Cook S, et al. Safety and efficacy of cladribine tablets in patients with relapsing–remitting multiple sclerosis: results from the randomized extension trial of the CLARITY study. *Mult Scler J.* 2017; doi: 10.1177/1352458517727603.
12. Leist TP, Comi G, Cree BA, et al. Effect of oral cladribine on time to conversion to clinically definite multiple sclerosis in patients with a first demyelinating event (ORACLE MS): a phase 3 randomised trial. *Lancet Neurol.* 2014;13:257–267.
13. Pakpoor J, Disanto G, Altmann DR, et al. No evidence for higher risk of cancer in patients with multiple sclerosis taking cladribine. *Neurol Neuroimmunol Neuroinflamm.* 2015;2:e158.
14. Subei AM, Cohen JA. Sphingosine 1-phosphate receptor modulators in multiple sclerosis. *CNS Drugs.* 2015;29:565–575.
15. David OJ, Kovarik JM, Schmouder RL. Clinical pharmacokinetics of fingolimod. *Clin Pharmacokinet.* 2012;51:15–28.
16. Selmaj K, Li DK, Hartung HP, et al. Siponimod for patients with relapsing-remitting multiple sclerosis (BOLD): an adaptive, dose-ranging, randomised, phase 2 study. *Lancet Neurol.* 2013;12:756–767.
17. Kappos L, Li DK, Stuve O, et al. Safety and efficacy of siponimod (BAF312) in patients with relapsing-remitting multiple sclerosis:

dose-blinded, randomized extension of the phase 2 BOLD study. *JAMA Neurol.* 2016;73:1089–1098.
18. Olsson T, Boster A, Fernandez O, et al. Oral ponesimod in relapsing-remitting multiple sclerosis: a randomised phase II trial. *J Neurol Neurosurg Psychiatry.* 2014;85:1198–1208.
19. Business Wire. Celgene announces positive results from phase III SUNBEAM trial of oral ozanimod in patients with relapsing multiple sclerosis [press release]. Summit, NJ: Celgene; 2017. Available at: http://www.businesswire.com/news/home/20170217005323/en/.
20. Business Wire. Celgene announces positive results from RADIANCE, the second pivotal phase III trial of oral ozanimod in patients with relapsing multiple sclerosis [press release]. Summit, NJ: Celgene; 2017. Available at: http://www.businesswire.com/news/home/20170522005603/en/.
21. Kappos L, Bar-Or A, Cree B, et al. Efficacy and safety of siponimod in secondary progressive multiple sclerosis—results of the placebo controlled, double-blind, phase III EXPAND study [abstract]. Presented at: ECTRIMS 2016, abstract 250. *Mult Scler.* 2016;22(S3)828–883.
22. Thone J, Linker RA. Laquinimod in the treatment of multiple sclerosis: a review of the data so far. *Drug Des Devel Ther.* 2016;10:1111–1118.
23. Varrin-Doyer M, Pekarek KL, Spencer CM, et al. Treatment of spontaneous EAE by laquinimod reduces Tfh, B cell aggregates, and disease progression. *Neurol Neuroimmunol Neuroinflamm.* 2016;3:e272.
24. Comi G, Jeffery D, Kappos L, et al. Placebo-controlled trial of oral laquinimod for multiple sclerosis. *N Engl J Med.* 2012;366:1000–1009.
25. Vollmer TL, Sorensen PS, Selmaj K, et al. A randomized placebo-controlled phase III trial of oral laquinimod for multiple sclerosis. *J Neurol.* 2014;261:773–783.
26. Business Wire. Teva and active biotech announce CONCERTO trial of laquinimod in RRMS did not meet primary endpoint [press release]. Petah Tikva, Israel: Teva; 2017. Available at: http://www.businesswire.com/news/home/20170505005740/en/.
27. Business Wire. Teva and active biotech announce discontinuation of higher doses of laquinimod in two multiple sclerosis trials [press release]. Petah Tikva, Israel: Teva; 2016. Available at: http://www.businesswire.com/news/home/20160104005710/en/.
28. Pender M, Csurhes P, Smith C, et al. Symptomatic and objective clinical improvement in progressive multiple sclerosis patients treated with autologous Epstein-Barr virus-specific T cell therapy: interim results of a phase I trial [abstract]. Presented at: AAN 2017; Boston, MA.
29. Walczak A, Siger M, Ciach A, et al. Transdermal application of myelin peptides in multiple sclerosis treatment. *JAMA Neurol.* 2013;70:1105–1109.
30. Lutterotti A, Yousef S, Sputtek A, et al. Antigen-specific tolerance by autologous myelin peptide-coupled cells: a phase 1 trial in multiple sclerosis. *Sci Transl Med.* 2013;5:3006168.
31. Lassmann H, van Horssen J, Mahad D. Progressive multiple sclerosis: pathology and pathogenesis. *Nat Rev Neurol.* 2012;8:647–656.

32. Sedel F, Papeix C, Bellanger A, et al. High doses of biotin in chronic progressive multiple sclerosis: a pilot study. *Mult Scler Relat Disord.* 2015;4:159–169.

33. Tourbah A, Lebrun-Frenay C, Edan G, et al. MD1003 (high-dose biotin) for the treatment of progressive multiple sclerosis: a randomized, double-blind, placebo-controlled study. *Mult Scler.* 2016;22:1719–1731.

34. Black JA, Liu S, Hains BC, et al. Long-term protection of central axons with phenytoin in monophasic and chronic-relapsing EAE. *Brain.* 2006;129:3196–3208.

35. Al-Izki S, Pryce G, Hankey DJ, et al. Lesional-targeting of neuroprotection to the inflammatory penumbra in experimental multiple sclerosis. *Brain.* 2014;137:92–108.

36. Raftopoulos R, Hickman SJ, Toosy A, et al. Phenytoin for neuroprotection in patients with acute optic neuritis: a randomised, placebo-controlled, phase 2 trial. *Lancet Neurol.* 2016;15:259–269.

37. Arun T, Tomassini V, Sbardella E, et al. Targeting ASIC1 in primary progressive multiple sclerosis: evidence of neuroprotection with amiloride. *Brain.* 2013;136:106–115.

38. McKee JB, Elston J, Evangelou N, et al. Amiloride clinical trial in optic neuritis (ACTION) protocol: a randomised, double blind, placebo controlled trial. *BMJ Open.* 2015;5:e009200.

39. Craner MJ, Damarjian TG, Liu S, et al. Sodium channels contribute to microglia/macrophage activation and function in EAE and MS. *Glia.* 2005;49:220–229.

40. Black JA, Liu S, Waxman SG. Sodium channel activity modulates multiple functions in microglia. *Glia.* 2009;57:1072–1081.

41. Saeedi Saravi SS, Arefidoust A, Dehpour AR. The beneficial effects of HMG-CoA reductase inhibitors in the processes of neurodegeneration. *Metab Brain Dis.* 2017;32:949–965.

42. Tsakiri A, Kallenbach K, Fuglo D, et al. Simvastatin improves final visual outcome in acute optic neuritis: a randomized study. *Mult Scler.* 2012;18:72–81.

43. Chataway J, Schuerer N, Alsanousi A, et al. Effect of high-dose simvastatin on brain atrophy and disability in secondary progressive multiple sclerosis (MS-STAT): a randomised, placebo-controlled, phase 2 trial. *Lancet.* 2014;383:2213–2221.

44. Simvastatin trial planned for secondary progressive multiple sclerosis [Press Release]. Multiple Sclerosis Trust, Letchworth Garden City, Hertfordshire, UK; 2017. Available at: https://www.mstrust.org.uk/news/news-about-ms/simvastatin-trial-planned-secondary-progressive-multiple-sclerosis.

45. Diem R, Molnar F, Beisse F, et al. Treatment of optic neuritis with erythropoietin (TONE): a randomised, double-blind, placebo-controlled trial-study protocol. *BMJ Open.* 2016;6:e010956.

46. Sadeghian M, Mastrolia V, Rezaei Haddad A, et al. Mitochondrial dysfunction is an important cause of neurological deficits in an inflammatory model of multiple sclerosis. *Sci Rep.* 2016;6:33249.

47. Sorbara CD, Wagner NE, Ladwig A, et al. Pervasive axonal transport deficits in multiple sclerosis models. *Neuron.* 2014;84:1183–1190.

48. Wong YC, Holzbaur EL. Autophagosome dynamics in neurodegeneration at a glance. *J Cell Sci.* 2015;128:1259–1267.

49. Wang J, He Z. NAD and axon degeneration: from the Wlds gene to neurochemistry. *Cell Adh Migr.* 2009;3:77–87.

50. Gerdts J, Summers DW, Milbrandt J, et al. Axon self-destruction: new links among SARM1, MAPKs, and NAD+ metabolism. *Neuron.* 2016;89:449–460.

51. Kaneko S, Wang J, Kaneko M, et al. Protecting axonal degeneration by increasing nicotinamide adenine dinucleotide levels in experimental autoimmune encephalomyelitis models. *J Neurosci.* 2006;26:9794–9804.

52. Vasek MJ, Garber C, Dorsey D, et al. A complement-microglial axis drives synapse loss during virus-induced memory impairment. *Nature.* 2016;534:538–543.

53. Liddelow SA, Guttenplan KA, Clarke LE, et al. Neurotoxic reactive astrocytes are induced by activated microglia. *Nature.* 2017;541:481–487.

54. Gordon-Lipkin E, Calabresi PA. Optical coherence tomography: a quantitative tool to measure neurodegeneration and facilitate testing of novel treatments for tissue protection in multiple sclerosis. *J Neuroimmunol.* 2017;304:93–96.

55. Bergles DE, Richardson WD. Oligodendrocyte development and plasticity. *Cold Spring Harb Perspect Biol.* 2015;8:a020453.

56. Chang A, Tourtellotte WW, Rudick R, et al. Premyelinating oligodendrocytes in chronic lesions of multiple sclerosis. *N Engl J Med.* 2002;346:165–173.

57. Mi S, Pepinsky RB, Cadavid D. Blocking LINGO-1 as a therapy to promote CNS repair: from concept to the clinic. *CNS Drugs.* 2013;27:493–503.

58. Mi S, Hu B, Hahm K, et al. LINGO-1 antagonist promotes spinal cord remyelination and axonal integrity in MOG-induced experimental autoimmune encephalomyelitis. *Nat Med.* 2007;13:1228–1233.

59. Cadavid D, Balcer L, Galetta S, et al. Safety and efficacy of opicinumab in acute optic neuritis (RENEW): a randomised, placebo-controlled, phase 2 trial. *Lancet Neurol.* 2017;16:189–199.

60. Cadavid D, Edwards KR, Hupperts R, et al. Efficacy analysis of opicinumab in relapsing multiple sclerosis: the phase 2b SYNERGY trial [abstract]. Presented at: ECTRIMS 2016; London, UK. *Mult Scler.* 2016;22(S3)7–87. Abstract 192.

61. Mellion M, Edwards KR, Hupperts R, et al. Efficacy results from the phase 2b SYNERGY study: treatment of disabling multiple sclerosis with the anti-LINGO-1 monoclonal antibody opicinumab [abstract]. Presented at: AAN 2017; Boston, MA. *Neurology.* 2017;88:S33.004.

62. Mei F, Fancy SP, Shen YA, et al. Micropillar arrays as a high-throughput screening platform for therapeutics in multiple sclerosis. *Nat Med.* 2014;20:954–960.

63. Najm FJ, Madhavan M, Zaremba A, et al. Drug-based modulation of endogenous stem cells promotes functional remyelination in vivo. *Nature.* 2015;522:216–220.

64. Green A, Gelfand J, Cree B, et al. Positive phase II double-blind randomized placebo-controlled crossover trial of clemastine [abstract]. Presented at: AAN 2016.

65. Goodman AD. Stem cell therapy for MS [abstract]. Presented at: ACTRIMS 2016; New Orleans, LA. *Mult Scler.* 2016;22(S1):8.

66. Cohen JA. Mesenchymal stem cell transplantation in multiple sclerosis. *J Neurol Sci.* 2013;333:43–49.

67. Harris VK, Vyshkina T, Sadiq SA. Clinical safety of intrathecal administration of mesenchymal stromal cell-derived neural progenitors in multiple sclerosis. *Cytotherapy.* 2016;18:1476–1482.

68. Cohen JA, Imrey PB, Planchon SM, et al. Pilot trial of intravenous autologous culture-expanded mesenchymal stem cell transplantation in multiple sclerosis. *Mult Scler.* 2017;1:1352458517703802.

69. Chew LJ, King WC, Kennedy A, et al. Interferon-gamma inhibits cell cycle exit in differentiating oligodendrocyte progenitor cells. *Glia.* 2005;52:127–143.

70. Back SA, Tuohy TM, Chen H, et al. Hyaluronan accumulates in demyelinated lesions and inhibits oligodendrocyte progenitor maturation. *Nat Med.* 2005;11:966–972.

71. Miron VE, Boyd A, Zhao JW, et al. M2 microglia and macrophages drive oligodendrocyte differentiation during CNS remyelination. *Nat Neurosci.* 2013;16:1211–1218.

72. Dombrowski Y, O'Hagan T, Dittmer M, et al. Regulatory T cells promote myelin regeneration in the central nervous system. *Nat Neurosci.* 2017;20:674–680.

17 | Overview of Rehabilitation in Multiple Sclerosis

Francois Bethoux

KEY POINTS FOR CLINICIANS

- Rehabilitation refers to a variety of interventions that aim at preserving or improving function and quality of life.
- In multiple sclerosis (MS), rehabilitation is a component of the comprehensive care approach and is a useful complement to disease-modifying and symptomatic therapies.
- The International Classification of Functioning, Disability, and Health (ICF) is increasingly used as a conceptual framework to describe the consequences of MS, and to assess the results of rehabilitation.
- The nature, intensity, and setting of rehabilitation interventions are determined on the basis of the patient's needs and on mutually agreed upon goals.

Rehabilitation refers to an array of skilled interventions which aim at optimizing function in patients with a variety of health conditions. The World Health Organization (WHO) defines rehabilitation as "a proactive and goal-oriented activity to restore function and/or to maximize remaining function to bring about the highest possible level of independence, physically, psychologically, socially and economically" (1). Often, rehabilitation is indicated after an acute injury (e.g., brain or spinal cord injury) or health event (e.g., stroke, surgery). The expectation is that the patient will achieve functional gains during the rehabilitation period, then will be returned to his or her usual environment, or to the appropriate setting (assisted living, nursing home), depending on the patient's ultimate functional status, personal characteristics, and environmental factors (such as physical environment and socioeconomic conditions).

Applying this traditional rehabilitation framework to MS requires an adjustment to this paradigm, as disability is expected to increase over time in a majority of patients. Therefore, delaying or slowing functional loss becomes a valuable goal of MS rehabilitation. In a consensus statement on rehabilitation in MS, a task force convened by the National Multiple Sclerosis Society defined rehabilitation as, "a process that helps a person achieve and *maintain* maximal physical, psychological, social and vocational potential, and quality of life consistent with physiologic impairment, environment, and life goals. Achievement and maintenance of optimal function are essential in a progressive disease such as MS" (2).

Even though rehabilitation is integrated as an important component of the comprehensive care of MS (3), obstacles to its implementation remain, and evidence to guide decision making remains insufficient (4). In this chapter, we introduce the rehabilitation process, instruments used to measure the results of rehabilitation and related conceptual framework, as well as practical applications of rehabilitation in MS.

THE REHABILITATION PROCESS

Referral

A patient's access to rehabilitation services is most often contingent upon a referral from the neurology treating team or primary care physician. Tables 17.1 and 17.2 describe the main goals for referring a patient to specific rehabilitation professionals and specialized rehabilitation services. To maximize the chances of a positive outcome, the main elements of the referral must be kept in mind:

1. To *which rehabilitation professional(s) should the patient be referred?* Rehabilitation is by nature a multidisciplinary specialty, but all professionals do not need to be involved in the care of a particular patient at all times. Even though there is a partial overlap in the expertise and problems addressed, it is important to refer the patient to the appropriate professional. The list provided in Table 17.1 is extensive, but not exhaustive. For example, psychologists, social workers,

recreation therapists, and music or art therapists also can be involved in the rehabilitation process. Another important component is the professional's knowledge and expertise in MS. Some MS centers offer rehabilitation services on site, but in many instances the patient needs to be referred to a therapist in the community. It is therefore important to establish a referral network, seeking therapists with neurorehabilitation training and expertise.

2. *What is the purpose/goal of the referral to rehabilitation services?* It is essential that the reason for the referral and the expected outcome be discussed with the patient (and family when appropriate) as precisely as possible. This promotes an understanding of how rehabilitation "fits" within the individualized MS management plan, gives patients an opportunity to talk about their own goals, increases their motivation, and helps set realistic expectations regarding the results of rehabilitation. This information should also be shared with the rehabilitation professional. Goals and expectations may be adjusted over time on the basis of feedback from the rehabilitation professionals and from the patient. Specialized rehabilitation services may be sought to address specific needs, such as adapted driving.

3. *What is the best rehabilitation setting to address the patient's needs?* In most cases, MS rehabilitation interventions are provided in an outpatient setting where space, setup, and equipment are often optimized. However, for patients who cannot drive or have adequate transportation, or when the goal is specifically to assess performance and work on functional tasks within the home environment, home rehabilitation services should be considered. Inpatient rehabilitation is indicated when patients have more complex needs and require more intensive rehabilitation involving several types of therapies. In most cases, patients are transferred to inpatient rehabilitation from a medical or surgical acute inpatient unit after a major health event (e.g., severe MS exacerbation, sepsis, surgery). Less commonly, admission to inpatient rehabilitation may also occur directly from home; for example, when patients experience a rapid functional decline within a

relatively short time frame, compromising their ability to function at home, but have a good potential to regain function. Thanks to technological advances, telehealth and telerehabilitation can now be offered more widely, and could help individuals with limited mobility or who live in remote areas have access to practitioners specialized in MS, although they are not yet widely used (8).

TABLE 17.1   Professionals Involved in MS Rehabilitation

REHABILITATION PROFESSIONALS	EXAMPLES OF INDICATIONS
Physiatrist (5)	Complex symptom management and functional issues requiring the coordination of multiple rehabilitation interventions (e.g., spasticity management)
Rehabilitation nurse, advanced practice nurse, physician assistant	
Physical therapist (6)	Lower extremity impairments Teaching of home exercise program Gait/balance training Mobility aides fitting/training
Occupational therapist (7)	Upper extremity impairments Limitation of self-care activities Fatigue management Upper extremity splinting Use of assistive devices for ADLs Home/work modifications
Speech language pathologist	Language and speech impairment Dysphagia
Orthotist	Fabrication and fitting of orthotics

ADLs, activities of daily living; MS, multiple sclerosis.

TABLE 17.2   Specialized Rehabilitation Services

SERVICE	MAIN GOALS
Driver rehabilitation	To assess driving performance (in the office and on the road, sometimes with a driving simulator) To provide on-the-road training To determine the need for vehicle adaptations (e.g., hand controls) and train patients to their use
Vocational rehabilitation	To help gain or maintain employment despite functional limitations
Wheelchair/seating clinic	To determine the most appropriate wheeled mobility device and seating arrangement for the patient, provide the information needed for reimbursement, train the patient, and assess the need for wheelchair/seating adjustments over time
Functional capacity evaluation	To assess the need for work accommodations To document physical performance for disability application
Cognitive rehabilitation	To perform exercises that aim at enhancing cognitive performance in daily activities To teach compensatory strategies

Assessment

Rehabilitation professionals share common concepts in order to describe a patient's current functional status and rehabilitation goals. Disablement models have refined the operational definitions of these concepts, which have been used for clinical practice, clinical research, and healthcare policy. In Nagi's disablement model, an active pathology results in impairments (abnormalities in body functions), leading to functional limitations (limitations in the performance of usual daily activities), and to disability (limitations in the fulfilment of personal and societal roles). In this model, the focus of care progresses from the disease process or injury, to body systems, to the person as a whole, and finally to the person within a community and a society (9). The National Center for Medical Rehabilitation Research (NCMRR) disablement model added to Nagi's model an emphasis on societal limitations, and more recently a focus on interventions to address or prevent limitations, particularly rehabilitation (10).

Currently, the most utilized framework for rehabilitation worldwide is the ICF, published by the WHO (11). This framework builds on the models mentioned earlier. The ICF classifies the consequences of medical conditions (disease, injury, malformation) in terms of body function and structure, activities, and participation. In addition, the ICF takes into account personal and environmental factors. The ICF is useful in identifying problems and goals relevant to rehabilitation. For example, a patient in the early stages of MS after an exacerbation with partial transverse myelitis, who works on an assembly line in a factory, may experience chronic weakness and spasticity in one leg (alteration of body function), resulting in difficulty walking and standing for long periods (activity limitation), and consequent inability to perform work duties full time (participation restriction). After rehabilitation, the patient's ability to work may be preserved by improving spasticity via stretching and symptomatic medication, by improving walking through physical therapy (PT) and the use of an ankle–foot orthosis, and by recommending modifications to the work environment.

Examples of assessment tools that can be used for rehabilitation are listed in Table 17.3. This list is not exhaustive, and more comprehensive information can be found in chapters 19–21, 25–30, and 36. The same instruments may be used to measure individual patient performance and to set quantitative goals for a course of rehabilitation, and to assess changes at the group level in clinical trials of rehabilitation.

While conceptual models such as the disablement model may seem remote from daily clinical practice, they are actually instrumental to perceptions and decision making at the level of the patients (and families), healthcare providers, payors, and healthcare policy stakeholders. One common practical example is the use of assistive devices to enhance mobility. In a traditional disease severity model, reflected in widely used outcome measures such as the Expanded Disability Status Scale, using a cane, walker, or wheelchair results in worse scores, and indeed the need for such devices reflects a progression in the overall disease course. However, at a given point in time, using an assistive device may allow individuals to improve their activity or participation limitations, thereby reducing their disability.

These models have also been used in MS rehabilitation research. In a study published by Klaren et al., measurements classified according to Nagi's disablement model were administered to 63 individuals with MS. Using path analysis, a statistical model was developed that provided an excellent fit for the data. In this statistical model, impairments (aerobic fitness and muscle strength) were indirectly associated with disability limitations (disability limitation subscale of the abbreviated Late Life Function and Disability Inventory [LL-FDI]) through lower extremity functional limitations (lower extremity function subscales of the LL-FDI), but not functional performance (Timed 25 Foot Walk) (12).

TABLE 17.3 Examples of Assessment Tools for MS Rehabilitation

ASSESSMENT TOOL	RATED BY	ICF LEVEL	COMMENTS
Global assessment			
Expanded Disability Status Scale	Clinician	Body function Activity	Scores based on neurological examination and ambulation status
Environmental Status Scale	Clinician	Participation	Scores based on the ability to perform complex activities (e.g., work, use of transportation, social life)
Functional Independence Measure	Clinician	Activity	Scores based on the level of assistance needed to perform daily activities
Incapacity Status Scale	Clinician	Body function Activity	Scores based on the need for assistive devices or physical assistance to perform activities and the functional impact of symptoms
MS Impact Profile	Patient	Body function Activity Participation	Assesses the perception of disability related to MS

(continued)

TABLE 17.3 Examples of Assessment Tools for MS Rehabilitation (*continued*)

ASSESSMENT TOOL	RATED BY	ICF LEVEL	COMMENTS
MS Impact Scale-29	Patient	Body function Activity Participation	Asks how much problems related to MS bothered the patient during the past 2 wk
NeuroQOL	Patient	Body function Activity Participation	Assesses the health-related quality of life of individuals with neurological disorders
Community Integration Questionnaire	Patient	Participation	Assesses limitations in the ability to perform social roles (home integration, social integration, productive activity)
Targeted Assessment			
Manual Muscle Testing, Dynamometry	Clinician	Body function	Measures strength
Ashworth Scale, Tardieu scale	Clinician	Body function	Measures spasticity
MS Spasticity Scale-88	Patient	Body function Activity Participation	Asks how much spasticity bothered the patient in the past 2 wk
Goniometry	Clinician	Body function	Measures range of motion
Timed walking tests (e.g., Timed 25 foot walk, 2- or 6-min walk, Timed up and go)	Clinician	Activity	These tests are frequently used in clinical practice and clinical trials of rehabilitation interventions
MS Walking Scale-12	Patient	Activity	Asks the patient how much MS has limited various aspects of walking in the past 2 wk
Balance scales (e.g., Berg Balance Scale, BESTest, Dynamic Gait Index, Functional Reach Test)	Clinician	Activity	Most of these scales consist of a series of tests assessing static and dynamic balance
Activities-specific Balance Confidence scale	Patient	Activity	Asks about the level of self-confidence about performing activities without losing balance
Timed upper extremity function tests (e.g., 9-hole peg test, Box and Block Test)	Clinician	Activity	These tests are easy and quick to administer
Modified Fatigue Impact Scale	Patient	Body function Activity Participation	Assesses the impact of fatigue on physical, cognitive, and psychosocial functioning

ICF, International Classification of Functioning, Disability, and Health; MS, multiple sclerosis.

OBSTACLES TO REHABILITATION IN MS

As the awareness of the role of rehabilitation grows among patients and healthcare providers, it is important to acknowledge limitations and obstacles and to take them into account when planning a referral. Some limitations stem from the disease itself. Fatigue and depression may decrease the patient's motivation to engage in a rehabilitation program. MS symptoms often worsen transiently with exertion, making it necessary to determine the right "dose" and type of exercises for each patient. Fluctuations in symptoms and functional performance over time require adjustments to the goals and contents of rehabilitation. Access to rehabilitation services may be compromised by the absence of neurorehabilitation specialists in the patient's area, by difficulty getting transportation, and by limits imposed by third-party payors (many patients have a limited number of PT and occupational therapy [OT] sessions covered per year, and maintenance of functional performance is generally not accepted as a valid indication to start or continue rehabilitation). Patient education, communication between

providers, and assistance with access problems all help overcome these obstacles.

FOR WHAT PURPOSE SHOULD REHABILITATION BE USED IN MS?

Education and Teaching of a Home Exercise Program

The development of an exercise program, to be performed by the patient at home or in a gym, independently or with a helper, is one of the goals of most rehabilitation programs. Randomized studies have demonstrated the benefits of exercise in MS on fitness, fatigue, muscle strength, mood, quality of life, and function. A meta-analysis based on results from 22 publications showed a small but significant improvement of walking performance after exercise training (13). Both aerobic (endurance) exercise and resistance training were shown to be effective (14).

In practice, it is often difficult for patients with MS to initiate a physical exercise routine on their own, owing to the obstacles discussed. This limitation further exposes them to physical deconditioning, and increases the risk of comorbidities such as osteoporosis and cardiovascular conditions. Therefore, a referral to a PT or OT is strongly recommended to optimize patients' exercise routines. At the early stages of MS, one visit may be sufficient to teach an individualized program. Later in the course of the disease, a series of sessions is often needed to initiate an adapted exercise routine. The general rule for exercise in MS is to begin with a short duration and low intensity, and to increase very gradually ("start low, go slow"). If overheating causes a transient worsening of symptoms, it can be avoided by using a fan or cooling garments, or by exercising in water. Although clinicians used to discourage patients from exercising because of fears of overheating, this is now recognized to only cause transient symptoms in a subset of patients and does not cause permanent neurologic injury.

Comprehensive Symptom Management

Rehabilitation can be integrated into the management of MS symptoms, particularly fatigue and spasticity. In fact, rehabilitation may at times be the first line of treatment, before medications or other interventions.

Fatigue is one of the most frequently reported symptoms by MS patients, and has a profound impact on functional performance and quality of life. The comprehensive management of MS fatigue includes behavioral changes aimed at improving and preserving energy, often initiated by OTs or PTs, and encompasses exercise, modification of daily activities, and the use of assistive devices. Detailed recommendations for the management of fatigue can be found in Chapter 19.

Spasticity is another frequent indication for referral to PT and OT, often in conjunction with other treatment modalities (see Chapter 29) (15). All patients with spasticity should initiate a stretching routine under the supervision of a rehabilitation professional, to ensure that the stretches will be performed with an effective and safe technique. In patients with severe disability, family members and home health aides need to be trained to perform stretching. Other rehabilitation modalities relevant to spasticity management are splinting, serial casting, brace fitting, and functional training. In addition, botulinum toxin therapy and intrathecal baclofen therapy are often managed by physiatrists (16).

Even though there is evidence suggesting that a rehabilitation approach is helpful in chronic pain management (17), specific evidence related to MS is lacking.

Task-Specific Rehabilitation

Task-specific rehabilitation is focused on training the patient to a specific function or activity, and can play an essential role in helping to maintain a patient's independence. The function that has been the most studied is walking, with treatment modalities including conventional gait training and the use of advanced technology such as body weight supported treadmill training and the use of robotics (see

Chapter 30). Other examples include balance and a variety of activities of daily living (ADLs; basic ADLs mostly represent self-care tasks, while instrumented ADLs [IADLs] refer to more complex activities such as cooking a meal and managing bills). Assessment and rehabilitation for dysphagia and dysphonia, performed by speech language pathologists, also fall into this category. Cognitive rehabilitation involves task-specific training, and aims at improving specific impairments (e.g., attention/concentration deficit) and teaching compensatory strategies (e.g., use of memory aids) (18). Driving is an essential activity for community mobility, and as a consequence a patient's ability to drive safely is a sensitive discussion topic. Driver rehabilitation specialists (often OTs) perform in-office and on-the-road (or via a driving simulator) assessments (19), and can help preserve a patient's ability to drive when indicated by providing training, and by recommending vehicle adaptations and modifications, such as hand controls. Another important goal of MS management is to preserve the patients' ability to work, as the disease affects them at the peak of their productive years. A functional capacity evaluation (FCE), usually performed by a PT or an OT, helps quantify a patient's physical ability in relation to employment (e.g., sedentary vs. more physically demanding work). FCEs are often used to support an application for disability, but may also help formulate recommendations for workplace accommodations. Vocational rehabilitation services (discussed in Chapter 36) can provide further assistance in maintaining a patient's ability to work.

Evaluation and Training for Assistive Devices and Orthotics

Even though a prescription from a physician, a physician assistant, clinical nurse specialist, or nurse practitioner is required to obtain assistive devices and orthotics, rehabilitation professionals play a key role in determining which type of equipment is most appropriate for the patient, in providing supporting information to obtain reimbursement (particularly for wheeled mobility devices), in helping with fitting and adjustments, and in training patients to use their devices efficiently and safely. A comprehensive description of orthoses and assistive devices that can be prescribed to patients with MS are discussed in Chapter 28. Extensive information about assistive technology, including suppliers, can be found at www.abledata.com. More specific information related to MS is available on the National Multiple Sclerosis Society website (https://www.nationalmssociety.org/Living-Well-With-MS/Work-and-Home/Technology).

Rehabilitation After MS Exacerbations

MS exacerbations resulting in new onset of functional limitations, or worsening of preexisting disability (particularly those resulting from lesions involving the spinal cord and brain stem) constitute a valid indication for rehabilitation. The loss of function typically occurs over a short time period, and even though some recovery is expected in the following weeks and months, residual disability from exacerbations is common (20,21). A randomized controlled trial of inpatient rehabilitation in 40 MS patients treated with intravenous (IV) steroids for an MS exacerbation showed improvement in neurological disability and functional performance at 3 months, compared to routine care (22). Another study of inpatient rehabilitation after treatment with corticosteroids for MS exacerbation, using an uncontrolled pre–post intervention design, showed improvement of Expanded Disability Status Scale scores and functional performance scores (Barthel Index, Functional Independence Measure) at the time of discharge (23). Contrasting with these findings, a randomized single-blind clinical trial of outpatient rehabilitation twice per week for 6 weeks, starting 4 weeks after IV methylprednisolone treatment for an exacerbation of MS, showed no significant between-group differences in Incapacity Status Scale and 36-Item Short Form Health Survey (SF-36) scores at 3 months or 1 year (24). These observations suggest that the intensity of rehabilitation plays a role in the efficacy of the intervention. In practice, the onset of rehabilitation may need to be delayed until the peak of the relapse has passed, to ensure that the patient is able to tolerate the therapies.

Rehabilitation for Progressive MS

An emphasis has been placed recently on finding treatments for progressive forms of MS (25). There is evidence suggesting that rehabilitation is effective in this patient population, although most of the studies were thought to be underpowered in a recent literature review (26). A randomized single-blind controlled trial of inpatient rehabilitation showed improvement of activity performance (FIM) and self-reported health status (SF-36) after 3 weeks in the treatment group, compared to a no-intervention group (approximately 80% of the subjects in each group had progressive MS) (27). Another

study of inpatient rehabilitation in patients with progressive MS showed improvement of disability, handicap, psychological status, and perceived physical health status, which was sustained for at least 6 months (28). Di Fabio et al. observed a significant decrease in symptom frequency and fatigue at 1 year, and a slower progression of disability in MS patients receiving outpatient rehabilitation, compared to no intervention (29). A more recent randomized controlled trial compared a 12-month comprehensive rehabilitation intervention (inpatient followed by outpatient) to usual care (wait list), and found a significant improvement of FIM-motor scores in the treatment group. A significantly greater proportion of patients in the control group exhibited a worsening of functional performance on the FIM (58.7% vs. 16.7%; $p < .001$). No significant benefit was observed on self-report measures (MS Impact Scale and General Health Questionnaire) (30). Altogether, these studies suggest that both inpatient and outpatient multidisciplinary rehabilitation improve or stabilize functional status in some patients with progressive MS, although the carryover of the benefit after the end of rehabilitation needs to be determined. Wheelchairbound individuals with MS are often not included in rehabilitation studies, although new studies are specifically targeting this subgroup of more disabled individuals (31).

CONCLUSION

Rehabilitation should be considered in the management of MS at all stages of the disease. The nature, intensity, and setting of rehabilitation interventions are determined on the basis of the patient's needs and on mutually agreed upon goals. As the success of rehabilitation relies on long-term behavioral modifications, it is important to initiate these interventions early, and to explain to the patient how they fit within the overall management plan for their disease. Ongoing communication is essential in ensuring that outcomes are optimized.

KEY POINTS FOR PATIENTS AND FAMILIES

- Rehabilitation is an important part of the comprehensive management of MS. Rehabilitation can be performed at home, in an outpatient office or clinic, or in a hospital as an inpatient, depending on your needs.

- Examples of rehabilitation professionals include physiatrists (physicians specialized in rehabilitation), physical therapists, occupational therapists, speech therapists, and many other professionals and services.

- The main goal of rehabilitation is to optimize a person's ability to function in daily life. Rehabilitation can be helpful all along the course of the disease, both to the persons with MS and to loved ones that are involved in their care.

- It is important to mention to your neurology team symptoms that prevent you from carrying out daily activities, so you can be referred to the appropriate rehabilitation professional or service when indicated.

- Specific goals need to be agreed upon with the person with MS before starting rehabilitation, so the effects of rehabilitation can be assessed.

REFERENCES

1. WHO Centre for Health Development. *A Older Persons. World Health Organization Centre for Development, Ageing and Health Glossary of Terms for Community Health Care and Services for Technical Report,* Vol 5. Geneva, Switzerland: World Health Organization; 2004. Available at: http://www.who.int/iris/handle/10665/68896.

2. Medical Advisory Board of the National Multiple Sclerosis Society. *Rehabilitation: Recommendations for Persons with Multiple Sclerosis.* National Multiple Sclerosis Society; 2004:10. Available at: https://www.nationalmssociety.org/NationalMSSociety/media/MSNationalFiles/Brochures/Opinion-Paper-Rehabilitation-Recommendations-for-Persons-with-MS.pdf.

3. *European-Wide Recommendations on Rehabilitation for People Affected by Multiple Sclerosis.* European Multiple Sclerosis Platform; 2008:63.

4. Haselkorn JK, Hughes C, Rae-Grant A, et al. Summary of comprehensive systematic review: rehabilitation in multiple sclerosis: Report of the Guideline Development, Dissemination, and Implementation Subcommittee of the American Academy of Neurology. *Neurology.* 2015;85(21):1896–1903.

5. McKee K, Bethoux F. Team focus: physiatrist. *Int J MS Care.* 2009;11:144–147.

6. Sutliff M. Team focus: physical therapist. *Int J MS Care.* 2008;10:127–132.

7. Forwell SJ, Zackowski KM. Team focus: occupational therapist. *Int J MS Care.* 2008;10:94–98.

8. Khan F, Amatya B, Kesselring J, et al. Telerehabilitation for persons with multiple sclerosis. A Cochrane review. *Eur J Phys Rehabil Med.* 2015;51(3):311–325.

9. Nagi S. Some conceptual issues in disability and rehabilitation. In: Sussman M, ed. *Sociology and Rehabilitation.* Washington, DC: American Sociological Association; 1965:100–113.

10. Eunice Kennedy Shriver National Institute of Child Health and Human Development, NIH, DHHS. *National Center for Medical Rehabilitation Research (NCMRR), NICHD, Report to the NACHHD Council.* Washington, DC: U.S. Government Printing Office; January 2006.

11. World Health Organization. *International Classification of Functioning, Disability and Health.* Geneva: World Health Organization; 2001.

12. Klaren RE, Pilutti LA, Sandroff BM, et al. Impairment and disability in persons with MS: do functional performance or functional limitations matter? *Psychol Health Med.* 2015;20(6):646–652.

13. Snook EM, Motl RW. Effect of exercise training on walking mobility in multiple sclerosis: a meta-analysis. *Neurorehabil Neural Repair.* 2009;23:108–116.

14. Dalgas U, Stenager E, Ingemann-Hansen T. Multiple sclerosis and physical exercise: recommendations for the application of resistance-, endurance- and combined training. *Mult Scler.* 2008;14(1):35–53.

15. Brar SP, Smith MB, Nelson LM, et al. Evaluation of treatment protocols on minimal to moderate spasticity in multiple sclerosis. *Arch Phys Med Rehabil.* 1991;72(3):186–189.

16. Bethoux F, Marrie RA. A Cross-sectional study of the impact of spasticity on daily activities in multiple sclerosis. *Patient.* 2016;9(6):537–546.

17. Sullivan AB, Scheman J, Venesy D, et al. The role of exercise and types of exercise in the rehabilitation of chronic pain: specific or nonspecific benefits. *Curr Pain Headache Rep.* 2012;16(2):153–161.

18. Goverover Y, Chiaravalloti ND, O'Brien A, et al. Evidenced based cognitive rehabilitation for persons with multiple sclerosis: an updated review of the literature from 2007 to 2016. *Arch Phys Med Rehabil.* September 25, 2017;pii: S0003-9993(17)31117-6.

19. Schultheis MT, Weisser V, Ang J, et al. Examining the relationship between cognition and driving performance in multiple sclerosis. *Arch Phys Med Rehabil.* 2010;91(3):465–473.

20. Bethoux F, Miller D, Kinkel R. Recovery following acute exacerbations of multiple sclerosis: from impairment to quality of life. *Mult Scler.* 2000;7:137–142.

21. Lublin FD, Baier M, Cutter G. Effect of relapses on development of residual deficit in multiple sclerosis. *Neurology.* 2003;61:1528–1532.

22. Craig J, Young CA, Ennis M, et al. A randomised controlled trial comparing rehabilitation against standard therapy in multiple sclerosis patients receiving steroid treatment. *J Neurol Neurosurg Psychiatry.* 2003;74:1225–1230.

23. Liu C, Playfird ED, Thompson AJ. Does neurorehabilitation have a role in relapsing remitting multiple sclerosis? *J Neurol.* 2003;250(10):1214–1218.

24. Bethoux F, Miller DM, Stough D. Efficacy of outpatient rehabilitation after exacerbations of multiple sclerosis. *Arch Phys Med Rehabil.* 2005;84:A10.

25. Fox RJ, Thompson A, Baaker D, et al. Setting a research agenda for progressive multiple sclerosis: the International Collaborative on Progressive MS. *Mult Scler.* 2012;18:1534–1540.

26. Campbell E, Coulter EH, Mattison PG, et al. Physiotherapy rehabilitation for people with progressive multiple sclerosis: a systematic review. *Arch Phys Med Rehabil.* 2016;97(1):141–151.

27. Solari A, Filippini G, Gasco P, et al. Physical rehabilitation has a positive effect on disability in multiple sclerosis patients. *Neurology.* 1999;52:57–62.

28. Freeman J, Langdon D, Hobart J, et al. Inpatient rehabilitation in multiple sclerosis: do the benefits carry over in the community? *Neurology.* 1999;52:50–56.

29. Di Fabio R, Soderberg J, Choi T, et al. Extended outpatient rehabilitation: its influence on symptom frequency, fatigue, and functional status for persons with progressive multiple sclerosis. *Arch Phys Med Rehabil.* 1998;79:141–146.

30. Khan F, Pallant JF, Brand C, et al. Effectiveness of rehabilitation intervention in persons with multiple sclerosis: a randomised controlled trial. *J Neurol Neurosurg Psychiatry.* 2008;79(11):1230–1235.

31. Freeman JA, Hendrie W, Creanor S, et al. Standing up in multiple sclerosis (SUMS): protocol for a multi-centre randomised controlled trial evaluating the clinical and cost effectiveness of a home-based self-management standing frame programme in people with progressive multiple sclerosis. *BMC Neurol.* 2016;16:62.

18 Relationship-Centered Care in a Multiple Sclerosis Comprehensive Care Center

Adrienne Boissy and Claire Hara-Cleaver

> The secret of the care of the patient is in caring for the patient (1).
>
> —*Dr. Francis Peabody*

KEY POINTS FOR CLINICIANS

- Multiple sclerosis (MS) comprehensive care centers have an opportunity to embrace relationship-centered care in their design.
- Beyond colocalization of services, MS comprehensive care centers create value by attending to access, communication, and research.
- Patient advisory councils enhance our delivery of what matters most to those we serve.
- Patient engagement in MS begins by understanding patient values and preferences.

RELATIONSHIP-CENTERED CARE

Patient-centered care has been evolving as a concept over the last decade. For many, patient-centered care is defined as healthcare delivery that is designed based on patient's values and preferences as captured in the Institute of Medicine's report *Crossing the Quality Chiasm* (2). At its core, patient-centered care involves knowing patients "in the context of their own social worlds, listened to, informed, respected, and involved in their care—their wishes honored" (3). Additional studies into what matters most to patients highlight access to the medical information and care teams, care based on values and preferences, involvement as partners in healthcare decisions, and continuity across care transitions. In addition, research has expanded to include patient reported outcomes (PROs), not simply objective measures. Even more recently there is ongoing interest in including patients in decision making, so-called shared decision making (SDM), as well as incorporating the use of aids which may help in this process. These aids can be embedded in the electronic medical record and visually represent the risks of a choice the patient is facing.

Of note, patient-centered care is core to patient experience efforts. In fact, many of the patient satisfaction surveys of today were designed based on quality metrics that were important in the patients' lens. What these surveys tell us is that there are ongoing opportunities in service, communication, access, and delays. Specifically, service is about the basics of having needs met and minimizing the challenges a patient faces, such as finding a parking space or getting a return call. Communication is interpersonal with the center itself, while access is often about appointments and scheduling issues. Finally, many patients spend unnecessary time waiting in waiting rooms to be seen and then even longer once in an exam room. These practical issues, although less about values and preferences, have a profound impact of the experience of any patient.

Patient-centeredness is a powerful concept which places the patient at the center of care. Given the chronicity of multiple sclerosis (MS), relationships and bonds form between the clinician and patient. Relationships in healthcare have therapeutic potential as patients and clinicians influence each other substantially. This is the core of relationship-centered care (RCC), which was first put forth by Beach and Inui (4). RCC advances beyond patient-centered care to include the healing power of relationships, dual expertise, and shared goals regarding health and well-being. The longevity of the disease and the relationships formed with MS patients make RCC feel more relevant for the care of MS patients and will be used to guide the chapter.

Although many patients share common needs, unique populations with unique needs also exist. These can be disease focused as we will discuss for MS, as well as based on demographics or functional status. The challenge to any healthcare system or practice is to align its services to the needs of the population it serves. A 30-year-old patient with primary progressive MS likely has different needs than a 75-year-old patient with secondary progressive MS. Likewise, someone who watched their mother die of the disease has different expectations and fears than a young mother who was blindsided by the diagnosis and never heard of it before. The future of RCC will align to specific preferences and values within a given patient.

MS is a disease that impacts nearly every aspect of a person's life: relationships, occupations, finances, self-perception, mental well-being, as well as physical functioning. Many comprehensive care centers offer a variety of services that touch each of these domains. In this chapter, we spend time discussing RCC and the role of a comprehensive care center, specifically in communication, access, and partnerships with patients and community. We use examples from the Mellen Center for MS at the Cleveland Clinic to illustrate how RCC can be promoted, acknowledging that similar initiatives are undertaken in other institutions.

COMPREHENSIVE CARE CENTER DESIGN

Especially important to note is that many MS patients get their care outside of a comprehensive care center. Sometimes, "centers without walls" are developed, using a network of providers from different facilities. Community neurologists, and at times primary care physicians, are very involved in the day-to-day management of MS patients. Although we focus on a comprehensive MS Center design, RCC can be implemented in all settings, although in different forms and using different resources.

Many of you may be familiar with a MS comprehensive care center or you are considering creating one. Appreciating how difficult accessing care can be for the MS patient means MS comprehensive care centers have an opportunity to deliver not just high-quality care, but empathic care. Enhanced access is accomplished through colocalization, team-based approach, and novel access mechanisms. Communication among team members and with the patient is optimized. Finally, high-quality research is incorporated into clinical practice and workflows. MS comprehensive care centers are well-positioned to deliver value to those they serve in a variety of ways highlighted in the next sections, and illustrated in Figure 18.1.

A. Enhanced Access

Foundationally, comprehensive care centers attend to all the needs of a given patient by leveraging multidisciplinary resources at a single site or in pulling resources from across an organization and community. Colocalization of services on site literally organizes care around the patient. In MS, this can be especially important given potential limitations in mobility or sight. Being able to visit the clinician, complete an MRI, and receive physical therapy (PT) or other necessary services saves MS patients time and energy. Even something as basic as parking on site makes the MS patient's life just a little easier.

Placing patients at the forefront of medical decision making requires providing them access to medical care and medical information. In order to do this in an MS comprehensive care center, a variety of programs must be created to meet the patient's need.

Patients desire and require access to their healthcare providers, especially when newly diagnosed or awaiting diagnosis, when their health is declining or they are experiencing an MS relapse.

Access to an MS specialist and an MS comprehensive care center in a timely manner is extremely important to the patient who is awaiting diagnosis. These patients are often traveling far and at great expense to obtain a definitive diagnosis. In order to expedite access, a program aimed at assessing and meeting the needs of this patient population was developed at the Cleveland Clinic Mellen Center for Multiple Sclerosis. Patients who have never been evaluated at the MS comprehensive care center but who are requesting to be seen are contacted ahead of time for a 30-minute phone triage visit. The phone visit is scheduled within 7 days of the initial contact. The scheduler sets up a time for the phone triage call with the patient and explains the purpose of the call: assess the patient's primary goals for the visit, obtain a brief medical history and a description of current symptoms, and identify potential ancillary services within or outside of the MS Center that would benefit the patient.

A skilled MS specialist, an Advanced Practice Clinician (APC) (a Nurse Practitioner [NP] or a Physician Assistant [PA]), conducts the phone interview. Once completed, this allows the clinician to instruct the patients on necessary records to bring with them, and to order services such as rehabilitation, spasticity management, and behavioral health psychology within the MS Center if a need is identified during the call. If symptoms and diagnosis outside of the MS spectrum exist (such as chronic pain, insomnia, headaches), orders may also be placed to arrange for the patient to see relevant specialists during their visit.

The in-person visit is then expedited and if requested by the patient, can occur within the same week. Thus, the patient is able to be evaluated when they wish, with the proper records and coordinated appointments. From the beginning, this program builds rapport and creates the foundation of the relationship between the patient and the MS comprehensive care center.

Another way to offer patients access to medical education and specialists is by shared

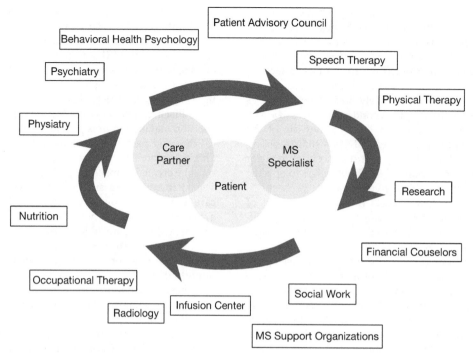

FIGURE 18.1 Relationship-centered MS comprehensive care center.

MS, multiple sclerosis.

medical appointments (SMA). Offering SMAs to newly diagnosed MS patients is a form of empowerment. In these visits, the patients may receive a short questionnaire asking for their priorities and current symptoms. An MS specialist (NP/PA), a behavioral health psychologist, a nurse coordinator, and anywhere from 5 to 10 newly diagnosed patients participate in the visit. These visits are an opportunity to educate the patients to the pragmatics of the MS Center and to the basic aspects of their disease. Additive benefits include an opportunity to introduce members of the MS team, how to reach each team member, and what to expect from future visits. Finally, and most importantly, SMAs allow patients to discuss their worries, fears, and symptoms with those who are experiencing a similar journey.

A behavioral health psychologist, specialized in MS, plays an integral role to the success of the visit, and discusses signs and symptoms of anxiety and depression, which are common in the newly diagnosed patient, and in MS in general. This offers participants emotional support and coping at a time when they are most vulnerable, and provides them with knowledge about resources that they can use throughout the course of their disease.

Comprehensive care centers often function in *teams* around the patient. The team may be made of an MS specialist and an APC, and of course, the patient. Other professionals within the MS comprehensive care center may include physical therapists, occupational

therapists, speech language pathologists, physiatrists, social workers, psychologists, neuropsychologists, nurses, and medical assistants. Often either the neurologist or the APC sees the patient independently, at times they see the patients as a team. Inherently team-based care offers enhanced communication and might be intuitive, Extending the team care concept to the entire center is of great value when an MS patient needs urgent evaluation and can be seen by any member of the practice.

Providing urgent/access appointments for patients experiencing a decline in their health or an MS relapse is critical. The priority is to enable the patient to be seen quickly by any qualified MS clinician (not necessarily from their usual team). In some comprehensive care centers, established patients call in and speak to an RN who triages calls and identifies the need for an immediate appointment. The visit occurs in a timely manner and the visit details are shared with the patient's usual care team afterward via the electronic medical record. The clinician seeing the patient will order additional testing, prescribe medications, and coordinate care. If treatment of the relapse is imminent, the treatment can be scheduled on the same day. The patient then returns for continuity of care to his or her usual team within 1 to 2 months. This process for providing urgent appointments reduces unnecessary emergency room (ER) visits and improves quality of care.

Novel methods of access have also emerged that enhance convenience and satisfaction. Virtual visits (telemedicine) are one such mechanism. Virtual visits can occur both for new and established MS patients and are especially attractive for the latter since the relationship is already established. Most patients have access to the technology needed for a virtual visit: a mobile device or laptop with a camera and an Internet connection. The visit can occur from the comfort of the patient's home. For patients who live in remote areas with little access to any MS specialists, or who are physically challenged, virtual visits are transformative.

Virtual visits may be an out-of-pocket cost to patient, although insurance coverage varies state by state. Virtual visits offer insight into the characteristics of the patients' living situation, including the accessibility of their home or facility, their refrigerator to understand their eating habits, and their physical (and human) environment. Again, innovative access meets the patients where they are, and allows the clinicians greater flexibility in their own schedule since virtual visits can be performed in various locations.

B. Communication

An important feature of MS comprehensive care centers, beyond the collection of information, is the ability to communicate this information effectively back to the patient and use it for SDM. Several models of effective communication exist (5–7), and relationship-centered communication skills can enhance the interaction between the clinician and the patient. Given the complexity of the issues navigated in diseases like MS, the uncertainty regarding prognosis, and the significant risks associated with some of the treatments, communication is critical.

Communication can make or break the relationships with MS patients, who are primarily *people* with MS. They want to be seen and known as human beings, especially as the disease has potential to rob them of their dignity, personhood, occupation, and identity. As noted earlier, effective models of communication talk about the importance of language in fostering these connections (5-7). Techniques such as collaborative agenda setting, prioritization of topics to be addressed, expressions of empathy, and SDM are skills every caregiver needs. Although these may not seem like key steps in enhancing treatment adherence, many patients behave differently if they have a strong relationship with their MS care team and might not only follow recommendations, but also communicate more readily when they have chosen to stop the medication for one reason or another.

Given the potential for severe neurological disability from MS, partnering around the right solution for a given patient in an honest way is not only the right thing to do, but also it likely impacts outcomes. The most valued decisional factor for patients in one study was the ability to take a single dose oral medication (8). Few studies have looked at SDM in MS. Carlin and colleagues have found that "no-drug" options are attractive to many patients, and side effects and severe relapse risk are essential decision drivers with any treatment option (9). So if patients may prefer to not be on a medicine, the ability to communicate the rationale for a medicine, and more importantly, exploring their values, expectations, and understanding of the severity of their MS and potentials risks and benefits of treatment, is a skill worth developing.

Furthermore, some patient satisfaction surveys specifically discuss whether SDM took place by asking not only whether side effects were reviewed, but also whether reasons to NOT take the medication were also discussed (acocahps.cms.gov/). There is often tremendous fear as patients face the realities and unknowns of MS. Asking about, understanding, and acknowledging the impact the disease has on a person's life is critical.

Difficult conversations also abound in MS. Beyond explaining why a medication is a better choice than another or the need to take it, effective communication skills are essential to optimize care. Sometimes patients are seeking an MS diagnosis when they do not actually have MS (10). In other circumstances, patients are not appropriately diagnosed, and the MS clinicians are explaining not just the new diagnosis of MS, but also what the patient may have been told before. Patients often see multiple other clinicians before arriving at a comprehensive care center and the likelihood of conflicting information is high. Important issues such as advance care planning, navigating insurance, disability choices, and the often difficult realities of the disease make effective, relational communication skills paramount for anyone caring for MS patients.

To make communication even more complex, electronic communication has replaced much of the patient/clinician phone communications. Many MS patients communicate with their care providers through the electronic medical record. These secure electronic communications allow for patient autonomy. Patients are able to view their test results, obtain medication refills, and communicate expeditiously with their care team. In return, clinicians are able to respond faster with timely documentation in the patient's chart. Various electronic portals can also be used to obtain second opinions or to answer more complicated questions when appropriate. Web-based portals for completion of PROs have been also deemed feasible, especially in patients who believe it will benefit their care (11). No matter the form, effective communication shapes the experience a patient has with the center and its people.

C. PROs and Research

Comprehensive care centers often have on site research and a collaborative environment to better recruit patients and manage the research efforts. Some centers have physically created rooms or spaces to collect PROs or encourage patients to contribute through online patient portals. The attentiveness through physical space design can impact patients' willingness and ability to spend time articulating what matters most to them and how they feel they are doing from their perspective.

The ability to collect MS data, specifically PROs and perform outcomes research is an integral part to any comprehensive MS research program. A mechanism to do so accurately and efficiently without taxing the patient and clinicians is an imperative. For example, the Multiple Sclerosis Performance Test (MSPT) is an iPad®-based assessment comprised of two patient-completed questionnaires and four objective performance assessments (12). The patient questionnaires are the MyHealth (MH) questionnaire and the Neuro-QoL (NQ) PRO scales (www.healthmeasures.net/explore-measurement-systems/neuro-qol). The objective performance assessments are the Manual Dexterity Test (MDT), the Low contrast Letter Acuity Test (LCLAT), the Processing Speed Test (PST), and the Walking speed Test (WST) (12). These tests are completed by audio instructions via headphones and the screen prompts guide the patient through the testing. The MSPT app and custom iPad enclosure were specifically developed for the purposes of neuro-performance testing. See Figure 18.2.

Goals of incorporating the MSPT into the work flow are the following:

1. To identify what specifically is important to the patient from the patient's perspective for the visit.
2. To enable routine structured data collection to inform individual patient care.
3. To minimize impact to clinical workflow through self-administered testing.
4. To allow aggregation of data that will facilitate research.

Within the MH questionnaire, the MS patient experience survey includes the questions listed in Table 18.1. The development of this program at the Mellen Center for Multiple Sclerosis was completed in partnership with patients to design a process that asks them about what is most important to them regarding their care in addition to how confident and motivated they are to manage their health. These latter questions assess a patient's activation level, which is required before any engagement can meaningfully occur. The clinician can review the answers prior or during the office visit with the patient and improve the patient–clinician relationship and value of the visit.

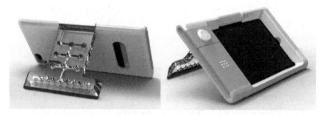

FIGURE 18.2 The MSPT device and custom enclosure.

Mspt, Multiple Sclerosis Performance Test.

TABLE 18.1 MS Patient Experience Survey in MyHealth Questionnaire

1) How important is it for you to have direct input in decisions about your MS management?
2) How confident are you that you have the tools and resources to manage your MS?
3) How motivated are you today to manage your MS?
4) What is the most important thing you want your care team to know today?

MS, multiple sclerosis.

By capturing patient data in this format, the Cleveland Clinic and others who use it have greater ability to enhance patient engagement, understand patient goals and priorities for office visits, improve clinical efficiency, and embrace innovation to drive higher quality MS care.

PATIENT ADVISORY COUNCILS AND CODESIGN

Beyond access, communication, and research, however, a comprehensive MS care center dedicated to the needs of the patient should have their voice at the table. Partnering with patients, families, and caregivers through advisory councils provides valuable insight to the needs of patients and can improve the efficiency of an MS Center, as well as the patient experience. A patient advisory council is comprised of a majority of patients, possibly family members or loved ones, several clinicians or care team members, and a representative from administration with the ability to implement changes decided on by the committee. The committee may meet a minimum of once per month or once a quarter and addresses issues put forth by the patients. These topics can be anything from long waiting lines when checking in, to more options for wellness programs, to better comprehensive care. Often, a discussion is needed to balance feasibility and value of these topics.

The committee purposefully gives the voice to the patient to define the priorities and assist in finding solutions for problem areas, or creating innovative programs. Several process improvement projects that centers have successfully implemented are improvement in communication efficiency between patients and providers, improvement of online medical resources specific to MS patients, implementation of wellness programs, and involvement in creating medical information for MS patients. Rather than a focus group, patient advisory councils should be actively working on projects that the center is committed to implement, in order to maximize engagement. Beyond advisory councils there is an increasing shift to involve patients on committees that have standing meetings to influence policy and programs institution wide.

True partnership with patients also means involving them in all aspects of the clinical care. The family members are also significantly involved. Any comprehensive care center should incorporate the voices of these stakeholders into the design of programs and services.

Opportunities are frequent and multiple including education, support services, and clinical care.

As stated earlier, the emotional stress and shock caused by disclosure of the diagnosis may make it difficult to convey educational information and for the patient to be able to receive digest and understand this information. Thus, it is often helpful to follow the initial conversation regarding the diagnosis with patient-directed education at a time that best suits her needs. Educational sessions run by clinicians for newly diagnosed patients are often quite different than those for patients at later stages of the disease. Partnering with patients regarding the content of those sessions, as well as any materials distributed to patients is an opportunity. Rather than having clinicians design and convey education, patients themselves can be invited to make videos to share their experiences with other patients. Patients and caregivers can equally participate in educational SMAs. This brings the actual patients and their experiences to the table and allows empathy and relationships to grow.

ENGAGEMENT

Relationship-centered comprehensive MS care centers effectively engage patients in managing their health. Patient engagement has many definitions and is a popular concept these days. The Center for Advancing Health defines it as the behaviors a patient would demonstrate to take greatest benefit from healthcare services available to them (13). The concept of patient engagement is often used interchangeably with patient empowerment and patient activation, which are more inclusive of confidence, skills, and motivation required to become engaged. Yet, it is worth considering patient engagement and how centers can best connect with the patients they serve. In MS, engagement is foundational to comprehensive care given that it is known to impact the patients' ability to take expensive medications, whose route of administration they often find less than ideal. Up to 39% of patients are not adherent with taking disease-modifying therapies (DMTs), often because they simply forget to take them (14). Yet, a review of the literature found that increased adherence and persistence with DMTs resulted in improved clinical outcomes, decreased relapses, fewer ER visits, and decreased healthcare resource utilization (15). Excluding cost of DMTs, this same review demonstrated a reduction of 22% in patient/year total care cost with adherence and persistence. The need to engage patients, to understand the barriers to taking DMTs, and the subsequent impact of DMTs on their overall health and financial burden is essential.

A 2015 report on patient engagement in MS identified five areas of focus in MS: education and confidence building, increasing importance of quality of life and patient concerns through PROs, providing credible sources of accurate information, encouraging adherence, and empowering patients through responsibility (16). Others include behaviors such as end-of-life planning and medication management (17). It is fair to say the process is complex, but should include the entire span of the disease course, from the moment a patient discovers they have MS to the end of life with the disease. These patient engagement strategies should also be built on what matters most to the patient, including at times not being engaged. For example, patients who are struggling with their diagnosis and do not want to be reminded of their disease should not be asked to download information regarding their walking performance every day. The most effective engagement of these patients means allowing them to live their life outside of MS fully, yet at the same time maintain an effective relationship with them that meets their needs.

In summary, RCC is at the core of a comprehensive MS care center. Clinicians must take great effort in understanding the patient as a unique person, understanding their social context, their priorities, and their healthcare perspectives. Doing so will optimize the care of the patient and the relationship between the patient and the clinician. The patient's engagement, likelihood to adhere to treatments, and follow through with both medical and nonmedical interventions will be enhanced. Using technology and novel approaches such as virtual visits, the collection of PROs, and patient advisory councils are all integral to a successful MS comprehensive care center. However, these approaches will only be successful if the model of care prioritizes care and interventions based on the patients' values and preferences. Because, at the core of any successful comprehensive care center, is the patient.

KEY POINTS FOR PATIENTS AND FAMILIES

- MS care is significantly improved when patients and families are partners in design.
- Articulating what matters most to you in your MS, but also in personal goals, helps us to better understand how we can achieve them together.
- You are an expert in your own body and can teach your MS care team, and other patients, about your experience.
- Forming relationships with patients and their loved ones often gives the MS care team meaning and value.

REFERENCES

1. Peabody FW. The care of the patient. *JAMA*. 2015;313(18):1868. doi:10.1001/jama.2014.11744.
2. Institute of Medicine. *Crossing the Quality Chiasm*. Washington, DC: National Academy Press; 2001. http://www.nap.edu/openbook.php?isbn=0309072808.
3. Epstein RM, Street RL, Jr. The values and value of patient-centered care. *Ann Fam Med*. 2011;9(2):100–103. doi:10.1370/afm.1239.
4. Beach MC, Inui T, Relationship-Centered Care Research Network. Relationship-centered care. a constructive reframing. *J Gen Intern Med*. 2006;21(suppl 1):S3–S8. doi:10.1111/j.1525-1497.2006.00302.x.
5. Baile WF, Buckman R, Lenzi R, et al. SPIKES-A six-step protocol for delivering bad news: application to the patient with cancer. *Oncologist*. 2000;5(4):302–311.
6. Frankel RM, Stein T. Getting the most out of the clinical encounter: the four habits model. *J Med Pract Manage*. 2001;16(4):184–191.
7. Windover AK, Boissy A, Rice TW, et al. The REDE model of healthcare communication: optimizing relationship as a therapeutic agent. *J Patient Exp*. 2014;1(1):8–13. doi:10.1177/237437431400100103.
8. Bottomley C, Lloyd A, Bennett G, et al. A discrete choice experiment to determine UK patient preference for attributes of disease modifying treatments in multiple sclerosis. *J Med Econ*. 2017;20(8):863–870. doi:10.1080/13696998.2017.1336099.
9. Carlin CS, Higuera L, Anderson S. Improving patient-centered care by assessing patient preferences for multiple sclerosis disease-modifying agents: a stated-choice experiment. *Perm J*. 2017;21. doi:10.7812/TPP/16-102.
10. Boissy AR, Ford PJ. A touch of MS: therapeutic mislabeling. *Neurology*. 2012;78(24):1981–1985. doi:10.1212/WNL.0b013e318259e0ec.
11. Engelhard MM, Patek SD, Sheridan K, et al. Remotely engaged: lessons from remote monitoring in multiple sclerosis. *Int J Med Inform*. 2017;100:26–31. doi:10.1016/j.ijmedinf.2017.01.006.
12. Rudick RA, Miller D, Bethoux F, et al. The multiple sclerosis performance test (MSPT): an iPad-based disability assessment tool. *J Vis Exp*. 2014;88:e51318. doi:10.3791/51318.
13. Center for Advancing Health. *A New Definition for Patient Engagement: What Is Engagement and Why Is It Important?* Washington, DC; 2010. http://www.cfah.org/file/CFAH_Engagement_Behavior_Framework_current.pdf.
14. Treadaway K, Cutter G, Salter A, et al. Factors that influence adherence with disease-modifying therapy in MS. *J Neurol*. 2009;256(4):568–576. doi:10.1007/s00415-009-0096-y.
15. Lizan L, Comellas M, Paz S, et al. Treatment adherence and other patient-reported outcomes as cost determinants in multiple sclerosis: a review of the literature. *Patient Prefer Adherence*. 2014;8:1653–1664. doi:10.2147/PPA.S67253.
16. Rieckmann P, Boyko A, Centonze D, et al. Achieving patient engagement in multiple sclerosis: a perspective from the multiple sclerosis in the 21st century steering group. *Mult Scler Relat Disord*. 2015;4(3):202–218. doi:10.1016/j.msard.2015.02.005.
17. Colligan E, Metzler A, Tiryaki E. Shared decision-making in multiple sclerosis. *Mult Scler*. 2017;23(2):185-190. doi:10.1177/1352458516671204.

Fatigue in Multiple Sclerosis

Matthew Plow and Aaron Nicka

KEY POINTS FOR CLINICIANS

- Fatigue is experienced by 75% to 90% of persons with multiple sclerosis (MS), of which 60% indicate it is one of their worst problems.
- The pathogenesis of fatigue continues to be unclear.
- Factors that contribute to fatigue include depression, sleep problems, medication side effects, deconditioning, chronic stressors, and comorbid conditions.
- The approach to fatigue management should be individual-centered, comprehensive, systematic, and sensitive to the individual's experience and priorities.
- It is helpful to use a four-phase iterative process (identifying the presence of fatigue, screening, comprehensively assessing, and implementing an appropriate intervention) when managing fatigue.

Fatigue is one of the most common and debilitating symptoms of MS. It is reported that 75% to 90% of people with MS have fatigue, and up to 60% describe it as their most disabling symptom (1–4). Fatigue can be a major problem for persons with MS across all types of MS and all life situations. MS fatigue can adversely affect physical, mental, and social function. It can be a profound barrier to participating in self-management behaviors, leisure activities, domestic roles, and employment. MS fatigue is different from how healthy individuals experience fatigue. MS fatigue comes on quickly and there can be a long recovery even after resting or sleeping. People describe MS fatigue as overwhelming, and they often cite it as a main reason for being unable to maintain employment, enjoy social activities, and engage in self-care activities (5–8). People with MS often express frustration because they feel that family members, friends, and healthcare providers do not fully understand the extent to which fatigue causes problems.

There are numerous definitions that have been used to describe MS fatigue. Some definitions address the duration and impact of fatigue, whereas other definitions address the chronic nature of fatigue (1,9) and the causes of fatigue (9) or the complexities of it (10). For the purpose of this chapter, we use the definition provided by The Multiple Sclerosis Council for Clinical Practice Guidelines: "a subjective lack of physical and/or mental energy that is perceived by the individual or caregiver to interfere with usual and desired activities" (1).

This chapter provides an overview of the issues related to MS fatigue, the factors that contribute to MS fatigue, and the ways in which to address MS fatigue. In the second edition of this book, we (Plow and Nicka) have revised and updated this chapter, which was originally written by Susan Forwell. Within the short amount of time since the first edition of this book was published, we note that progress has been made on understanding MS fatigue. Advances in neuroimaging have facilitated insight into primary causes of fatigue, while survey studies have facilitated further insight into secondary causes of fatigue and the impact of fatigue on physical, mental, and social function.

Although our understanding of the factors that contribute to MS fatigue has improved, we also note that few advances have been made on improving the effectiveness of treatments for MS fatigue. Thus, sections on addressing fatigue in this chapter have largely been unedited from the previous edition. We believe Susan Forwell's principles and processes for addressing MS fatigue in this chapter are not only relevant in guiding healthcare providers for managing fatigue, but can also serve as a blueprint for researchers who are trying to identify more effective ways to reduce fatigue.

PATHOPHYSIOLOGY AND CLASSIFICATION OF MS FATIGUE

The negative impact of MS fatigue on individuals and their families has significant implications for their functional status and use of healthcare services. MS fatigue is associated with a higher number of emergency room (ER) visits and hospitalizations (11,12). The costliest components of treating MS are disease-modifying therapies (DMTs), managing multiple comorbidities, and reducing the impact of exacerbations (13). MS fatigue decreases adherence to DMTs, contributes to the development of multiple comorbidities, and is related to the onset of exacerbations (14–17). This, in turn, makes DMTs less effective and accelerates functional decline (18). Consistently, studies have demonstrated the relationships between MS fatigue and physical, mental, and social function.

Physical function. The effects of fatigue on physical function have been well documented (19). Increases in fatigue are associated with decreases in physical function. Many of the first studies on MS fatigue focused on the relationship between fatigue and muscle function (20). These studies typically found a small relationship between perceived fatigue and objective measures of muscular endurance and strength. This suggests that MS fatigue cannot be entirely explained by muscle weakness.

Mental function. A growing number of studies are now documenting the negative impact of MS fatigue on mental function (21,22). Cognitive fatigue is similar to physical fatigue; that is, cognitive fatigue increases as more time is spent engaging in a cognitive task. The functional consequences of cognitive fatigue include trouble concentrating, organizing, and/or remembering things (23). Cognitive fatigue can subside with rest and self-management strategies (23).

Social Function. MS fatigue is referred to as a "hidden" disability because of the difficulties in visually observing it and objectively measuring it. Family members and friends can mistake MS fatigue simply as a lack of motivation to participate in daily chores and/or leisure activities (24). MS fatigue can make it difficult to maintain social relationships, which can lead to reduced autonomy and to depression. Furthermore, societal norms pertaining to productivity can make it difficult to engage in self-management behaviors (e.g., activity pacing), which can reduce the negative impact of fatigue on social function.

> *The impact of MS fatigue can be described through its effects on physical, mental, and social function.*

Pathogenesis

Although the pathophysiology of MS fatigue remains unclear, most researchers now conclude that fatigue is caused by multiple factors. Researchers have typically distinguished between primary and secondary factors that contribute to MS fatigue (25). Primary factors pertain to MS pathology and adaptive responses, such as brain lesions, axonal damage, and cortical reorganization (26–30). Studies using neuroimaging to understand potential anatomical correlates of MS fatigue show no correlation with T2 lesion load, but otherwise lack consensus in their findings (25,31). More recent evidence has found that distinctive clusters of lesions and atrophy at different locations, mostly bifrontal or in subcortical structures, are associated with fatigue (21). A functional cortico-subcortical disconnection due to widespread microstructural damage in "normal appearing white matter" has recently been found to be associated with fatigue (32). Other studies indicate that increased inflammation may also contribute to fatigue. However, most studies finding associations between cytokines like interleukin (IL)-1 and tumor necrosis factor (TNF)-alpha and fatigue are in vitro (21). Preliminary evidence comparing healthy controls to people with MS indicates that IL-6 may play a role in MS fatigue (33).

Secondary factors that contribute to fatigue pertain to personal characteristics not specific to the disease processes of MS. Secondary factors include depression, sleep problems, medication side effects, deconditioning, chronic stressors, comorbid medical conditions, and mobility impairments. Secondary factors can typically be addressed, by prescribing appropriate therapies when applicable, and by encouraging self-management behaviors, such as physical activity. Thus, it is important to screen and identify secondary factors that are contributing to MS fatigue.

Depression plays a significant role in MS fatigue (34,35), and when depression is effectively treated the reported experience of fatigue is reduced (36,37). Although there is overlap between fatigue and depression in people with MS, they are considered separate entities (38).

Sleep problems are common in people with MS (39). Poor sleep quality is associated with fatigue, and when sleep disorders are treated there can be improvement in fatigue (40,41). Unfortunately, sleep problems are often underdiagnosed in people with MS (42).

Medication side effects of fatigue are common for persons with MS. This includes DMTs as well as drugs used for symptomatic management, such as those prescribed for neuropathic pain and spasticity (43).

Deconditioning has been shown to be a contributor to MS fatigue. Persons with MS are less active and the presence of muscle weakness and decreased endurance requires more energy to engage in daily activities (44). Physical activity and exercise programs can reduce the impact of MS fatigue (45).

Chronic stressors have been linked to MS fatigue (46). Stressful events can increase fatigue, which then results in more stress. Interventions that empower people with MS to reduce stressors in their environment may also reduce fatigue (47). Furthermore, recent research has indicated that reducing stress may prevent new brain lesions (48,49).

Comorbid medical conditions present a host of complications for persons with MS, among them fatigue (50,51). A recent study found that depression, anxiety, irritable bowel syndrome, and migraines were independently associated with MS fatigue (52). Treating these comorbid conditions may help improve MS fatigue.

Mobility impairments are related to MS fatigue due in part to increased energy expenditure (44,53,54).

Maximizing efficient ambulation and encouraging more efficient ways to perform daily chores can have an impact on reducing fatigue (54).

> *Secondary factors contributing to MS fatigue should be systematically assessed, since many can be addressed.*

Types of Fatigue in MS

While there have been many different labels for the various experiences and factors contributing to fatigue in MS, six types of fatigue are described here. Some of these are overlapping, some discrete, and all are relevant in the overall picture of MS fatigue.

Central fatigue (also called generalized fatigue) refers to the overall exhausted feeling that is a full body experience and has both a physical and a mental component (55). Simple resting does not remediate central fatigue.

Peripheral fatigue (also called motor fatigue) is the depletion, fatiguing, or progressive weakening of a muscle group with prolonged use (55). Sufficient rest is typically therapeutic for this type of peripheral fatigue (55).

Primary MS fatigue refers to the fatigue experience that is directly related to the MS disease process such as demyelination, autoimmune phenomenon, or axonal loss (25).

Nonprimary MS fatigue refers to fatigue that is not directly related to the MS disease process and is considered to represent additional factors that contribute to fatigue in MS. Subtypes of nonprimary MS fatigue are secondary, acute, and chronic fatigue.

Secondary fatigue, a subset of nonprimary fatigue, refers to the fatigue resulting from or secondary to other symptoms of MS. For example, with increased walking challenges due to weakness or spasticity, more energy is required to move around.

Acute fatigue, another subset of nonprimary MS fatigue, refers to fatigue that occurs for a short period. It emerges as a result of a short-term condition or circumstance such as acute infection (e.g., the common cold) or stressful events (e.g., moving residence) (1).

Chronic fatigue, the final subset of nonprimary MS fatigue, refers to fatigue that lasts more than 6 months and emerges with long-term issues (1) such as depression and comorbid conditions.

MANAGEMENT OF MS FATIGUE

Approach to Addressing Fatigue in MS

The diverse impact and factors related to fatigue clearly underscore the complex nature of the problem and the need for a targeted yet comprehensive approach. The principles of this approach are 4-fold: individual-centered, comprehensive, systematic, and sensitive.

Individual-centered refers to ensuring the individual with MS identifies their priorities, preferences, and constraints related to fatigue, and its impact on their life. Their priorities may be as diverse as maintaining employment to attending a child's soccer game, while preferences may be related to valuing physical exercise or an interest in social activities. Constraints will also differ. For example, economic issues may present a barrier for some, while time to integrate suggestions is a concern for others.

Comprehensiveness refers to identifying and addressing not only the primary fatigue related to MS, but also factors the secondary factors that contribute to fatigue. As the number of contributing factors increases, so does the severity of fatigue (22).

Systematic refers to using a process that sequences assessment and intervention and allows for reevaluation and monitoring of all aspects and factors of the fatigue experience. Using the four-phase process described here follows this principle.

The principle of *sensitivity* refers to addressing the area of fatigue in MS thoughtfully, recognizing that psychosocial attitudes, values, and experiences have shaped the individual's perception of normalcy, acceptability, stigma, and usefulness of reporting and addressing the issues of fatigue.

> *The individual's priorities, preferences, and constraints should be taken into account when designing a fatigue management plan.*

Process for Addressing Fatigue in MS

Mindful of these principles, a four-phase iterative process is provided that includes identifying the presence of fatigue, screening, comprehensively assessing, and implementing an appropriate program of intervention. For additional information on treatment algorithms for fatigue, we also refer the reader to a publication by Veauthier et al. (56).

1. **Identify the presence of fatigue**. This phase establishes whether the person with MS has fatigue that interrupts or impacts everyday life. Questions to ask might include: "Is fatigue a problem for you?" or "Does fatigue get in the way of doing the things you need and want to do?"

   It is also critical to establish whether addressing the issue of fatigue is a priority or something the patient would like to deal with. While fatigue may be considerable and have a profound impact, other aspects of life or symptoms of MS may be a priority.

2. **Screen for severity of fatigue**. If fatigue is an issue and priority for the individual, then moving onto screening for the severity of fatigue is recommended. The reason for screening is to
   • Determine the level or severity of fatigue
   • Ensure fatigue is targeted for treatment, if appropriate

- Account for fatigue when treating other issues of MS or other chronic conditions
- Identify an outcome measure to establish a baseline and attest to the efficacy of intervention for fatigue

There are no clinical laboratory tests or imaging techniques for screening of fatigue. Rather, the measures that screen for the presence and severity of fatigue in MS are usually self-report questionnaires completed using paper and pencil, mobile technology (e.g., smartphone), or computers. These measures are usually valid and reliable, include between one and 40 items, and are typically statements evaluated on Likert scales (e.g., 0–4) or visual analog scales (e.g., marking a point on a line from least to most fatigue).

It is recommended that when screening for MS fatigue that measures developed for or tested with the MS population be used. Table 19.1 provides examples of such measures. In a consensus conference (57) with a multidisciplinary group of clinicians and researchers in MS, it was shown that most measures included in Table 19.1 address issues of impact on activities and participation, are time efficient, have established psychometrics for MS, and are self-administered. It is useful to select one of these measures and have it readily available, to be used as needed, during clinical visits.

Completing phases 1 and 2 can be done efficiently, and in most cases does not take more than 15 minutes. Even at this screening phase, however, there may be an opportunity to provide targeted interventions. For example, if heat is identified as impacting fatigue tolerance, there might be consideration for trying a cooling garment.

3. **In-depth assessment of fatigue in MS**. After screening for the level of MS fatigue, completing an in-depth assessment is essential. The comprehensive assessment provides information to
   - Identify and ascertain the scope of potential factors contributing to fatigue
   - Ensure factors contributing to fatigue are addressed
   - Guide intervention decisions

Studies have shown that factors that may contribute to nonprimary MS fatigue are present for 72% to 74% of persons with MS who experience fatigue and that this subgroup experiences a higher level of fatigue (67,68). Furthermore, some of these factors can be treated, or at least

TABLE 19.1 Measures to Screen for Fatigue in MS

MEASURE	NUMBER OF ITEMS	FORMAT	SCORING	DESCRIPTION	SOURCE
Short measures (5–7 min to complete)					
Fatigue Severity Scale	9	Likert scale; 1–7 for each item	Sum values and divide by 9. Score is out of 7. Higher score = worse fatigue	Items are phrases related to severity and impact on activities	(58)
Daily Fatigue Impact Scale	8	Likert scale; 0–4 for each item	Sum score. Score is out of 32. Higher score = worse fatigue	Items are phrases related to current daily changes in life attributable to fatigue	(59)
PROMIS v1.0 Fatigue Short Form	7	Likert scale; 1–5	Sum score. Score is out of 35 with higher score = worse fatigue	Items are phrases related to feelings of tiredness and sense of exhaustion that decrease the ability to execute daily activities and family/social roles	(60) www. nihpromisorg/ assessment
Visual Analog Scale for fatigue	1	100-mm line	Divide the line into one-thirds—mild, moderate, and severe fatigue	Ends of line are "Not fatigued at all" and "Extremely fatigued"	(58)
Categorical					
Fatigue Impact Scale	36	Likert scale; 0–4 for each item	Summed scores. Score is out of 144 with higher scores = worse fatigue	3 three dimensions: cognitive (10 items), physical (10 items), social (16 items)	(3)

(continued)

TABLE 19.1   Measures to Screen for Fatigue in MS (*continued*)

MEASURE	NUMBER OF ITEMS	FORMAT	SCORING	DESCRIPTION	SOURCE
Modified Fatigue Impact Scale	21	Likert scale; 0–4 for each item	Summed scores; Score is out of 84 with higher scores = worse fatigue	3 three subscales: cognitive (10 items), physical (nine items), psycho-social (two items)	(61)
Multicomponent Fatigue Scale	15	Likert scale; 0–4 for each item	Summed scores. Score is out of 60 with higher scores = worse fatigue	3 two subscales: cognitive (seven items), physical (eight items)	(62)
Fatigue Scale for Motor & Cognitive Functions	20	Likert scale; 0–4 for each item	Summed scores. Score is out of 80 with higher scores = worse fatigue	3 two subscales: cognitive (10 items), physical (10 items)	(63)
Noncategorical					
Fatigue Assessment Instrument	29	Likert scale; 1–7 for each item	Sum values. Score ranges from 29 to 203. Higher score = worse fatigue	Items are phrases capturing quantitative and qualitative components of fatigue	(64)
Würzburg Fatigue Inventory for MS	17	Likert scale; 0–4 for each item	Sum values. Score is out of 68 with higher score = worse fatigue	Items are phrases related severity and impact on activities and cognition	(65)
Rochester Fatigue Diary	24	24 lines (one for each hour of the day). Ends are "Energetic, no fatigue" to "Exhausted, severe fatigue"	Divide the line into one-thirds—mild, moderate, and severe fatigue	Place a mark on the line rating average energy for each hour. If asleep, the line is not marked for that hour.	(66)

MS, multiple sclerosis.

partially alleviated, such as depression, sleep problems, mobility challenges, and medication side effects.

A comprehensive assessment of fatigue in MS can begin with a series of self-report questionnaires that assess factors which may contribute to the severity of fatigue. Because these questionnaires cover a broad spectrum of issues, they take time to complete. These questionnaires can be forwarded to the individual to be completed in advance of the appointment with the healthcare provider. In an unhurried setting, the questionnaires can then be completed more thoughtfully, with less stress, and may allow for input from others who know them well, all of which increase the ecological validity of responses. The completed questionnaires are then reviewed at the next visit by the healthcare provider, who can quickly see the issues and target discussion and intervention priorities.

Preliminary work has been completed on a Comprehensive Fatigue Assessment Battery for MS that assesses the presence of comorbid conditions, fatigue and self-efficacy, pain, sleep, stress, depression, anxiety, mobility, environment, nutrition, and fatigue management history (69). To review the completed questionnaires, the healthcare provider and patient will take, on average, 10 to 30 minutes depending on the number of issues identified and the clarifying discussion that follows. Along with this information, it may be necessary to complete performance-based assessments related to mobility. It is important to remember that clinically observed performance does not necessarily correlate MS fatigue.

It is important to formally identify MS fatigue, measure its severity, and assess contributing factors, prior to designing an intervention.

4. **Intervention**. In the fourth phase, it is important that interventions target both primary and secondary factors that contribute to fatigue. This can be done concurrently or in a sequence.

   a. **Addressing secondary factors of fatigue**. Most often, several secondary factors contribute to MS fatigue, and fortunately many of these factors have intervention pathways, either through referral or directly attending to the issue. For example,
      - Depression can be treated with counseling, psychotherapy, medication, or group interventions.
      - Fatiguing side effects of medications can be identified through a review of the medications, and adjustments might then be made to the administration schedule, type, or dosage of drug.
      - Sleep problems, depending on the nature, may be addressed through educating on sleep hygiene principles, providing strategies to manage the social environment that interrupts sleep, medications, and in some cases referral to a sleep specialist to assess and treat possible sleep disorders.
      - Inefficient mobility or deconditioning is typically managed through the use of mobility devices and/or an appropriate exercise or physical activity program.

   b. **Addressing primary factor of fatigue**. The intervention plan for addressing primary factors of MS fatigue usual follows a multipronged approach. There are three types of interventions: (a) Pharmacotherapy, (b) behavior change interventions, and (c) complementary and alternative strategies.
      i. **Pharmacotherapy**. Table 19.2 lists the agents that have been tested, their dosage, and the results. Of these, amantadine and modafinil have shown the greatest promise. However, meta-analyses show that fatigue medications have a small and nonsignificant pooled effect size on reducing MS fatigue (77,78). In fact, meta-analyses show that self-management interventions may be more effective than medications in reducing fatigue (77). We also note that although methylphenidate is a commonly prescribed medication to treat MS fatigue, there is limited evidence that it is effective (79).
      ii. **Behavior change interventions** can reduce MS fatigue (77). These interventions have typically focused on promoting fatigue self-management strategies or promoting physical activity and exercise (80). Several of these interventions have targeted self-efficacy or confidence to overcome barriers to use fatigue self-management strategies or engage in physical activity.

TABLE 19.2 Evidence for Pharmacotherapy for Treating Fatigue in MS

AUTHOR	DOSAGE	MEASURE	METHOD	RESULT
Amantadine				
(70) (n = 32)	100 mg twice a day	Fatigue Assessment Scale	Double-blind, controlled study	Moderate—marked improvement
(71) (n = 115)	100 mg twice daily	VAS and ADLs	Crossover design	Small but significant improvement
(72) (n = 22)	100 mg twice daily	5-point scales for energy, strength, cognition, and well-being	Double-blind, controlled study	Higher self-report ratings
(73) (n = 93)	100 mg twice daily	MS-specific FSS; FSS	Randomized, double-blind, placebo-controlled study	Significant improvement
3,4 diaminopyridine				
(74) (n = 8)	50–60 mg/according to body size, taken for 3 wk	FSS	Open label clinical trial	Improvement observed
Modafinil				
(75) (n = 72)	200 mg/d for 2 wk followed by 400 mg/d for 2 wk	FSS, MFIS, fatigue VAS	Single blind, pilot study	Significant improvement
(76) (n = 115)	200 mg/d for 1 wk based on tolerance, increased to: 300 mg/d in wk 2 400 mg/d in wk 3	MFIS	5 week randomized, double-blind, placebo-controlled	No difference

ADLs, activities of daily living; FSS, fatigue severity scale; MFIS, modified fatigue impact scale; VAS, visual analog scale.

a. Fatigue self-management interventions facilitate the learning of strategies and skills that can reduce the impact of fatigue on daily activities. These interventions are typically delivered by occupational therapist and can include content on the importance of rest or activity pacing, communication skills, body mechanics, environmental modifications, goal setting, self-monitoring, and reappraisal of standards and priorities. The fatigue self-management intervention entitled *Managing Fatigue: A Six-week Course for Energy Conservation* has been found to be effective in reducing fatigue across a variety of delivery formats including face-to-face formats, teleconference, and online (81–83). A series of 5, 15- to 25-minute videos entitled, "Fatigue: Take Control," has also shown a positive effect on reducing the impact of fatigue (84).

b. Engaging in regular physical activity and exercise can also reduce the impact of fatigue. Vestibular training (85), treadmill training (86), elliptical exercise (87), and progressive resistance training (88) may reduce fatigue. Meta-analyses have found that exercise programs have significant and moderate effects on reducing MS fatigue (45,70). However, the best types of exercise programs to reduce fatigue remains unknown.

iii. **Complementary and alternative strategies**. The use of complementary and alternative methods (CAM) is widely accepted among persons with MS, with 65% to 90% using at least one kind of CAM (89,90). People with MS frequently report positive benefits from CAMs (91). Preliminary research indicates that yoga (92), hippotherapy (93), hydrotherapy (94), tai chi (95), and mindfulness training (96) may be beneficial. CAM that showed no effect were hyperbaric oxygen, polyunsaturated fatty acid diets, dental amalgam removal, and bee venom therapy (68).

Self-management interventions may be more effective than medications in reducing fatigue, based on meta-analyses.

CONCLUSION

MS fatigue can make it difficult to participate in meaningful activities, such as employment and family roles, which can adversely impact well-being and quality of life. Fortunately, our understanding of MS fatigue has significantly progressed in the last 20 years. There are now numerous screening measures available and we have a greater understanding of the factors that contribute to fatigue. However, current treatments only have a small-to-moderate effect on reducing fatigue. To improve current treatments for fatigue, comparative effectiveness research is needed to identify better ways of tailoring treatments to the characteristics of patients. At the time of writing this chapter, such research is now being conducted. The most effective treatment will most likely be a tailored approach that targets both primary and secondary factors of fatigue that are specific to each patient. These types of tailored fatigue interventions will require a comprehensive assessment of fatigue as well as a repertoire of intervention strategies as outlined in this chapter.

KEY POINTS FOR PATIENTS AND FAMILIES

- While fatigue is very common with MS and has a significant impact on quality of life, it is also one of the "hidden symptoms" of MS.
- Although the cause of MS fatigue has not been fully elucidated, many contributing factors have been identified.
- Some of the factors that contribute to MS fatigue can be addressed, such as mood and sleep issues, medication side effects, lack of physical activity, and other health problems.
- Questionnaires have been developed to measure the severity and impact of fatigue, and to measure the results of fatigue management.
- Interventions that may help with MS fatigue include educational programs, exercise programs, medications, as well as complementary and alternative strategies.
- Prioritizing activities and planning rest periods are important steps in managing energy throughout the day.
- It is essential to communicate with your health care provider about your fatigue; for example, how fatigue affects you, if your fatigue has worsened, and whether treatments for fatigue were effective or not.

REFERENCES

1. Multiple Sclerosis Council for Clinical Practice Guidelines. *Fatigue and Multiple Sclerosis: Evidence-based Management Strategies for Fatigue in Multiple Sclerosis*. Washington DC: Paralyzed Veterans of American; 1998.

2. Branas P, Jordan R, Fry-Smith A, et al. Treatments for fatigue in multiple sclerosis: a rapid and systematic review. *Health Technol Assess*. 2000;4(27):1–61.

3. Fisk J, Pontefract A, Ritvo P, et al. The impact of fatigue on patients with multiple sclerosis. *Can J Neurol Sci*. 1994;21(1):9–14.

4. Freal JE, Kraft GH, Coryell JK. Symptomatic fatigue in multiple sclerosis. *Arch Phys Med Rehabil*. 1984;65(3):135–138.

5. Finlayson M, Winkler Impey M, Nicolle C, et al. Self-care, productivity and leisure limitations of people with multiple sclerosis in Manitoba. *Can J Occu Ther*. 1998;65(5):299–308.

6. Flensner G, Ek AC, Soderhamn O. Lived experience of MS-related fatigue—a phenomenological interview study. *Int J Nurs Stud*. 2003;40(7):707–717.

7. Krupp L. Fatigue is intrinsic to multiple sclerosis (MS) and is the most commonly reported symptom of the disease. *Mult Scler*. 2006;12(4):367–368.

8. Schwid SR, Murray TJ. Treating fatigue in patients with MS: one step forward, one step back. *Neurology*. 2005;64(7):1111–1112.

9. Induruwa I, Constantinescu CS, Gran B. Fatigue in multiple sclerosis—a brief review. *J Neurol Sci*. 2012;323(1-2):9–15.

10. Braley TJ, Chervin RD. Fatigue in multiple sclerosis: mechanisms, evaluation, and treatment. *Sleep*. 2010;33(8):1061–1067.

11. Asche CV, Singer ME, Jhaveri M, et al. All-cause health care utilization and costs associated with newly diagnosed multiple sclerosis in the United States. *J Manag Care Pharm*. 2010;16(9):703–712.

12. Jones E, Pike J, Marshall T, et al. Quantifying the relationship between increased disability and health care resource utilization, quality of life, work productivity, health care costs in patients with multiple sclerosis in the US. *BMC Health Serv Res*. 2016;16(1):294.

13. Brown MG, Murray TJ, Sketris IS, et al. Cost-effectiveness of interferon beta-1b in slowing multiple sclerosis disability progression. *Int J Technol Assess Health Care*. 2000;16(03):751–767.

14. Remington G, Rodriguez Y, Logan D, et al. Facilitating medication adherence in patients with multiple sclerosis. *Int J MS Care*. 2013;15(1):36–45.

15. Crawford A, Jewell A, Mara H, et al. Managing treatment fatigue in patients with multiple sclerosis on long-term therapy: the role of multiple sclerosis nurses. *Patient Prefer Adherence*. 2014;8:1093–1099.

16. Fiest KM, Fisk JD, Patten SB, et al. Fatigue and comorbidities in multiple sclerosis. *Int J MS Care*. 2016;18(2):96–104.

17. Runia TF, Jafari N, Siepman DA, et al. Fatigue at time of CIS is an independent predictor of a subsequent diagnosis of multiple sclerosis. *J Neurol Neurosurg Psychiatry*. 2015;86(5):543–546.

18. Tan H, Cai Q, Agarwal S, et al. Impact of adherence to disease-modifying therapies on clinical and economic outcomes among patients with multiple sclerosis. *Adv Ther*. 2011;28(1):51–61.

19. Newton G, Griffiths A, Soundy A. The experience of fatigue in neurological patients with multiple sclerosis: a thematic synthesis. *Physiotherapy*. 2016.

20. Krupp LB, Alvarez LA, LaRocca NG, et al. Fatigue in multiple sclerosis. *Arch Neurol*. 1988;45(4):435–437.

21. Patejdl R, Penner IK, Noack TK, et al. Multiple sclerosis and fatigue: a review on the contribution of inflammation and immune-mediated neurodegeneration. *Autoimmun Rev*. 2016;15(3):210–220.

22. Spiteri S, Hassa T, Claros-Salinas D, et al. eds. *Functional MRI Changes Illustrating Cognitive Fatigue in Patients with Multiple Sclerosis in 25 Rehabilitationswissenschaftliches Kolloquium*; 2016.

23. Sandry J, Genova HM, Dobryakova E, et al. Subjective cognitive fatigue in multiple sclerosis depends on task length. *Front Neurol*. 2014;5:214.

24. Stuifbergen AK, Rogers S. The experience of fatigue and strategies of self-care among persons with multiple sclerosis. *Appl Nurs Res*. 1997;10(1):2–10.

25. Kos D, Kerckhofs E, Nagels G, et al. Origin of fatigue in multiple sclerosis: review of the literature. *Neurorehabil Neural Repair*. 2008;22(1):91–100.

26. Colombo B, Martinelli Boneschi F, Rossi P, et al. MRI and motor evoked potential findings in nondisabled multiple sclerosis patients with and without symptoms of fatigue. *J Neurol*. 2000;247(7):506–509.

27. Tartaglia MC, Narayanan S, Francis SJ, et al. The relationship between diffuse axonal damage and fatigue in multiple sclerosis. *Arch Neurol*. 2004;61(2):201–207.

28. Filippi M, Rocca MA. Cortical reorganisation in patients with MS. *J Neurol Neurosurg Psychiatry*. 2004;75(8):1087–1089.

29. Gottschalk M, Kumpfel T, Flachenecker P, et al. Fatigue and regulation of the hypothalamo-pituitary-adrenal axis in multiple sclerosis. *Arch Neurol*. 2005;62(2):277–280.

30. Tellez N, Comabella M, Julia E, et al. Fatigue in progressive multiple sclerosis is associated with low levels of dehydroepiandrosterone. *Mult Scler*. 2006;12(4):487–494.

31. Mainero C, Faroni J, Gasperini C, et al. Fatigue and magnetic resonance imaging activity in multiple sclerosis. *J Neurol*. 1999;246(6):454–458.

32. Bisecco A, Caiazzo G, d'Ambrosio A, et al. Fatigue in multiple sclerosis: the contribution of occult white matter damage. *Mult Scler*. 2016;22(13):1676–1684.

33. Malekzadeh A, Van de Geer-Peeters W, De Groot V, et al. Fatigue in patients with multiple sclerosis: is it related to pro-and anti-inflammatory cytokines? *Dis Markers*. 2015;2015.

34. Wood B, van der Mei I, Ponsonby A-L, et al. Prevalence and concurrence of anxiety, depression and fatigue over time in multiple sclerosis. *Mult Scler*. 2013;19(2):217–224.

35. Greeke EE, Chua AS, Healy BC, et al. Depression and fatigue in patients with multiple sclerosis. *J Neurol Sci*. 2017;380:236–241.

36. Turner AP, Hartoonian N, Sloan AP, et al. Improving fatigue and depression in individuals with multiple sclerosis using telephone-administered physical activity counseling. *J Consult Clin Psychol*. 2016;84(4):297.

37. Mohr DC, Hart SL, Goldberg A. Effects of treatment for depression on fatigue in multiple sclerosis. *Psychosom Med*. 2003;65(4):542–547.

38. Gunzler DD, Perzynski A, Morris N, et al. Disentangling multiple sclerosis and depression: an adjusted depression screening score for patient-centered care. *J Behav Med*. 2015;38(2):237–250.

39. Veauthier C, Paul F. Sleep disorders in multiple sclerosis and their relationship to fatigue. *Sleep Med*. 2014;15(1):5–14.

40. Strober LB. Fatigue in multiple sclerosis: a look at the role of poor sleep. *Front Neurol*. 2015;6:21.

41. Veauthier C, Gaede G, Radbruch H, et al. Treatment of sleep disorders may improve fatigue in multiple sclerosis. *Clin Neurol Neurosurg*. 2013;115(9):1826–1830.

42. Brass SD, Li C-S, Auerbach S. The underdiagnosis of sleep disorders in patients with multiple sclerosis. *J Clin Sleep Med*. 2014;10(9):1025.

43. Rottoli M, La Gioia S, Frigeni B, et al. Pathophysiology, assessment and management of multiple sclerosis fatigue: an update. *Expert Rev Neurother*. 2017;17(4):373–379.

44. Motl RW, Goldman M. Physical inactivity, neurological disability, and cardiorespiratory fitness in multiple sclerosis. *Acta Neurol Scand*. 2011;123(2):98–104.

45. Pilutti LA, Greenlee TA, Motl RW, et al. Effects of exercise training on fatigue in multiple sclerosis: a meta-analysis. *Psychosom Med*. 2013;75(6):575–580.

46. Powell DJ, Moss-Morris R, Liossi C, et al. Circadian cortisol and fatigue severity in relapsing-remitting multiple sclerosis. *Psychoneuroendocrinology*. 2015;56:120–131.

47. Plow MA, Finlayson M, Gunzler D, et al. Correlates of participation in meaningful activities among people with multiple sclerosis. *J Rehabil Med.* 2015; 47(6):538–545.

48. Burns MN, Nawacki E, Kwasny MJ, et al. Do positive or negative stressful events predict the development of new brain lesions in people with multiple sclerosis? *Psychol Med.* 2014;44(2):349–359.

49. Mohr DC, Lovera J, Brown T, et al. A randomized trial of stress management for the prevention of new brain lesions in MS. *Neurology.* 2012;79(5):412–419.

50. Marrie RA, Horwitz RI. Emerging effects of comorbidities on multiple sclerosis. *Lancet Neurol.* 2010;9(8):820–828.

51. Berrigan LI, Fisk JD, Patten SB, et al. Health-related quality of life in multiple sclerosis direct and indirect effects of comorbidity. *Neurology.* 2016;86(15):1417–1424.

52. Fiest KM, Fisk JD, Patten SB, et al. Fatigue and comorbidities in multiple sclerosis. *Int J MS Care.* 2016;18(2):96–104.

53. Garg H, Bush S, Gappmaier E. Associations between fatigue and disability, functional mobility, depression, and quality of life in people with multiple sclerosis. *Int J MS Care.* 2016;18(2):71–77.

54. Sutliff MH. Contribution of impaired mobility to patient burden in multiple sclerosis. *Curr Med Res Opin.* 2010;26(1):109–119.

55. Chaudhuri A, Behan PO. Fatigue in neurological disorders. *Lancet.* 2004;363(9413):978–988.

56. Veauthier C, Hasselmann H, Gold SM, et al. The Berlin Treatment Algorithm: recommendations for tailored innovative therapeutic strategies for multiple sclerosis-related fatigue. *EPMA J.* 2016;7:25.

57. Hutchinson B, Forwell SJ, Bennett S, et al. Toward a consensus on rehabilitation outcomes in MS: gait and fatigue. *Int J MS Care.* 2009;11(2):67–78.

58. Krupp LB, LaRocca NG, Muir-Nash J, et al. The fatigue severity scale. Application to patients with multiple sclerosis and systemic lupus erythematosus. *Arch Neurol.* 1989;46(10):1121–1123.

59. Benito-León J, Martínez-Martín P, Frades B, et al. Impact of fatigue in multiple sclerosis: the fatigue impact scale for daily use (D-FIS). *Mult Scler.* 2007;13(5):645–651.

60. Cella D, Riley W, Stone A, et al. The Patient-Reported Outcomes Measurement Information System (PROMIS) developed and tested its first wave of adult self-reported health outcome item banks: 2005-2008. *J Clin Epidemiol.* 2010;63(11):1179–1194.

61. Ritvo P, Fischer JS, Miller DM, et al. *Multiple Sclerosis Quality of Life Inventory: A User's Manual.* New York, NY: National Multiple Sclerosis Society; 1997:1–65.

62. Paul RH, Beatty WW, Schneider R, et al. Cognitive and physical fatigue in multiple sclerosis: relations between self-report and objective performance. *Appl Neuropsychol.* 1998;5(3):143–148.

63. Penner I, Raselli C, Stöcklin M, et al. The Fatigue Scale for Motor and Cognitive Functions (FSMC): validation of a new instrument to assess multiple sclerosis-related fatigue. *Mult Scler.* 2009;15(12):1509–1517.

64. Schwartz JE, Jandorf L, Krupp LB. The measurement of fatigue: a new instrument. *J Psychosom Res.* 1993;37(7):753–762.

65. Flachenecker P, Meissner H. Fatigue in multiple sclerosis presenting as acute relapse: subjective and objective assessment. *Mult Scler.* 2008;14(2):274–277.

66. Schwid SR, Covington M, Segal BM, et al. Fatigue in multiple sclerosis: current understanding and future directions. *J Rehabil Res Dev.* 2002;39(2):211–224.

67. Forwell SJ, Brunham S, Tremlett H, et al. Primary and nonprimary fatigue in multiple sclerosis. *Int J MS Care.* 2008;10(1):14–20.

68. Stewart TM, Tran ZV, Bowling A. Factors related to fatigue in multiple sclerosis. *Int J MS Care.* 2007;9(2):29–34.

69. Forwell SJ, Ghahari S. *Comprehensive Fatigue Assessment Battery for Multiple Sclerosis: Clinico-metric Properties.* Stockholm, Sweden: Council of Occupational Therapists from the European Countries (COTEC); 2012.

70. Murray TJ. Amantadine therapy for fatigue in multiple sclerosis. *Can J Neurol Sci.* 1985;12(3):251–254.

71. A randomized controlled trial of amantadine in fatigue associated with multiple sclerosis. The Canadian MS Research Group. *Can J Neurol Sci.* 1987;14(3):273–278.

72. Cohen RA, Fisher M. Amantadine treatment of fatigue associated with multiple sclerosis. *Arch Neurol.* 1989;46(6):676–680.

73. Krupp LB, Coyle PK, Doscher C, et al. Fatigue therapy in multiple sclerosis: results of a double-blind, randomized, parallel trial of amantadine, pemoline, and placebo. *Neurology.* 1995;45(11):1956–1961.

74. Sheean GL, Murray NM, Rothwell JC, et al. An open-labelled clinical and electrophysiological study of 3,4 diaminopyridine in the treatment of fatigue in multiple sclerosis. *Brain.* 1998;121(pt 5):967–975.

75. Rammohan K, Rosenberg J, Lynn D, et al. Efficacy and safety of modafinil (Provigil®) for the treatment of fatigue in multiple sclerosis: a two centre phase 2 study. *J Neurol Neurosurg Psychiatry.* 2002;72(2):179–183.

76. Stankoff B, Waubant E, Confavreux C, et al. Modafinil for fatigue in MS: a randomized placebo-controlled double-blind study. *Neurology.* 2005;64(7):1139–1143.

77. Asano M, Finlayson ML. Meta-analysis of three different types of fatigue management interventions for people with multiple sclerosis: exercise, education, and medication. *Mult Scler Int.* 2014;2014:798285.

78. Mücke M, Cuhls H, Peuckmann-Post V, et al. Pharmacological treatments for fatigue associated with palliative care. *The Cochrane Library.* 2015.

79. Cameron MH, McMillan G. Methylphenidate is likely less effective than placebo for improving imbalance, walking, and fatigue in people with multiple sclerosis. *Mult Scler.* 2017;23(13):1799–1801. doi:10.1177/1352458517692421.

80. Ehde DM, Elzea JL, Verrall AM, et al. Efficacy of a telephone-delivered self-management intervention for persons with multiple sclerosis: a randomized controlled trial with a one-year follow-up. *Arch Phys Med Rehabil.* 2015;96(11):1945–1958. e2.

81. Finlayson M, Preissner K, Cho C, et al. Randomized trial of a teleconference-delivered fatigue management program for people with multiple sclerosis. *Mult Scler.* 2011;17(9):1130–1140.

82. Ghahari S, Packer T. Effectiveness of online and face-to-face fatigue self-management programmes for adults with neurological conditions. *Disabil Rehabil.* 2012;34(7):564–573.

83. Lindstrom K, Mogush A, Mathiowetz V. Effects of one-to-one fatigue management course for persons with chronic conditions and fatigue. *Am J Occup Ther.* In press.

84. Hugos CL, Copperman LF, Fuller BE, et al. Clinical trial of a formal group fatigue program in multiple sclerosis. *Mult Scler.* 2010;16(6):724–732.

85. Hebert JR, Corboy JR, Manago MM, et al. Effects of vestibular rehabilitation on multiple sclerosis-related fatigue and upright postural control: a randomized controlled trial. *Phys Ther.* 2011;91(8):1166–1183.

86. Pilutti LA, Lelli DA, Paulseth JE, et al. Effects of 12 weeks of supported treadmill training on functional ability and quality of life in progressive multiple sclerosis: a pilot study. *Arch Phys Med Rehabil.* 2011;92(1):31–36.

87. Huisinga JM, Filipi ML, Stergiou N. Elliptical exercise improves fatigue ratings and quality of life in patients with multiple sclerosis. *J Rehabil Res Dev.* 2011;48(7):881–890.

88. Dalgas U, Stenager E, Jakobsen J, et al. Fatigue, mood and quality of life improve in MS patients after progressive resistance training. *Mult Scler.* 2010;16(4):480–490.

89. Olsen SA. A review of complementary and alternative medicine (CAM) by people with multiple sclerosis. *Occup Ther Int.* 2009;16(1):57–70.

90. Bowling AC. Complementary and alternative medicine in multiple sclerosis: dispelling common myths about CAM. *Int J MS Care.* 2005;7(2):42–44.

91. Shinto L, Yadav V, Morris C, et al. The perceived benefit and satisfaction from conventional and complementary and alternative medicine (CAM) in people with multiple sclerosis. *Complement Thr Med.* 2005;13(4):264–272.

92. Oken BS, Kishiyama S, Zajdel D, et al. Randomized controlled trial of yoga and exercise in multiple sclerosis. *Neurology.* 2004;62(11):2058–2064.

93. Vermöhlen V, Schiller P, Schickendantz S, et al. Hippotherapy for patients with multiple sclerosis: a multicenter randomized controlled trial (MS-HIPPO). *Mult Scler.* 2017:doi:135245851 7721354.

94. Castro-Sánchez AM, Matarán-Peñarrocha GA, Lara-Palomo I, et al. Hydrotherapy for the treatment of pain in people with multiple sclerosis: a randomized controlled trial. *Evid Based Complementary Altern Med.* 2011;2012.

95. Zou L, Wang H, Xiao Z, et al. Tai chi for health benefits in patients with multiple sclerosis: a systematic review. *PLOS ONE.* 2017;12(2):e0170212.

96. Ulrichsen KM, Kaufmann T, Dorum ES, et al. Clinical utility of mindfulness training in the treatment of fatigue after stroke, traumatic brain injury and multiple sclerosis: a systematic literature review and meta-analysis. *Front Psychol.* 2016;7:912.

20 Emotional Disorders in Multiple Sclerosis

Elias A. Khawam and Matthew Sacco

KEY POINTS FOR CLINICIANS

- Emotional disorders are common in multiple sclerosis (MS) and cause significant disturbances in patients' quality of life and compliance with treatment.
- Depression is the most common psychiatric comorbidity encountered in MS and can affect up to 54% of patients. The etiology of major depression in MS is multifactorial and includes both biological and psychological factors. Early recognition and treatment is essential to decrease morbidity and mortality.
- Screening tools are available to identify depressed patients. The Hospital Anxiety and Depression Scale and the Beck Depression Inventory-Fast Screen have been validated for MS patients.
- Treatment for psychiatric disorders in MS should be individualized and involve psychopharmacology, psychotherapy, or combined treatment.
- The suicide rate in MS is elevated compared to the general population. Patients' suicidal ideations should be taken seriously. If the patient appears at high risk, a psychiatric evaluation should be immediately requested.
- Pseudobulbar affect (PBA) causes significant distress and has a negative impact on patients and caregivers. The Center for Neurologic Study-Lability Scale (CNS-LS) is a useful tool for the assessment of PBA. Medications are available to effectively treat this condition.

MS is a chronic and disabling demyelinating disorder of the central nervous system. It causes multiple neuropsychiatric disturbances including mood, affect, behavior, and cognitive abnormalities. Psychiatric conditions cause significant disturbances in patients' social life, occupation, and family structure, in addition to affecting compliance with treatment.

Despite their higher prevalence in MS compared to the general population (1,2) and their negative effect on quality of life (3), psychiatric disorders remain underdiagnosed and undertreated.

While depression has been the most studied, other psychiatric disorders, such as anxiety disorders, bipolar disorder, euphoria, PBA, and psychotic disorders, received less attention. We review in this chapter the most common psychiatric disorders in MS. Cognitive disorders are discussed in Chapter 21.

MAJOR DEPRESSION IN MS

Depression disorder is the most common psychiatric comorbidity encountered in MS. Its prevalence in MS is 2- to 3-folds that of the general population (Table 20.1). Depression causes significant personal suffering and adversely affects physical activity, fatigue, pain, and quality of life.

Diagnosis of Depression

Physicians should be able to differentiate between depressed mood as a symptom and major depressive disorder (MDD), which represents a cluster of symptoms and necessitates treatment.

The *Diagnostic and Statistical Manual of Mental Disorders*, fifth edition (*DSM-V*) criteria for major depressive episode require the presence of five or more of the following symptoms within a 2-week period with at least one

TABLE 20.1 Prevalence and Common Psychopharmacological Treatment for Emotional Disorders in MS

EMOTIONAL DISORDERS	PREVALENCE	PSYCHOPHARMACOLOGICAL TREATMENT
Major depressive disorder	12 mo: 15.7% (1) Life time: 27%–54% (1,4,5)	SSRIs, SNRIs, bupropion, mirtazapine, TCAs
Bipolar disorder	2.4%–13% (6,7)	Lithium, Depakote, carbamazepine, atypical antipsychotics
Euphoria	Up to 13% (8)	None
Anxiety disorders	35.7% (2)	SSRIs, SNRIs, buspirone
Psychotic disorders	2%–3% (9)	Atypical antipsychotics, typical antipsychotics

MS, multiple sclerosis; SNRI, serotonin norepinephrine reuptake inhibitors; SSRI, selective serotonin reuptake inhibitors; TCA, tricyclic antidepressant.

symptom being either depressed mood or loss of interest or pleasure:

- Depressed mood
- Loss of interest or pleasure in all or almost all activities
- Weight loss or weight gain
- Insomnia or hypersomnia
- Psychomotor retardation or agitation
- Fatigue or loss of energy
- Feelings of worthlessness, or excessive inappropriate guilt
- Diminished ability to think or concentrate
- Recurrent thoughts of death

Symptoms are present most of the day, nearly every day and cause significant functioning impairment.

Diagnosing major depression in MS based on *DSM-V* criteria could be challenging because of an overlap between neurological impairments and the vegetative symptoms of MDD. Symptoms such as fatigue, insomnia, and decreased concentration and appetite occur in many MS patients in the absence of depression. The presence of inappropriate guilt, self-blaming, and passive thoughts of death or active suicidal ideations should not be considered a normal reaction to a chronic illness. Symptoms such as anger, irritability, worry, and discouragement have been associated with depression in MS. Isolation, hopelessness, helplessness, and worthlessness are often associated with MDD.

Some features that may help physicians differentiate between somatic symptoms related to depression versus MS symptoms are the following:

- Persistent low mood and loss of interest or pleasure beyond what is expected as a normal reaction to stress, even after the resolution of such stress
- Worsening mood despite neurological improvement
- Initial or middle insomnia are more prevalent in MS than in depression
- Fatigue tends to get worse as the day progresses in MS compared to some improvement or fluctuation of energy level in depressed patients
- Dramatic worsening of fatigue and concentration, compared to baseline level, in association with depressed mood

Early recognition and treatment of MDD in MS patients are essential to decrease morbidity and mortality and to improve quality of life. Physicians are encouraged to use screening tools (Table 20.2) to identify depressed patients, keeping in mind that the clinical

TABLE 20.2 Screening Tools for Depression in MS

Hospital Anxiety and Depression Scale (HADS) (10)	14-item scale self-report questionnaire split equally between anxiety and depression questions. A threshold score of 8 or greater has 90% sensitivity and 87.3% specificity for the depression subscale.
Beck Depression Inventory-Fast Screen (BDI-FS) (11)	Self-report questionnaire that consists of seven items: dysphoria, anhedonia, suicide, and four items that measure nonsomatic criteria for major depressive disorder.
Beck Depression Inventory (BDI) (12)	21-item self-report inventory that has been used widely for depression screening in MS. A cutoff score of 13 has 71% sensitivity and 79% specificity for depression.
PHQ-9 (13)	The PHQ-9 uses the *DSM-IV* criteria for depression and asks the patient to rate them from "0" (not at all) to "3" (nearly every day). A score ≥10 had 88% sensitivity and 88% specificity for major depression. Scores of 5, 10, 15, and 20 correlate respectively with mild, moderate, moderately severe, and severe depression.
Center for Epidemiologic Studies-Depression Scale (CES-D) (14)	Depression screening tool that has been used in epidemiological studies.
Chicago Multiscale Depression Inventory (CMDI) (15)	This inventory is divided into three depression scales which help differentiating mood, vegetative, and depressive cognitive symptoms.
Inventory for Depressive Symptomatology (IDC) (16)	Combines a clinician-rated (IDS-C) and a self-report (IDS-SR) scale.

DSM-IV, Diagnostic and Statistical Manual of Mental Disorders, fourth edition; MS, multiple sclerosis; PHQ-9, Patient Health Questionnaire-9.

interview remains the golden standard to diagnose major depression. The American Academy of Neurology identified Beck Depression Inventory (BDI) and a two-question screen (2QS) as potentially effective in screening MDD in MS patients (17). The Hospital Anxiety and Depression Scale (HADS) (10) and the BDI-Fast Screen (11) minimally reflect somatic symptoms and both have been validated for MS patients. We have found that the Patient Health Questionnaire-9 (PHQ-9) items are a useful screening tool for depression in our center.

The Goldman algorithm (18,19) recommends a regular screening for depression for all MS patients by either the 2QS, the BDI, or the PHQ-9. In case of positive screening, a diagnostic interview for depression is recommended, including an assessment for suicidality. Referral to psychiatry is warranted if severe depression is identified. Otherwise, the neurologist should discuss the treatment options, including pharmacotherapy, psychotherapy (supportive, interpersonal, or cognitive behavioral therapy [CBT]), or both, in addition to setting up a follow-up assessment.

Etiology of Depression in MS

The etiology of major depression in MS is multifactorial and includes biological, psychological, and social factors (Table 20.3). Structural neuroimaging studies highlighted the association between depression in MS and an increase in lesion load in the left suprainsular region, the right temporal lobe (20), and the superior frontal and parietal white matter, as well as atrophy affecting the frontal lobe, the third and lateral ventricles (21).

A growing body of evidence suggests an association between brain inflammation, autoimmune dysregulation, and endocrine dysfunction in MS-related depression. Lower $CD8^+$ cell numbers and higher CD4/CD8 ratio were linked to increased depression in chronic progressive MS patients. The production of the cytokine interferon (IFN) gamma in relapsing–remitting MS is related to depression, and its production was reduced in association with depression treatment. Several other studies confirmed the association between elevated cytokine levels and depression (22).

TABLE 20.3 Factors Associated With Depression in MS

- Brain lesion location
- Autoimmune dysregulation
- Endocrine abnormalities
- MS somatic symptoms (pain, fatigue, etc.)
- Cognitive impairment
- Unpredictability of disease progression
- Psychosocial stressors
- MS effects on social life, occupation, and family
- Limited support system
- Poor coping strategies

MS, multiple sclerosis.

Fassbender et al. (23) studied the relationship between depressive symptoms and hypothalamic–pituitary–adrenal (HPA) axis function in MS patients. When compared to a control group, MS patients failed to suppress corticotropin releasing hormone (CRH)-induced corticotrophin and cortisol response after dexamethasone administration. A higher level of depression and anxiety is associated with increased serum cortisol level following a dexamethasone CRH Suppression Test.

Treatment for Major Depression

Treatment for depression in MS should be individualized and involve psychopharmacology, psychotherapy, or combined treatment (18). Despite the common use of antidepressants among depressed MS patients and empirical evidence of its clinical effectiveness, rigorous evidence is lacking.

There are only two published randomized controlled trials (RCTs) so far studying the effectiveness of antidepressants on major depression in MS. In a 5-week small RCT ($N = 28$), desipramine was found to be more effective when compared to control group (24). Side effects including postural hypotension, constipation, and dry mouth, limited desipramine dose increase. Paroxetine was compared to placebo in a double-blind 12-week RCT ($N = 42$) (25). Patients who were treated with paroxetine showed improvement of depressive symptoms. However, patients in both trials did not achieve full remission of depression. The effectiveness of antidepressants was also documented in uncontrolled trials (sertraline, duloxetine, and moclobemide) and case reports (fluoxetine).

The effectiveness of psychotherapy for the treatment of depression in MS has been assessed in a number of studies. Individual cognitive behavior therapy (CBT) has been compared to supportive expressive group psychotherapy (SET) and to sertraline. CBT and sertraline were found to be equally effective, and superior to SET, in the treatment of major depression (26). CBT delivered by telephone was found to be valuable and more beneficial compared to telephone-delivered SET (27).

The combination of psychopharmacology and psychotherapy was found to be superior to either one delivered alone. Patients receiving combined treatments of desipramine and individual psychotherapy showed more improvement than psychotherapy and placebo (24). A meta-analysis from the general psychiatry literature also supports the advantage of combining psychotherapy and psychopharmacology versus medication alone (28).

When choosing an antidepressant, four principles should be taken into consideration. The optimum choice is an antidepressant that

- Has minimum potential side effects
- Has low potential for drug–drug interactions
- Targets multiple depressive symptoms (insomnia, decreased appetite, and energy)
- Targets other MS symptoms (pain, fatigue, etc.)

Selective serotonin reuptake inhibitors (SSRIs) are often the first choice of treatment for major depression in MS given their favorable side-effect profile, low number of contraindications, and lower chance of drug–drug interaction. However, other antidepressants could be used as first-line therapy on the basis of the need to target other MS symptoms (Table 20.4).

What if the first medication fails to achieve full remission despite a good therapeutic trial? Evidence on how to proceed is generated from the general psychiatry literature. The two most commonly used strategies are augmentation with another antidepressant, or switching to a different medication. Results from the sequenced treatment alternatives to relieve depression (STAR*D) trial suggest that patients who did not achieve complete response after 12 weeks or more of therapy might benefit more from augmentation therapy compared to switching medication (29).

There are probable safety concerns when using antidepressants that may prolong the QTc interval, particularly citalopram, and the disease-modifying therapy (DMT) fingolimod. The initiation of fingolimod is associated with transient bradycardia and increased risk of QTc prolongation. As a result, antidepressants with risk of QTc prolongation may need to be stopped prior to initiation of fingolimod. However, there was no increased incidence of QTc changes when antidepressants were used during initiation of fingolimod or coadministered over 16 weeks after starting this medication (30,31).

Electroconvulsive therapy (ECT) is an effective treatment for refractory depression. It should be considered for severely depressed, suicidal, or psychotic MS patients who failed to respond to psychopharmacology and psychotherapy (32). There are no randomized controlled studies on ECT in MS but case reports suggest improvement in psychiatric conditions. Obtaining brain MRI prior to ECT treatment should be considered due to concerns of ECT exacerbating MS symptoms in patients with active brain lesions. ECT is probably safe in patients without active disease on brain MRI. The use of transcranial direct current stimulation (tDCS) and transcranial magnetic stimulation (rTMS) have been reported with mixed results (32,33).

SUICIDE

Epidemiological studies report various rates of suicide, but all show an elevated suicidal rate in MS patients when compared to the general population. Suicidal risk in MS was at least twice as greater than the general population rate (34). Feinstein et al. reported that the lifetime prevalence of suicidal intent in MS is 28.6% (35). Suicide was identified as the cause of 15% of deaths in an MS clinic in a Canadian study (36) and the suicidal rate was 7.5 times greater compared to age-matched controls from the general population in a Danish study (37). Suicide risk factors include male gender, young age of onset of MS symptoms (34), severity of depression, social isolation, recent functional deterioration, and alcohol abuse (35). Even though only a minority of patients complete suicide, patients' suicidal ideations should be taken seriously. If the patient appears at high risk, a psychiatric evaluation should be immediately requested.

ADJUSTMENT DISORDER

Patients with adjustment disorder develop a group of symptoms involving emotions, such as depressed mood or anxiety, or behavior. These symptoms occur within 3 months of the onset of an identifiable stress. The prevalence of adjustment disorder with depressed mood was 22% in patients who were examined within 2 months of an MS diagnosis (13). Adjustment disorder does not necessarily require long-term psychopharmacological therapy except in severe cases. However, short-term medication management targeting specific symptoms, such as insomnia and anxiety, would be beneficial. Psychotherapy is usually the primary treatment modality.

TABLE 20.4 Medication for Depression That Is Associated With Other Comorbid Conditions

ANTIDEPRESSANTS	COMMON ADDITIONAL USES AND BENEFITS	CAUTIONS AND COMMON SIDE EFFECTS
SNRIs (venlafaxine, duloxetine)	Neuropathic pain Comorbid anxiety	Increased risk of serotonin syndrome if combined with SSRI Discontinuation syndrome
Bupropion	No sexual side effects No weight gain Improved energy Smoking cessation Could alleviate sexual side effects caused by SSRIs	Lowers seizure threshold
Mirtazapine	Loss of appetite Sleep disturbance	Sedation Worsening fatigue
TCAs	Sleep disturbance Neuropathic pain Nocturia	Sedation Cardiovascular side effects Anticholinergic side effects including urinary retention Avoid abrupt discontinuation

SNRI, serotonin norepinephrine reuptake inhibitors; SSRI, selective serotonin reuptake inhibitors; TCA, tricyclic antidepressants.

BIPOALAR DISORDER

The association between MS and bipolar disorder has been documented in multiple case reports. The prevalence of bipolar disorder in MS is higher than in the general population (9,10) (Table 20.1). Mania has been reported as an initial presentation of MS. The relation between MS brain lesions and bipolar disorder has been reviewed in a few MRI studies which suggest that mania is likely associated with the severity of demyelination (38).

There have been no studies on the treatment of bipolar disorder in MS. Anecdotal reports suggest successful management of mania with mood stabilizers, antipsychotics, and benzodiazepines. Lithium has been used to treat acute mania and has been associated with reducing suicide risk. Patients who are treated with lithium for bipolar disorder should maintain adequate hydration, which might be a problem in MS patients, as they sometimes restrict their fluid intake owing to bladder dysfunction. Carbamazepine and valproate sodium are effective but they should be monitored closely because of potential side effects such as tremor, weight gain, and drug–drug interactions. Lamotrigine is approved for maintenance therapy of bipolar depression and does not prevent manic episodes.

All atypical antipsychotics are used for the treatment of bipolar mania. Lurasidone and quetiapine have been approved for bipolar depression. Antipsychotics should be monitored closely because of risks of extrapyramidal symptoms (EPS), metabolic syndrome, and worsening of fatigue. The use of antidepressants alone should be avoided in bipolar depression as they might precipitate a manic or mixed episode.

EUPHORIA

Euphoria is defined as a fixed mental state of well-being and optimism despite the presence of severe physical disability. It is similar to mania in that euphoric patients have elevated mood, but other manic symptoms are lacking. Patients with euphoria usually have significant neurological disability, severe cognitive impairment, enlarged ventricles, cerebral atrophy, and a high lesion load, often with an extensive frontal lobe involvement (39). There is no treatment for this condition that does not cause suffering to patients but might cause caregiver distress.

ANXIETY DISORDERS

Although anxiety disorders are common in MS, they have received less attention in the literature and often have been overlooked in clinical practice. The lifetime prevalence of any anxiety disorder in MS is higher compared to the general population (Table 20.1). Generalized anxiety disorder (GAD) was identified as the most common among anxiety disorders with a prevalence rate of 18.6%. Panic disorder and obsessive compulsive disorder prevalence rates were 10% and 8.6%, respectively. Injection phobia affects up to 50% of patients who use self-injectable DMTs.

Patients with anxiety disorders are more likely to be female (2,40), and to have a history of major depression and alcohol abuse. They are more likely to report greater social stress, a limited support system, and a higher rate of suicidal intent and self-harm attempts (2). The risk of anxiety disorder is higher in newly diagnosed MS patients, and in patients who experience pain, fatigue, and sleep disruption. It was noted that a psychiatric diagnosis has been previously given to one-third of these patients, but none were previously diagnosed with anxiety disorder. Moreover, more than one-half of anxiety disorder patients did not receive any type of treatment. Anxiety has not been linked to specific brain lesions (41).

Early identification of anxiety disorder would improve quality of life and medications adherence and reduce the unnecessary use of healthcare resources. The use of the GAD-7 or the HADS screening instruments can be used for anxiety screening in MS clinics (42).

Treatment for anxiety disorders has not been studied in the MS population. Most of the body of knowledge is obtained from studies conducted in general psychiatry. Multiple medications have been approved for the treatment of anxiety disorders. SSRIs are safe and reliable; however, they do not have a rapid onset of action. Serotonin norepinephrine reuptake inhibitors (SNRIs) and buspirone are other effective options for the treatment of GAD. Short-term treatment with benzodiazepines in combination with SSRIs or SNRIs might be considered for quick relief of anxiety symptoms. However, clinicians should be aware of the potential side-effect profile of benzodiazepines. Side effects include sedation, cognitive decline, worsening of fatigue, and increased risk of falls. Psychotherapy is also effective in anxiety disorders, with or without medication. Patients should be educated on all options and encouraged to participate in both types of treatment in cases of moderate-to-severe anxiety disorders.

PSYCHOTIC DISORDERS

An elevated rate of psychosis was reported in MS compared to the general population (12) (Table 20.1). However, the majority of the data is derived from case reports. Multiple types of psychotic symptoms have been reported in MS, including hallucinations, paranoid delusion, Capgras syndrome, erotomanic delusion, and delusion of mercury poisoning.

The treatment is similar for MS-related psychosis and psychotic disorders diagnosed in general population. Antipsychotic medications should be considered, starting initially with small doses, to target psychotic symptoms. Close monitoring is advised because of potential side effects such as EPS, metabolic syndrome, and worsening fatigue.

PSEUDOBULBAR AFFECT

PBA describes a disconnection between the patient's affect and mood. Patients may laugh or cry spontaneously, out of proportion to, or in the absence of, specific feelings. PBA causes significant distress and has a negative impact on patients and caregivers. It is often overlooked or underdiagnosed.

PBA has been also referred to as pathological laughing and crying, emotional incontinence, and involuntary emotional expressive disorder (IEED). It has been recognized in MS for many years and affects approximately 10% of MS patients (43). The etiology is unclear and PBA has been considered as a disconnection syndrome resulting from the loss of brain stem inhibition of the putative center for laughing and crying. PBA has been recently linked to lesions in the frontal, parietal, and brain stem regions (44). PBA is associated with cognitive impairment, particularly on tasks that are mediated by the frontal lobe, increased physical disability, and chronic progressive forms of MS.

The CNS-LS is a useful tool for the assessment of PBA. It is short (seven questions) and should be completed by patients. The CNS-LS has been validated for the screening of PSA in MS (45), and has been used in clinical and research settings.

SSRIs are recommended as first-line therapy for PBA and patients usually respond quickly within a few days (1–3 days). Other treatment options include SNRIs, mirtazapine, tricyclic antidepressants (TCAs), lamotrigine, amantadine, and levodopa. Dextromethorphan/quinidine (DM/Q) was shown to be effective in the treatment of PBA in a RCT (46), with improved quality of life, quality of relationship, and pain intensity scores. Dizziness was the only side effect that occurred more often in the DM/Q group. Headache and nausea were also reported, but the difference between the DM/Q and the placebo group was not significant.

PSYCHIATRIC EFFECTS OF MS TREATMENTS

There have been concerns that disease-modifying agents cause depression. This concern was initially raised after reports of increased suicidal risk during the IFN beta-1b trial. However, data from the same study showed a decrease in the rate of depression in the treatment group (47). An increase in depression has been reported in clinical trials during the first 2 to 6 months of treatment with IFN beta-1a and IFN beta-1b. However, this increase in depression symptoms appears to be related to a prior history of depression disorder rather than to the treatment itself (48). Several studies showed no difference in depression rates (49), whereas other studies showed improvement of mood with IFN treatment (50).

History of depression prior to initiation of IFN is the main risk factor for worsening depression during IFN therapy. Therefore, in the presence of severe depression, the use of another agent should be considered. If a patient develops depression after IFN therapy initiation, it is not necessarily an indication to discontinue IFN, but rather to initiate treatment for depression.

Corticosteroids can be associated with mood instability. Mania and depression symptoms represent 75% of cases. It has been reported that a quarter of patients receiving high dose corticosteroid for MS relapses develop depression symptoms and approximately a third of them experience (hypo) mania (51).

Other corticosteroid side effects include insomnia, irritability, anxiety, psychosis, and delirium. Treatment of neuropsychiatric symptoms includes tapering corticosteroids and administering an antidepressant, lithium, or an antipsychotic in case of mania or psychosis.

Psychotherapy

Psychotherapy can be an effective intervention for treating a wide range of psychological and emotional difficulties, including difficulties arising from the diagnosis of a chronic health condition like MS. Psychotherapy as it pertains to the treatment of individuals diagnosed with MS often focuses on issues related to adjustment to diagnosis, change in disease state or disability status, impact on family and work, and mood and anxiety issues in addition to a wide range of other issues. There is limited research investigating the effects of psychotherapy as it specifically relates to MS (52). However, there are many studies that have more generally looked at the effectiveness of psychotherapy for treating symptoms associated with depression and anxiety among other psychological and emotional difficulties (53). Multiple studies have shown that with an effective therapist, psychotherapy has significant and enduring positive effects that are cost effective and lead to fewer recurrences than medication use alone (54).

CBT is one of the most common types of psychotherapy utilized in the treatment of individuals with chronic or complex medical conditions. CBT can consist of a variety of techniques including and not limited to relaxation training, systematic desensitization, assertiveness training, social skills training, and goal setting. CBT often is marked by a more active approach that can begin with the identification of problematic patterns of thinking, how these patterns are reinforced and maintained, and the interplay with the person's environment and health. There is often increased emphasis on irrational/maladaptive patterns of thinking including automatic thoughts, emotional reasoning, catastrophic thinking, and more. Often, patients diagnosed with MS have specific beliefs about how MS symptoms (i.e., fatigue, spasticity, memory problems) will affect their lives (55). These beliefs can lead to negative internal emotional experiences that in turn can lead to maladaptive coping behaviors (i.e., avoidance of activities, isolation, periods of over activity followed by marked periods of underactivity). CBT can play a significant role in breaking this cycle and teaching new and more adaptive strategies to deal with the impact of MS symptoms on day-to-day living (52,56).

Since the 1990s, the traditional sense of CBT has undergone a marked shift in alignment away from conventional theoretical underpinnings and an offshoot has gained significant traction. This is often referred to as "third wave" approaches include the adoption of mindfulness training and acceptance from Eastern philosophies, as opposed to the more active and seemingly confrontational approach that is often noted in more traditional CBT. Studies have demonstrated that individuals who learned mindfulness training reported improvements in her emotional symptoms of anxiety and depression as well as fatigue and reported overall improvements in quality of life (57). Mindfulness has also been shown to be effective for reducing stress, improving pain as well as for improving sleep (58,59).

CONCLUSION

MS has a high association with a wide spectrum of emotional disorders which can profoundly affect the quality of life and overall well-being of patients and their family. While depression has been widely studied in MS, other psychiatric disturbances cause significant suffering and deserve more attention. Screening and recognition of emotional disturbances is essential, and effective treatment is available for almost all emotional issues. Our knowledge of the psychiatric disorders in MS has improved over the years; however, further research is still needed, particularly regarding their pathophysiology and the effectiveness of various treatment strategies.

KEY POINTS FOR PATIENTS AND FAMILIES

- Emotional distress, including depressive and anxious symptoms, often occurs as a result of being diagnosed with MS.
- Depression is very common and can affect almost one half of all MS patients. Anxiety symptoms are often encountered as well and occur more frequently in MS patients when compared to others.
- Treatments for depression, anxiety, and other emotional disturbances are available and include both medication management and psychotherapy.
- Working with a behavioral health practitioner is an effective way to learn to cope with the emotional challenges and changes in life that often accompany living with MS.

REFERENCES

1. Schubert DS, Foliart RH. Increased depression in multiple sclerosis patients: a meta analysis. *Psychosomatics.* 1993;34:124–130.
2. Korostil M, Feinstein A. Anxiety disorders and their clinical correlates in multiple sclerosis patients. *Mult Scler.* 2007;13:67–72.
3. Amato MP, Ponziani G, Rossi F, et al. Quality of life in multiple sclerosis: the impact of depression, fatigue and disability. *Mult Scler.* 2001;7:340–344.
4. Patten SB, Beck CA, Williams JV, et al. Major depression in multiple sclerosis: a population based perspective. *Neurology.* 2003;61:1524–1527.
5. Minden SL, Orav J, Reich P. Depression in multiple sclerosis. *Gen Hosp Psychiatry.* 1987;9:426–434.
6. Marrie RA, Horwitz R, Cutter G, et al. The burden of mental comorbidity in multiple sclerosis: frequent, underdiagnosed, and undertreated. *Mult Scler.* 2009;15(3):385–392.
7. Joffe RT, Lippert GP, Gray TA, et al. Mood disorder and multiple sclerosis. *Arch Neurol.* 1987;44:376–378.
8. Diaz-Olavarrieta C, Cummings JL, Velazquez J, et al. Neuropsychiatric manifestations of multiple sclerosis. *J Neuropsychiatry Clin Neurosci.* 1999;11:51–57.
9. Patten SB, Svenson LW, Metz LM. Psychotic disorders in MS: population-based evidence of an association. *Neurology.* 2005;65:1123–1125.
10. Honarmand K, Feinstein A. Validation of the hospital anxiety and depression scale for use with multiple sclerosis patients. *Mult Scler.* 2009;15:1518–1524.
11. Benedict RH, Fishman I, McClellan MM, et al. Validity of the beck depression inventory-fast screen in multiple sclerosis. *Mult Scler.* 2003;9:393–396.
12. Sullivan MJ, Weinshenker B, Mikail S, et al. Screening for major depression in the early stages of multiple sclerosis. *Can J Neurol Sci.* 1995;22(3):228–231.
13. Kroenke K, Spitzer RL, Williams JB. The PHQ-9: validity of a brief depression severity measure. *J Gen Intern Med.* 2001;16(9):606–613.
14. Verdier-Taillefer MH, Gourlet V, Fuhrer R, et al. Psychometric properties of the center for epidemiologic studies-depression scale in multiple sclerosis. *Neuroepidemiology.* 2001;20(4):262–267.
15. Nyenhuis DL, Rao SM, Zajecka JM, et al. Mood disturbance versus other symptoms of depression in multiple sclerosis. *J Int Neuropsychol Soc.* 1995;1(3):291–296.
16. Rush AJ, Gullion CM, Basco MR, et al. The Inventory of Depressive Symptomatology (IDS): psychometric properties. *Psychol Med.* 1996;26(3):477–486.
17. Minden SL, Feinstein A, Kalb RC, et al. Evidence-based guideline: assessment and management of psychiatric disorders in individuals with MS: Report of the Guideline Development Subcommittee of the American Academy of Neurology. *Neurology.* 2014;82:174–181.
18. Goldman Consensus Group. The Goldman Consensus Statement on depression in multiple sclerosis. *Mult Scler.* 2005;11:328–337.
19. Schiffer RB. Depression in neurological practice: diagnosis, treatment, implications. *Semin Neurol.* 2009;29:220–233.
20. Berg D, Supprian T, Thomae J, et al. Lesion pattern in patients with multiple sclerosis and depression. *Mult Scler.* 2000;6:156–162.
21. Bakshi R, Czarnecki D, Shaikh ZA, et al. Brain MRI lesions and atrophy are related to depression in multiple sclerosis. *Neuroreport.* 2000;11:1153–1158.
22. Schiepers OJ, Wichers MC, Maes M. Cytokines and major depression. *Prog Neuropsychopharmacol Biol Psychiatry.* 2005;29:201–217.

23. Fassbender K, Schmidt R, Mossner R, et al. Mood disorders and dysfunction of the hypothalamic-pituitary-adrenal axis in multiple sclerosis. *Arch Neurol*. 1998;55:66–72.

24. Schiffer RB, Wineman NM. Antidepressant pharmacotherapy of depression associated with multiple sclerosis. *Am J Psychiatry*. 1990;147:1493–1497.

25. Ehde DM, Kraft GH, Chwastiak L, et al. Efficacy of paroxetine in treating major depressive disorder in persons with multiple sclerosis. *Gen Hosp Psychiatry*. 2008;30(1):40–48.

26. Mohr DC, Boudewyn AC, Goodkin DE, et al. Comparative outcomes for individual cognitive-behavioral therapy, supportive-expressive group psychotherapy and sertraline for the treatment of depression in multiple sclerosis. *J Consult Clin Psychology*. 2001;69:942–949.

27. Mohr DC, Hart SL, Julian L, et al. Telephone-administered psychotherapy for depression. *Arch Gen Psychiatry*. 2005;62:1007–1014.

28. Pampallona S, Bollini P, Tibaldi G, et al. Combined pharmacotherapy and psychological treatment for depression: a systematic review. *Arch Gen Psychiatry*. 2004;61:714–719.

29. Gaynes BN, Dusetzina SB, Ellis AR, et al. Treating depression after initial treatment failure: directly comparing switch and augmenting strategies in STAR*D. *J Clin Psychopharmacol*. 2012;32(1):114–119.

30. Bayas A, Schuh K, Baier M, et al. Combination treatment of fingolimod with antidepressants in relapsing-remitting multiple sclerosis patients with depression: a multicentre, open-label study—REGAIN. *Ther Adv Neurol Disord*. 2016;9:378–388.

31. Bermel RA, Hashmonay R, Meng X, et al. Fingolimod first-dose effects in patients with relapsing multiple sclero-sis concomitantly receiving selective serotonin-reuptake inhibitors. *Mult Scler Relat Disord*. 2015;4(3):273–80.

32. Steen K, Narang P, Lippmann S. Electroconvulsive therapy in multiple sclerosis. *Innov Clin Neurosci*. 2015;12(7-8):28–30.

33. Palm U, Ayache SS, Padberg F, et al. Non-invasive brain stimulation therapy in multiple sclerosis: a review of tDCS, rTMS and ECT results. *Brain Stimul*. 2014;7(6):849–854.

34. Brønnum-Hansen H, Stenager E, Nylev Stenager E, et al. Suicide among Danes with multiple sclerosis. *J Neurol Neurosurg Psychiatry*. 2005;76(10):1457–1459.

35. Feinstein A. An examination of suicidal intent in patients with multiple sclerosis. *Neurology*. 2002;59:674–678.

36. Sadovnik AD, Eisen RN, Ebers GC, et al. Cause of death in patients attending multiple sclerosis clinics. *Neurology*. 1991;41:1193–1196.

37. Stenager EN, Stenager E, Koch-Henriksen N, et al. Suicide and multiple sclerosis: an epidemiological investigation. *J Neurol Neurosurg Psychiatry*. 1992;55:542–545.

38. Murphy R, O'Donoghue S, Counihan T, et al. Neuropsychiatric syndromes of multiple sclerosis. *J Neurol Neurosurg Psychiatry*. 2017;88:697–708.

39. Rabins PV. Euphoria in multiple sclerosis. In: Rao SM, ed. *Neurobehavioral Aspects of Multiple Sclerosis*. New York, NY: Oxford University Press; 1990:180–185.

40. Feinstein A, O'Connor P, Gray T, et al. The effects of anxiety on psychiatric morbidity in patients with multiple sclerosis. *Mult Scler*. 1999;5:323–326.

41. Zorzon M, de Masi R, Nasuelli D, et al. Depression and anxiety in multiple sclerosis. A clinical and MRI study in 95 subjects. *J Neurol*. 2001;248:416–421.

42. Terrill AL, Hartoonian N, Beier M, et al. The 7-item generalized anxiety disorder scale as a tool for measuring generalized anxiety in multiple sclerosis. *Int J MS Care*. 2015;17(2):49–56.

43. Feinstein A, Feinstein K, Gray T, et al. Prevalence and neurobehavioral correlates of pathological laughing and crying in multiple sclerosis. *Arch Neurol*. 1997;54:1116–1121.

44. Ghaffar O, Chamelian L, Feinstein A. The neuroanatomy of pseudobulbar affect. *J Neurol*. 2008;255(3):406–412.

45. Smith RA, Berg JE, Pope LE, et al. Validation of the CNS emotional lability scale for pseudobulbar affect (pathological laughing and crying) in multiple sclerosis patients. *Mult Scler*. 2004;10(6):679–685.

46. Panitch HS, Thisted RA, Smith RA, et al. Randomized, controlled trial of dextromethorphan/quinidine for pseudobulbar affect in multiple sclerosis. *Ann Neurol*. 2006;59:780–787.

47. University of British Columbia MS/MRI Analysis Group. IFNB Multiple Sclerosis Study Group, Interferon beta-1b in the treatment of multiple sclerosis: final outcome of the randomized controlled trial. *Neurology*. 1995;45:1277–1285.

48. Polman CH, Thompson AJ, Murray TJ, et al. eds. *Multiple Sclerosis: The Guide to Treatment and Management*. 5th ed. New York, NY: Demos Publishing; 2001:7–43.

49. Patten SB, Metz LM. SPECTRIMS Study Group. Interferon beta 1a and depression in secondary progressive MS: data from the SPECTRIMS trial. *Neurology*. 2002;59:744–746.

50. Feinstein A, O'Connor P, Feinstein K. Multiple sclerosis, interferon beta-1b and depression: a prospective investigation. *J Neurol*. 2002;249:815–820.

51. Morrow SA, Barr J, Rosehart H, et al. Depression and hypomania symptoms are associated with high dose corticosteroids treatment for MS relapses. *J Affect Disord*. November 15, 2015;187:142–146.

52. Hind D, Cotter J, Thake A, et al. Cognitive behavioural therapy for the treatment of depression in people with multiple sclerosis: a systematic review and meta-analysis. *BMC Psychiatry*. 2014;14:5.

53. Seligman ME. The effectiveness of psychotherapy. The Consumer Reports study. *Am Psychol*. 1995;50(12):965–974

54. Hollon SD. The efficacy in effectiveness of psychotherapy relative to medications. *Am Psychol*. 1996;51(10):1025–1030.

55. Skerrett TN, Moss-Morris R. Fatigue and social impairment in multiple sclerosis: the role of patients' cognitive and behavioral responses to her symptoms. *J Psychosom Res*. 2006;61:587–593.

56. Van der Werf SP, Evers A, Jongen PJ, et al. The role of helplessness as mediator between neurological disability, emotional instability, experienced fatigue and depression in patients with multiple sclerosis. *Mult Scler*. 2003;9:89–94.

57. Grossman P, Kappos L, Gensicke H, et al. MS quality of life, depression, and fatigue improve after mindfulness training: a randomized trial. *Neurology*. 2010;75:1141–1149

58. Garland EL, Howard Mo. Mindfulness–oriented recovery enhancement reduces pain attentional bias in chronic pain patients. *Psychother Psychosom*. 2013;82:311–318.

59. Gross CR, Kreitzer MJ, Reilly-Spong M, et al. Mindfulness–based stress reduction versus pharmacotherapy for chronic primary insomnia: a randomized controlled clinical trial. *Explore (NY)*. 2011;7:76–87.

21 Cognitive Dysfunction in Multiple Sclerosis

Stephen M. Rao

KEY POINTS FOR CLINICIANS

Cognitive dysfunction …

- Occurs in 43% to 65% of patients with multiple sclerosis (MS)
- Is often under recognized or misdiagnosed as depression, stress, or personality disorder
- Is assessed with neuropsychological testing with the most common deficits observed on measures of recent memory and information processing speed
- Contributes significantly to unemployment, motor vehicle accidents, impairment in activities of daily living, and loss of social contacts
- Is strongly related to the extent of white matter lesion volume and brain atrophy on MRI
- May be treated with disease-modifying and symptomatic treatments with modest success

---

INTRODUCTION

Cognitive function is often impaired in MS patients (for recent comprehensive reviews of this literature, see (1,2)). Nearly 43% to 65% of MS patients exhibit some degree of impairment on standardized neuropsychological (NP) tests (3). Cognitive impairment can have devastating consequences for the MS patient in the areas of employment (4,5), driving skills and safety (6), social activities (4), personal and community independence (4,5), and the likelihood of benefiting from rehabilitation (7). Not surprisingly, it is a major source of caregiver strain (8).

Cognitive dysfunction occurs in half of all MS patients

Cognitive impairment is the direct result of MS-related cerebral pathology. Brain abnormalities, as visualized by various MRI techniques, correlate moderately with NP tests (for recent reviews (9–11)). Cognitive deficits have been shown to correlate with T2- and T1-weighted white matter lesions as well as lesions in gray matter; brain atrophy; and microscopic pathology, as visualized by magnetization transfer, diffusion tensor, and proton spectroscopy, in both lesions and normal appearing brain tissue.

Furthermore, longitudinal studies have shown that deteriorating cognitive function is associated with increased lesion burden and atrophy (12–14).

Secondary progressive MS patients typically perform more poorly on NP testing than do patients with relapsing–remitting or primary progressive MS (15). Surprisingly, NP test scores correlate only weakly with disease duration and neurologic disability (16). The weak cross-sectional correlations between cognitive dysfunction and disease duration may be due to the high variability in symptom presentation in MS: some patients exhibit cognitive dysfunction as an early presentation of the disease, whereas other patients may never exhibit problems with cognition.

Neurologic disability, as typically assessed by the Expanded Disability Standard Scale (EDSS), correlates only modestly with degree of cognitive dysfunction (17). The EDSS tends to emphasize disability associated with ambulation. As a consequence, lesions affecting primarily brain regions associated with higher cognitive functions may not have an impact on the EDSS; likewise, lesions of the spinal cord may impact ambulation and the EDSS score, but have no effect on cognitive functions.

Most common deficits are in the areas of recent memory and information processing speed

Not all cognitive functions are equally susceptible to disruption by MS. Deficits in learning and recall of new information (episodic memory) and in information processing speed and working memory (i.e., the ability to simultaneously buffer and manipulate information) are the most common (18). Less common, but significant deficits are observed on visuospatial abilities and executive functions (including reasoning, problem solving, and planning/sequencing) (18). In contrast, very few MS patients exhibit deficits on measures of auditory attention span and language abilities, although recent natural history studies suggest that deficits in these domains become evident when cohorts are followed for longer periods of time (5). The severity and pattern of cognitive deficits may vary considerably across individual MS patients (19). This heterogeneity of NP impairment can best be appreciated when large samples of patients are administered a comprehensive NP test battery.

The natural history of MS-related cognitive impairment has been reported from studies (5,20–22) conducted prior to the appearance of disease-modifying drugs (see Table 21.1). Progression rates vary considerably across patients and across cognitive functions, but on average, approximately 5% to 9% of patients will experience deterioration on NP tests annually. In general, cognitive impairment is unlikely to remit to any significant extent, but cognitive deficits may remain stable for long periods of time before worsening. Acute exacerbations and remissions involving cognitive functions can be seen (see Figure 21.1).

In recent years, there has become a greater appreciation that MS can occur in pediatric populations (23). Cognitive deficits have been identified in approximately one third of children and adolescents, with the most prominent deficits in motor and cognitive processing speed as

TABLE 21.1 Indicators of Cognitive Dysfunction in MS

- Need for help with activities of daily living not attributable to physical disability
- Underemployment or unemployment not attributable to physical disability
- Change in mood or behavior (e.g., increased irritability, disinhibition) not attributable to anxiety or depression
- Withdrawal from usual social activities not attributable to anxiety or depression
- MRI showing global atrophy and a high lesion load on T2-weighted imaging

MS, multiple sclerosis.

well as in attention, verbal and visual memory, expressive and receptive language, and visuo-motor integration (24–27).

EVALUATION

Cognitive dysfunction is typically evaluated by a board-certified clinical neuropsychologist. The purposes of such an evaluation can be varied and involve questions of differential diagnosis (depression vs. cognitive dysfunction), disability assessment (e.g., Social Security), design of cognitive rehabilitation interventions, and clinical management with symptomatic and disease-modifying drugs. Comprehensive assessment will necessarily involve several measures that capture different cognitive domains. An example of a comprehensive for monitoring MS patients is the Minimal Assessment of Cognitive Function in MS (MACFIMS) (28) (see Table 21.2). The MACFIMS takes approximately 90 minutes to

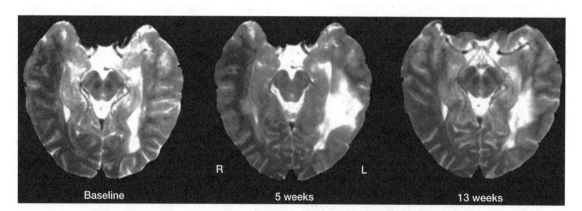

FIGURE 21.1 Female RRMS patient (age 37) had normal cognitive functions at baseline NP testing. At 5 weeks, she developed a selective impairment in verbal episodic memory in association with the development of a large white matter hyperintensity in the left temporal lobe on T2-weighted MRI imaging. The white matter lesion had decreased in size at 13 weeks postbaseline with an improvement in verbal episodic memory, although her test performance did not return to baseline. Her performance on NP tests of visuospatial episodic memory and information processing speed were unchanged during the three examinations.

NP, neuropsychological; RRMS, relapsing–remitting MS.

TABLE 21.2   Minimal Assessment of Cognitive Function in MS

TEST	ESTIMATED ADMINISTRATION TIME
Information Processing Speed	
Paced Auditory Serial Addition Test (PASAT)	10 min
Symbol Digit Modalities Test (SDMT)	5 min
Episodic Memory	
California Verbal Learning Test-II (CVLT-2)	25 min
Brief Visuospatial Memory Test-Revised (BVMT-R)	10 min
Executive Functions	
California Sorting Test (CST)	25 min
Visuospatial Perception	
Judgment of Line Orientation Test (JLO)	10 min
Language/Other	
Controlled Oral Word Association Test (COWAT)	5 min

MS, multiple sclerosis.
Source: Jennekens-Schinkel A, Laboyrie PM, Lanser JBK, et al. Cognition in patients with multiple sclerosis. After four years. *J Neurol Sci.* 1990;99:229–247.

administer and was created on the basis of a consensus panel of neuropsychologists. The Brief Repeatable NP Battery (BRB) (29) and the Brief International Cognitive Assessment for MS (BICAMS) (30,31) are alternative batteries that focus exclusively on the assessment of processing speed and episodic memory and take less than 30 minutes to administer.

NP evaluations are needed to gauge the severity and pattern of cognitive deficits

A major challenge in clinical practice is the identification of MS patients who would benefit from a comprehensive NP evaluation. Numerous studies have shown that self-report of cognitive dysfunction is frequently inaccurate. Patients with depression may over report cognitive symptoms but perform normally on NP testing. Conversely, patients with significant cognitive dysfunction determined from objective NP testing may lose self-awareness and minimize the report of their cognitive deficits. Likewise, because the cognitive deficits in MS typically do not involve language or communication deficits, physicians who specialize in MS are not typically able to identify cognitive dysfunction from the mental status examination. Furthermore, screening examinations for dementia, such as the Mini Mental State Examination, are insensitive to the cognitive dysfunction in MS.

Self-report of cognitive impairment can be unreliable

Single test screening examinations using measures of processing speed, like the Paced Auditory Serial Addition Test (PASAT) or the Symbol Digit Modalities Test (SDMT), are capable of identifying 45% to 74% of patients diagnosed with cognitive dysfunction relative to results derived from a comprehensive NP battery (18,32). This approach, however, will be insensitive to MS patients with cognitive dysfunction in other domains (e.g., episodic memory). In addition, even brief tests like the 90-second SDMT are infrequently administered in busy clinical practices due to personnel time constraints associated with administration, scoring, conversion of raw scores using normative data, and entering results into the electronic medical record.

To address these concerns, we developed the Multiple Sclerosis Performance Test (MSPT) (33), a self-administered, iPad-based computerized battery of cognitive, vision, and motor tasks that is currently integrated in several large MS clinics. The cognitive measure from the MSPT is called the Processing Speed Test (PST), which closely resembles the SDMT. The PST has excellent retest reliability, demonstrates a strong correlation with the SDMT, was slightly more sensitive than SDMT in discriminating MS from healthy control groups, and correlated better with cerebral T2 lesion load than did the SDMT (34). Finally, PST performance was no different with or without a technician present in the testing environment, a key element in validating the self-administration approach (34).

Modest success has been shown in treating cognitive dysfunction with disease modifying drugs

MANAGEMENT

Disease-Modifying Medications. As the prevalence and functional consequences of MS-related cognitive dysfunction became recognized, several randomized, placebo-controlled trials of disease-modifying medications for relapsing–remitting MS and progressive MS incorporated NP outcome measures. Tables 21.3 (relapsing–remitting MS) and 21.4 (progressive MS) provide an overview of these trials. The studies indicate that the beneficial effects of disease-modifying therapies can extend to cognitive function, although these effects may be subtle (for a review (46)). Statistically significant NP effects were most often observed on composite NP outcome measures.

Symptomatic Therapy. Table 21.5 summarizes clinical trials designed to assess the efficacy of medications designed to

TABLE 21.3   Randomized Clinical Trials of Disease-Modifying Medications With NP Outcome Assessment: Relapsing–Remitting MS

TRIAL	INITIAL SAMPLE	NP MEASURES AND DESIGN	NP OUTCOME
Betaseron (rIFNß-1b) (35,36)	372 patients EDSS = 0.0–5.5	Focused battery (WMS Logical Memory and Visual Reproduction, Trails A & B, Stroop) at 2 y and 4 y only (n = 30 at a single site)	Treatment effect on Delayed Visual Reproduction, favoring high-dose group, with a similar trend on Trails B
Copaxone (glatiramer acetate) (37,38)	248 patients EDSS = 0.0–5.0	Focused battery (10/36 SRT, PASAT, SDMT, and Word List Generation) at Baseline, 12 mo, and 24 mo	No significant treatment effects
Avonex (IFNß-1a) (39,40)	166 patients EDSS = 0.0–3.5	Broad-spectrum battery at Baseline and 2 y, and focused battery every 6 mo × 24 mo	Significant treatment effects on memory and information processing, with a trend on visuospatial abilities and executive functions
Tysabri (natalizumab) (41,42)	942 patients EDSS = 0–5.5	PASAT-3″ (as component of MS Functional Composite) at baseline, then every 3 mo × 24 mo	Sustained worsening was 7% in natalizumab group and 12% in placebo group

EDSS, Expanded Disability Standard Scale; IFNß-1b, interferon β; MS, multiple sclerosis; NP, neuropsychological; PASAT, Paced Auditory Serial Addition Test; SDMT, Symbol Digit Modalities Test; SRT, Selective Reminding Test; WMS, Wechsler Memory Scale.

symptomatically treat cognitive impairment (for reviews of the literature (46,56)). Patients enrolling in these symptomatic trials were required to have documented cognitive deficits or at minimum subjective cognitive complaints. The typical trial involved a relatively small number of patients (n < 70) and was conducted at a single site, although larger (n > 100), multisite trials have begun to appear in the literature (54,55). Results of these trials have been mixed. Medications approved for the treatment of Alzheimer's disease (donepezil, rivastigmine, memantine) show either no clinical benefit or a very modest benefit in treating MS-related cognitive dysfunction. Likewise, *Ginkgo biloba* does not appear to be effective for treatment of cognitive dysfunction. Surprisingly, L-amphetamine sulfate, a stimulant, appears to have a promising effect on verbal and visuospatial episodic memory, but no effect on measures of information processing speed and attention. Also promising is the effect of modafinil on measures of simple attention and working memory.

Some symptomatic therapies involving drugs and cognitive rehabilitation show improved cognitive function

Cognitive rehabilitation techniques are designed to either restore functions or develop strategies to compensate for cognitive dysfunction. In recent years, rigorous randomized controlled trials have begun to appear in the literature supporting the use of these interventions in MS (for recent reviews (57–59). A recent randomized controlled trial (60), for example, provided class I evidence that a behavioral intervention (i.e., modified Story Memory Technique) improved learning and memory as well as reported everyday life functioning. Several other authors have shown similar improvements from behavioral interventions in persons with MS focusing on attention,

TABLE 21.4   Randomized Clinical Trials of Disease-Modifying Medications With NP Outcome Assessment: Progressive MS

TRIAL	INITIAL SAMPLE	NP MEASURES AND DESIGN	NP OUTCOME
Methotrexate (43)	60 CPMS patients EDSS = 3.0–6.5	Broad-spectrum battery at Baseline, 12 mo, 24 mo (n = 40); focused NP battery every 6 wk × 24 wk to a subset of patients	Trend toward beneficial overall treatment effect, due primarily to effects on PASAT; effect on PASAT was evident early in treatment
Betaferon (IFNß-1b) (44, Langdon, unpublished data)	718 SPMS patients EDSS = 3.0–6.5	Broad-spectrum battery (10/36 SRT, PASAT, SDMT, Word List Generation) at baseline, 12 months, 24 months, and 36 months	No significant treatment effect; secondary analyses indicated that fewer IFNß-1b patients met criteria for Anew or worsened cognitive impairment at 24 mo
Avonex (IFNß-1a) (45)	436 SPMS patients EDSS = 3.5–6.5	PASAT (as component of MS Functional Composite) at 3 baseline visits, then every 3 mo × 24 mo	Trend toward beneficial treatment effect on PASAT

CPMS, Chronic Progressive Multiple Sclerosis; EDSS, Expanded Disability Standard Scale; IFNß-1b, interferon β; MS, multiple sclerosis; NP, neuropsychological; PASAT, Paced Auditory Serial Addition Test; SDMT, Symbol Digit Modalities Test; SPMS, secondary progressive MS; SRT, Selective Reminding Test.

TABLE 21.5 Placebo-Controlled Clinical Trials of Symptomatic Medications for Cognitive Dysfunction in Patients With Documented or Subjective Cognitive Deficits at Entry

STUDY	SAMPLE/STUDY DESIGN	NP MEASURES	OUTCOME
IV physostigmine (47)	Four patients (EDSS 3.0–6.0) with documented memory impairment; 6-wk placebo-controlled crossover (no washout)	Focused battery (Buschke SRT and Digit Span Forward) at baseline, then weekly × 6 wk	Significant treatment effects on selected Buschke SRT variables (LTS, LTR, STR) and consistent trends on others; no effect on Digit Span
Donepezil hydrochloride (10 mg/d) (48)	N = 69 MS patients with documented cognitive impairment; 24-wk randomized, double-blind, parallel group	Broad-spectrum battery (Brief Repeatable Battery, Tower of Hanoi) at baseline and 24 wk	Significant treatment effect on primary outcome measure, Buschke SRT; nonsignificant trend for PASAT; no effect on 10/36, SDMT, Word List Generation, and Tower of Hanoi
Donepezil hydrochloride (10 mg/d) (49)	N = 120 MS patients with documented cognitive impairment; 24-wk randomized, multicenter, double-blind, parallel group	Primary outcomes included SRT and self-reported change in memory functioning	No significant treatment effects
Ginkgo biloba (240 mg/d) (50)	N = 39 MS patients with documented impairment on PASAT or CVLT-II; 12-wk randomized, double-blind, parallel group	Broad-spectrum battery (PASAT, CVLT-II, Stroop, Symbol Digit, Useful Field of View Test) at baseline and 12 wk	No significant treatment effects; a trend for improved function in the drug group on the Stroop test; more impaired patients at baseline demonstrated a stronger treatment effect
Modafinil (200 mg/d × 16 wk) (51)	N = 49 RRMS patients with documented impairment on attention measures; 6-wk randomized, single-blind, parallel group	Broad-spectrum battery (PASAT, CPT, CVLT, Trails, ANAM, Digit Span, Digit Symbol, verbal and visuospatial fluency)	Significant treatment effects on measures of simple attention span, working memory, and verbal fluency; nonsignificant trends on measures of sustained attention and episodic memory
Rivastigmine (6 mg/d × 12 wk) (52)	N = 60 MS patients (19 RR, 31 SP, 10 PP) with documented impairment on Wechsler Memory Scales; 12 wk, randomized, double-blind, parallel group	Focused Battery (subtests of Wechsler Memory Scales)	No significant treatment effects observed on the Wechsler Memory Scale General Memory score or subtest scores
Rivastigmine (9 mg/d) (53)	N = 15 MS patients (12 RR and 3 SP) with subjective complaints of cognitive impairment; 32-wk randomized, single-blind, crossover (no washout)	Broad-spectrum battery (Brief Repeatable Battery, Stroop, N-Back) at baseline, 16 and 32 wk	Nonsignificant trend on BRB for improved cognitive function on vs. off rivastigmine; no performance effects of drug on Stroop and N-Back
L-amphetamine sulfate (30 mg/d) (54)	N = 151 MS patients with documented impairment on Symbol Digit or CVLT-II or PASAT; 28 d, randomized, double-blind, parallel group (2:1 drug:placebo)	Broad-spectrum battery (Symbol Digit, CVLT-II, Brief Visual Memory Test, PASAT) at baseline and at 29 d	No significant effect on primary NP outcome measure (Symbol Digit); significant treatment effects observed on memory measures
Memantine (20 mg/d × 16 wk) (55)	N = 114 MS patients (RR, PP, and SP) with documented impairment on PASAT or CVLT-II; 16-wk randomized, double-blind, parallel group	Broad-spectrum battery (PASAT, CVLT-II, Stroop, Symbol Digit, COWAT, DKEFS) at baseline and 16 wk	No significant treatment effects observed on the primary (PASAT, CVLT-II) and secondary NP outcome measures

BRB, Brief Repeatable NP Battery; COWAT, Controlled Oral Word Association Test; CVLT-2, California Verbal Learning Test-II; EDSS, Expanded Disability Standard Scale; IV, intravenous; LTR, Long Term Retrieval; LTS, Long Term Storage; MS, multiple sclerosis; NP, neuropsychological; PASAT, Paced Auditory Serial Addition Test; PP, primary progressive; RR, relapsing–remitting; RRMS, relapsing–remitting MS; SDMT, Symbol Digit Modalities Test; SP, secondary progressive; SRT, Selective Reminding Test; STR, Short Term Retrieval.

working memory, and executive functions. Several recent studies have successfully used computerized programs for retraining attention dysfunction (61,62).

Another avenue of treatment for cognitive dysfunction involves physical activity. Recent reviews of this burgeoning literature (63,64) suggest that increasing activity levels has a promising overall positive effect on cognition, but the definitive evidence for this effect is lacking.

PATIENT CASE A married male with 15 years of education was diagnosed with MS at the age of 45. At age 48, his primary symptoms and signs included: spastic paraparesis, ataxic gait (requiring the use of a cane), dysarthria, bilateral upper extremity numbness, back pain, and bladder dysfunction. His clinical course was progressive with am EDSS score of 3.5. The patient was performing most activities of daily living without difficulty and was working full-time as a computer technician. He denied memory or other cognitive symptoms; his wife, however, reported that he was experiencing mild recent memory disturbance.

Question: What evaluation is needed?

Answer: Self-report of cognitive deficits is generally less reliable than those of close relatives and friends. The wife's report of memory disturbance would suggest referral for a neuropsychological (NP) evaluation and a cranial MRI. NP testing indicated that the patient obtained a Verbal IQ of 101, which is in the average range but perhaps lower than expected for his educational background. Cognitive deficits were confined to measures of verbal and nonverbal recent memory. Performance was normal on an executive function task involving conceptual reasoning. MRI showed multiple confluent and focal periventricular areas with high signal intensity on T2-weighted images throughout the cerebral white matter, left cerebellum, and pons. In addition, the corpus callosum was abnormally thin. Lesion volume in the frontal lobes was relatively minimal.

The patient was reevaluated 3 years later. He was wheelchair bound as a result of increased truncal and lower extremity ataxia; EDSS score increased to 6.5. He also demonstrated more pronounced dysarthria and a reduction in fine motor control of the upper extremities. The patient was no longer able to work. His wife expressed concerns over a change in his cognitive and personality functioning, characterized by impaired judgment, anger outbursts, recent memory loss, word-finding difficulties, and decreased self-awareness. The patient nearly drowned in the family pool when he decided to swim without a life vest. He also experienced two cases of heat exhaustion when he failed to protect himself from overexposure to the sun.

Question: What do you do now?

Answer: Both neuropsychological (NP) testing and MRI were repeated. NP testing was relatively unchanged on measures of verbal intelligence, recent memory, and language. In contrast, a prominent decrement in performance was observed on an executive function task, with the patient experiencing a large number of perseverative responses suggesting cognitive inflexibility. MRI demonstrated a marked increase in white matter lesions within the frontal lobes (360% increase in frontal white matter lesion volume; by contrast, only a 29% increase was observed in *non*frontal lesion volume). This case illustrates the point that the location and severity of intracranial lesions can have an important influence on the expression of cognitive deficits.

KEY POINTS FOR PATIENTS AND FAMILIES

Cognitive (thinking and memory) problems …

- Occur in about half of people diagnosed with MS
- Result because MS can affect areas of the brain that control the speed in which problems are solved or the way memories are retrieved
- Can sometimes be made worse with depression and stress
- Are assessed with neuropsychological tests administered by a clinical neuropsychologist
- Can affect an MS person's ability to work, drive a car, and be able to perform daily activities
- May be treated or prevented with approved drugs for MS

REFERENCES

1. Benedict RHB, DeLuca J, Enzinger C, et al. Neuropsychology of multiple sclerosis: looking back and moving forward. *J Int Neuropsychol Soc.* 2017;23:832–842.
2. Sumowski JF, Benedict RH, Enzinger C, et al. Cognition in multiple sclerosis: state of the field and priorities for the future. *Neurology.* In press.
3. Bobholz JA, Rao SM. Cognitive dysfunction in multiple sclerosis: a review of recent developments. *Curr Opin Neurol.* 2003;16(3):283–288.
4. Rao SM, Leo GJ, Ellington L, et al. Cognitive dysfunction in multiple sclerosis: II. Impact on social functioning. *Neurology.* 1991;41:692–696.
5. Amato MP, Ponziani G, Siracusa G, et al. Cognitive dysfunction in early-onset multiple sclerosis: a reappraisal after 10 years. *Arch Neurol.* 2001;58(10):1602–1606.
6. Schultheis MT, Garay E, DeLuca J. The influence of cognitive impairment on driving performance in multiple sclerosis. *Neurology.* 2001;56(8):1089–1094.
7. Langdon DW, Thompson AJ. Multiple sclerosis: a preliminary study of selected variables affecting rehabilitation outcome. *Mult Scler.* 1999;5(2):94–100.
8. Chipchase SY, Lincoln NB. Factors associated with carer strain in carers of people with multiple sclerosis. *Disabil Rehabil.* 2001;23(17):768–776.
9. Mollison D, Sellar R, Bastin M, et al. The clinico-radiological paradox of cognitive function and MRI burden of white matter lesions in people with multiple sclerosis: a systematic review and meta-analysis. *PLOS ONE.* 2017;12(5):e0177727.
10. van Munster CE, Jonkman LE, Weinstein HC, et al. Gray matter damage in multiple sclerosis: impact on clinical symptoms. *Neuroscience.* 2015;303:446–461.
11. Rocca MA, Amato MP, De Stefano N, et al. Clinical and imaging assessment of cognitive dysfunction in multiple sclerosis. *Lancet Neurol.* 2015;14(3):302–317.
12. Hohol MJ, Guttmann CR, Orav J, et al. Serial neuropsychological assessment and magnetic resonance imaging analysis in multiple sclerosis. *Arch Neurol.* 1997;54(8):1018–1025.
13. Sperling RA, Guttmann CR, Hohol MJ, et al. Regional magnetic resonance imaging lesion burden and cognitive function in multiple sclerosis: a longitudinal study. *Arch Neurol.* 2001;58(1):115–121.
14. Zivadinov R, Sepcic J, Nasuelli D, et al. A longitudinal study of brain atrophy and cognitive disturbances in the early phase of relapsing-remitting multiple sclerosis. *J Neurol Neurosurg Psychiatry.* 2001;70(6):773–780.
15. Fischer JS. Using the Wechsler Memory Scale-Revised to detect and characterize memory deficits in multiple sclerosis. *ClinNeuropsychologist.* 1988;2:149–172.
16. Beatty WW, Goodkin DE, Hertsgaard D, et al. Clinical and demographic predictors of cognitive performance in multiple sclerosis: do diagnostic type, disease duration, and disability matter? *ArchNeurol.* 1990;47:305–308.
17. Whitaker JN, McFarland HF, Rudge P, et al. Outcomes assessment in multiple sclerosis clinical trials: a critical analysis. *Mult Scler.* 1995;1(1):37–47.
18. Rao SM, Leo GJ, Bernardin L, et al. Cognitive dysfunction in multiple sclerosis. I. Frequency, patterns, and prediction. *Neurology.* 1991;41(5):685–691.
19. Beatty WW, Wilbanks SL, Blanco CR, et al. Memory disturbance in multiple sclerosis: reconsideration of patterns of performance on the selective reminding test. *J Clin Exp Neuropsychol.* 1996;18(1):56–62.
20. Amato MP, Ponziani G, Pracucci G, et al. Cognitive impairment in early-onset multiple sclerosis. Pattern, predictors, and impact on everyday life in a 4-year follow-up. *ArchNeurol.* 1995;52(2):168–172.
21. Jennekens-Schinkel A, Laboyrie PM, Lanser JBK, et al. Cognition in patients with multiple sclerosis. After four years. *J Neurol Sci.* 1990;99:229–247.
22. Kujala P, Portin R, Ruutiainen J. The progress of cognitive decline in multiple sclerosis. A controlled 3-year follow-up. *Brain.* 1997;120(pt 2):289–297.
23. Wassmer E, Chitnis T, Pohl D, et al. International Pediatric MS Study Group Global Members Symposium report. *Neurology.* 2016;87(9)(suppl 2):S110–116.
24. Till C, Racine N, Araujo D, et al. Changes in cognitive performance over a 1-year period in children and adolescents with multiple sclerosis. *Neuropsychology.* 2013;27(2):210–219.
25. Amato MP, Goretti B, Ghezzi A, et al. Neuropsychological features in childhood and juvenile multiple sclerosis: five-year follow-up. *Neurology.* 2014;83(16):1432–1438.
26. Charvet LE, O'Donnell EH, Belman AL, et al. Longitudinal evaluation of cognitive functioning in pediatric multiple sclerosis: report from the US Pediatric Multiple Sclerosis Network. *Mult Scler.* 2014;20(11):1502–1510.
27. Pardini M, Uccelli A, Grafman J, et al. Isolated cognitive relapses in multiple sclerosis. *J Neurol Neurosurg Psychiatry.* 2014;85(9):1035–1037.
28. Benedict RH, Fischer JS, Archibald CJ, et al. Minimal neuropsychological assessment of MS patients: a consensus approach. *Clin Neuropsychol.* 2002;16(3):381–397.
29. Rao SM, Group NCFS. *A manual for the Brief Repeatable Batter of Neuropsychological Test in Multiple Sclerosis.* New York, NY: National MS Society; 1990.
30. Benedict RH, Amato MP, Boringa J, et al. Brief International Cognitive Assessment for MS (BICAMS): international standards for validation. *BMC Neurol.* 2012;12:55.
31. Langdon DW, Amato MP, Boringa J, et al. Recommendations for a brief international cognitive assessment for multiple sclerosis (BICAMS). *Mult Scler.* 2012;18(6):891–898.
32. Rosti E, Hamalainen P, Koivisto K, et al. PASAT in detecting cognitive impairment in relapsing-remitting MS. *Appl Neuropsychol.* 2007;14(2):101–112.
33. Rudick R, Miller D, Bethoux F, et al. The multiple sclerosis performance test (MSPT): an iPad-based clinical disability assessment tool. *Mult Scler Journal.* 2013;19(11):356–357.
34. Rao SM, Losinski G, Mourany L, et al. Processing speed test: validation of a self-administered, iPad®-based tool for screening cognitive dysfunction in a clinic setting. *Mult Scler.* 2017;23(14):1929–1937. doi:10.1177/1352458516688955.
35. Group TIMSS. Interferon beta-1b is effective in relapsing-remitting multiple sclerosis: I. Clinical results of a multicenter, randomized, double-blind, placebo-controlled trial. *Neurology.* 1993;43:655–661.
36. Pliskin NH, Hamer DP, Goldstein DS, et al. Improved delayed visual reproduction test performance in multiple sclerosis patients receiving interferon beta-1b. *Neurology.* 1996;47(6):1463–1468.
37. Johnson KP, Brooks BR, Cohen JA, et al. Copolymer 1 reduces relapse rate and improves disability in relapsing-remitting multiple sclerosis: results of a phase III multicenter, double-blind placebo-controlled trial. The Copolymer 1 Multiple Sclerosis Study Group. *Neurology.* 1995;45(7):1268–1276.
38. Weinstein A, Schwid SI, Schiffer RB, et al. Neuropsychologic status in multiple sclerosis after treatment with glatiramer. *Arch Neurol.* 1999;56(3):319–324.
39. Jacobs LD, Cookfair DL, Rudick RA, et al. Intramuscular interferon beta-1a for disease progression in relapsing multiple sclerosis. The Multiple Sclerosis Collaborative Research Group (MSCRG). *Ann Neurol.* 1996;39(3):285–294.
40. Fischer JS, Priore RL, Jacobs LD, et al. Neuropsychological effects of interferon beta-1a in relapsing multiple sclerosis. Multiple Sclerosis Collaborative Research Group. *Ann Neurol.* 2000;48(6):885–892.
41. Polman CH, O'Connor PW, Havrdova E, et al. A randomized, placebo-controlled trial of natalizumab for relapsing multiple sclerosis. *N Engl J Med.* 2006;354(9):899–910.
42. Polman CH, Rudick RA. The multiple sclerosis functional composite: a clinically meaningful measure of disability. *Neurology.* 2010;74(suppl 3):S8–15.

43. Goodkin DE, Rudick RA, VanderBrug Medendorp S, et al. Low-dose (7.5 mg) oral methotrexate reduces the rate of progression in chronic progressive multiple sclerosis. *Ann Neurol.* 1995;37(1):30–40.

44. Placebo-controlled multicentre randomised trial of interferon beta-1b in treatment of secondary progressive multiple sclerosis. European Study Group on interferon beta-1b in secondary progressive MS. *Lancet.* 1998;352(9139):1491–1497.

45. Cohen JA, Cutter GR, Fischer JS, et al. Benefit of interferon beta-1a on MSFC progression in secondary progressive MS. *Neurology.* 2002;59(5):679–687.

46. Roy S, Benedict RH, Drake AS, et al. Impact of pharmacotherapy on cognitive dysfunction in patients with multiple sclerosis. *CNS Drugs.* 2016;30(3):209–225.

47. Leo GJ, Rao SM. Effects of intravenous physostigmine and lecithin on memory loss in multiple sclerosis: report of a pilot study. *J Neurol Rehabil.* 1988;2:123–129.

48. Krupp LB, Christodoulou C, Melville P, et al. Donepezil improved memory in multiple sclerosis in a randomized clinical trial. *Neurology.* 2004;63(9):1579–1585.

49. Krupp LB, Christodoulou C, Melville P, et al. Multicenter randomized clinical trial of donepezil for memory impairment in multiple sclerosis. *Neurology.* 2011;76(17):1500–1507.

50. Lovera J, Bagert B, Smoot K, et al. Ginkgo biloba for the improvement of cognitive performance in multiple sclerosis: a randomized, placebo-controlled trial. *Mult Scler.* 2007;13(3):376–385.

51. Wilken JA, Sullivan C, Wallin M, et al. Treatment of multiple sclerosis-related cognitive problems with adjunctive modafinil: rationale and preliminary supportive data. *Int J MS Care.* 2008;10:1–10.

52. Shaygannejad V, Janghorbani M, Ashtari F, et al. Effects of rivastigmine on memory and cognition in multiple sclerosis. *Can J Neurol Sci.* 2008;35(4):476–481.

53. Cader S, Palace J, Matthews PM. Cholinergic agonism alters cognitive processing and enhances brain functional connectivity in patients with multiple sclerosis. *J Psychopharmacol.* 2009;23(6):686–696.

54. Morrow SA, Kaushik T, Zarevics P, et al. The effects of L-amphetamine sulfate on cognition in MS patients: results of a randomized controlled trial. *J Neurol.* 2009;256(7):1095–1102.

55. Lovera JF, Frohman E, Brown TR, et al. Memantine for cognitive impairment in multiple sclerosis: a randomized placebo-controlled trial. *Mult Scler.* 2010;16(6):715–723.

56. He D, Zhang Y, Dong S, et al. Pharmacological treatment for memory disorder in multiple sclerosis. *Cochrane Database Syst Rev.* 2013;(12):CD008876.

57. das Nair R, Martin KJ, Lincoln NB. Memory rehabilitation for people with multiple sclerosis. *Cochrane Database Syst Rev.* 2016;3:CD008754.

58. Rosti-Otajarvi EM, Hamalainen PI. Neuropsychological rehabilitation for multiple sclerosis. *Cochrane Database Syst Rev.* 2014;(2):CD009131.

59. Sandry J, Akbar N, Zuppichini M, et al. Cognitive rehabilitation in multiple sclerosis. In: Sun M-K, ed. *Research Progress in Alzheimer's Disease and Dementia.* Vol 6. New York, NY: Nova Science Publisher; 2016:195–233.

60. Chiaravalloti ND, Moore NB, Nikelshpur OM, et al. An RCT to treat learning impairment in multiple sclerosis: The MEMREHAB trial. *Neurology.* 2013;81(24):2066–2072.

61. Amato MP, Goretti B, Viterbo RG, et al. Computer-assisted rehabilitation of attention in patients with multiple sclerosis: results of a randomized, double-blind trial. *Mult Scler.* 2014;20(1):91–98.

62. Cerasa A, Gioia MC, Valentino P, et al. Computer-assisted cognitive rehabilitation of attention deficits for multiple sclerosis: a randomized trial with fMRI correlates. *Neurorehabil Neural Repair.* 2013;27(4):284–295.

63. Morrison JD, Mayer L. Physical activity and cognitive function in adults with multiple sclerosis: an integrative review. *Disabil Rehabil.* 2017;39(19):1909–1920.

64. Sandroff BM, Motl RW, Scudder MR, et al. Systematic, evidence-based review of exercise, physical activity, and physical fitness effects on cognition in persons with multiple sclerosis. *Neuropsychol Rev.* 2016;26(3):271–294.

22 | Epilepsy, Sleep Disorders, and Transient Neurological Events in Multiple Sclerosis

Burhan Z. Chaudhry and Alexander D. Rae-Grant

KEY POINTS FOR CLINICIANS: EPILEPSY AND MULTIPLE SCLEROSIS

- Seizures occur in about 3% of multiple sclerosis (MS) patients.
- Seizures of all types have been described.
- Seizures may be refractory in some patients.
- Seizures may resolve as relapses or lesions regress.
- Treatment is as per standard epilepsy protocols.
- Carbamazepine and phenytoin may increase MS symptoms.
- Some medicines used in MS treatment may make seizures more likely.
- Insomnia is best treated with nonpharmacological approaches, including sleep hygiene, avoidance of caffeine and stimulants, and treatment of depression.

In MS, symptoms vary widely from patient to patient. Relapses in MS are typically well recognized and do not lead to much clinical confusion (e.g., optic neuritis, brain stem syndromes, and spinal cord syndromes). However, there are other paroxysmal events that occur in MS which may be less expected. These may lead to an extensive and potentially unnecessary investigation for what is a known problem in MS. In this chapter, we focus on a variety of paroxysmal events in MS which may not receive much attention but which can be disruptive to patients. These include the occurrence of epilepsy or sleep disorders, both of which occur at an increased frequency in the MS population and may have implications for therapy. We discuss the common, sometimes weird, and often under-recognized phenomena of transient neurological events (including tonic spasms) which may be distressing to patients. The hope of this chapter is to help clinicians recognize and treat this fascinating set of issues in MS and perhaps both save patients unneeded investigations and expedite their pathway to effective intervention.

EPILEPSY AND MS

Epidemiology

Kelley and Rodriguez in 2009 performed a systematic review of the literature on seizures in the MS population (1). The best data came from six population-based studies.

Overall, these studies included 1,843 patients of whom 3.8% had epilepsy. Taken together, they indicated a prevalence rate in the MS population of 3% to 4%, which is approximately three times that expected in the general population (1). Hospital-based series, which would be expected to show a higher risk because of more severely affected patients, actually showed a similar risk, with estimates ranging from 1.8% to 7.5%. Prevalence is highest in electroencephalography (EEG) cohorts, likely because of selection bias (2).

Types of Seizures

Patients with MS and seizures had a variety of seizure types, including simple partial, complex partial, secondary generalized seizures, as well as convulsive status epilepticus (3). Specific case reports of musicogenic epilepsy (4), aphasic status epilepticus (5), and epilepsia partialis continua (6) attest to the variety of seizure types that can occur in the setting of MS.

Relationship With Clinical and Paraclinical Measures

Seizures have been reported throughout the course of MS, with occasional case reports of MS presenting with seizures (1). One study using a prospective MS database showed an increased risk of epilepsy among progressive forms of MS (7). Seizures during a relapse are in the minority in published cases (3). There is limited prognostic data on the course of epilepsy other than to say that it varies (3). In some cases, seizures resolve spontaneously or with treatment of an acute relapse, whereas in others they can persist (8). Some case series suggested that seizures may continue to occur in many patients with MS (9).

A variety of studies looking at EEG findings in MS patients with seizures have been published. Study design, timing of EEG, and other parameter differences make comparison of this data difficult. The prevalence of EEG changes varied from 60% to 100%, with focal or generalized slowing being the most common finding (10). Epileptiform discharges (both interictal and ictal) have been reported in such studies. The absence of EEG change does not rule out seizure, a finding similar to that of epilepsy in general.

MRI findings also vary. In one case control study, Truyen et al., found a higher cortical–subcortical lesion burden in MS patients with seizures than those without (11). One study using double inversion recovery (DIR) (which improves detection of cortical plaques) showed an increase in intracortical lesions in those with epilepsy (12). Confounding this issue is that cortical lesions are common but frequently not visible on standard MRI studies (13). Newer techniques such as DIR MRI and higher field strength magnets may increase the yield for such cortical lesions (14).

Pathogenesis of Seizures in MS

Pathological data have emphasized the early (15) and frequent (16) involvement of cortical regions in MS. This likely underlies some seizures in MS. Of course, some patients may have epilepsy based on genetic factors or other causes similar to the general population. Medicines used in MS may also precipitate seizures. For example, patients suddenly withdrawing from baclofen can have status epilepticus (usually seen in baclofen pump patients) (17). The use of extended-release dalfampridine is associated with an increased risk of seizures (18), likely due to its stimulatory effect on demyelinated axons. Individual case reports of focal cortical epilepsy have shown a lesion/seizure focus correlation (13). However, most patients with MS have multiple cortical and subcortical lesions making specific lesional diagnosis problematic.

Treatment of Seizures in the MS Population

No randomized controlled trials of antiepileptic medicines have been done in this population (19). Because seizures may resolve spontaneously, particularly in the setting of resolution of acute relapse or acute new MRI lesion formation, many clinicians wait until repeated seizures to occur to treat patients. There is no clear data to guide selection of individual antiepileptic medicines. There is some theoretical risk with the use of sodium channel blocking agents based on animal model experience, but it is not clear if this is an issue in humans (20,21). There is also case report literature of symptomatic worsening with the use of carbamazepine in the MS population. Solaro et al. showed frequent "relapse-like" events with carbamazepine with fewer events related to gabapentin and none related to lamotrigine use in MS (22). A case report showed improvement of refractory tonic clonic seizures after treatment with natalizumab, but there is limited data about the use of immune therapies for MS-related seizures (23).

KEY POINTS FOR PATIENTS: EPILEPSY AND MULTIPLE SCLEROSIS

- Seizures occur in some patients with MS.
- They can usually be treated with medications.
- They likely occur because of MS affecting the surface of the brain (cortex).

KEY POINTS FOR CLINICIANS: SLEEP AND MULTIPLE SCLEROSIS

- Sleep disorders are common in MS and should be considered particularly when patients have fatigue, complaints of sleep disruption, or cognitive deficits.
- Consider formal sleep study and consultation where there is sleep disruption or excess fatigue.
- Restless leg syndrome (RLS) and rapid eye movement (REM) sleep behavior disorders can be treated per standard protocol (ropinirole for RLS, clonazepam for REM behavior disorder).

(continued)

(continued)

- Rarer sleep disorders occurring in MS include narcolepsy, Kleine–Levin syndrome, and REM behavior disorder.
- Narcolepsy has been correlated with hypothalamic lesions and low CSF hypocretin-1 levels in MS patients in one study.
- Insomnia is best treated with nonpharmacological approaches, including sleep hygiene, avoidance of caffeine and stimulants, and treatment of depression.

SLEEP EVENTS AND MS

Introduction

Traditionally, sleep disorders have not been among the phenomena that MS clinicians recognize in their MS patients. Although fatigue is very commonly seen in MS, it has been thought to be part of the MS spectrum and based on mechanisms such as cytokine activation, increased brain activation for a functional task, medication effect, or depression (24). In fact, recent studies have shown an increase in frequency of sleep disorders in the MS population. Case reports have also highlighted a variety of unusual manifestations of sleep disease in the MS population of which healthcare practitioners should be aware. Finally, some studies have shown a correlation between daytime fatigue and sleep disorders in MS patients, prompting clinicians to look further for sleep disorders in this population.

Epidemiology

PREVALENCE OF SLEEP DISORDERS IN MS POPULATION
Studies of the prevalence of sleep disorders naturally vary depending on the patient population (neurology clinic, MS clinic, sleep lab, population, etc.) and ascertainment methodology (e.g., clinical evaluation, sleep questionnaires, sleep studies, etc.). Clark et al. in 1992 studied a selected outpatient MS population using the Minnesota Multiphasic Personality Inventory (MMPI) and found that patients reported sleep problems more frequently than controls on three sleep-related items, especially the statement "Is my sleep fitful and disturbed?" (25). Tachibana et al. studied 28 outpatients with MS from an MS clinic using clinical parameters, all-night oximetry, and polysomnography (PSG) in a small subset (26). They found sleep disorders in more than one-half, including frequent awakenings due to spasms or leg discomfort, difficulty initiating or maintaining sleep, habitual snoring, and nocturia. One small PSG study of MS patients found evidence of reduced sleep efficiency and more frequent awakenings compared

to controls but otherwise normal sleep latency and sleep architecture (27).

Stanton et al. assessed a convenience sample of patients attending an outpatient MS clinic in London, United Kingdom, using the Fatigue Severity Scale (FSS), Epworth Sleepiness Scale (ESS), and a 7-day sleep diary (28). They showed a significant association between the FSS score and number of days in which the subjects reported "middle insomnia" (waking at least two times per night). More than one-half of the patients reported problems on two or more nights a week with falling asleep, waking during the night, or early waking.

A study of outpatient and inpatient MS patients from a Berlin MS clinic assessed mobile outpatient PSG in a subgroup of 66 patients (29). Seventy-four percent of this group was found to have a "clinically relevant" sleep disorder which could cause daytime sleepiness. Another study compared 15 patients with MS and fatigue with 15 MS patients without fatigue from an MS clinic using actigraphy (30) and showed that in the fatigued patients, two had a delayed sleep phase disorder and 10 had disrupted sleep. Twelve of 15 nonfatigued patients had normal sleep recordings, one had an irregular sleep phase, and two had disrupted sleep. The authors concluded that sleep disturbance was correlated with fatigue in the MS population.

A large self-report mail survey of individuals recruited through a National MS society chapter (Washington state) compared responses to those of participants in a postmenopausal women's study (31). MS participants had more sleep-related difficulties than controls. In addition, women with MS were more likely than men to report sleep disorders, and the overall prevalence of moderate-to-severe sleep disturbances was 51.5%.

Kaminska et al. evaluated MS patients without known sleep disorders and healthy controls with PSG and multiple sleep latency tests (MSLTs) (32). They found obstructive sleep apnea (OSA) in 36 of 62 MS and 15 of 32 controls (no significant difference). They found that fatigue was correlated with OSA in MS but not controls.

TYPES OF SLEEP DISORDERS IN MS POPULATION

Insomnia appears to be common in the MS population (38). In one study, 40% of those studied had insomnia with difficulty initiating and maintaining sleep (26). Factors associated with this insomnia include muscle spasms, pain, periodic limb movements, restless leg syndrome (RLS), nocturia, medication effects, and psychiatric syndromes such as depression. Particularly of note is the occasional use of stimulant medications during the day for fatigue, which may inadvertently compromise nighttime sleeping.

OSA appears to be similar in frequency to the general population, but may not be immediately apparent on clinical questioning and may be correlated with fatigue in the MS population (32).

Nocturnal movement disorders appear to be more common in the MS population than the general population (27,39). In one study, RLS was seen in 36% of participants versus estimates of 5% to 15% in the general population (27).

Nocturia and pain frequently interrupt sleep in MS patients. Nocturia affects as many as 70% to 80% of MS patients (40). Pain can disrupt sleep causing daytime somnolence and worsening fatigue, as well as reducing pain threshold (41).

RARER SLEEP DISORDERS REPORTED IN MS

Narcolepsy. A handful of case reports have noted the presence of narcolepsy in a few patients with MS. Whether this is a chance association is unclear. Most reported cases have an older age of onset than sporadic narcolepsy (23.4 and 24.4 years in two large population-based studies) (42),

suggesting an association with MS and not simply representing sporadic narcolepsy (see Table 22.1).

Klein–Levin Syndrome. There is a single case report of Klein–Levin syndrome at onset of MS (43). A 20-year-old male presented with two episodes of daytime hypersomnia, orthostatic hypotension, compulsive masturbation, and hyperphagia, with well-defined MS-like brain lesions and CSF oligoclonal bands. Whether cases of hypersomnolence in MS represent part of this spectrum or vice versa is unclear, but such cases probably share hypothalamic involvement.

REM Behavior Disorders. Patients with REM sleep behavioral disorder (RBD) have been described in the MS population in some case reports (44,45). A large case control study of 135 MS patients and 118 controls assessed by history found four patients in the MS group with RBD, and none in the control group (46).

Ondine's Curse. Two case reports in patients with sudden death during sleep showed multiple medulla oblongata lesions (47). Lesions overlying the ventral nuclear complex of respiratory control were present in both cases.

Practical suggestions for clinicians:

- Inquire about sleep disorders in the MS population;
- Consider formal sleep study and consultation where there is sleep disruption or excess fatigue;
- RLS and RBD can be treated per standard protocol (ropinarole for RLS, clonazepam for RBD);
- Insomnia is best treated with nonpharmacological approaches including sleep hygiene, avoidance of caffeine and stimulants, and treatment of depression

TABLE 22.1 Narcolepsy and MS Case Reports

SOURCE	AGE/SEX	AGE ONSET MS/ NARCOLEPSY	IMAGING	COMMENT
(33)	M/31	31/23	No imaging	
(33)	F/42	33/31	No imaging	
(34)	M/48	26/28	No imaging	Noted familial clustering of MS
(34)	F/52	38/26	No imaging	
(34)	F/40	20/29	No imaging	
(35)	F/62	31/56	CT atrophy	Monozygotic twin, twin not affected
(36)	M/46	40/17	T2 lesions paraventricular and peduncular	MSLT SOREMP
(36)	F/46	13/45	Right frontal, paraventricular	MSLT SOREMP
(37)	F/45	Not reported	Hypothalamic lesion	Hypocretin less than 40 pg/mL
(37)	F/21	Not reported	Hypothalamic lesion	Hypocretin less than 40 pg/mL
(37)	F/54	Not reported	Hypothalamic lesion	Hypocretin 184 pg/mL
(37)	M/61	Not reported	Hypothalamic lesion	Hypocretin 173 pg/mL

MS, multiple sclerosis; MSLT, multiple sleep latency test; SOREMP, sleep onset rapid eye movement periods.
Note: Hypocretin less than 40 to 110 pg/mL markedly reduced, 110 to 200 pg/mL markedly reduced

---

KEY POINTS FOR PATIENTS: MULTIPLE SCLEROSIS AND SLEEP DISORDERS

- Sleep disorders occur commonly in MS and may require treatment;
- Snoring, frequent awakening at night, and fatigue in the morning may be symptoms of a sleep disorder;
- Insomnia is common in MS and is best treated with nonmedication approaches

MS, multiple sclerosis.

TRANSIENT NEUROLOGICAL EVENTS (PAROXYSMAL EVENTS) IN MS

Case

A 49-year-old male delivery man presents with recurrent events of speech arrest. He notices an odd sensation in his throat, followed a few seconds later by tingling on his right face. For the next 30 to 60 seconds he stutters, and has trouble getting his words out. He may have episodes two to three times a day, and they occur more frequently when he is working as a volunteer toastmaster. His health has been good other than treated hypertension. MRI with and without contrast shows multiple paraventricular and infratentorial lesions on fluid-attenuated inversion recovery (FLAIR) and T2 imaging without enhancing lesions (Figure 22.1). CSF shows oligoclonal banding and a mild lymphocytic pleocytosis. Over the ensuing year the patient develops some gait spasticity, fatigue, paraesthesia of the legs, and new nonenhancing MRI lesions. His episodes spontaneously resolve after 4 months.

Overview

Clinicians caring for patients with MS are well aware of relapses of MS, as well as of the progressive nature of MS in many patients. However, many MS patients describe transient, stereotyped, even bizarre sounding events lasting seconds that do not conform to a typical relapse or epileptic, migranous, or sleep phenomena. Such events have been called various things (tonic spasms, painful tonic spasms, paroxysmal attacks, paroxysmal symptoms). However, none of these terms capture the full group of phenomena that have the following general characteristics that distinguish them from others.

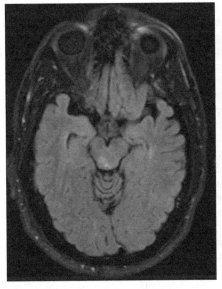 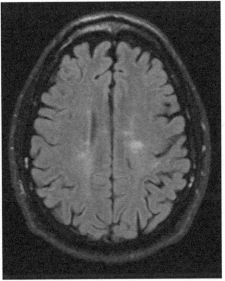

FIGURE 22.1   FLAIR axial views showing callosal, paraventricular, and mesencephalic lesions consistent with demyelination.

KEY POINTS FOR CLINICIANS: TRANSIENT NEUROLOGICAL EVENTS IN MULTIPLE SCLEROSIS

Transient neurological events

- Occur in setting of MS or other demyelinating syndrome
- Last usually seconds (typically less than 60 seconds) rather than minutes or hours
- Are stereotyped
- May have a combination of different types of sensory, motor, or visual activity or sensation (e.g., blurred vision due to nystagmus, dysarthria, focal sensory symptoms)
- May occur multiple times a day up to hundreds of times a day
- Are more common early in MS but may occur any time during the course of the disease
- Do not conform to more usual descriptions of focal seizures or migrainous events
- May last for a few weeks and resolve spontaneously, sometimes in the setting of acute relapse
- Typically respond to antiepileptic medicines. Antiepileptic medications are usually effective. We tend to taper these off after a few months if possible

---

Although clinicians may under-recognize these events, for patients and their families, they are very disruptive and a source of concern and anxiety. They may lead to a fruitless search for epilepsy or sleep disorders, and result in extensive testing.

PATHOPHYSIOLOGICAL CONCEPTS

Many MS symptoms are likely related to conduction block, slowed conduction, loss of axons, reduced safety factor, and other disruption of neural transmission. Positive symptoms such as paroxysmal events may have a variety of underlying mechanisms. Positive symptoms such as paresthesias, Lhermitte's phenomenon, and tonic spasms may be caused by spontaneously generated trains of spurious impulses arising in an area of demyelination and propagating along axons in both directions (48). In experimental models of central demyelination, newly demyelinated axons do not seem to have this property, but develop it after a week or two (49). Different patterns of spontaneous bursting have been seen in demyelinated fibers, including trains of evenly spaced impulses at frequencies of 10 to 50 Hz for periods of 0.1 to 5 seconds, and bursts of impulses (50). These patterns may have differing mechanisms based on sodium or potassium channel activity, but the exact correlations in experimental models are unclear. "Spontaneous bursting" patterns can sometimes be provoked by stimulating axons at physiological frequencies, providing a model for the precipitation of Lhermitte's phenomenon with neck movement. In addition, positive phenomena are often enhanced by hyperventilation (51) which increases axonal excitability by reducing membrane surface charge due to reduced extracellular free calcium (52). Other mechanisms have been proposed for positive phenomena in MS. In a demyelinated fiber, conduction may be slow enough to re-excite

backward the normal area which has recovered from the refractory period (53). Impulse conduction may activate adjacent fibers via ephaptic transmission (54). Clinically, it is unclear which of these mechanisms, if any, are causing positive symptoms but some or all are likely to underlie the phenotypic expression of symptoms.

CLINICAL DESCRIPTION

Events lasting a few seconds that are apparent to patients with MS have been described for years, but often go under-recognized by patients and physicians. The description of these events varies and many neurologists recognize some but not all of the paroxysmal events in MS. Most neurologists separate such paroxysmal events from epilepsy by their brevity, high frequency, absence of change in awareness, and lack of typical seizure aura, but it is unclear whether this separation is artificial as the mechanisms of paroxysmal symptoms in MS are not fully worked out. No prospective study has been done in an MS population to define the frequency of transient neurological events.

Paroxysmal events in MS usually last seconds and can be stereotyped. They may occur hundreds of times a day or only on occasion. Sometimes their time course overall is clustered in a few weeks, similar to the time course of a relapse. The relationship between paroxysmal events and relapse has not been fully elucidated. They appear to occur more frequently early in the disease course, and may be related to the time of a relapse. However, they can occur throughout the disease and independent of an acute relapse.

The phenomenology of paroxysmal events varies as much as other manifestations of MS. Essentially, any part of the central neuraxis can be affected. Sensory symptoms (usually a spreading sensation of some kind), motor symptoms (tonic spasms, transient inhibition of motor function, or ataxia), brain stem symptoms (dysarthria, blurred vision or diplopia, vertigo), or gustatory symptoms (altered taste, taste hallucination) can all be seen (see Table 22.2).

Tonic Spasms

The original description of tonic spasms in MS was by Matthews in 1958 (61). Since that time, multiple publications have described this most well defined of paroxysmal events in MS. Tonic spasms can be triggered by movement, hyperventilation, or other stimuli. They may be accompanied or preceded by sensory symptoms such as tingling, burning, or itching, suggesting involvement of nearby sensory fibers during the event. When unilateral, they are often generated by a focal plaque in the contralateral corticospinal pathways, most typically the cerebral peduncle or internal capsule (55,62). They have also been

referred to as tonic seizures; however, this term may imply a cortical localization for their generation, which may not be correct.

Matthews characterized "tonic seizures" as (58,61)

- Brief (duration up to 90 seconds)
- Frequent (up to hundreds per day)
- Usually intensely painful or uncomfortable
- Limbs on one side adopt a tetanic posture
- Often precipitated by movement or sensory stimulation
- Remit completely in weeks

Matthews and others have noted that such tonic spasms are neither accompanied by surface EEG changes nor by altered consciousness.

Other types of transient neurological events are as noted in Table 22.3, which is by no means exhaustive. What characterize these events are their brevity, repetition, and

TABLE 22.2   Types of Transient Neurological Events, System Involved, and Localization

SYMPTOM	SIGN	SYSTEM INVOLVED	LOCALIZATION (IF KNOWN)	COMMENTS
Tonic spasm (55)	Movement with dystonic component lasting seconds	Motor	Posterior internal capsule, cerebral peduncle, spinal cord	May be triggered by movement, hyperventilation
Bilateral tonic spasm (56)	Bilateral tonic movements	Motor	Medulla	
Paroxysmal dysarthria (57)	Transient slurred speech often with ataxia	Cerebellar connections, corticobulbar fibers	Various	
Paroxysmal itching, other paresthesia (56)	None	Sensory afferents	Unknown	May last minutes to hours
Paroxysmal akinesia (58)	Transient loss of motor function	Unclear		Usually lower limb involved
Kinesigenic choreoathetosis (59)	Complex movement of limb with or without other signs	Unclear	Unclear	
Paroxysmal diplopia (56)		Unclear		Responded to carbamazepine
Ocular convergence spasm (60)	Convergence spasm	Convergence system midbrain	Brainstem lesion MLF	

MLF, medial longitudinal fasciculus

TABLE 22.3   Descriptions of Transient Neurological Events

"'Cramp' in the left leg followed by sensation heat without pain, lasting 1 minute, up to 15 times per day" (56)

"Sudden sensation of right knee 'locked' . . . lost tone muscles right leg . . . seconds . . . 30 times a day . . . lasted 6 months" (56)

"Attacks in which she felt as if her eyes were turning in. Her head would turn slightly to the right and the left eye would adduct. These attacks lasted about 10 seconds and were extremely distressing . . ." (58)

"Sensation of quivering in the right side of the face, spreading to the right arm, index finger, and thumb . . . last for a few seconds . . . highly unpleasant" (58)

"Warning sensation of 'dullness,' quickly followed by diplopia, difficulty pronouncing words . . . stiffness and unsteadiness of legs" (63)

"Lose color in one eye" (39)

"Sensation of 'heaviness' and 'stiffness' right leg and arm. Almost simultaneously she experienced double vision, ataxia and dysarthria . . . a few moments later she felt a sensation of heat in the left forearm" (56)

stereotypy. Table 22.3 lists some descriptions of episodes from the neurological literature, which emphasize the variation of symptomatology across individuals.

One study (55) looked at MRI in two patients with unilateral painful tonic limb spasms. They found focal lesions in the cerebral peduncle and upper pons in these cases. Spissu et al. reviewed five cases of tonic spasms and found lesions in the posterior limb of the internal capsule in four and of the cerebral peduncle in two (62).

Treatment of tonic spasms and other transient neurological events has been described in either case studies or case series. Anecdotally, many patients do not require treatment once symptoms are explained, but for others, particularly when events are uncomfortable or affect function, intervention may be necessary. Twomey et al. described using carbamazepine with "good response" in five of seven treated patients among a series of 14 patients with paroxysmal symptoms (64). Osterman described multiple patients treated with carbamazepine with reduction or cessation of episodes (56). In Matthews's case series of 28 episodes of paroxysmal symptoms, 12 stopped spontaneously, phenobarbital or phenytoin "appeared to arrest the paroxysms" in six, and carbamazepine was used "effectively" in six. In four patients, there was no response to these medicines (58). Sakurai et al. described treating patients with "positive MS symptoms" with orally administered mexiletine with reduction of episodes (65). Symptoms which patients described included paroxysmal Lhermitte's sign, paroxysmal pain, or itching. Solaro et al. in 1998 described an open label trial of gabapentin in doses ranging from 600 to 1,200 mg/day in 21 patients with a variety of paroxysmal events (66). Eighteen experienced resolution or amelioration of their symptoms during this uncontrolled trial. Restivo et al. in 2003 described the use of botulinum toxin for painful tonic spasms in five patients not obtaining relief from a variety of anticonvulsant medicines and reduced pain scores at 30-day follow-up after botulinum injection (67). Importantly, these syndromes are often confused with spasticity and treated with baclofen and other antispasticity medications, typically without beneficial response.

Treating tonic spasms and other transient neurological events in MS patients can be the most rewarding of therapeutic exercises. The patient often presents having up to hundreds of episodes per day, has defied diagnosis and treatment by others, and is cured within hours of starting an antiepileptic medication. Initial treatment has traditionally involved carbamazepine or phenytoin, although new antiepileptic therapies may be similarly effective. Serum drug levels are rarely needed, as dosing is guided by treatment response and side effects.

REFERENCES

1. Kelley BJ, Rodriguez M. Seizures in patients with multiple sclerosis. *CNS Drugs.* 2009;23:805–815.
2. Koch M, Uyttenboogaart M, Polman S, et al. Seizures in multiple sclerosis. *Epilepsia.* 2008;49:948–953.
3. Catenoix H, Marignier R, Ritleng C, et al. Multiple sclerosis and epileptic seizures. *Mult Scler.* 2011;17(1):96–102.
4. Newman P, Saunders M. A unique case of musicogenic epilepsy. *Arch Neurol.* 1980;37(4):244–245.
5. Spatt J, Goldenberg G, Mamoli B. Simple dysphasic seizures as the sole manifestation of relapse in multiple sclerosis. *Epilepsia.* 1994;35(6):1342–1345.
6. Hess DC, Sethi KD. Epilepsia partialis continua in multiple sclerosis. *Int J Neurosci.* 1990;50(1-2):109–111.
7. Martinez-Juarez IE, Lopez-Meza E, Gonzalez-Arragon MD, et al. Epilepsy and multiple sclerosis: increased risk among progressive forms. *Epilepsy Res.* 2009;84:250–253.
8. Spatt J, Chaix R, Mamoli B. Epileptic and non-epileptic seizures in multiple sclerosis. *J Neurol.* 2001;248(1):2–9.
9. Kinnunen E, Wilkström J. Prevalence and prognosis of epilepsy in patients with multiple sclerosis. *Epilepsia.* 1986;27:729–733.
10. Nyquist PA, Cascino GD, Rodriguez M. Seizures in patients with multiple sclerosis seen at Mayo Clinic, Rochester, Minn, 1990-1998. *Mayo Clin Proc.* 2001;76:983–986.
11. Truyen L, Barkhof F, Frequin ST, et al. Magnetic resonance imaging of epilepsy in multiple sclerosis: a case control study. *Mult Scler.* 1996;1:213–217.
12. Calabrese M, De Stefano N, Atzori M, et al. Extensive cortical inflammation is associated with epilepsy in multiple sclerosis. *J Neurol.* 2008;255:581–586.
13. Geurts JJ, Bo L, Pouwels PJ, et al. Cortical lesions in multiple sclerosis: combined postmortem MR imaging and histopathology. *Am J Neuroradiol.* 2005;26:572–577.
14. Ciccarelli O, Chen JT. MS cortical lesions on double inversion recovery: few but true. *Neurology.* 2012;78:296–297.
15. Luchinetti CF, Bogdan FG, Popescu MD, et al. Inflammatory cortical demyelination in early multiple sclerosis. *N Engl J Med.* 2011;365:2188–2197.
16. Peterson JW, Bo L, Mork S, et al. Transected neurites, apoptotic neurons, and reduced inflammation in cortical multiple sclerosis lesions. *Ann Neurol.* 2001;50:389–400.
17. Schuele SU, Kellinghaus C, Shook SJ, et al. Incidence of seizures in patients with multiple sclerosis treated with intrathecal baclofen. *Neurology.* 2005;64:1086–1087.
18. Goodman AD, Brown TR, Edwards KR, et al. A phase 3 trial of extended release oral dalfampridine in multiple sclerosis. *Ann Neurol.* 2010;68:494–502.
19. Koch MW, Polman SK, Uyttenboogaart M, De Keyser J. Treatment of seizures in multiple sclerosis. *Cochrane Database Syst Rev.* July 8, 20098;(3):CD007150.
20. Waxman SG. Axonal conduction and injury in multiple sclerosis: the role of sodium channels. *Nat Rev Neurosci.* 2006;7:932–941.
21. Dan P. The role of ion channels in neurodegeneration. *Modulator.* 2008;22:14–17.
22. Solaro C, Brichetto G, Battaglia MA, et al. Antiepileptic medications in multiple sclerosis: adverse effects in a three-year follow-up study. *Neurol Sci.* 2005;25:307–310.
23. Sotgiu S, Murrighile MR, Constantin G. Treatment of refractory epilepsy with natalizumab in a patient with multiple sclerosis. Case report. *BMC Neurol.* 2010;10:84.
24. Krupp LB, Alvarez LA, LaRocca NG, et al. Fatigue in MS. *Arch Neurol.* 1988;11:78–83.
25. Clark CM, Fleming JA, Li D, et al. Sleep disturbance, depression and lesion site in patients with multiple sclerosis. *Arch Neurol.* 1992;49:641–643.
26. Tachibana N, Howard RS, Hirsch NP, et al. Sleep problems in multiple sclerosis. *Eur Neurol.* 1994;34:320–323.
27. Ferini-Strambi L, Filippi M, Martinelli V, et al. Nocturnal sleep study in multiple sclerosis: correlations with clinical and brain magnetic resonance imaging findings. *J Neurol Sci.* 1994;125:194–197.
28. Stanton BR, Barnes F, Silber E. Sleep and fatigue in multiple sclerosis. *Mult Scler.* 2006;12:481–486.
29. Veauthier C, Radbruch H, Gaede G, et al. Fatigue in multiple sclerosis is closely related to sleep disorders: a polysomnographic cross-sectional study. *Mult Scler.* 2011;17(5):613–622.

30. Attarian HP, Brown KM, Duntley SP, et al. The relationship of sleep disturbances and fatigue in multiple sclerosis. *Arch Neurol.* 2004;61:525–528.

31. Barner AM, Johnson KL, Amtmann D, et al. Prevalence of sleep problems in individuals with multiple sclerosis. *Mult Scler.* 2008;14:1127–1130.

32. Kaminska M, Kimoff RJ, Benedetti A, et al. Obstructive sleep apnea is associated with fatigue in multiple sclerosis. *Mult Scler.* 2012;18(8):1159–1169.

33. Berg O, Hanley J. Narcolepsy in two cases of multiple sclerosis. *Acta Neurol Scand.* 1963;39(3):252–257.

34. Ekbom K. Familial multiple sclerosis with narcolepsy. *Arch Neurol.* 1966;15(4):337–344.

35. Schrader H, Gotlibsen OB, Skomedal GN. Multiple sclerosis and narcolepsy/cataplexy in a monozygotic twin. *Neurology.* 1980;30:105–108.

36. Younger DS, Pedley TA, Thorpy MJ. Multiple sclerosis and narcolepsy: possible similar genetic susceptibility. *Neurology.* 1991;41:447–448.

37. Kanbayashi T, Shimohata T, Nakashima I, et al. Symptomatic narcolepsy in patients with neuromyelitis optica and multiple sclerosis. *Arch Neurol.* 2009;66(12):1563–1566.

38. Fleming WE, Pollak CP. Sleep disorders in multiple sclerosis. *Semin Neurol.* 2005;25:64–68.

39. Rae-Grant AD, Eckert NJ, Bartz S, et al. Sensory symptoms of multiple sclerosis: a hidden reservoir of morbidity. *Mult Scler.* 1999;5:179–183.

40. Amarenco G, Kerdraon J, Denys P. Bladder and sphincter disorders in multiple sclerosis: clinical, urodynamic and neurophysiological study of 225 cases (in French). *Rev Neurol (Paris).* 1995;151:722–730.

41. Onen SH, Alloui A, Gross A, et al. The effects of total sleep deprivation, selective sleep interruption and sleep recovery on pain tolerance thresholds in health subjects. *J Sleep Res.* 2001;10:35–42.

42. Dauvilliers Y, Montplaisir J, Molinari N. Age at onset of narcolepsy in two large populations of patients in France and Quebec. *Neurology.* 2001;57(11):2029–2033.

43. Testa S, Oppotuno A, Gallo P, Tavolato B. A case of multiple sclerosis with an onset mimicking the Klein-Levin syndrome. *Ital J Neurol Sci.* 1987;8:151–155.

44. Plazzi G, Montagna P. Remitting REM sleep behavior disorder as the initial sign of multiple sclerosis. *Sleep Med.* 2002;3(5):437–439.

45. Tippmann-Peikert M, Boeve BF, Keegan BM. REM sleep behavior disorder initiated by acute brainstem multiple sclerosis. *Neurology.* 2006;66:1277–1279.

46. Gomez-Choco MJ, Iranzo A, Blanco Y, et al. Prevalence of restless legs syndrome and REM sleep behavior disorder in multiple sclerosis. *Mult Scler.* 2007;13:805–808.

47. Auer RN, Rowlands CG, Perry SF, et al. Multiple sclerosis with medullary plaques and fatal sleep apnea (Ondine's curse). *Clin Neuropathol.* 1996;15:101–105.

48. Baker M, Bostock H. Ectopic activity in demyelinated spinal root axons of the rat. *J Physiol.* 1992;451:539–552.

49. Smith KJ, McDonald WI. The pathophysiology of multiple sclerosis? The mechanisms underlying the production of symptoms and the natural history of the disease. *Phil Trans R Soc Lond B.* 1999;354:1649–1673.

50. Felts PA, Kapoor R, Smith KJ. A mechanism for ectopic firing in central demyelinated axons. *Brain.* 1995;118:1225–1231.

51. Davis FA, Becker FO, Michael JA, Sorensen E. Effect of intravenous sodium bicarbonate, disodiumedetate and hyperventilation on visual and oculomotor signs in multiple sclerosis. *J Neurol Neurosurg Psychiatry.* 1970;33:723–732.

52. Burke D. Microneurography, impulse conduction, and paresthesias. *Muscle Nerve.* 1993;16:1025–1032.

53. Burchiel KJ. Abnormal impulse generation in focally demyelinated trigeminal roots. *J Neurosurg.* 1980;53:674–688.

54. Raminsky M. Hyperexcitability of pathologically myelinated axons and positive symptoms in multiple sclerosis. In: Waxman SG, Ritchie JM, eds. *Demyelinating Diseases: Basic and Clinical Electrophysiology.* New York, NY: Raven Press; 1981:289–297.

55. Rose MR, Ball JA, Thompson PD. Magnetic resonance imaging in tonic spasms of multiple sclerosis. *J Neurol.* 1993;241:115–117.

56. Osterman PO, Westerberg C-E. Paroxysmal attacks in multiple sclerosis. *Brain.* 1975;98:189–202.

57. Andermann F, Cosgrove JBR, Lloyd-Smith D, et al. Paroxysmal dysarthria and ataxia in multiple sclerosis. *Neurology.* 1959;9:211–215.

58. Mathews WB. Paroxysmal symptoms in multiple sclerosis. *J Neurol Neurosurg Psychiatry.* 1975;38:617–623.

59. Roos RA, Wintzen AR, Vielvoye G, Polder TW. Paroxysmal kinesigenic choreoathetosis as a presenting symptom of multiple sclerosis. *J Neurol Neurosurg Psychiatry.* 1991;54:657–658.

60. Postert T, McMonagle U, Buttner T, et al. Paroxysmal convergence spasm in multiple sclerosis. *Acta Neurol Scand.* 1996;94:35–37.

61. Matthews WB. Tonic seizures in disseminated sclerosis. *Brain.* 1958;81:193–201.

62. Spissu A, Cannas A, Ferrigno P, et al. Anatomic correlates of painful tonic spasms in multiple sclerosis. *Mov Disord.* 1999;14:331–335.

63. Espir MLE, Watkins SM, Smith HV. Paroxysmal dysarthria and other transient neurological disturbances in disseminated sclerosis. *J Neurol Neurosurg Psychiatry.* 1966;29:323–330.

64. Twomey JA, Espir MLE. Paroxysmal symptoms as the first manifestations of multiple sclerosis. *J Neurol Neurosurg Psychiatry.* 1980;43:296–304.

65. Sakurai M, Kanazawa I. Positive symptoms in multiple sclerosis: their treatment with sodium channel blockers, lidocaine, and mexiletine. *J Neurol Sci.* 1999;162:162–168.

66. Solaro C, Lunardi GL, Capello E, et al. An open-label trial of gabapentin treatment of paroxysmal symptoms in multiple sclerosis patients. *Neurology.* 1998;51:609–611.

67. Restivo DA, Tinazzi M, Patti F, et al. Botulinum toxin treatment of painful tonic spasms in multiple sclerosis. *Neurology.* 2003;61:719–720.

23 Eye Symptoms, Signs, and Therapy in Multiple Sclerosis

Collin M. McClelland and Steven L. Galetta

KEY POINTS FOR CLINICIANS

- Demyelinating optic neuritis (DON) is a hallmark manifestation of multiple sclerosis (MS) and is marked by acute or subacute onset of vision loss, eye pain, and a relative afferent pupillary defect (RAPD) in unilateral cases.

- Intravenous steroids do not alter the long-term visual outcome of isolated DON but expedite visual recovery and show a protective effect against MS development for 2 years.

- Neuromyelitis optica (NMO)-associated optic neuritis may present similar to DON. Providers should maintain a low threshold for serum NMO antibody testing in cases of DON as NMO requires a different long-term treatment.

- Optical coherence tomography (OCT) is a noninvasive imaging test that can be used clinically to aid in the diagnosis of MS by detecting subtle optic nerve atrophy. It can be used in the management of MS by serially measuring retinal nerve fiber layer thickness as a structural correlate of optic nerve disease in MS patients.

- Maculopathies, including fingolimod-associated macular edema, often have subtle fundus findings and can mimic DON. Unlike DON, they characteristically lack pain and often do not demonstrate an RAPD.

- Demyelination rarely causes isolated ocular motor (cranial nerve [CN] III, IV, and VI) palsies. Alternative etiologies should always be carefully evaluated.

MS frequently affects both the afferent visual system and the efferent ocular motor system. An estimated one third of MS patients develop DON during their disease course, whereas up to three out of four suffer from abnormalities of ocular movement. A basic understanding of neuro-ophthalmology is important for all providers who manage MS patients.

The neuro-ophthalmic effects of MS include highly characteristic features such as DON and internuclear ophthalmoplegia (INO), as well as other manifestations such as nystagmus, cranial nerve (CN) palsies, uveitis, and saccadic abnormalities. Vision loss may also arise from treatment complications including fingolimod-associated macular edema (ME), corticosteroid-induced central serous chorioretinopathy (CSR), and natalizumab-associated progressive multifocal leukoencephalopathy (PML). This chapter reviews high-yield clinical knowledge pertinent to the diagnosis and management of MS-associated visual impairment.

EVALUATION: AFFERENT PATHOLOGY

A hallmark feature of MS, DON occurs in about 50% of MS patients during the course of the disease and may be the presenting feature in about 20%. While the term *optic neuritis* is often used as a synonym for DON associated with MS, the term *optic neuritis* also refers to optic nerve inflammation that complicates other inflammatory and infectious conditions. Referring to MS-associated optic neuritis as idiopathic DON lessens the ambiguity.

The optic neuritis treatment trial (ONTT) defined the presenting characteristics (1), optimal treatment (2), visual prognosis (3), and long-term risk of MS in patients with DON (4). MS and DON share similar patient demographics; DON is common in young patients (mean age = 31.8), whites (85%), and females (F:M = 3:1) (1). The diagnosis of DON remains clinical and is characterized by vision loss over hours to days, eye pain, and the presence of a RAPD in unilateral cases. Visual impairment can affect central vision, peripheral vision, and color vision; a thorough exam for suspected DON should assess all these aspects of visual function. In most clinical settings, visual acuity is tested on a high-contrast distance Snellen acuity chart or a near card using the patient's glasses correction for the distance tested. If a patient's glasses are not available, use of a pinhole occluder is one means to estimate the best corrected visual acuity for both near and distance vision testing. Presenting visual acuity in DON ranges from normal to no light perception, with severe vision loss occurring in a minority of patients (Table 23.1) (1).

> *DON is characterized by acute vision loss, eye pain, and a relative afferent pupillary defect (in unilateral cases).*

Dyschromatopsia, or abnormal color perception, occurs in most DON cases (88%–94%) and can be tested easily in clinic using pseudoisochromatic color plates (e.g., Ishihara color plates) or subjective red desaturation testing using a red bottle top (1). Visual field loss on formal perimetry testing occurs in nearly all patients with symptomatic DON. Although confrontation testing techniques are helpful for large visual field defects, more subtle defects require formal visual field testing. Automated static threshold perimetry (e.g., Humphrey visual field testing) was used in the ONTT, which found that the most common pattern (45%) was a diffuse depression or a large central scotoma (1). The study found that virtually any pattern of visual field loss may occur with DON and there is no specific pattern that strongly suggests DON. Unfortunately, the presenting features of vision loss in DON are nonspecific and occur in many other optic neuropathies and retinopathies. Diagnosis, therefore, often relies on more distinguishing features such as eye pain, fundus appearance, and the presence of visual recovery.

TABLE 23.1   Presenting Features of Vision Loss in DON

VISION	PERCENTAGE (%)
VA: 20/20 or greater	10.5
VA: 20/25–20/40	24.8
VA: 20/50–20/190	28.8
VA: 20/200–20/800	20.3
VA: Finger counting or lesser	15.6

Note that 20/200 or worse vision in both eyes typically defines the legal VA criteria for blindness. VA worse than 20/200 in an eye is considered a functionally blind eye.
DON, demyelinating optic neuritis; VA, visual acuity.
Source: The clinical profile of optic neuritis. Experience of the optic neuritis treatment trial. Optic neuritis study group. *Arch Ophthalmol*. 1991;109(12):1673-1678.

Eye pain is described in about 92% of DON cases, may vary from mild to severe, is not typically associated with conjunctival injection, and is often worse with eye movement (1). The pain may precede or follow vision loss and usually subsides in 3 to 5 days. DON without eye pain is atypical and raises concern for alternative diagnoses (Table 23.2). Almost all DON cases will exhibit an RAPD on the swinging flashlight test (**Video 23.1**). The absence of an RAPD raises concern (Table 23.2) for bilateral DON, retinopathy-mimicking DON, or prior insult to the contralateral optic nerve. About two thirds of DON cases have normal-appearing optic nerves, whereas the other one third typically show only mild optic disc edema (1). Hemorrhages around the optic nerve head (peripapillary) and retinal exudates caused by swelling and lipid deposition associated with severe disc edema occur in about 5% of cases and suggest "atypical optic neuritis" related to infectious or nondemyelinating inflammatory disorders (Table 23.2). While laboratory tests for DON mimics (e.g., sarcoidosis, lupus, antineutrophil cytoplasmic antibodies (ANCA) vasculitides) are rarely helpful in classic presentations of DON, the presence of peripapillary hemorrhages, retinal exudates, or severe disc edema should prompt a targeted evaluation.

VIDEO 23.1

> *The presence of peripapillary hemorrhages, retinal exudates, or severe disc edema in the setting of acute optic nerve dysfunction should prompt a targeted evaluation for causes of atypical optic neuritis.*

Optic disc edema accompanied by macular exudates forming a sunburst-like pattern surrounding the fovea (Figure 23.1) is highly suggestive of neuroretinitis, a diagnosis not associated with MS. While most cases of neuroretinitis are idiopathic, specific etiologies (Table 23.2) should be considered and tested for depending on clinical context.

> *On fundus examination, most cases of demyelinating optic neuritis (DON; two thirds) have normal-appearing optic nerves. The other one third usually shows mild disc edema.*

While neuroimaging is not usually necessary to diagnose DON, MRI of the brain is indicated to assess characteristic white matter lesions in patients without known MS (see the section on management). In cases when DON

TABLE 23.2 Clues to Alternative Diagnoses in Presumed DON

ATYPICAL FEATURE	ALTERNATIVE DIAGNOSES TO CONSIDER
Severe disc swelling (including peripapillary hemorrhages or exudates)	"Atypical optic neuritis": Autoimmune-associated (lupus, Sjogren's, sarcoid, inflammatory bowel disease), infectious (syphilis, HIV, Lyme disease, tuberculosis), papilledema, hypertensive retinopathy, anterior ischemic optic neuropathy (nonarteritic and giant cell arteritis)
Macular star of exudates	Neuroretinitis (cat-scratch disease, Lyme disease, syphilis, toxoplasmosis, sarcoid, tuberculosis, numerous viral etiologies)
Lack of visual recovery	Neuromyelitis optica-associated optic neuritis, compressive lesions (malignancy or aneurysm), sarcoidosis, ischemic optic neuropathy, maculopathies (CSR, ME, choroidal neovascular membrane, retinal vascular occlusion, etc.), nutritional/toxic (B_{12} deficiency, vitamin A deficiency, folate deficiency, cigarette smoking), metabolic (Leber hereditary optic neuropathy)
Severe photophobia	Nondemyelinating optic neuritis associated with uveitis: Sarcoid-, syphilis-, Lyme disease-, Behcet-, tuberculosis-, and inflammatory bowel disease-associated optic neuritis
Optic nerve sheath enhancement on MRI	"Optic perineuritis": Orbital pseudotumor, sarcoid, inflammatory bowel disease, Lyme disease, syphilis, Wegener's disease, and optic nerve sheath meningioma
Lack of pain	Ischemic optic neuropathy, neuromyelitis optica-associated optic neuritis, Leber hereditary optic neuropathy, numerous maculopathies (CSR, ME, choroidal neovascular membrane, retinal vascular occlusion, etc.). Consider retrochiasmatic visual loss.
Lack of a relative afferent pupillary defect	Numerous maculopathies (CSR, ME, choroidal neovascular membrane, retinal vascular occlusion, etc.), bilateral optic neuropathy (including bilateral DON), media opacities (e.g., posterior subcapsular cataract, corneal pathology, vitreous hemorrhage)
Metamorphopsia	Numerous maculopathies (CSR, ME, choroidal neovascular membrane, retinal vascular occlusion, etc.)
Receiving TNF-I	TNF-I-associated optic neuritis. TNF-Is are known to occasionally incite inflammation throughout the CNS.

CNS, central nervous system; CSR, central serous chorioretinopathy; DON, demyelinating optic neuritis; ME, macular edema; TNF-I, tumor necrosis factor inhibitor.

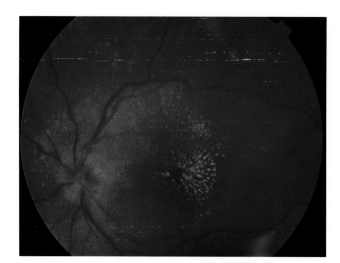

FIGURE 23.1 Color fundus photograph of the left eye demonstrating characteristic features of neuroretinitis in a patient with cat-scratch fever. There is moderate to severe optic nerve swelling with macular exudates forming a "star" pattern. The patient with typical papillitis may have a similar disc appearance, without the retinal exudates.

is difficult to distinguish clinically from nonarteritic anterior ischemic optic neuropathy (NAION), dedicated orbital MRI sequences may be beneficial (5). DON demonstrates optic nerve enhancement in nearly all cases (>90%) while it is rarely seen in NAION (about 7%) (5). In cases with acute painful vision loss, RAPD, and orbital signs (e.g., proptosis, conjunctival injection/chemosis, or restricted motility), MRI of the orbits may be helpful to evaluate for orbital pseudotumor or idiopathic orbital inflammatory syndrome. Usually idiopathic and considered within the spectrum of orbital pseudotumor, optic perineuritis is primarily a radiographic diagnosis characterized by peripheral enhancement of the optic nerve (6). Peripheral vision loss tends to predominate in optic perineuritis, although central acuity can be affected and mimic DON. Distinction from DON is important because optic perineuritis is exquisitely sensitive to steroids (intravenous [IV] or oral) and is not associated with MS.

Some maculopathies may mimic DON. Fingolimod (Gilenya) has been shown to cause ME in 0.5% to 0.6% of patients (7). ME is associated with painless central vision loss in one or both eyes, typically with normal pupillary function (no RAPD). The result of a breakdown of the blood retinal barrier, ME frequently occurs in association with diabetes, uveitis, and retinal vein occlusions. The fundus findings of ME are often subtle, and diagnosis relies heavily on ocular coherence tomography (OCT) (Figure 23.2) and fluorescein angiography (FA). The greatest risk for ME occurs in the first 3 to 4 months of fingolimod treatment. Patients should receive a baseline pretreatment ophthalmic exam followed by a repeat exam 3 to 4 months after starting fingolimod (7). If no ME is

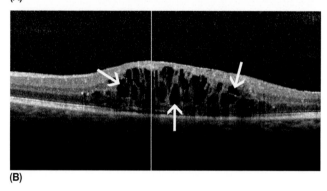

FIGURE 23.2 (A) SD-OCT slice demonstrating normal macular contour with the foveal pit located centrally. (B) SD-OCT slice showing cyst-like spaces of fluid within the retina (arrows) characteristic of ME, which can be associated with fingolimod (Gilenya) therapy.

SD-OCT, spectral domain ocular coherence tomography.

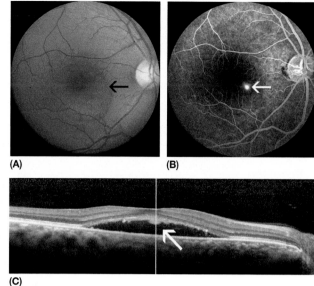

FIGURE 23.3 Color fundus photograph of the right eye showing subtle findings of a neurosensory retinal detachment including a hyperpigmented macular patch (arrow) that would be slightly elevated on stereoscopic view. Arteriovenous phase FA image showing a hyperfluorescent "dot" inferonasal to the fovea (arrow). (B) The complete FA sequence (not shown) reveals an "expansile dot" pattern of leakage diagnostic of CSR. (C) SD-OCT slice demonstrating macular subretinal fluid (arrow) consistent with serous retinal detachment due to CSR.

CSR, central serous chorioretinopathy; FA, fluorescein angiography; SD-OCT, spectral domain ocular coherence tomography

present after 4 months on therapy, patients may resume routine once yearly eye care. Patients with risk factors for ME (such as diabetes and uveitis) may require closer follow-up.

> *Fingolimod-associated macular edema typically causes painless central vision loss and when it occurs it typically occurs in the first 4 months of treatment.*

CSR is a maculopathy marked by painless detachment of the neurosensory retina (8). CSR causes subacute onset of central vision loss that may mimic DON. CSR is important to MS providers because it can be triggered by glucocorticoid administration and, unlike DON, will worsen with prolonged steroid therapy (9). Patients are classically middle aged (mean = 41 years), predominantly male (M:F = 6:1), and exhibit type A personalities (8).

Exam findings are often subtle (Figure 23.3A) and include mild elevation of the detached macula, an absence of the normal foveal light reflex, and abnormal macular coloration. Diagnosis is facilitated by FA (Figure 23.3B) and OCT (Figure 23.3C).

In addition to corticosteroids and fingolimod, there are other medications used in the treatment of MS that can have visual and ocular side effects (Table 23.3). Both CSR- and fingolimod-associated ME are maculopathies most easily distinguished from unilateral DON by the lack of pain and absence of an RAPD. Metamorphopsia, or the wavy distortion of straight lines, is a specific symptom of maculopathies not usually described in optic neuropathies.

> *Maculopathies, unlike DON, are usually painless and may lack a RAPD. OCT and FA often aid in the diagnosis of maculopathies.*

TABLE 23.3 Visual/Ocular Side Effects of Drugs Used to Treat MS

DRUG	SIDE EFFECT	CLINICAL PEARLS
Corticosteroids	CSR	Vision loss that worsens with corticosteroids may indicate CSR, particularly when the vision loss is central, painless, and not associated with a new ipsilateral APD.
Fingolimod	ME	Patients require a baseline eye exam and a repeat exam 4 months after starting drug. ME causes painless, central blurring without an APD. Macular OCT is a sensitive and specific test for ME.
Natalizumab	Cortical vison loss from PML	MS rarely causes symptomatic homonymous hemianopic visual field defects from plaques involving the optic radiations or visual cortex. Occurring with current or recent use of natalizumab, this raises concern for PML.
Alemtuzumab	Thyroid eye disease	Up to 30% of patients on drug develop autoimmune thyroid disease. Ocular features parallel idiopathic Graves ophthalmopathy and include periocular skin and conjunctival swelling and redness, eye pain, proptosis, ocular motility deficits, and double vision.
IFN-B	Retinal microvasculopathy	Rarely IFN may be associated with retinal microvasculopathy including cotton wool spots, microaneurysms, and small hemorrhages causing mild vision impairment. Findings and symptoms resolve with drug cessation.

APD, afferent pupillary defect; CSR, central serous chorioretinopathy; IFN-B, interferon-beta; ME, macular edema; MS, multiple sclerosis; OCT, optical coherence tomography; PML, progressive multifocal leukoencephalopathy.

EVALUATION: EFFERENT PATHOLOGY

The symptoms of MS-related eye movement abnormalities include visual fatigue, blurred vision, diplopia (double vision), and oscillopsia (subjective movement of visual targets). In most cases, these abnormalities reflect demyelinating lesions of the brain stem and cerebellum. The motility disturbance INO is highly characteristic of MS and indicates disruption of interneurons traveling through the medial longitudinal fasciculus (MLF) from the abducens nucleus in the pons to the contralateral medial rectus oculomotor subnucleus in the midbrain. INO results in dysconjugate horizontal eye movements in which the speed and strength of the adducting eye are impaired relative to the abucting eye. INO is detectable clinically in up to one third of patients with MS (10). Findings of INO include ipsilateral impairment of adduction often combined with a compensatory jerk nystagmus of the contralateral eye in abduction (**Video 23.2**). Subtle cases of INO may be symptomatic yet easily missed on exam, because the motility in the adducting eye may appear full yet there is a delay in adducting saccades in the eye ipsilateral to the MLF lesion. Patients with MS who complain of transient double vision or blurring upon quick lateral gaze may harbor a subtle INO. Asking patients to repeatedly alternate fixation from a target in far left gaze to a target in far right gaze helps to expose the slow adducting saccades in subtle cases of INO.

VIDEO 23.2

Patients with transient double vision or blurring upon quick lateral gaze may have a subtle INO.

In most cases of INO, the eyes are horizontally aligned in primary gaze. Not unusual in MS, bilateral INO may lead to a large exotropia in primary gaze called "wall-eyed" bilateral INO (WEBINO).

MS accounts for about 34% of INO cases and is second to ischemia as the most common cause. INO due to stroke is more commonly unilateral and is less apt to recover compared to demyelinating INO, which recovers completely in about 60% of cases (11). Proton density imaging (PDI) MRI sequences may be more sensitive than either T2-weighted or fluid-attenuated inversion recovery (FLAIR) sequences for detecting MLF lesions (12).

Nystagmus, or abnormal rhythmic eye movements, occurs in about 30% of MS patients. The underlying pathophysiology is complex but can be simplified to the failure of one or more gaze-stabilizing systems including visual fixation, vestibular function, and gaze-holding mechanisms (13). Pendular nystagmus, characterized by a back-and-forth slow phase of equal velocity in the absence of a fast corrective phase, can occur in MS and may be asymmetric with more prominent nystagmus in the eye with worse visual acuity. Pendular nystagmus can occur in association with lesions throughout the brain stem or cerebellum (14).Gaze-evoked nystagmus, occurring in up to 26% of MS patients, is characterized by a jerk nystagmus that beats in the direction of attempted eccentric gaze (15). Fortunately, this nystagmus does not typically manifest in primary gaze, so it is less debilitating than pendular nystagmus.

Isolated ocular motor CN palsies occur infrequently in MS patients. Demyelination of either the nuclei or fascicles of CN III, IV, and VI can present with binocular diplopia. MS patients with a new onset isolated CN III, IV, or VI palsy should be considered for other etiologies including compressive lesions, diabetes, hypertension, stroke, and infection. This is particularly true in patients with isolated CN III palsy, which may be a harbinger of impending rupture of a posterior communicating artery aneurysm. Only about 1% of CN III palsies are attributable to MS (16). Demyelinating CN IV palsies occur even less frequently comprising an estimated 0.06% of all CN IV palsies (17). MS-associated CN VI palsy is more common than CN III or CN IV palsy and responsible for about 7% of all CN VI palsies (18); the estimated rate is higher (24%) when considering younger patients (aged 15–50) without trauma (19).

Isolated cranial nerve (CN) III and IV nerve palsies are uncommon in MS. Alternative etiologies should be considered carefully before attributing these deficits to MS.

Saccadic dysmetria, a common finding in MS and associated with cerebellar dysfunction, occurs when the eyes undershoot (hypometria) or overshoot (hypermetria) the target of fixation and can result in subjective complaints of difficulty focusing or tracking. Testing for saccades can be performed by asking the patient to alternate fixation repeatedly from a target in left gaze to a target in right gaze; dysmetria is evident when small corrective saccades are necessary to fixate the target after it was missed on initial attempts. Other saccadic abnormalities, such as delay and intrusions, also occur in MS patients.

MANAGEMENT: AFFERENT DEMYELINATION

Most cases of DON recover well without treatment. IV methylprednisolone 250 mg 4 times daily followed by oral prednisone 1 mg/kg a day for 11 days has been shown to expedite visual recovery in DON. In practice, most clinicians use a dose of 1,000 mg a day for 3 days followed by the oral prednisone taper. There is no evidence, however, that corticosteroids change long-term visual outcomes (2). In most cases, visual improvement in DON begins after 2 to 3 weeks and maximal recovery usually occurs within months. Ten years following DON, the majority of patients have excellent vision with 74% retaining 20/20 vision and 90% retaining 20/40 or even better vision (3). Failure to abide by this timeline for progression and recovery should raise suspicion for alternative diagnoses including neuromyelitis optica (NMO). NMO presents with unilateral optic neuritis in up to 63% of cases and is often indistinguishable from MS-associated DON (20). A common theme differentiating NMO and MS relapses, NMO-associated optic neuritis tends to be more severe at onset and less apt to recover compared to MS-associated DON (21). Only about 43% of NMO-associated optic neuritis cases experience complete recovery. The combination of limited recovery and high recurrence rate leads to a dismal visual prognosis. About 60% to 70% of patients with NMO have severe

unilateral vision loss (less than 20/200) in 7 to 11 years (20,22). A recent study found that about 32% of apparent DON cases with severe vision loss (<20/200) at presentation were NMO antibody positive (23). Treatment for NMO frequently requires immunosuppressive therapy and preliminary evidence suggests that interferon beta (IFN-B) may exacerbate NMO, making early distinction important (21). For these reasons, testing for anti-aquaporin-4 antibodies should be considered in all apparent idiopathic DON cases, especially cases with bilateral, recurrent, or severe presentation and in cases with poor visual recovery. Recently, antimyelin oligodendrocyte glycoprotein (anti-MOG) antibodies have been identified in patients with a variety of demyelinating diseases including acute disseminated encephalomyelitis (ADEM), isolated DON, isolated transverse myelitis, recurrent optic neuritis, and aquaporin-4 antibody seronegative NMO (24). While the clinical spectrum of anti–MOG-associated demyelinating disease remains incompletely understood at this time, antibody testing may become more clinically important in the near future.

Serum neuromyelitis optica (NMO) antibody testing should be considered in all idiopathic demyelinating optic neuritis (DON) cases. In cases that are negative, testing for MOG antibodies should be considered in patients with an NMO phenotype or recurrent optic neuritis.

Although vision usually recovers well, many patients with prior DON complain of persistent "faded" vision. Common permanent findings of prior DON include optic atrophy, OCT nerve fiber layer thinning, diminished contrast sensitivity, visual field defects, color vision deficits, and prolonged latency on visual evoked potential (VEP) testing. In both active and recovered DON, patients may complain of temporary visual blurring related to body temperature elevation. Coined "Uhthoff's phenomenon," visual loss occurs owing to heat-related slowing of impulse conduction in ganglion cell axons. Upon normalization of body temperature, the vision recovers within minutes to hours. Despite patient fears, Uhthoff's phenomenon will not precipitate recurrent DON nor result in additional optic nerve damage.

Temporary vision loss related to elevated body temperature is called Uhthoff's phenomenon and is a nonspecific feature of DON.

OCT has quickly transitioned from a research-oriented tool to a valuable clinical test in the care of patients with DON and MS (25). OCT has the ability to accurately measure retinal nerve fiber layer thickness, allowing clinicians to detect subclinical optic atrophy that may not be detectable on vision testing or fundus exam. Eyes that suffer a clinical event of DON will often demonstrate a subtle initial relative thickening of retinal nerve fiber layer (RNFL) at the onset of vision loss. In cases of retrobulbar DON, this acute swelling is impossible to discern on exam but OCT with comparison to the contralateral optic nerve RNFL thickness facilitates diagnosis. The acute relative thickening of RNFL transitions to relative thinning around 2 months and reaches maximal thinning by 3 to 6 months. Interestingly, in MS patients who suffer from unilateral DON, the contralateral "healthy" eye also often demonstrates RNFL thinning as compared to age-matched controls indicating that not all retinal ganglion cell loss in MS occurs as a result of clinically apparent DON. In patients with possible MS, the detection of RNFL thinning in one or both eyes may be a valuable tool in its ability to detect subtle optic nerve atrophy. OCT may also be used as a longitudinal structural correlate of disease burden and may be considered in the long-term treatment decisions of a given MS patient. Similar to new MRI white matter lesions, a pattern of persistent and significant (more than 5 microns) RNFL loss on serial OCTs in medically treated MS patients should raise concern for disease progression from medication failure. Studies have shown a strong correlation between low-contrast visual acuity and RNFL thickness. For every 5 microns of average RNFL thinning, low-contrast visual acuity deteriorates by about one line. Similarly, a change in 5 microns of average RNFL between OCT scans over time may signify disease progression while a new difference in 5 microns of average RNFL between the two eyes may suggest an optic nerve lesion on the side with the lower RNFL value.

> *Thinning of 5 microns of average RNFL:*
>
> - *In one eye compared to the other indicates probable prior optic nerve injury in MS suspects*
> - *In one eye over serial OCTs indicates disease progression in MS patients*
> - *In an eye correlates to about 1 line of low contrast visual acuity loss in MS patients*

In addition to expediting recovery, the ONTT suggested that sequential IV and oral steroid treatment for acute DON is protective against the development of MS for 2 years (7.5% of treated patients vs. 16.7% of untreated controls developed MS) (26). Accordingly, either IV steroids or observation may be considered in low-risk patients with acute DON and a normal brain MRI depending on the severity of vision loss and the patient's functional needs. In DON patients with characteristic white matter changes of MS on MRI, however, IV steroids should be administered for the potential protective effect. While controversial, oral steroids are avoided by most clinicians for the first episode of DON

after the ONTT found that they incur a higher risk of optic neuritis recurrence than no treatment at the 5-year mark (27).

The risk for MS development in patients with isolated DON can be predicted by the presence of characteristic white matter changes on MRI (see Chapter 8). According to the ONTT, the long-term risk of MS in DON patients with a normal brain MRI is 25% whereas the risk is 72% with an abnormal MRI (4). While other risk factors for MS development after clinically isolated syndrome have been identified, MRI remains the most utilized predictor (see Chapters 8 and 9). Early recognition of high-risk patients is important considering the proven safety and efficacy of disease-modifying therapies in preventing the development of MS (see Chapter 11). Patients with DON and characteristic white matter changes should be considered for preventive MS therapy.

Although most patients with DON recover well, relapses and incomplete recovery can lead to debilitating, permanent vision loss. Management in these cases focuses on symptom relief and maximizing residual visual function. Low vision specialists assist patients with moderate-to-severe vision loss and often substantially improve quality of life by offering individualized guidance on vision-enhancing tools such as handheld magnifiers, telescopes, and glare-reducing glasses.

MANAGEMENT: EFFERENT DEMYELINATION

Acute onset diplopia or nystagmus is debilitating and warrants corticosteroid therapy similar to other MS relapses (see Chapter 12). The management of permanent efferent sequelae is challenging and symptom dependent.

Medical treatment for nystagmus remains suboptimal. Nevertheless, some patients will enjoy dampening of nystagmus and visual improvement with medication. While numerous medications have been reported to help MS-associated pendular nystagmus, controlled trials suggest that gabapentin and memantine are the most promising (13). Gabapentin is also reported to be effective in many other nystagmus forms. Other nystagmus forms seen occasionally in MS have been shown to benefit from the following treatments: baclofen for acquired periodic alternating nystagmus; 3,4-diaminopyridine or 4-aminopyridine for downbeat nystagmus; and clonazepam for seesaw nystagmus (13). Prisms can dampen nystagmus that improves with convergence, although this feature is more typical of infantile nystagmus rather than MS-related nystagmus. Although eye muscle surgery has an important role in patients with infantile nystagmus, there is little evidence to support its use in acquired MS-related nystagmus. In the future, an experimental electro-optical device using image stabilization optics to neutralize oscillopsia in pendular nystagmus may become widely available (28).

> *Gabapentin and memantine are first-line medications for the treatment of MS-associated pendular nystagmus.*

Chronic diplopia is a debilitating MS manifestation. Single binocular vision in primary-gaze and down-gaze is most important for daily function and is the goal of both prism therapy and strabismus surgery. Occasionally, the motility disturbance is complex and patching one eye is the only reasonable solution.

Prisms bend light entering the eye to varying amounts, creating single vision for patients with small-angle strabismus. For incomitant strabismus, where the ocular misalignment varies depending on gaze direction, prisms help to create a window of single vision (typically in primary gaze) but may not correct diplopia in all directions. Temporary "stick-on" prisms are inexpensive, lightweight, and easy to apply. Owing to mild visual blurring, however, they are poorly tolerated as a long-term solution. Prisms may also be "ground in" to glasses, providing excellent visual clarity, but are considerably more expensive than temporary prisms. Increased visual distortion and weight inherent with higher power prism glasses (>10–15 prism diopters of total prismatic correction) limit patient satisfaction.

For patients who have chronic large ocular deviations and are dissatisfied with prisms, strabismus surgery may be considered to improve both appearance and binocular function. Similar to prism therapy, strabismus surgery may only achieve a window of single binocular vision in a particular gaze (usually primary gaze). In practice, strabismus surgery is rarely performed in MS patients because of the risk of subsequent events that may produce diplopia again.

SPECIAL CONSIDERATIONS

Retrochiasmatic Demyelination

Demyelination less commonly affects the retrochiasmal visual pathways and is typically asymptomatic. Rarely, large plaques can cause visual field defects. As opposed to DON, retrochiasmatic lesions will present with painless homonymous visual field defects (in both eyes), normal visual acuity, and often occur concomitantly with other neurological deficits. Similar to other MS relapses, recovery of visual field loss is expected. Because visually symptomatic retrochiasmal disease is rare, other MS mimics should be considered including neurosarcoidosis, Lyme disease, syphilis, malignant glioma, and PML. A brain infection attributed to the John Cunningham (JC) virus and occurring mostly in the immunocompromised and those receiving certain immunotherapies, PML frequently involves the retrogeniculate visual pathway. Homonymous hemianopia was the presenting feature in 35% to 45% of PML cases before the HIV epidemic and decreased to an estimated 17% since (29,30). PML is associated with the use of natalizumab and several other MS disease-modifying therapies. While natalizumab-associated PML most commonly presents with cognitive, motor, and language deficits, one study showed that the presenting features included visual impairment in eight of 28 (29%) and hemianopia in 28 (18%) (31). Given these trends, new onset homonymous field defects in MS patients on recent or active natalizumab and other MS disease-modifying therapies should raise concerns for PML (Table 23.4).

TABLE 23.4 Referral Guidelines for Vision Problems in MS[a]

COMPLAINT OR FINDING	APPROPRIATE SPECIALIST	EXPECTED INTERVENTION
Monocular diplopia	General ophthalmologist	Evaluation and treatment for dry eye, cataract, uncorrected astigmatism, and epiretinal membrane
Acute binocular diplopia (if diagnosis unclear)	Neuroophthalmologist	Diagnosis and treatment is case specific
Chronic binocular diplopia with ocular misalignment	Pediatric ophthalmologist or neuroophthalmologist	Alignment measurements for possible prism therapy or rarely strabismus surgery
Acute eye pain, redness, photophobia, and/or new floaters	General ophthalmologist or retinal specialist	Evaluation and treatment for uveitis, posterior vitreous detachment, or retinal detachment
Atypical fundus findings in presumed DON (e.g., severe disc edema or macular pathology)	Neuroophthalmologist, general ophthalmologist, or retinal specialist	Careful dilated examination evaluating for intraocular causes of vision loss including maculopathies
Absence of a relative afferent pupillary defect in presumed DON	Neuroophthalmologist, general ophthalmologist, or retinal specialist	Careful dilated examination evaluating for intraocular causes of vision loss including maculopathies
Metamorphopsia	Neuroophthalmologist, general ophthalmologist, or retinal specialist	Careful dilated examination evaluating for intraocular causes of vision loss including maculopathies
Failure of visual recovery in presumed DON (if diagnosis unclear)	Neuroophthalmologist	Evaluation for DON mimics
Any patient with moderate or severe permanent vision loss limiting activities	Low vision specialist	Low-vision refraction and patient-tailored education on low vision aides
Mild insidious blurred vision that improves with pinhole	Optometrist or general ophthalmologist	Refraction and glasses prescription

[a]These are guidelines. Specialists may vary considerably in scope of practice.
DON, demyelinating optic neuritis.

New-onset homonymous field defects in multiple sclerosis (MS) patients on natalizumab and other MS disease-modifying therapies is suspicious for progressive multifocal leukoencephalopathy (PML).

Uveitis in MS

Intraocular inflammation, or uveitis, occurs 10 times more commonly in MS patients than in the general population. There is an estimated incidence of 1% to 2% in the MS population (32,33). Uveitis may precede or follow the diagnosis of MS. While MS-associated uveitis may affect any segment of the eye, idiopathic intermediate uveitis, or pars planitis, is the most characteristic form (34). Up to 15% of pars planitis cases are associated with MS, and both share an associated human leukocyte antigen (HLA) type (HLA-DR15). Most MS-associated pars planitis is bilateral and occurs in young (aged 20–50) white females. In general, symptoms of uveitis include photophobia, eye pain, blurred vision, and conjunctival injection, or redness. Pars planitis, in contrast, tends to present with a slow, painless increase in floaters and blurred vision. Complications of pars planitis include retinal neovascularization, cystoid ME, epiretinal membrane, cataracts, and retinal detachment. Topical, local, and oral steroids are the mainstay of therapy and allow most patients to retain good vision.

Photophobia, new floaters, and eye irritation are the characteristic symptoms of uveitis.

KEY POINTS FOR PATIENTS AND FAMILIES

- Eye symptoms in MS include loss of vision in one eye (optic neuritis), double vision, a rare red eye due to inflammation of the eye (uveitis), and other visual symptoms.

- Optic neuritis is often treated by a course of high-dose steroids. While this does not affect the long-term outcome, it does speed recovery of visual function.

- Double vision and nystagmus (eye "jumpiness") usually resolves over time but when chronic, it may improve by placing prisms in the glasses or with certain medications.

- Careful ophthalmological screening and follow-up is important for patients using fingolimod (Gilenya) for MS to avoid possible visual changes due to a condition known as macular edema.

REFERENCES

1. The clinical profile of optic neuritis. Experience of the Optic Neuritis Treatment Trial. Optic Neuritis Study Group. *Arch Ophthalmol.* 1991;109(12):1673–1678.
2. Beck RW, Cleary PA. Optic neuritis treatment trial. One-year follow-up results. *Arch Ophthalmol.* 1993;111(6):773–775.
3. Beck RW, Trobe JD, Moke PS, et al. High- and low-risk profiles for the development of multiple sclerosis within 10 years after optic neuritis: experience of the optic neuritis treatment trial. *Arch Ophthalmol.* 2003;121(7):944–949.
4. Optic Neuritis Study Group. Multiple sclerosis risk after optic neuritis: final optic neuritis treatment trial follow-up. *Arch Neurol.* 2008;65(6):727–732.
5. Rizzo JF 3rd, Andreoli CM, Rabinov JD. Use of magnetic resonance imaging to differentiate optic neuritis and nonarteritic anterior ischemic optic neuropathy. *Ophthalmology.* 2002;109(9):1679–1684.
6. Purvin V, Kawasaki A, Jacobson DM. Optic perineuritis: clinical and radiographic features. *Arch Ophthalmol.* 2001;119(9):1299–1306.
7. Jain N, Bhatti MT. Fingolimod-associated macular edema: incidence, detection, and management. *Neurology.* 2012;78(9):672–680.
8. Ross A, Ross AH, Mohamed Q. Review and update of central serous chorioretinopathy. *Curr Opin Ophthalmol.* 2011;22(3):166–173.
9. Bouzas EA, Karadimas P, Pournaras CJ. Central serous chorioretinopathy and glucocorticoids. *Surv Ophthalmol.* 2002;47(5):431–448.
10. Muri RM, Meienberg O. The clinical spectrum of internuclear ophthalmoplegia in multiple sclerosis. *Arch Neurol.* 1985;42(9):851–855.
11. Keane JR. Internuclear ophthalmoplegia: unusual causes in 114 of 410 patients. *Arch Neurol.* 2005;62(5):714–717.
12. Frohman EM, Frohman TC, O'Suilleabhain P, et al. Quantitative oculographic characterisation of internuclear ophthalmoparesis in multiple sclerosis: the versional dysconjugacy index Z score. *J Neurol Neurosurg Psychiatry.* 2002;73(1):51–55.
13. Thurtell MJ, Leigh RJ. Therapy for nystagmus. *J Neuroophthalmol.* 2010;30(4):361–371.
14. Lopez LI, Bronstein AM, Gresty MA, et al. Clinical and MRI correlates in 27 patients with acquired pendular nystagmus. *Brain.* 1996;119(pt 2):465–472.
15. Serra A, Derwenskus J, Downey DL, et al. Role of eye movement examination and subjective visual vertical in clinical evaluation of multiple sclerosis. *J Neurol.* 2003;250(5):569–575.
16. Keane JR. Third nerve palsy: analysis of 1400 personally-examined inpatients. *Can J Neurol Sci.* 2010;37(5):662–670.
17. Thomke F, Lensch E, Ringel K, et al. Isolated cranial nerve palsies in multiple sclerosis. *J Neurol Neurosurg Psychiatry.* 1997;63(5):682–685.
18. Patel SV, Mutyala S, Leske DA, et al. Incidence, associations, and evaluation of sixth nerve palsy using a population-based method. *Ophthalmology.* 2004;111(2):369–375.
19. Peters GB 3rd, Bakri SJ, Krohel GB. Cause and prognosis of nontraumatic sixth nerve palsies in young adults. *Ophthalmology.* 2002;109(10):1925–1928.
20. Merle H, Olindo S, Bonnan M, et al. Natural history of the visual impairment of relapsing neuromyelitis optica. *Ophthalmology.* 2007;114(4):810–815.

21. Morrow MJ, Wingerchuk D. Neuromyelitis optica. *J Neuroophthalmol.* 2012;32(2):154–166.

22. Wingerchuk DM, Hogancamp WF, O'Brien PC, et al. The clinical course of neuromyelitis optica (Devic's syndrome). *Neurology.* 1999;53(5):1107–1114.

23. Lai C, Tian G, Takahashi T, et al. Neuromyelitis optica antibodies in patients with severe optic neuritis in China. *J Neuroophthalmol.* 2011;31(1):16–19.

24. Peschl P, Bradl M, Höftberger R, et al. Myelin oligodendrocyte glycoprotein: deciphering a target in inflammatory demyelinating diseases. *Front Immunol.* 2017;8(8):529.

25. Nolan RC, Narayana K, Galetta SL, et al. Optical coherence tomography for the neurologist. *Semin Neurol.* October 2015;35(5):564–577.

26. Beck RW, Cleary PA, Trobe JD, et al. The effect of corticosteroids for acute optic neuritis on the subsequent development of multiple sclerosis. The Optic Neuritis Study Group. *N Engl J Med.* 1993;329(24):1764–1769.

27. Optic Neuritis Study Group. The 5-year risk of MS after optic neuritis. Experience of the optic neuritis treatment trial. *Neurology.* 1997;49(5):1404–1413.

28. Smith RM, Oommen BS, Stahl JS. Application of adaptive filters to visual testing and treatment in acquired pendular nystagmus. *J Rehabil Res Dev.* 2004;41(3A):313–324.

29. Brooks BR, Walker DL. Progressive multifocal leukoencephalopathy. *Neurol Clin.* 1984;2(2):299–313.

30. Berger JR, Pall L, Lanska D, et al. Progressive multifocal leukoencephalopathy in patients with HIV infection. *J Neurovirol.* 1998;4(1):59–68.

31. Clifford DB, De Luca A, Simpson DM, et al. Natalizumab-associated progressive multifocal leukoencephalopathy in patients with multiple sclerosis: lessons from 28 cases. *Lancet Neurol.* 2010;9(4):438–446.

32. Chen L, Gordon LK. Ocular manifestations of multiple sclerosis. *Curr Opin Ophthalmol.* 2005;16(5):315–320.

33. Edwards LJ, Constantinescu CS. A prospective study of conditions associated with multiple sclerosis in a cohort of 658 consecutive outpatients attending a multiple sclerosis clinic. *Mult Scler.* 2004;10(5):575–581.

34. Zein G, Berta A, Foster CS. Multiple sclerosis-associated uveitis. *Ocul Immunol Inflamm.* 2004;12(2):137–142.

24 Bulbar and Pseudobulbar Dysfunction in Multiple Sclerosis

Devon S. Conway

KEY POINTS FOR CLINICIANS

- Corticobulbar and pseudobulbar pathology can be seen in multiple sclerosis (MS) and often go unrecognized.
- Neurogenic dysphagia can put patients at risk for aspiration pneumonia or other life-threatening complications.
- Noninvasive techniques are available for dysphagia management, but physicians may also want to consider surgical myotomy of the cricopharyngeal muscle, or chemical myotomy with botulinum toxin.
- Paroxysmal ataxia and dysarthria can be treated with agents such as carbamazepine, lamotrigine, or levetiracetam.
- Selective serotonin reuptake inhibitors, amitriptyline, and levodopa have all shown promise in treating pseudobulbar affect (PBA) in MS patients, but data for these agents are limited.
- Dextromorphan/quinidine was shown to be an effective treatment for PBA in MS in a large, randomized, placebo-controlled trial.

The corticobulbar tracts originate in the motor cortex and innervate the motor nuclei of cranial nerves V, VII, IX, X, XI, and XII. Corticobulbar dysfunction can occur in a variety of neurological conditions, including amyotrophic lateral sclerosis (ALS), stroke, and MS. Common symptoms of corticobulbar dysfunction in neurological disease are listed in Table 24.1.

PBA refers to pathological displays of emotion and can affect the MS patient. Other names commonly used to refer to PBA include pathological laughter and crying (PLC), emotional lability, and emotional incontinence. Although the exact anatomic etiology of PBA is unknown, a recent MRI study found patients with PBA were more likely to have lesions affecting the brainstem, bilateral medial

inferior frontal regions, and the bilateral inferior parietal regions (1). It is thought that such lesions may result in impaired inhibition of emotional display, thereby resulting in the characteristic features of PBA.

Corticobulbar and pseudobulbar dysfunction often go unrecognized in MS patients. It is important to remain mindful of these complications, as there are a number of possible interventions that may improve quality of life.

DYSPHAGIA

Swallowing is a complex motor task that involves moving food from the oral cavity to the stomach while simultaneously providing airway protection from aspiration. It is typically described as comprising four phases based on the location of the bolus: oral preparatory, oral, pharyngeal, and esophageal. Neurogenic dysphagia can occur in MS and can result in a number of complicating factors such as weight loss and decreased quality of life. Of special concern in MS patients with dysphagia is the risk of aspiration pneumonia. In one study, 62% of patients dying from a known complication of MS died from pneumonia (2).

TABLE 24.1   Common Corticobulbar Symptoms in Neurological Disease

- Dysphagia
- Dysarthria
- Laryngospasm
- Weakness of the facial muscles and tongue

Neurogenic dysphagia can cause life-threatening complications.

A number of brain structures are involved in the process of chewing and swallowing. These include the sensorimotor and premotor cortex, which project through the corticobulbar tracts to the nuclei of the trigeminal, facial, glossopharyngeal, vagal, and hypoglossal cranial nerves (3). The nucleus tractus solitarius and the nucleus ambiguus are the most important portions of the brainstem in the facilitation of normal swallowing. Proper swallowing depends on the interaction of sensory and motor functions as well as the interaction of voluntary and involuntary aspects of the process (4).

A number of groups have attempted to quantify the prevalence of dysphagia in MS patients. An early study of 525 patients (Expanded Disability Status Scale [EDSS] scores from 0 to 9.5) found that 43% had neurogenic dysphagia (5). A later study of 143 MS patients by Calcagno et al. found dysphagia in 49 of them (34.3%) (6). Interestingly, severe brainstem involvement from MS was associated with increased risk of dysphagia (odds ratio [OR] = 3.24, confidence interval [CI] = 1.44–7.31). Also, those with an EDSS score above 6.5 had increased risk of dysphagia compared to less affected patients (OR = 2.99, CI = 1.36–6.59). In the 46 patients with mild or moderate dysphagia, compensatory strategies such as postural changes and modifying the volume, quantity, and speed of food presentation were sufficient to avoid aspiration.

Brainstem involvement and greater disability levels are associated with dysphagia.

Thomas and Wiles surveyed 79 MS patients admitted to the hospital (24 at the diagnostic admission and 55 with established disease) (7). A standardized water swallowing test was administered and 43% of the MS patients were found to have abnormal swallowing. This constituted 29% of the newly diagnosed patients and 49% of those with established MS. While certain survey questions strongly predicted the presence of dysphagia (e.g., "episodes of coughing after eating or drinking" or "food going down the wrong way"), there were a number of false negative responses as well, suggesting that some patients might be unaware of their swallowing dysfunction.

A more recent study enrolled 308 consecutive patients with relapsing–remitting (RR), secondary progressive (SP), and primary progressive (PP) MS (8). Participants were only considered dysphagic if they had permanent dysphagia, meaning dysphagia outside of an acute relapse.

Permanent dysphagia was detected in 73 (24%) patients. Again, patients with greater disability were more likely to have dysphagia. It was present in 35.4% of those with an EDSS of 8.0 and 95% of those with an EDSS of 9.0. However, permanent dysphagia was observed in patients with an EDSS as low as 2.0.

Dysphagia prevalence in MS has been estimated between 24% and 43%.

Poorjavad et al. attempted to determine the prevalence of different types of swallowing disorders in MS patients (9). Participants were screened with the Northwestern Dysphagia Patient Check Sheet, which can be used to differentiate between pharyngeal or oral stage disorders and can detect aspiration and pharyngeal delay (10). In their cohort of 101 consecutive MS patients, 32 (31.7%) were found to have dysphagia. Pharyngeal stage disorders were found in 28.7% of the cohort, aspiration in 6.9%, oral stage disorders in 5%, and pharyngeal delay in 1%. Dysphagia was significantly more prevalent in patients with a longer disease duration, more cerebellar dysfunction, and in those with higher EDSS scores.

Potential interventions for patients with dysphagia are summarized in Table 24.2. A number of noninvasive techniques are available that may be of use in MS patients with dysphagia. For instance, repetitive exercises that focus on important aspects of swallowing such as mastication, cheek tonization, and movements of the tongue and larynx may be helpful with regard to restitution of the swallowing function (11). Postural changes and swallowing techniques are also available that facilitate swallowing and protection of the airway. For instance, holding the breath while swallowing and exhaling strongly immediately afterward helps to close the vocal cords and prevent aspiration. Finally, modification of the diet may also be useful. For instance, soft textured foods can be used in patients with difficulty in the oral preparation phase of swallowing. Also, use of cooled drinks or thickened liquids may be helpful in those who have choking with thin liquids (11).

TABLE 24.2 Management Options for Dysphagia in MS

- Repetitive exercises focusing on important aspects of swallowing
- Postural changes
- Swallowing techniques that facilitate airway protection
- Diet modification
- Cricopharyngeal muscle myotomy
- Chemical myotomy of the cricopharyngeal muscle with botulinum toxin
- Electrical stimulation of the pharynx

MS, multiple sclerosis.

Speech therapists can teach noninvasive techniques that may improve neurogenic dysphagia.

More invasive options are also available. As indicated, the most prevalent cause of dysphagia in MS patients is incomplete relaxation or defective opening of the upper esophageal sphincter. This can lead to hypopharyngeal retention of the food bolus, putting the patient at risk for aspiration (4). Myotomy of the cricopharyngeal muscle of the upper esophageal sphincter has been described as an effective method of management in patients with neurogenic dysphagia from causes other than MS (12).

A less invasive approach to upper esophageal sphincter dysfunction is chemical myotomy of the cricopharyngeal muscle with botulinum toxin (BTX). One study identified 25 MS patients with dysphagia (13). Video fluoroscopy was performed and demonstrated that 14 of them had signs of upper esophageal sphincter hyperactivity, such as reduced pharyngeal clearance and incomplete cricopharyngeal opening. Following BTX injection, patients were reassessed using video fluoroscopy and other tools. Dysphagia completely resolved in 10 of the patients and significantly improved in the remaining four. Injections were repeated every 3 to 4 months with sustained benefit. Work has also been done suggesting that electromyography (EMG) can predict which patients with neurogenic dysphagia are most likely to respond to cricopharyngeal muscle BTX injections (4).

Another approach to MS-related dysphagia is treatment with electrical stimulation. A randomized controlled pilot study of pharyngeal stimulation in 20 MS patients with severe dysphagia has been conducted (14). The participants received either 10 minutes of electrical stimulation of the pharynx or 10 minutes of sham stimulation for 5 consecutive days. Significant reductions in the penetration/aspiration scale were observed among the participants receiving electrical stimulation, but not among the control group. The difference was most pronounced immediately after the stimulation, but an effect was still seen 4 weeks later. Larger studies are necessary to verify this benefit and establish electrical stimulation as a treatment option for MS patients with dysphagia.

DYSARTHRIA

Dysarthria is dysfunction in the initiation, control, or coordination of speech. Speech production requires coordination of the lips, tongue, mandible, soft palate, vocal cords, and diaphragm and all of these actions can be impacted by MS. Three types of dysarthria are common in MS: spastic dysarthria (characterized by a harsh and strained vocal quality), ataxic dysarthria (characterized by vocal tremor and variable loudness), and mixed dysarthria, which has features of both spastic and ataxic dysarthrias.

The prevalence of dysarthria in MS has not been well studied. Shibasaki et al. characterized the initial neurological symptoms of 204 British and 60 Japanese patients with probable MS at the time of presentation (15). In this series, 3% of the patients presented with a speech disturbance. A later study was conducted with 77 MS patients including a mix of PPMS, SPMS, and RRMS (16). EDSS scores varied between 1.0 and 9.0. Participants underwent the clinical dysarthria test procedure, which assesses respiration, phonation, oral motor performance, articulation, prosody, and intelligibility (17). The study found that no patients had profound dysarthria, 8% had moderate-to-severe dysarthria, 37% had mild or moderate dysarthria, and 55% had none or minimal speech deviation. After correcting for dropouts, the true prevalence of dysarthria in MS patients was estimated to be 51%.

There is scarce evidence about the value of interventions for dysarthria in MS. However, a recent study evaluated the benefits of clear (exaggerated or hyperarticulation), loud, and slow speech in MS patients with mild dysarthria. Loud and clear speech were found to significantly improve intelligility relative to baseline (18). Early speech therapy, to educate patients on such techniques, is recommended (19).

Dysarthria may have a prevalence as high as 51% in MS.

Patients with MS are also at risk for developing paroxysmal dysarthria (20). Paroxysmal dysarthria typically lasts for a few seconds, and can occur frequently throughout the day. It is often accompanied by episodic ataxia, in which case it is referred to as paroxysmal dysarthria and ataxia (PDA). Most case reports of these conditions have described a midbrain lesion, which is the presumed etiology (20,21).

Paroxysmal events in MS are poorly understood but are thought to be secondary to ephaptic spread affecting the damaged neurons. Given this, membrane stabilizers such as carbamazepine have been used to treat PDA. One case series of three patients with paroxysmal dysarthria or PDA showed resolution of attacks after administration of carbamazepine 200 to 400 mg daily (20). Another case series with two patients found a similar benefit for carbamazepine (21). However, in both case series, the resolution occurred on the order of weeks to months and may simply reflect repair of the causative lesion.

MS patients may develop paroxysmal dysarthria and ataxia, which may respond to carbamazepine or lamotrigine.

A similar case of a 36-year-old woman with a 14-year history of MS has been reported (22). The patient developed paroxysmal dysarthria that became more frequent despite treatment with methylprednisolone. After treatment with carbamazepine 600 mg/d for 10 days led to no improvement, the patient was converted to lamotrigine 100 mg/d. Lamotrigine led to substantial reduction in her paroxysmal events and nearly complete resolution in 2 weeks. Successful treatment of PDA with levetiracetam has also been described (23).

PSEUDOBULBAR AFFECT

PBA is characterized by involuntary and inappropriate outbursts of emotional expression that do not properly align with the patient's emotional state. It is observed in a number of neurological conditions including stroke, ALS, traumatic brain injury, and MS (24). The pathophysiology of PBA is incompletely understood. According to one prominent theory, dysfunction in a corticopontinecerebellar circuit is the cause of PBA symptoms (25). Via this circuit, emotional expression is controlled by the cerebellum, which appropriately modulates the level of emotional response according to the situation. Disruption of the corticopontinecerebellar connections lowers the threshold for emotional response, and can predispose the individual to inappropriate outbursts (26).

Few studies have investigated the prevalence of PBA in MS. Further, comparison between studies can be confounded by inconsistent definitions of what constitutes PBA and the numerous competing terms for the syndrome such as PLC, emotional incontinence, and emotional lability. The most commonly cited investigation enrolled 152 consecutive outpatients that were screened by two neurologists for the presence of PLC (27). To receive this diagnosis, patients had to display a sudden loss of emotional control on multiple occasions in response to nonspecific stimuli and without a matching mood state. Fifteen of the subjects had PLC, a point prevalence of 9.9%. The patients with PLC were more likely to be in the progressive phase of MS and to have more physical disability (mean EDSS 6.0 vs. 4.7, $p = .03$). Also, patients with PLC were not more likely than controls to have a premorbid or a family history of mental illness. A Croatian study used the Center for Neurologic Stability Lability Scale to detect PBA in 79 MS patients undergoing inpatient rehabilitation. The study found a PBA prevalence of 41.8% in their inpatient population, with it occurring more commonly in women and patients with SPMS (28).

PBA is believed to have a prevalence of about 10% in MS patients.

A number of treatments have been proposed for PBA in patients with neurological disease, including selective serotonin reuptake inhibitors (SSRIs). One case series followed 10 patients: four with ALS, four with MS, and two with stroke (29). All included patients had more than 30 affective outbursts daily prior to study entry. The patients were treated with 100 mg of the SSRI fluvoxamine daily. Within 2 to 6 days, all patients' affective outbursts had decreased to five or less per day.

Levodopa has also been considered for the treatment of PLC in neurological disease. One study enrolled 25 patients with pathological crying, pathological laughing, or both (30). The cause was cerebrovascular disease in 23 patients and brain trauma in the remaining two. In 10 of the 25 patients treated with levodopa, there was complete resolution of PLC. All but four of the remaining patients had a partial response to the levodopa.

Finally, amitriptyline has been compared to placebo in a double-blind crossover trial. Seventeen MS patients with PLC were enrolled but only 12 completed the study (31). Patients were randomly assigned to receive 30 days of placebo or amitriptyline at a goal dose of 75 mg. This was followed by a 1 week washout period and then 30 days of the alternative option. A spouse or close family member kept a daily count of the number of episodes of inappropriate emotional outbursts. In eight patients, the number of episodes of PLC was reduced to zero while on active treatment, whereas four patients had more episodes on drug than off.

Case series have shown efficacy of SSRIs, levodopa, and amitriptyline in treating MS-associated PBA.

While these and similar studies provide promising preliminary results for the treatment of PBA/PLC in neurological disease, they suffer from a number of methodological problems. Most studies have had a limited sample size that includes patients with neurological diseases other than MS. Also, for the most part, the studies were not randomized placebo-controlled trials and instead involved a pre–post analysis. Hence, the results may not be specific to MS and the studies are prone to bias.

The largest randomized controlled trial of a PBA treatment in an exclusively MS population involved dextromethorphan/quinidine (DMQ) (32). A prior study of DMQ showed it to be effective in a combined sample of 326 MS and ALS patients (24). Dextromethorphan is a sigma-1 receptor agonist as well as a noncompetitive antagonist of the N-methyl-D-aspartate receptor (32). Through its activity, glutamate influence is attenuated. Dextromethorphan is rapidly metabolized to dextrorphan by cytochrome P450 2D6. Quinidine is a cytochrome P450 2D6 inhibitor, and is included to allow for steady concentrations of dextromethorphan.

The inclusion criteria included a diagnosis of MS and a clinical diagnosis of PBA. Participants were also required to have a score of 13 or more on the Center for Neurologic Study—Lability Scale (CNS-LS). This scale provides a score for PBA ranging from 7 to 35 and has been validated in MS (33).

A total of 150 participants were enrolled and were randomized 1:1 to either DMQ or placebo. The primary efficacy variable was mean reduction in the CNS-LS score, which was assessed four times between 15 and 85 days from treatment initiation. The mean reduction was 7.7 points for the active treatment group and 3.3 points for the placebo group ($p < .0001$). Secondary outcomes included quality of life, quality of relationships, and pain intensity, all assessed using visual analog scales. There was significant benefit in all three of these outcomes for the active treatment group versus placebo.

> *Dextromethorphan/quinidine was shown to be an effective treatment for PBA in MS in a large, randomized, placebo-controlled trial.*

With respect to safety, the most commonly reported adverse events from three large trials of DMQ included dizziness (18.2%–26.3%) and nausea (12.7%–32.9%) (34). When prescribing DMQ, one should consider whether the patient is already on a cytochrome P4502D6 inhibitor such as fluoxetine. In such cases, it may be appropriate to prescribe dextromethorphan alone given that quinidine's only role is to inhibit the same enzyme (35).

A summary of treatment options for PBA in MS is provided in Table 24.3, along with the level of evidence supporting each medication.

TABLE 24.3   Treatment Options and Evidence Level for PBA in MS

MEDICATION	GOAL DOSE	EVIDENCE LEVEL
Fluvoxamine	100 mg daily	Level 3
Levodopa	0.6–1.5 g daily	Level 3
Amitriptyline	75 mg daily	Level 3
Dextromethorphan/quinidine	30 mg/30 mg twice daily*	Level 1

*The commercially available formulation, Nuedexta, contains dextromethorphan 20 mg and quinidine 10 mg and is dosed twice daily.

MS, multiple sclerosis; PBA, pseudobulbar affect.

PATIENT CASE   A 24-year-old woman with no significant medical history comes to the clinic complaining of 1 week of transient episodes of slurred speech. She has never had a neurological episode previously.

Question: What evaluation is needed?

Answer: The case is concerning for transient ischemic attack. An MRI/magnetic resonance angiography (MRA) of the brain would be recommended both to rule out stroke and to evaluate for any flow limiting stenoses. Given the patient's age, the MRI would also be helpful in evaluating for demyelinating disease and it would be reasonable to administer gadolinium.

Question: The MRI is negative for stroke and the MRA is normal. However, the MRI does show a mild-to-moderate lesion burden of ovoid periventricular lesions and juxtacortical lesions. There is an enhancing midbrain lesion near the right red nucleus. What should the next step be?

Answer: The patient appears to have multiple sclerosis (MS) and is likely experiencing paroxysmal dysarthria as a result of her midbrain lesion. Given the active enhancement, a course of intravenous (IV) methylprednisolone, 1,000 mg daily for 3 to 5 days followed by a prednisone taper would be reasonable.

Question: After treatment with corticosteroids, the patient continues to experience paroxysmal dysarthria. What management options are available?

Answer: Treatment with carbamazepine or lamotrigine may help to resolve the episodes.

KEY POINTS FOR PATIENTS AND FAMILIES

- Corticobulbar dysfunction can affect many key functions such as swallowing and speaking.

- Speech therapy is an important and effective mechanism for counteracting the effects of corticobulbar dysfunction.

- For patients with swallowing difficulties despite speech therapy, more invasive options that involve surgery or injections can be considered.

- Some multiple sclerosis patients may develop intermittent episodes of incoordination and slurred speech. This is treatable with medications.

- Pseudobulbar affect can affect multiple sclerosis patients and causes them to express emotions that may be inappropriate and do not correspond to how they are actually feeling.

- A number of medications may help pseudobulbar affect, of which dextromethorphan/ quinidine has the best evidence.

REFERENCES

1. Ghaffar O, Chamelian L, Feinstein A. Neuroanatomy of pseudobulbar affect : a quantitative MRI study in multiple sclerosis. *J Neurol*. 2008;255(3):406–412.

2. Sadovnick AD, Eisen K, Ebers GC, et al: Cause of death in patients attending multiple sclerosis clinics. *Neurology*. 1991;41(8):1193–1196.

3. Tassorelli C, Bergamaschi R, Buscone S, et al. Dysphagia in multiple sclerosis: from pathogenesis to diagnosis. *Neurol Sci*. 2008;29(suppl 4):S360–S363.

4. Alfonsi E, Merlo IM, Ponzio M, et al. An electrophysiological approach to the diagnosis of neurogenic dysphagia: implications for botulinum toxin treatment. *J Neurol Neurosurg Psychiatry*. 2010;81(1):54–60.

5. Abraham S, Scheinberg LC, Smith CR, et al. Neurologic impairment and disability status in outpatients with multiple sclerosis reporting dysphagia symptomatology. *J Neuro Rehab*. 1997;11(1):7–13.

6. Calcagno P, Ruoppolo G, Grasso MG, et al. Dysphagia in multiple sclerosis—prevalence and prognostic factors. *Acta Neurol Scand*. 2002;105(1):40–43.

7. Thomas FJ, Wiles CM. Dysphagia and nutritional status in multiple sclerosis. *J Neurol*. 1999;246(8):677–682.

8. De Pauw A, Dejaeger E, D'hooghe B, et al. Dysphagia in multiple sclerosis. *Clin Neurol Neurosurg*. 2002;104(4):345–351.

9. Poorjavad M, Derakhshandeh F, Etemadifar M, et al. Oropharyngeal dysphagia in multiple sclerosis. *Mult Scler*. 2010;16(3):362–365.

10. Logemann JA, Veis S, Colangelo L. A screening procedure for oropharyngeal dysphagia. *Dysphagia*. 1999;14(1):44–51.

11. Prosiegel M, Schelling A, Wagner-Sonntag E: Dysphagia and multiple sclerosis. *Int MS J*. 2004;11(1):22–31.

12. Duranceau A. Criocpharyngeal myotomy in the management of neurogenic and muscular dysphagia. *Neuromuscul Disord*. 1997;7(suppl 1):S85–S89.

13. Restivo DA, Marchese-Ragona R, Patti F, et al. Botulinum toxin improves dysphagia associated with multiple sclerosis. *Eur J Neurol*. 2011;18(3):486–490.

14. Restivo DA, Casabona A, Centonze D, et al. Pharyngeal electrical stimulation for dysphagia associated with multiple sclerosis: a pilot study. *Brain Stimul*. 2013;6(3):418–423.

15. Shibasaki H, McDonald WI, Kuroiwa Y. Racial modification of clinical picture of multiple sclerosis: comparison between British and Japanese patients. *J Neurol Sci*. 1981;49(2):253–271.

16. Hartelius L, Runmarker B, Andersen O. Prevalence and characteristics of dysarthria in a multiple-sclerosis incidence cohort: relation to neurological data. *Folia Phoniatr Logop*. 2000;52(4):160–177.

17. Hartelius L, Svensson P. *Dysarthria Test*. Stockholm, Sweden: Psykologiforlaget; 1990.

18. Tjaden K, Sussman JE, Wilding GE. Impact of clear, loud, and slow speech on scaled intelligibility and speech severity in Parkinson's disease and multiple sclerosis. *J Speech Lang Hear Res*. 2014;57(3):779–792.

19. Langhorne P, Bernhardt J, Kwakkel G. Stroke rehabilitation. *Lancet*. 2011;377(9778):1693–1702.

20. Blanco Y, Compta Y, Graus F, et al. Midbrain lesions and paroxysmal dysarthria in multiple sclerosis. *Mult Scler*. 2008;14(5):694–697.

21. Li Y, Zeng C, Luo T. Paroxysmal dysarthria and ataxia in multiple sclerosis and corresponding magnetic resonance imaging findings. *J Neurol*. 2011;258(2):273–276.

22. Valentino P, Nistico R, Pirritano D, et al. Lamotrigine therapy for paroxysmal dysarthria caused by multiple sclerosis: a case report. *J Neurol*. 2011;258(7):1349–1350.

23. Goodwin SJ, Carpenter AF. Successful treatment of paroxysmal ataxia and dysarthria in multiple sclerosis with levetiracetam. *Mult Scler Relat Disord*. 2016;1079–1081.

24. Pioro EP, Brooks BR, Cummings J, et al. Dextromethorphan plus ultra low-dose quinidine reduces pseudobulbar affect. *Ann Neurol*. 2010;68(5):693–702.

25. Parvizi J, Coburn KL, Shillcutt SD, et al. Neuroanatomy of pathological laughing and crying: a report of the American Neuropsychiatric Association Committee on Research. *J Neuropsychiatry Clin Neurosci*. 2009;21(1):75–87.

26. Miller A, Pratt H, Schiffer RB. Pseudobulbar affect: the spectrum of clinical presentations, etiologies and treatments. *Expert Rev Neurother*. 2011;11(7):1077–1088.

27. Feinstein A, Feinstein K, Gray T, et al. Prevalence and neurobehavioral correlates of pathological laughing and crying in multiple sclerosis. *Arch Neurol*. 1997;54(9):1116–1121.

28. Vidovic V, Rovazdi MC, Kraml O, et al. Pseudobulbar affect in multiple sclerosis patients. *Acta Clin Croat*. 2015;54(2):159–163.

29. Iannaccone S, Ferini-Strambi L. Pharmacologic treatment of emotional lability. *Clin Neuropharmacol*. 1996;19(6):532–535.

30. Udaka F, Yamao S, Nagata H, et al. Pathologic laughing and crying treated with levodopa. *Arch Neurol*. 1984;41(10):1095–1096.

31. Schiffer RB, Herndon RM, Rudick RA. Treatment of pathologic laughing and weeping with amitriptyline. *N Engl J Med*. 1985;312(23):1480–1482.

32. Panitch HS, Thisted RA, Smith RA, et al. Randomized, controlled trial of dextromethorphan/quinidine for pseudobulbar affect in multiple sclerosis. *Ann Neurol*. 2006;59(5):780–787.

33. Smith RA, Berg JE, Pope LE, et al. Validation of the CNS emotional lability scale for pseudobulbar affect (pathological laughing and crying) in multiple sclerosis patients. *Mult Scler*. 2004;10(6):679–685.

34. Schoedel KA, Morrow SA, Sellers EM. Evaluating the safety and efficacy of dextromethorphan/quinidine in the treatment of pseudobulbar affect. *Neuropsychiatr Dis Treat*. 2014;10:1161–1174.

35. McGrane I, VandenBerg A, Munjal R. Treatment of pseudobulbar affect with fluoxetine and dextromethorphan in a woman with multiple sclerosis. *Ann Pharmacother*. 2017;1060028017720746.

25 Pain Management in Multiple Sclerosis

John F. Foley, Ryan R. Metzger, Kara Menning, Cortnee Roman, and Emily N. Stuart

---

KEY POINTS FOR CLINICIANS

- Pain is a common symptom in multiple sclerosis (MS).
- Pain may occur with primary demyelination as well as indirect musculoskeletal compromise.
- Acute MS relapses may produce pain (e.g., optic neuritis, dysesthesia, or Lhermitte's sign).
- Central neuropathic pain (CNP) occurs in up to 28% of MS patients, and most commonly involves the lower extremities.
- CNP is often associated with spinal cord plaque, and is most often amenable to treatment similar to that used to treat peripheral neuropathic pain.
- Trigeminal neuralgia is related to demyelination in the trigeminal nerve root entry zone, and is amenable to medical and surgical interventions.

PREVALENCE AND IMPACT OF PAIN IN MULTIPLE SCLEROSIS

Once thought to be an uncommon symptom in MS, we now know that pain is frequently reported by patients living with this disease. Pain may occur as a result of an acute relapse, or on a chronic daily basis as a result of long-standing neurological insult. It may represent the central presenting symptom of MS, or it may develop much later in the disease course. The estimated prevalence of pain in MS patients reported in the literature ranges from 29% to 86% (1–7). It has been estimated that almost one-half of MS patients report chronic pain, with some studies showing that its occurrence increases with age and disease duration (6,8,9). One study found pain to be present twice as often in women with relapsing-remitting MS (RRMS) compared to healthy women, with pain intensity over 7 days twice as high (10). A systematic review of 28 studies (7,101 subjects) estimated overall pain prevalence to be 63% in MS, with additional estimates of specific pain syndromes as follows: headache 43%, neuropathic extremity pain 26%, back pain 20%, Lhermitte's sign 16%, painful spasms 15%, and trigeminal neuralgia (TN) 3.8% (6). This is reflected in clinical practice, as well, with many office visits centering on evaluating and treating a patient's pain.

There is no doubt that pain adversely affects quality of life. For many MS patients, pain is often widespread, chronic, severe, and frequently interferes with sleep, occupational performance, and recreation (1,8). There also appears to be a connection between higher pain levels and worsened fatigue and depression (10–12). Pain also creates an economic burden resulting from direct medical expenses and productivity loss. One year's financial expenditure for patients with neuropathic pain is up to three times higher than those without pain, with far more frequent office visits per year (13).

MECHANISMS OF PAIN IN MS AND CLINICAL PRESENTATIONS

Multiple potential pain generators exist with MS. Pain can occur as a primary result of demyelination along the neuraxis, and is often mediated by dorsal root neurons radiating via the spinothalamic tract to the thalamus. Projections from the thalamus include the medial system with radiations to the locus coeruleus, periaquaductal gray matter, thalamic nuclei, insula, secondary somatosensory cortex, hippocampus, amygdala, and hypothalamus (14). This system processes the emotional and cognitive aspects of pain. The lateral system processes the sensory discriminative elements of the signal and flows through the lateral thalamus, somatosensory cortex, parietal operculum, and insula (14).

Abnormal amplification of normal axonal pain transmission can produce enhanced pain perception. MS plaque may interrupt descending inhibitory pain fibers (15). The immune process may also directly produce a central pain response (16,17). Generation of pain produced by activation of nonpain sensory receptors is called *allodynia*. Exaggeration of painful stimuli is known as *hyperalgesia*. This central sensitization phenomenon is poorly understood. Secondary pain syndromes can be related to asymmetric load carrying or hypertonicity-producing musculoskeletal activation of peripheral pain receptors. Headache seems to also occur with increased frequency in MS, though pathophysiological mechanisms remain poorly understood and certain disease-modifying treatments may increase prevalence (18–21). Recognition of pain type by the clinician is important for appropriate intervention, keeping in mind that different pain types often coexist in the same patient. Specific pain syndromes are listed in Table 25.1.

TABLE 25.1 Pain Syndromes Associated With MS

PAIN SYNDROME	CHARACTERISTICS
Central neuropathic pain	Chronic, worsened with relapse
Dysesthetic extremity pain	Generally chronic
Trigeminal/Glossopharyngeal/ Occipital neuralgia	Generally paroxysmal
Lhermitte's phenomenon	Paroxysmal
Pseudoradicular pain	Chronic or paroxysmal
Musculoskeletal	Chronic
Visceral pain	Chronic or paroxysmal
Headache	Chronic or paroxysmal
Optic neuritis pain[a]	Associated with relapse
Painful tonic spasm[a]	Generally paroxysmal

MS, multiple sclerosis.
[a]Discussed in other chapters.

ASSESSMENT OF PAIN IN MS

The management of MS-related pain can be a challenge, and often requires patient-specific tailoring, trial and error, and frequent reassessment. When assessing pain severity in patients, quantification is helpful, even if the responses obtained are ultimately subjective. A number of simple pain scales exist to help with the quantification of a patient's pain perception, such as the pain Visual Analogue Scale (VAS), Numeric Rating Scale, and Verbal Rating Scale (22). Questionnaires such as the Brief Pain Inventory and the McGill Pain Assessment Questionnaire can be utilized to assess in more detail the characteristics of the pain (23). In addition, patient-reported outcome (PRO) surveys that address how pain impacts quality of life and everyday functioning can help the clinician better ascertain the degree to which the patient is affected by their pain. Such instruments include PROMIS (Patient-Reported Outcomes Measurement Information System) measures, the Medical Outcomes

36-Item Short-Form Health Survey (SF-36), and the Pain Effects Scale (PES) (24). The PES is a six-item self-report questionnaire that can be completed by the patient within a few minutes (see Figure 25.1). This scale provides insight into the way pain interferes with mood, mobility, sleep, and activities of daily living, and can be readministered to assess changes over time (25). Patients with upper extremity or visual impairments can have questionnaires administered as an interview.

CENTRAL NEUROPATHIC PAIN

The prevalence of CNP in the MS population may be as high as 28% (26). In one study, among those reporting CNP, pain occurred in the lower extremities in 87% of cases, and in the upper extremities for 31%. Pain was bilateral in most cases (76%), and occurred daily in the far majority (88%) (26). Dysesthesias are described as a constant, burning discomfort, which can be symmetric or asymmetric, usually affecting the lower limbs, and can also present as increased sensitivity to touch. Paresthesias are most often described as a "pins and needles" sensation, but can also present as aching, throbbing, stabbing, shooting, tightness, or numbness (24). Dysesthesias and paresthesias are most commonly felt in the limbs, but may also occur elsewhere.

CNP management requires frequent assessments, managing expectations, and finding a regimen that is effective without causing too many treatment-related debilitating side effects. Nonpharmacological interventions may also be beneficial. Physical therapy, regular exercise, relaxation, stretching, massage therapy, hypnotherapy, and psychological intervention should be introduced where felt appropriate. Most therapeutic agents utilized for treatment of CNP have been coopted from the peripheral pain trials, or from studies in other central nervous system conditions. Dysesthesias and paresthesias can usually be treated with antiepileptics or tricyclic antidepressants. Sometimes, combinations of medications with different mechanisms of action are needed to adequately control pain symptoms without causing side effects such as sedation (23). Figure 25.2 describes the treatment algorithm utilized by our clinic.

Of particular importance, the use of opioids for treatment of pain should be reserved for third-line pharmacological therapy due to the significant potential for drug dependence, overdose, and impact on quality of life. Furthermore, when prescribing opioids, it is suggested that clinicians follow the most up-to-date recommendations for best practices that have been developed in response to the recent opioid-related public health emergency. Such guidelines include elements to help ensure safe and effective therapy such as a patient treatment agreement, screening for prior or current substance abuse or misuse, screening for depression, tracking pain and function to recognize tolerance and effectiveness, and tracking

INSTRUCTIONS

Individuals with MS can sometimes experience unpleasant sensory symptoms as a result of their MS (e.g., pain, tingling, burning). The next set of questions covers pain and other unpleasant sensations, and how they affect you. Please circle the one number (0, 1, 2, ...) that best indicates the extent to which your sensory symptoms (including pain) interfered with that aspect of your life during the past 4 weeks. If you need help in marking your responses, tell the interviewer the number of the best response (or what to fill in). Please answer every question. If you are not sure which answer to select, please choose the one answer that comes closest to describing you. The interviewer can explain any words or phrases that you do not understand.

During the past 4 weeks, how much did these symptoms interfere with your...

		Not at all	A little	Moderately	Quite a bit	To an extreme degree
1.	mood	1	2	3	4	5
2.	ability to walk or move around	1	2	3	4	5
3.	sleep	1	2	3	4	5
4.	normal work (both outside your home and at home)	1	2	3	4	5
5.	recreational activities	1	2	3	4	5
6.	enjoyment of life	1	2	3	4	5

FIGURE 25.1 MOS pain effects scale. MOS, medical outcomes study; MS, multiple sclerosis.

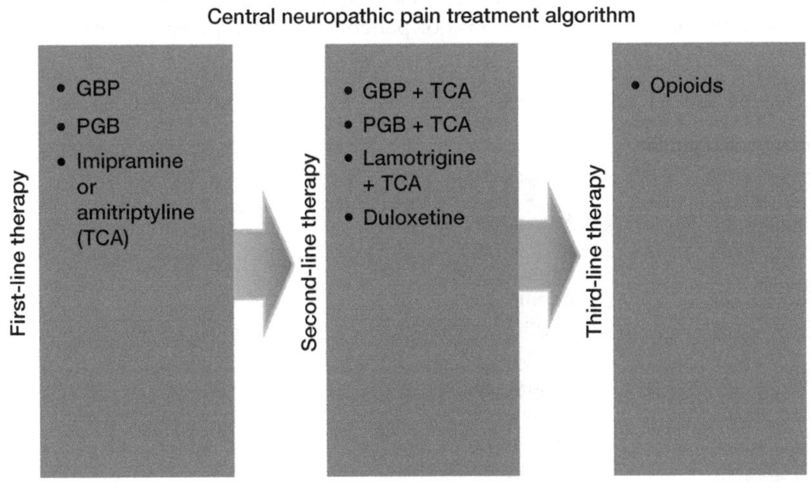

Central neuropathic pain treatment algorithm

First-line therapy
- GBP
- PGB
- Imipramine or amitriptyline (TCA)

Second-line therapy
- GBP + TCA
- PGB + TCA
- Lamotrigine + TCA
- Duloxetine

Third-line therapy
- Opioids

FIGURE 25.2 Algorithm for the pharmacological management of CNP in MS. CNP, central neuropathic pain; GBP, gabapentin; MS, multiple sclerosis; PGB, pregabalin, TCA, tricyclic antidepressant.

daily morphine-equivalent doses using an online dosing calculator (27).

Currently, class 1 clinical trials for pharmacological management of MS-related CNP by cannabinoid therapies are being conducted (28–32). Though there are greater than 60 cannabinoid compounds present in *Cannabis sativa* (cannabis), the main psychoactive ingredient, tetrahydrocannabinol (THC), and the nonpsychoactive ingredient, cannabidiol (CBD), are the current agents of medical interest for MS (33,34). Between 2004 and 2015, four out of five clinical trials investigating the impact of THC/CBD on CNP in MS reported a statistically significant reduction in pain (28–32). However, this does not necessarily mean cannabinoids are a suitable therapy for CNP. Although the reductions in CNP observed with cannabinoid treatment reached statistical significance in these trials, the actual clinical reduction of pain was small, and likely no better than that achieved by other agents currently utilized for pain

(28,30–32,35). In addition, methodological issues were present in many of these studies, including small sample size, nonstandard follow-up periods, large placebo effect, and a wide range of doses utilized (35). And though serious adverse effects were rare in these studies, cannabinoids may still carry a significant risk of cognitive impairment and psychotic illness (36,37). Thus, the American Academy of Neurology currently supports continued rigorous research to evaluate the safety and effectiveness of cannabinoid therapies, but does not advocate for the use of such therapies for neurological disorders such as MS at this time (38).

Trigeminal Neuralgia

TN occurs more frequently (typically 2%–4%) (3,6,39) and more often is bilateral (up to 18%) (40) in the MS population. TN may be the presenting symptom at the time of MS diagnosis (41). Lesions in the region of the trigeminal nerve root entry zone (REZ), and possibly the nerve nucleus itself, are felt to be causal to the condition, and vascular compression may further complicate the pathophysiology. Lesions in the REZ may also remain asymptomatic or produce only dysesthesia or hyperalgesia without classic TN (42). Clinical symptoms of TN may include hyperesthesia or hyperalgesia of one or several facial nerve segments. The pain occurs unilaterally along the path of the trigeminal nerve (V1–V3 distribution), and is described as lancinating, burning, shock-like, stabbing, or electrical pain. It is often precipitated by an external stimulus such as a puff of air to the face, chewing, drinking, shaving, brushing one's teeth, or touching the affected side. The pain is typically extremely short in duration, although lower level dysesthesia may persist in the same distribution as the more severe shock-like sensations. TN is one of the most severe pain syndromes of MS.

The mainstay of pharmacological treatment remains carbamazepine, though pain control may diminish with long-term use. If partial control is achieved, the addition of baclofen, imipramine, or valproate to the regimen is sometimes useful. Alternative therapies may include oxcarbamazepine, phenytoin, lamotrigine, or benzodiazepines. In patients refractory to pharmacological therapy, the options of radiofrequency or glycerol rhizotomy can sometimes provide lasting relief (42). In very unusual cases, nerve decompression may also be of benefit (see Figure 25.3).

Lhermitte's Sign

Jean Lhermitte presented the review paper on this phenomenon to the Neurological Society of Paris entitled *Pain of an Electric Character Discharge Following Head Flexion in Multiple Sclerosis* (43). Lhermitte's sign is described as a brief, electric, shock-like sensation extending down the spine, sometimes into the lower extremities, typically triggered by forward flexion of the head. It is a common complaint in the MS population, occurring with a frequency of 9% to 41% (6,44,45). It is generally felt to be related to a lesion of the ascending spinothalamic tract at the cervical level, with MRI showing a cervical spinal cord plaque in more than 95% of patients (45). An increase in pressure

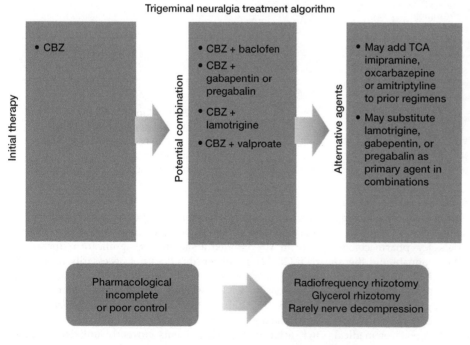

Trigeminal neuralgia treatment algorithm

Initial therapy
- CBZ

Potential combination
- CBZ + baclofen
- CBZ + gabapentin or pregabalin
- CBZ + lamotrigine
- CBZ + valproate

Alternative agents
- May add TCA imipramine, oxcarbazepine or amitriptyline to prior regimens
- May substitute lamotrigine, gabepentin, or pregabalin as primary agent in combinations

Pharmacological incomplete or poor control → Radiofrequency rhizotomy / Glycerol rhizotomy / Rarely nerve decompression

FIGURE 25.3 Algorithm for the management of TN in MS. CBZ, carbamazepine; MS, multiple sclerosis; TCA, tricyclic antidepressant; TN, trigeminal neuralgia.

on the dorsal columns with neck flexion is postulated to produce a transient conduction block, resulting in the dysesthetic sensation radiating down the spine. Therapy involves treatment of the primary MS cervical plaque with steroids if the plaque is acute or subacute, and treatment of the disease with immunomodulators. Symptomatic therapy is generally of limited utility.

PSEUDORADICULAR PAIN

A diagnosis of pseudoradiculopathy related to MS is a diagnosis of exclusion. Careful radiographic evaluation of the spine to rule out root compression is essential. The clinical syndrome in presentation is very similar to that of acute disc herniation. It occurs most typically in lumbar root transition zones, but has been noted in both cervical and thoracic regions (46). It may occur as the first manifestation of MS or years after the diagnosis. It may be constant or paroxysmal, and may be associated with trauma. Intravenous methylprednisolone may help ameliorate symptoms in acute or subacute presentations. CNP modulators are sometimes of assistance in more chronic presentations.

HEADACHE

Headache appears to occur more commonly in the MS population, with the studies done to date recently summarized by O'Connor (13) and Moisset et al. (18). Rolak and Brown (19) found that 52% of MS patients reported headache, with 31% classified as muscle contraction headache and 21% as migraine. Generally, headaches did not correlate with MS relapse. Headache can rarely occur as the presenting symptom in MS. MS-related headache is treated in the same fashion as idiopathic headache and is not further addressed in this chapter.

MUSCULOSKELETAL PAIN

Musculoskeletal pain can present as lower back, joint, or neck pain, and is most often a secondary manifestation of the disease process, exacerbated by poor posture, and body mechanics. If a patient has weakness of one limb, pain can be caused by inadequate attempts to stabilize the trunk with the opposite leg or either the knee or hip joint (23). Wheelchair-bound patients may present with chronic neck or back pain due to immobilization, spasticity, osteoporosis, or malposition. Increased biomechanical stress as well as a shifting of weight to accommodate a weak limb can cause sore muscles, joint pain, neuralgic pain such as occipital neuralgia, or radiculopathy. Orthopedic conditions such as osteoarthritis and osteoporosis, to which MS can indirectly contribute, should be ruled out and managed adequately. Spasticity is another problem frequently seen in this patient population and is addressed in Chapter 29.

In general, musculoskeletal pain is first treated with physical therapy (23) including exercise routines that contain frequent stretching and strengthening activities. Consultation with a physical therapist who is familiar with MS is generally immensely helpful in assessing each patient's needs. Use of durable medical equipment such as limb braces, canes, walkers, and electrical stimulation devices may improve energy conservation and reduce strain. Pharmacological treatment of musculoskeletal pain usually consists of nonsteroidal anti-inflammatory drugs (NSAIDs). Antidepressants and opioids have some support from randomized controlled trials but their long-term efficacy is not widely agreed upon (3). Local infiltrations of steroids and analgesics can be helpful. Orthopedic surgery can be performed if needed (e.g., for severe osteoarthritis), but indications and goals should be carefully assessed, ideally by concertation between the orthopedic surgeon, rehabilitation professionals, and the neurological team (see Figure 25.4).

VISCERAL PAIN

Visceral pain is an infrequent manifestation of MS, occurring in up to 2% of the population, and generally described as aching, bloating, or cramping generally related to constipation (39). This is a diagnosis of exclusion, and standard medical evaluation of the abdomen should be completed prior to settling on this diagnosis. Standard anti-constipation regimens will sometimes improve this problem (see Chapter 27).

Iatrogenic Pain. Treatment-related pain is common. Interferon-related pain may include myalgias, headache, and/or spasticity. By increasing hydration, administering anti-inflammatory medications pre- and postinjection, some discomfort may be minimized or even avoided. Subcutaneous injections can cause site pain, including swelling, tenderness, and bruising. Medications used for symptom management can be contributing factors to secondary pain, mainly headache and gastrointestinal pain, and may require medication adjustment or additional intervention.

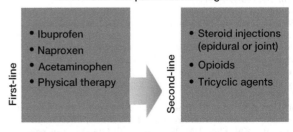

FIGURE 25.4 Algorithm for the management of musculoskeletal pain in MS. MS, multiple sclerosis.

SUMMARY

Pain is a pervasive symptom in MS and often is a major issue compromising quality of life. It is often undertreated and can present in many different fashions. It often is amplified in the setting of comorbid psychiatric disease, frequently seen with MS, and may occur at any stage in the disease. Adequate management requires precise characterization of the pain, realistic goal setting, periodic assessments, and a standardized treatment approach that optimizes pain control and minimizes polypharmacy.

PATIENT CASE A 44-year-old white female presented with a history of multiple sclerosis (MS) since 2003. At that time, she developed a sensation of spiders crawling on her feet and scalp, followed shortly thereafter by severe left-sided facial pain. The pain in the lower extremities evolved to a sensation of "stabbing and burning." The facial pain was described as "knife-like," very brief in duration, recurring multiple times. She had previously been treated with gabapentin, which had produced excessive fatigue. She was started on carbamazepine, which proved partially effective. Dose escalation failed to control the problem. Baclofen and valproate were tried with little efficacy. She was started on oxycarbamazepine 300 mg three times daily with generally fair control. In 2010, she had a relapse of trigeminal pain requiring intravenous (IV) hydromorphone in the emergency room, then oxycodone. He received 3 days of IV methylprednisolone with good improvement. Central neuropathic pain (CNP) in the lower extremities persisted but was attenuated with lamotrigine. In 2008, she experienced significant worsening in her left facial pain and underwent glycerol neurolysis. This resulted in pain freedom until 2010 when she noted electrical jolting pain into the left maxilla. Light touch to the face could bring on the pain. A repeat glycerol neurolysis was undertaken with excellent pain amelioration. She is currently stable with both her lower extremity pain and trigeminal neuralgia.

KEY POINTS FOR PATIENTS AND FAMILIES

- MS may generate a variety of pain syndromes.
- MS-related pain is treatable. Your neurologist can help with finding the right medications and other treatments for you.

REFERENCES

1. Hirsch AT, Turner AP, Ehde DM, et al. Prevalence and impact of pain in multiple sclerosis: physical and psychologic contributors. *Arch Phys Med Rehabil.* 2009;90(4):646–651.
2. Piwko C, Desjardins OB, Bereza BG, et al. Pain due to multiple sclerosis: analysis of prevalence and economic burden in Canada. *Pain Res Manage.* 2007;12(4):259–265.
3. Solaro C, Brichetto G, Amato MP, et al. The prevalence of pain in multiple sclerosis. *Neurology.* 2004;63:919–921.
4. O'Connor AB, Schwid SR, Herrmann DN, et al. Pain associated with multiple sclerosis: systematic review and proposed classification. *Pain.* 2008;137(1):96–111.
5. Truini A, Barbanti P, Pozzilli C, et al. A mechanism-based classification of pain in multiple sclerosis. *J Neurol.* 2013;260(2):351–367.
6. Foley PL, Vesterinen HM, Laird BJ, et al. Prevalence and natural history of pain in adults with multiple sclerosis: systematic review and meta-analysis. *Pain.* 2013;154(5):632–642.
7. Seixas D, Foley P, Palace J, et al. Pain in multiple sclerosis: a systematic review of neuroimaging studies. *NeuroImage Clin.* 2014;5:322–331.
8. Stenager E, Knudsen L, Jensen K. Acute and chronic pain syndromes in multiple sclerosis. *Acta Neurol Scand.* 1991;84(3):197–200.
9. Alschuler KN, Ehde DM, Kratz A, et al. Prevalence of pain and associations with functioning and quality of life in individuals newly-diagnosed with multiple sclerosis. *J Pain.* 2016;17(4):S18–S19.
10. Newland PK, Naismith RT, Ullione M. The impact of pain and other symptoms on quality of life in women with relapsing remitting multiple sclerosis. *J Neurosci Nurs.* 2009;41(6):322–328.
11. Feinstein A, Magalhaes S, Richard JF, et al. The link between multiple sclerosis and depression. *Nat Rev Neurol.* 2014;10(9):507–517.
12. Alschuler KN, Ehde DM, Jensen MP. The co-occurrence of pain and depression in adults with multiple sclerosis. *Rehabil Psychol.* 2013;58(2):217–221.
13. O'Connor AB. Neuropathic pain: quality of life impact, cost and cost effectiveness of therapy. *Pharmacoeconomics.* 2009;27(2):95–112.
14. Scherder E, Wolters E, Polman C, et al. Pain in Parkinson's disease and multiple sclerosis: its relation to the medial and lateral pain systems. *Neurosci Biobehav Rev.* 2005;29(7):1047–1056.
15. White SR, Vyas D, Bieger D, et al. Monoamine-containing fiver plexus in spinal cord of guinea pigs during paralysis, recovery and relapse stages of chronic relapsing experimental allergic encephalomyelitis. *J Neuroimmunol.* 1989;22(3):211–221.
16. Zhang JH, Huang YG. The immune system: a new look at pain. *Chin Med J.* 2006;119:930–938.
17. Wieseler F, Maier SF, Watkins LR. Central proinflammatory cytokines and pain enhancement. *Neurosignals.* 2005;14(4):166–174.
18. Moisset X, Ouchchane L, Guy N, et al. Migraine headaches and pain with neuropathic characteristics: comorbid conditions in patients with multiple sclerosis. *Pain.* 2013;154(12):2691–2699.
19. Rolak L, Brown S. Headaches in multiple sclerosis: a clinical study and review of the literature. *J Neurol.* 1992;237:300–302.

20. La Mantia L, Prone V. Headache in multiple sclerosis and autoimmune disorders. *Neurol Sci.* 2015;36(1):75–78.

21. Terlizzi R, Merli E, Buccellato E, et al. P037. Headache in multiple sclerosis: prevalence and clinical features in a case control-study. *J Headache Pain.* 2015;16(S1):A83.

22. Williamson A, Hoggart B. Pain: a review of three commonly used pain rating scales. *J Clin Nurs.* 2005;14(7):798–804.

23. Fillingim RB, Loeser JD, Baron R, et al. Assessment of chronic pain: domains, methods, and mechanisms. *J Pain.* 2016;17(9):T10–T20.

24. Kenner M, Menon U, Elliot DG. Multiple sclerosis as a painful disease. *Int Rev Neurobiol.* 2007;79:303–321.

25. Ritvo P, Fischer J, Miller D, et al. *MSQLI: Multiple Sclerosis Quality of Life Inventory: A User's Manual.* New York, NY: Nat'l MS Society;1997. https://www.nationalmssociety.org/For-Professionals/Researchers/Resources-for-Researchers/Clinical-Study-Measures/MOS-Pain-Effects-Scale-(PES). Accessed November 1, 2017.

26. Osterberg A, Boivie J, Thuomas KA. Central pain in multiple sclerosis-prevalence and clinical characteristics. *Euro J Pain.* 2005;9(5):531–542.

27. Franklin GM. Opioids for chronic noncancer pain: a position paper of the American Academy of Neurology. *Neurology.* 2014;83(14):1277–1284.

28. Svendsen KB, Jensen TS, Bach FW. Does the cannabinoid dronabinol reduce central pain in multiple sclerosis? Randomised double blind placebo controlled crossover trial. *BMJ.* 2004;329(7460):253.

29. Wade DT, Makela P, Robson P, et al. Do cannabis-based medicinal extracts have general or specific effects on symptoms in multiple sclerosis? A double-blind, randomized, placebo-controlled study on 160 patients. *Mult Scler.* 2004;10(4):434–441.

30. Rog DJ, Nurmikko TJ, Friede T, et al. Randomized, controlled trial of cannabis-based medicine in central pain in multiple sclerosis. *Neurology.* 2005;65(6):812–819.

31. Langford RM, Mares J, Novotna A, et al. A double-blind, randomized, placebo-controlled, parallel-group study of THC/CBD oromucosal spray in combination with the existing treatment regimen, in the relief of central neuropathic pain in patients with multiple sclerosis. *J Neurol.* 2013;260(4):984–997.

32. Turcotte D, Doupe M, Torabi M, et al. Nabilone as an adjunctive to gabapentin for multiple sclerosis-induced neuropathic pain: a randomized controlled trial. *Pain Med.* 2015;16(1):149–159.

33. Mecha M, Feliú A, Carrillo-Salinas FJ, et al. Cannabidiol and multiple sclerosis. In: Preedy V, ed. *Handbook of Cannabis and Related Pathologies.* Cambridge, MA: Elsevier;2017:893–903.

34. Hill KP. Medical marijuana for treatment of chronic pain and other medical and psychiatric problems: a clinical review. *JAMA.* 2015;313(24):2474–2483.

35. Meng H, Johnston B, Englesakis M, et al. Selective cannabinoids for chronic neuropathic pain: a systematic review and meta-analysis. *Anesth Analg.* 2017;125(5):1638–1652.

36. Murray RM, Quigley H, Quattrone D, et al. Traditional marijuana, high-potency cannabis and synthetic cannabinoids: increasing risk for psychosis. *World Psychiatry.* 2016;15(3):195–204.

37. Mizrahi R, Watts JJ, Tseng KY. Mechanisms contributing to cognitive deficits in cannabis users. *Neuropharmacology.* 2017;124:84–88.

38. American Academy of Neurology. Position statement: use of medical marijuana for neurologic disorders. 2014. www.aan.com/policy-and-guidelines/policy/position-statements/medical-marijuana/. Accessed May 30, 2018.

39. Moulin D. Pain in central and peripheral demyelinating disorders: multiple sclerosis and Guillain-Barre syndrome. *Neurol Clin.* 1998;16(4):889–893.

40. Zorro O, Lobato-Polo J, Kano H, et al. Gamma knife radiosurgery for multiple sclerosis-related trigeminal neuralgia. *Neurology.* 2009;73(14):1149–1154.

41. Fallata A, Salter A, Tyry T, et al. Trigeminal neuralgia commonly precedes the diagnosis of multiple sclerosis. *Int J MS Care.* 2017;19(5):240–246.

42. Hooge JP, Redekop WK. Trigeminal neuralgia in multiple sclerosis. *Neurology.* 1995;45(7):1294–1296.

43. Lhermitte J, Bollack J, Nicolas M. Les douleurs à type de décharge électrique à la flexion céphalique dans la sclérose en plaques. *Rev Neurol (Paris).* 1924;2:36–52.

44. Kanchandani R, Howe JG. Lhermitte's sign in multiple sclerosis: a clinical survey and review of the literature. *J Neurol Neurosurg Psychiatry.* 1982;45:308–312.

45. Al-Araji A, Oger J. Reappraisal of Lhermitte's sign in multiple sclerosis. *Mult Scler.* 2005;11:398–402.

46. Ramirez-Lassepas M, Tulloch JW, Quinones MR, et al. Acute radicular pain as a presenting symptom in multiple sclerosis. *Arch Neurol.* 1992;49(3):255–258.

26 | Upper Extremity Function in Multiple Sclerosis

Christine Smith and Kathleen M. Zackowski

KEY POINTS FOR CLINICIANS

- Upper extremity (UE) dysfunction is a common issue for individuals with multiple sclerosis (MS).

- Adequately measuring and treating UE dysfunction is critical for improving function in MS.

- Areas of assessment of the UE which should be considered include strength, sensation, coordination, manual dexterity, and range of motion.

- An occupational therapist can work with individuals to help them maintain their independence and participation in daily tasks and as well as reduce the effects of disability caused by the symptoms of MS.

- Patient/caregiver education is paramount in the successful management of UE dysfunction.

INTRODUCTION

UE dysfunction is a common yet often overlooked issue for individuals with MS. In a study by Kister et al. (1), 60% of participants reported that impaired function of the hand was the most frequently reported symptom in the first year of the disease. UE dysfunction may be present in up to 80% of individuals with MS, yet it is frequently not addressed in the clinical setting (2). This is at least in part due to the weight placed on ambulation and lower limb dysfunction in clinical rating scales such as the Kurtzke Expanded Disability Status Scale (EDSS) (3,4). Dysfunction of the UE is multifactorial, including weakness, spasticity, ataxia, tremor, sensory loss, and pain. When faced with one or more of these symptoms, individuals with MS often present with difficulty performing their activities of daily livings (ADLs) due to the primary or secondary symptoms that affect UE movement and coordination.

It has been shown that the degree of UE dysfunction correlates to an individual's level of independence, negatively impacting quality of life (5). These difficulties may arise even in the initial time following a diagnosis of MS. MS symptoms change with time, affecting the unique capacity each person has for activity and participation. Symptoms fluctuate due to exacerbations or they can

progressively worsen without fluctuations, and this occurs amid changing demands due to age and personal circumstances (i.e., the need to work, care for kids, make meals, drive, etc.). People with MS can have one or both UE affected, and to different degrees of severity. This clinical heterogeneity limits the effectiveness of a standard intervention and highlights the need for client-centered interventions. Often, it is difficult to ascertain the root of the dysfunction as it can be due to impairments of the motor system, sensory system, or a combination of the two. Accurately measuring and treating UE dysfunction is of critical importance for improving function in MS. However, the UE is involved with complex multidimensional tasks (e.g., reaching, grasping, stabilizing the body, and manipulating objects); therefore, it is important to consider several issues before assessing or treating dysfunction. A primary issue is that there are a wide variety of UE assessment measures to choose from, many of which are ordinal in nature and consequently are broad and not well defined for detection of subtle deficits (e.g., EDSS). A second issue is that assessment measures are often most sensitive within a particular window of disability; therefore, one assessment measure may not be appropriate throughout the disability continuum. A third problem is that people with MS typically have multiple symptoms and these combinations make it difficult to determine the best choice of intervention to target their symptoms and improve disability. There is currently no cure for MS, and thus rehabilitation for symptom management is a viable choice to maintain and improve UE functional status.

Identifying symptoms and quantifying their severity as well as their impact on function is essential to medical management. Areas which should be considered include strength; sensation; coordination; manual dexterity; range of motion of the shoulder, elbow, wrist, and finger joints; and endurance and sustained activity (2). Accurate evaluation and effective rehabilitation for people with MS is challenging. In this chapter, we discuss some of the causes of UE dysfunction as well as provide rehabilitation strategies which can be used to address them. Rehabilitation strategies will include direct intervention to improve function and decrease symptoms as well as compensatory strategies to maximize independence in ADLs.

SPASTICITY IN UE MS AND ITS IMPACT ON FUNCTION

Spasticity, often described as stiffness, is a common and often challenging problem in individuals with MS. Spasticity is defined by Lance as "a motor disorder characterized by a velocity-dependent increase in tonic stretch reflexes (muscle tone) with exaggerated tendon jerks, resulting from hyper-excitability of the stretch reflex" (6). The symptoms of spasticity, a component of the upper motor neuron (UMN) syndrome, can vary widely from one individual to the next and can fluctuate within that individual over the course of the day. UMN symptoms can range from mild stiffness or muscular tightness to painful spasms, weakness, and lack of dexterity. While spasticity is more commonly noted in the lower extremities, it can present in the UEs as well (7). Musculature from the shoulder girdle distally through the digits may be impaired causing interference in the ability to complete daily activities such as opening containers, shampooing hair, handling medication, freely utilizing smartphones, and managing fasteners on clothing.

Spasticity can lead to both body function and structure alterations (impairments) and activity limitations if not well managed. Some alterations of body function can include muscle shortening or soft tissue contractures, which can diminish an individual's ability to complete purposeful movements and engage in everyday tasks as well as increase the risk of developing skin breakdown and ulcers. These issues can lead to an individual experiencing poor self-esteem or poor body image. Additionally, increased spasticity can set in motion limitations to activity and participation in activities such as driving, eating, or using a keyboard. Reduced intimacy with a partner and social isolation are also factors to be considered when an individual is dealing with increased spasticity. This being said, in other people a certain amount of spasticity can be functional, affording necessary stability to maintain the capacity to

complete various ADL such as using an affected hand as a stabilizer when opening a zippered bag. Regardless of whether the spasticity is functional or detrimental, when spasticity is present it means that an individual requires additional effort to complete their ADL, which leads to increased fatigue over the course of the day.

Unmanaged upper extremity spasticity can lead to increasing functional limitations in individuals with MS.

In the presence of noxious stimuli, spasticity can worsen. These stimuli can include increased core temperature, pain/discomfort, skin breakdown, or infection. Individuals with MS, as well as all members of the healthcare team, need to be aware of this so when a change from typical presentation of spasticity is noted these factors can be considered and appropriately addressed.

Assessment of UE Spasticity

Assessment of UE spasticity should not only include addressing the fundamental symptoms of the spasticity but consideration should also be given to the concerns of the individual and their caregivers towards the changes to quality of life and participation in meaningful activities. The clinician should consider the significance, not the severity of the spasticity when working with individuals to establish an appropriate treatment plan.

Two commonly used tools to measure spasticity through clinical evaluation are the Ashworth (Modified Ashworth) Scale and the Tardieu (Modified Tardieu) Scale (8–11). Both of these tools measure resistance during passive soft tissue stretching. Neither of these techniques incorporates the patient's experience of spasticity, nor how it affects their daily lives. There are also self-report measures of spasticity and they include the Numeric Rating Scale of spasticity, the MS Spasticity Scale-88, and the Spasm Frequency scale that have been used to ascertain the effects of spasticity on an individual's function (12–14).

Assessment of spasticity should incorporate standardized tools and a measure of the patient's experience.

Treatment of UE Spasticity

Spasticity in and of itself is not the reason for providing treatment. Addressing someone's spasticity often occurs when the spasticity is at the level where it begins to affect functional abilities or if there is pain associated with the spasticity that requires intervention. It is this impact on a person's well-being that drives the need for treatment. When intervention is considered, it is imperative to recognize that the decrease in spasticity may change the individual's ability to complete functional tasks and this must be weighed against the benefit of decreasing spasticity. A team approach between the patient, caregivers, and the healthcare team provides an effective treatment approach as both pharmacologic and nonpharmacologic approaches can be utilized as a part of a well-rounded treatment plan.

Focal spasticity in the UE can be treated effectively with botulinum toxin injected into specific muscles; this can then be coupled with splinting as needed to provide successful muscle relaxation and prevention of contractures (15). Figure 26.1(A–D) shows examples of how spasticity may appear in hand and arm. Flexion contractures are common in the fingers, wrist, and elbow joints. Using orthoses or braces will help to maintain a functional or natural position of the treated UE. Numerous prefabricated splints are readily available; however, an occupational therapist can fabricate static, static-progressive, or dynamic splints that provide a customized support tailored for the specific needs of the individual.

Stretching and range of motion exercises are integral portions to any treatment plan for spasticity, as they can minimize muscle shortening that is associated with spasticity. Stretching can be performed independently by the individual who has MS or it can be provided by a caregiver. For optimal effect, stretching must be performed daily. A stretch must be sustained in order to impact spasticity; some practitioners suggest holding a stretch for greater than 1 minute, while others suggest that a prolonged stretch (hours) must be maintained by using a splint or a brace (Consortium of MS Centers clinical practice guideline on Spasticity 2005) (16).

Whatever the treatment approach, patient/caregiver education is paramount in the successful management of spasticity. Individuals need to be independent in their home exercise program in order to improve adherence to the program.

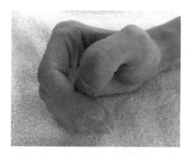

FIGURE 26.1A Picture of a hand posture with increased tone in the thumb musculature. Increased tone in the thumb makes it difficult to achieve functional pincer positions which enable fine motor tasks to be completed. Functional examples of these activities include picking up coins, buttoning a shirt, and grasping a glass of water.

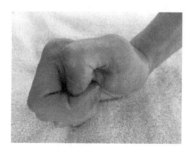

FIGURE 26.1C Picture of a hand with flexion contractures. When contractures are present functional use of the hand becomes challenging. Another concern when contractures are present is the increased risk of skin infections and wounds as it becomes difficult to complete adequate hygiene of the area.

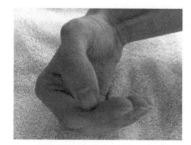

FIGURE 26.1B Picture of a hand posture of increased muscle tone in the wrist flexor muscles. Increased muscle tone in the wrist flexors makes it difficult to complete tasks which require active grasping. Functional examples of these activities include holding a toothbrush, maintaining a strong grasp on a walker, and squeezing shampoo out of a bottle.

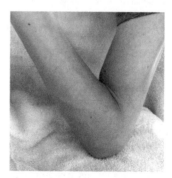

FIGURE 26.1D Picture of an elbow with flexion contractures. Contractures add to difficulty with ADLs such as dressing which becomes increasingly difficult for people with MS and their caregivers. Sleep can also become disrupted due to difficulty with arm and hand positioning for comfort.

UE WEAKNESS IN MS AND ITS IMPACT ON FUNCTION

The clinical manifestations of muscle weakness are a primary symptom of MS. Weakness is a clinically distinct impairment that can affect arm and hand function and the performance of ADL. Although most studies of weakness in MS focus on lower extremity limitations recent studies show that weakness of the UE is also very common in people with MS. One study shows that 60% of individuals with MS report weakness of their hand or arm (1). Grip strength, for example, in healthy adults has been shown to be a predictor of health status, functional independence, and increased morbidity and mortality (17,18). The impact of muscle weakness on physical functioning is substantial, leading to difficulty with walking, balance, dexterity, grip, and arm function.

Weakness can vary among individuals with MS, ranging from very mild to severe and even leading, in extreme cases, to a fully flaccid extremity(ies), though typically this type of extreme weakness occurs after 10 or more years of having MS symptoms. The muscles affected by MS can also vary. Individuals may have weakness in individual hand muscles only, or solely in proximal arm muscles on one side, or bilaterally. Weakness in individual hand muscles can cause functional limitations in tasks such as typing, writing, or playing an instrument, thus affecting a person's work performance. By contrast, weakness in larger arm muscles may cause difficulties with gross motor tasks such as carrying things, cleaning, or driving. Weakness is often reported as a feeling of heaviness in the limb or in terms of slowed movement, making it difficult to move quickly and accurately to complete fine or gross motor tasks. In addition to weakness, an individual may experience sensory changes in their arm that result in tingling or a feeling of numbness that varies by the time of day, and further impedes function. An individual may report, for example, that getting dishes down from a shelf is more difficult after a long day of work, so much so that he/she will stop and rest for a minute before getting the dishes down. These small events are often hardly noticed at first, but typically become more frequent and worsen over time and patients may not begin telling a clinician until they are affecting function on a regular basis. Some patients describe having cramping or moments of dystonic posturing of the hand or arm after completing a particularly strenuous task. These types of symptoms may be exacerbated by weakness even if they are not the primary cause of the weakness. It is important for clinicians to be aware of and ask about function so as to determine if strength is the impairment that needs to be addressed. Individual descriptions of weakness are important to listen to as they typically indicate what type of functional loss the individual is experiencing, and can be informative for goal setting. Be sure to ask the patient questions beyond what is required for their job, including questions about home chores, child care, and recreational activities. Weakness in a person with MS may not be obvious when observing an individual in a clinic, but becomes clear when accompanied with fatigue or when something has to be done quickly or accurately. Overall activity levels change dramatically in many people from morning to night, especially after a busy day.

Weakness rarely comes in isolation, and the combination of symptoms contributes to impaired function.

In addition to the functional impact of weakness, the location and severity of weakness may progress over the course of the disease. As with so many symptoms, muscle weakness does not follow a typical pattern but may increase in severity and functional impact over time. Lower and UE muscles may show symptoms on the right or left or both sides of the body. Goal setting is an important part of the process of identifying what is important to the patient and how it will be addressed. The patient and caregiver should both be consulted during this process. It is important to determine, for example, whether the patient is primarily interested in modifying bathing tasks or if the patient really enjoys painting and this can be a focus to achieve improvements in both areas. Being aware of the often competing needs of the patient and caregiver is critical for goal making and for decisions on what tools are best for assessment and intervention.

Assessment of UE Weakness

Assessment of UE muscle weakness should focus on appropriate measurement of muscle strength and the functional impact that weakness has on the individual's ADL and participation in meaningful activities. Assessments used should be responsive to muscle weakness as well as reliable and valid in MS.

Two commonly used tools to measure weakness are Manual Muscle Testing (MMT) and Dynamometry. Both tools are specific for measuring the amount of resistance a person can produce against a known force. Neither of these tools evaluates the effects of weakness on an individual's activity or participation in real-life tasks. Patient reported outcomes and timed functional task tests are most commonly used to assess overall UE function. There are no functional tasks that specifically measure how strength alone impacts function; however, the effect of weakness on self-care activities is discussed in the section titled UE Coordination and its Impact On Function.

The MMT scale is one of the most commonly used clinical methods to assess UE strength (19–22). It is easy to use, does not require any specialized equipment, and can be done by occupational therapists, physical therapists, nurses or physicians, and other healthcare professionals. MMT is designed to evaluate individual muscles from the upper and lower extremities. Each muscle is tested against the resistance of the clinician and subsequently graded against the patient's strength on a scale from 0 to 5. Scoring is subjective, based on the clinician's perception. Proper technique must be used during testing to ensure a reliable and valid measure. Important limitations to be aware of include (a) the test is dependent on patient effort which may be poor in the presence of pain or psychological issues; (b) the patient must not be wearing restrictive clothing; (c) muscles should first be tested in a gravity-eliminated plane and modified accordingly for individuals who cannot engage the muscles against gravity; (d) the less affected side should be tested first for comparison with the more effected side; and (e) discrimination between a 0 and a 1 is done by instructing the patient to contract the muscle while the clinician places their hand gently on the muscle being tested. This grading system classifies strength levels but does not directly quantify strength.

Alternatively, quantitative tools used to evaluate and track muscle strength over time can provide a useful method for clinical management in MS. Quantitative methods of strength assessment use a strain gauge or other measuring device, typically a hand-held dynamometer or grip dynamometer, or use a fixed apparatus to measure isokinetic or isometric strength (23). Dynamometry offers a more precise measurement of the force that a muscle produces and offers the sensitivity to track changes over time that a clinician may not subjectively notice using MMT. These methods can be used to evaluate grip strength, pinch strength, as well as the strength of wrist, elbow, and shoulder musculature. Dynamometry has been found to be fast, objective, clinically accessible, and valid in MS, and there are normative values available for comparison (24–27). Proper technique is also important for reliable measurement. Dynamometry also has limitations the clinician should keep in mind: (a) equipment is necessary for measurement; (b) not all muscles can be tested (e.g., lumbricals, and other small hand muscles); and (c) not all clinicians use the same equipment, and thus there is limited availability of comparable measurements to clinicians across specialties and clinic settings.

> *Assessment should include quantitative measures of strength for reliable tracking of strength changes but equally important is consideration of how strength limitations affect the patients function.*

Treatment of UE Muscle Weakness

Once it is determined that UE weakness is a significant problem, deciding which treatment intervention to use is the next step. Given that weakness across the lifespan may fluctuate over time or following exacerbations, it is important for the clinician to decide which intervention is appropriate now, and to reassess frequently to determine if the individual is gaining or at least maintaining strength. Common secondary symptoms such as pain, fatigue, or depression may impact an individual's ability to continue with the intervention and should be monitored carefully. Adaptations to any intervention may be necessary given the many additional symptoms an individual with MS experiences. Clinicians need to be sure to communicate with caregivers of the patient to determine how interventions are tolerated at home, identify problems with carry over, and to track functional improvements or declines in function. Tailoring of interventions for individuals with MS is common.

There are several studies that have evaluated the feasibility of UE strengthening programs in MS (28). One study showed that UE endurance training is tolerable and beneficial for improving arm strength even in severely impaired MS patients (29,30). For this study, the participants received 4 weeks of inpatient rehabilitation and a comparison group received tailored upper body strengthening exercises. Details about the tailored exercises that were used can be found at Sorensen et al. (31). Results showed the greatest improvements in the group that received the tailored strengthening exercises. A separate study used manual wheelchair propulsion as exercise training over 3 months resulting in improvements in UE strength and function (32). Inpatient and outpatient exercise progressions have also been shown to be effective to improve UE strength in MS (31).

Alternative methods of improving UE strength have been studied, but only using small sample sizes. We highlight here published preliminary findings that support the use of novel strengthening methods in MS. One study demonstrated the feasibility of combining functional electrical stimulation (FES) with mechanical robotic support (33). In this study, patients rested their most affected arm in a robotic support splint and were given FES to the anterior deltoid and biceps muscles while making reaching movements. Iterative learning control methods were used to facilitate voluntary effort while controlling the amount of FES needed to make precise reaching movements. Individuals were given 18 treatment sessions over 10 weeks and results showed significant improvements in arm control and a reduction in the extent of FES required for the movements. It is possible that combining strengthening with mechanical support or electrical stimulation may be useful in improving UE function. Aquatic exercise has also been shown to have positive effects on UE strength. A small study focused on the use of a specific type of aquatic exercise called Ai Chi and showed positive results following 8 weeks of exercises (34). Ai Chi uses the fundamentals of Tai Chi combining balance, strength, relaxation, flexibility, and breathing as progressive resistance training while standing in shoulder-deep water (35,36). Exercises are slow and rhythmic and accompanied with deep diaphragmatic breathing, and have shown improved strength and function in populations such as Parkinson's Disease (35). This type of aquatic training may prove to be an interesting alternative to traditional UE resistance training in MS.

Although research is limited in terms of guidance for what intervention, dose, and intensity are most beneficial for improving UE strength, it is clear that there are options for clinicians to choose from. In order for an exercise program to be successful, exercises need to be individualized and meaningful to the patient. It is perhaps most important for the clinical professional to identify an intervention that the patient is interested in pursuing, can be done within the resources available, and is focused on reaching the patient's goals.

> *There is not one exercise program that improves strength for people with MS.. It is important to individualize the exercise program based on assessment, observation, and feedback from the patient so as to meet the needs and capabilities of the patient*

UE COORDINATION AND ITS IMPACT ON FUNCTION

UE coordination problems are common in MS and are considered a core deficit (37). The clinical manifestations include reports of clumsiness and difficulty manipulating objects which affect the performance of ADL, participation in work and leisure activities affecting individuals' overall quality of life. In MS, a combination of symptoms including weakness, spasticity/sensory deficits, tremor, and ataxia typically contribute to UE coordination deficits, and this makes treatment planning difficult. One study reports that, in a cohort of mildly impaired individuals with MS, 76% had measurable problems with manual dexterity that, combined with, cognition, walking, energy, and mood contribute to a decreased quality of life (38).

UE coordination deficits can vary among individuals with MS ranging from mild reports of occasional clumsiness to severe cases where tremor and ataxia are completely debilitating. UE coordination deficits are thought to arise from deficits in the cerebellum, basal ganglia, and cortex or impairment of their connections (39). As is so characteristic of MS, there is no typical pattern for predicting coordination severity or progression. It has been reported that cerebellar relapses account for approximately 10% of all MS relapses (40) and poor relapse recovery is characteristic of cerebellar and brainstem relapses. Individuals with MS may present with either acute coordination problems relating to a relapse or chronic issues related to progressive disease. These are clues that can be gathered from a patient's chart and may provide the clinician with added information for prognosis. Since coordination derives from such a variety of sources, it is important for the clinician to focus their goals on what the patient reports as their biggest issue in combination with results from the clinical evaluation, and discussions with caregivers.

Assessment of Coordination

Assessment of UE coordination deficits should focus on measurement of UE function with a particular emphasis on tools that are most sensitive to the individual's deficit areas. The choice of tools should be based on those that are systematic and valid for MS as well as measurable and responsive for the individual's level of ability. For example, an individual with severe tremor may be unable to complete a fine motor assessment, but could complete a gross motor dexterity test to establish a baseline. We describe two timed tests for assessment of UE function: the nine hole peg test (NHPT) and the action research arm test (ARAT); however, there are many other tests used in the literature. We focus on the NHPT and ARAT because they are frequently used in studies of MS and have established standardized procedures.

The NHPT, originally developed by Kellor et al. in 1971, evaluates fine motor coordination and requires the individual to place nine pegs into nine holes then remove them from the holes and place them in an attached bowl, as quickly as possible (41). The test is timed and the score is the amount of time it takes the individual to place and remove all nine pegs. Alternative scoring can be done where the tester records the number of pegs removed per second. Feys et al. (37) provides a very useful review of the NHPT and its history as well as its implementation guidelines in MS. Reliability, sensitivity, and clinically detectable change of the NHPT has been evaluated and reported in MS (42). The NHPT shows strong reliability in MS, over a 1-week period. Clinically important change, measured as a minimal detectable change (MDC), has been established but differs depending on how scoring is done, time or speed, and which hand is used, dominant or nondominant. The MDC of the dominant hand for speed is 18.6% and for time is 19.4%; by contrast, for the nondominant hand the MDC for speed is 20.5% and for time is 29.1%. The MDC for speed is smaller than that for time, which is important to keep in mind when using this test (42). These values can be used by the clinician to measure if NHPT performance change over time is clinically meaningful or associated with measurement error. These standards are valuable guidelines for the clinician; however, it should be used in combination with reports from the patient as to whether they notice a valuable difference in function.

The ARAT is a clinical test that evaluates UE function using observational methods. The ARAT has 19 items organized into four sections: grasp, grip, pinch, and gross movements, allowing assessment of proximal and distal UE function (43). For the test, the individual is seated at a table and instructed by the tester to complete a series of specific tasks. Each test is given a score of 0 to 3 with higher values indicating better UE function. The ARAT score is determined by summing the 19 scores (43). Yozbatiran et al. and others have published instruction manuals for performance and scoring of the ARAT (43,44). A well-known limitation to the described tests earlier are that they do not provide more specific detail about the quality of the movements that may prove to be essential for measuring subtle changes over time. For this reason there has been growing interest in the use of wearable accelerometer and gyroscope devices (i.e., inertial sensors) that can quantify subtle changes in movement control. These devices are inexpensive, easy to use, and allow for objective measurement and characterization of movements, outside of a laboratory. Carpinella et al. (45) developed an instrumented ARAT in which individuals with MS used a single wrist worn inertial sensor while doing the ARAT. Their small study revealed that the instrumented method is valid in MS, in that it was able to discriminate between individuals with MS and controls, revealed subtle changes in arm movements that were not detectable from the ARAT score, and that this type of testing can be done in a clinical setting. It is possible that the use of sensors on individual fingers could provide further detail about hand function that is clinically useful.

Rating scales, though often time consuming, are appealing because they provide a single number to describe overall disability and require little if any equipment. Disability rating scales such as the EDSS are commonly used in MS clinical trials. The EDSS relies heavily on motor dysfunction, particularly walking; however, disturbances of functional systems such as visual function and UE motor and ataxia signs are also assessed and can contribute to the overall score (3,4).

> When assessing UE coordination it is important to consider the patient's level of function, as well as the floor and ceiling limits of the assessment tool.

Treatment for UE Coordination Deficits

Despite the global effects of UE coordination deficits, there are relatively few treatment interventions and there is limited scientific evidence. This may be because coordination deficits can result from a variety of impairments; thus, interventions specific to impairments are often used and modified to fit the needs of the individual. Nonpharmacological approaches are commonly used, and given the limited evidence specific to MS, borrowing interventions that are designed for individuals with other pathologies such as spinal cord injury or stroke are a viable option. Impaired coordination can limit function

dramatically; therefore, the use of weighted utensils or modifying feeding techniques to limit the number of joints that need to be controlled (e.g., resting the elbow on the table to minimize tremor) are commonly used. These treatments need to be used carefully on a case-by-case basis. It is important to keep in mind that the use of treatments that modify how tasks are done can be fatiguing and frustrating for the patient.

When making goals and planning which intervention to start with it is important to keep in mind that MS is a progressive disease and disability typically fluctuates depending on exacerbations, fatigue, and body temperature. A recent review of UE interventions in MS evaluated 11 published studies that used a variety of interventions including strength training, endurance training, functional activities including whole body activities, client-centered goal-directed training, overload training, use of real objects versus instrumented, context-specific training, and feedback-focused motor learning (28). Overall, there were improvements in the context of the training with limited measurable functional improvement, suggesting specificity of training is important. The review also reports that progression of an exercise program is a key element in the studies, resulting in the most improvement in function. In clinical practice, this suggests that using a variety of training components may be important to gain the best rehabilitation outcomes.

SELF-CARE DEFICITS ASSOCIATED WITH UE DYSFUNCTION

In a survey through the North American Research Committee on MS (NARCOMS) it was reported that 60% of individuals surveyed are affected by upper limb impairment. Of those reporting limitations in hand function, weakness was cited as the most common reason, followed by tremor, numbness, and spasticity (46). These symptoms, whether experienced individually or in conjunction with one another, negatively affect the individual's ability to participate in daily activities and maintain independence.

Occupational therapists are unique members of the healthcare team whose function is to help individuals maintain independence and participation in chosen tasks and roles as well as to reduce the effects of disability (47). This can be achieved through patient education, for example, energy management strategies, exercise programs such as individualized stretching programs, and utilizing activity analysis in order to recommend the use of assistive devices and modifications to the task at hand. Even in early MS, subtle UE dysfunction may be present and cause functional difficulties. As many as one third of participants mentioned earlier NARCOMS survey reported limitations in their ADL, (46) and as the level of disability progresses, the UE impairment can not only affect tasks associated with the use of one's hands and arms but it can translate to their ability to properly utilize mobility aides such as canes, walkers, and wheelchairs (2).

Individuals with UE limitations will often modify their lifestyle to compensate for their impaired function. They may do this by changing the way that they approach a task or though modifications to the tools needed in order to complete a task successfully. Recommendations by an occupational therapist for the use of adaptive equipment/ techniques may include

- Choosing a new stove with controls at the front so reaching around hot pots and pans can be avoided
- Utilizing weighted or built up utensils to counteract the effects of tremor or muscular weakness in the hands
- Changing the hardware on difficult to manage doors. Changing round doorknobs to lever style handles to facilitate opening and closing
- Wearing clothes with larger buttons or Velcro closures or utilizing a buttonhook to manipulate smaller buttons
- Reviewing the settings on an individual's computer in order to accommodate for UE limitations such as changing the sensitivity of the mouse to accommodate for tremor
- Energy management strategies and work simplification strategies are commonly addressed within occupational therapy sessions. Examples of these strategies include:
  - Putting commonly used items within an easily reached zone, typically described as at a height somewhere between the knees and the top of the head. These techniques will lessen reaching and bending thus minimizing fatigue
  - Plotting works centers within the home where an individual can sit with all necessary items for the task at hand readily available. Within these work centers items may be stored in a variety of ways such as in file cabinets, hanging baskets, on pegboards, and on rolling carts

- Adjusting the height of a desk may provide improved stability to UEs, which may minimize tremor and in turn improve coordination and independence
- Recommending the use of precut/prewashed produce when engaging in cooking tasks if the individual experiences challenges with decreased control, weakness, or fatigue

> *Self-care deficits are most commonly addressed by occupational therapists, who have specific expertise of the upper extremity that allows them to assist individuals in maximizing their independence.*

CONCLUSION

UE dysfunction is common in MS, yet there is limited guidance for how to effectively treat patients who experience UE limitations. We have highlighted several areas that commonly affect the UE in MS, spasticity, weakness, dyscoordination, and limitations to self-care independence and then provide evaluation and treatment suggestions. Overall, successful management of UE dysfunction requires assessment and treatment from members of the multidisciplinary team. Despite the important role the occupational therapist plays in the care of individuals with MS, studies show that the majority of people with MS have not utilized the services of an occupational therapist and of those who had worked with an occupational therapist, most reported positive experiences despite having multiple areas of limitations (48).

KEY POINTS FOR PATIENTS AND FAMILIES

- If you notice changes in the way that you can use your arms and/or hands, speak with your medical professional about getting a referral to work with an occupational therapist or a physical therapist. They can assess changes in your coordination, strength, and overall function and make recommendations to help ease daily life.
- Appropriate management of spasticity is necessary for long-term comfort and independence.
- Talking with a healthcare provider, such as an occupational therapist (OT) or a physical therapist (PT) about an appropriate UE exercise program is an important way to manage symptoms such as weakness and spasticity.
- Difficulty moving and using your arm or hand may be a result of a combination of symptoms, including spasticity, weakness, and dyscoordination. Your healthcare provider can help determine which intervention may work best for you.
- If you find yourself having increasing difficulty completing self-care activities, talk to an occupational therapist and they can work with you to assess ways to make yourself more independent.

REFERENCES

1. Kister I, Bacon TE, Chamot E, et al. Natural history of multiple sclerosis symptoms. *Int J MS Care*. 2013;15(3):146–158.
2. Kraft GH, Amtmann D, Bennett SE, et al. Assessment of upper extremity function in multiple sclerosis: review and opinion. *Postgrad Med*. September 2014;126(5):102–108.
3. Kurtzke JF. Rating neurologic impairment in multiple sclerosis: an expanded disability status scale (EDSS). *Neurology*. November 1983;33(11):1444–1452.
4. Kurtzke JF. A new scale for evaluating disability in multiple sclerosis. *Neurology*. August 1955;5(8):580–583.
5. Yozbatiran N, Baskurt F, Baskurt Z, et al. Motor assessment of upper extremity function and its relation with fatigue, cognitive function and quality of life in multiple sclerosis patients. *J Neurol Sci*. July 15, 2006;246(1-2):117–122.
6. Lance JW. Symposium synopsis: In: Feldmann RG, Young RR, Koella WP, eds. *Spasticity: Disordered Motor Control*. Chicago, IL: Yearbook Med Publishers; 1980.
7. Bethoux F. A cross-sectional study of the impact of spasticity on daily activities in multiple sclerosis. *Patient*. 2016;9(6):537–546.
8. Bohannon RW, Smith MB. Interrater reliability of a modified Ashworth scale of muscle spasticity. *Phys Ther*. February 1987;67(2):206–207.
9. Gracies JM, Marosszeky JE, Renton R, et al. Short-term effects of dynamic lycra splints on upper limb in hemiplegic patients. *Arch Phys Med Rehabil*. December 2000;81(12):1547–1555.
10. Pandyan AD, Johnson GR, Price CI, et al. A review of the properties and limitations of the Ashworth and modified Ashworth Scales as measures of spasticity. *Clin Rehabil*. October 1999;13(5):373–383.
11. Glinsky J. Tardieu scale. *J Physiother*. October 1, 2016;62(4):229.
12. Hobart JC, Riazi A, Thompson AJ, et al. Getting the measure of spasticity in multiple sclerosis: the Multiple Sclerosis Spasticity Scale (MSSS-88). *Brain J Neurol*. January 2006;129(pt 1):224–234.
13. Snow BJ, Tsui JKC, Bhatt MH, et al. Treatment of spasticity with botulinum toxin: a double-blind study. *Ann Neurol*. October 1, 1990;28(4):512–515.
14. Farrar JT, Troxel AB, Stott C, et al. Validity, reliability, and clinical importance of change in a 0-10 numeric rating scale measure of spasticity: a post hoc analysis of a randomized, double-blind, placebo-controlled trial. *Clin Ther*. May 2008;30(5):974–985.
15. Schapiro RT. Team approach to complex symptomatic management in multiple sclerosis. *Int J MS Care*. 2011;13(suppl 4):12–16.
16. Matchar MD, McCrory DC, Rutschmann O, et al. The chair and members of the Spasticity Management Guideline Development Panel express. 2005;28(2):167–199.
17. Bohannon RW. Hand-grip dynamometry predicts future outcomes in aging adults. *J Geriatr Phys Ther*. 2001;31(1):3–10.
18. Kaehrle P, Maljanian R, Bohannon RW, et al. Factors predicting 12-month outcome of elderly patients admitted with hip fracture to an acute care hospital. *Outcomes Manag Nurs Pract*. September 2001;5(3):121–126.
19. Brandsma JW, Van Brakel WH, Anderson AM, et al. Intertester reliability of manual muscle strength testing in leprosy patients. *Lepr Rev*. September 1998;69(3):257–266.
20. Great Lakes ALS Study Group. A comparison of muscle strength testing techniques in amyotrophic lateral sclerosis. *Neurology*. December 9, 2003;61(11):1503–1507.
21. Ciesla N, Dinglas V, Fan E, et al. Manual muscle testing: a method of measuring extremity muscle strength applied to critically ill patients. *J Vis Exp*. April 12, 2011;50:2632.
22. Naqvi U, Sherman Al. Muscle strength grading. In: StatPearls [Internet]. Treasure Island (FL): StatPearls Publishing; May 26, 2017. Available at: http://www.ncbi.nlm.nih.gov/books/NBK436008/.
23. Symonds T, Campbell P, Randall JA. A review of muscle- and performance-based assessment instruments in DM1: a review of PerfO's in DM1. *Muscle Nerve*. July 2017;56(1):78–85.
24. Keller JL, Fritz N, Chiang CC, et al. Adapted resistance training improves strength in eight weeks in individuals with multiple sclerosis. *J Vis Exp*. January 29, 2016;(107). Available at: http://www.jove.com/video/53449/adapted-resistance-training-improves-strength-eight-weeks-individuals.
25. Newsome SD, Wang JI, Kang JY, et al. Quantitative measures detect sensory and motor impairments in multiple sclerosis. *J Neurol Sci*. June 2011;305(1-2):103–111.
26. Fritz NE, Marasigan RER, Calabresi PA, et al. The impact of dynamic balance measures on walking performance in multiple sclerosis. *Neurorehabil Neural Repair*. January 1, 2015;29(1):62–69.
27. Van Harlinger W, Blalock L, Merritt JL. Upper limb strength: study providing normative data for a clinical handheld dynamometer. *PM R*. February 2015;7(2):135–140.
28. Spooren AI, Timmermans AA, Seelen HA. Motor training programs of arm and hand in patients with MS according to different levels of the ICF: a systematic review. *BMC Neurol*. 2012;12(1):49.
29. Skjerbaek AG, Naesby M, Lützen K, et al. Endurance training is feasible in severely disabled patients with progressive multiple sclerosis. *Mult Scler J*. 2014;20(5):627–630.
30. Dalgas U, Stenager E. Progressive resistance therapy is not the best way to rehabilitate deficits due to multiple sclerosis: no. *Mult Scler*. 2014;20(2):141.
31. Sørensen J, Lee A, Løvendahl B, et al et al. Study protocol: to investigate effects of highly specialized rehabilitation for patients with multiple sclerosis. A randomized controlled trial of a personalized, multidisciplinary intervention. *BMC Health Serv Res*. 2012;12(1):306.
32. Rice IM, Rice LA, Motl RW. Promoting physical activity through a manual wheelchair propulsion intervention in persons with multiple sclerosis. *Arch Phys Med Rehabil*. October 2015;96(10):1850–1858.
33. Sampson P, Freeman C, Coote S, et al. Using functional electrical stimulation mediated by iterative learning control and robotics to improve arm movement for people with multiple sclerosis. *IEEE Trans Neural Syst Rehabil Eng*. February 2016 ;24(2):235–248.
34. Bayraktar D, Guclu-Gunduz A, Yazici G, et al. Effects of Ai-Chi on balance, functional mobility, strength and fatigue in patients with multiple sclerosis: a pilot study. *NeuroRehabilitation*. 2013;33(3):431–437.
35. Pérez de la Cruz S. Effectiveness of aquatic therapy for the control of pain and increased functionality in people with Parkinson's disease: a randomized clinical trial. *Eur J Phys Rehabil Med*. June 19, 2017; 53:825–832.
36. Kurt EE, Büyükturan B, Büyükturan Ö et al., Effects of Ai Chi on balance, quality of life, functional mobility, and motor impairment in patients with Parkinson's disease. *Disabil Rehabil*. 2018 Apr;40(7):791–797.
37. Feys P, Lamers I, Francis G, et al. The Nine-Hole Peg Test as a manual dexterity performance measure for multiple sclerosis. *Mult Scler*. 2017;23(5):711–720.
38. Johansson S, Ytterberg C, Claesson IM, et al. High concurrent presence of disability in multiple sclerosis: associations with perceived health. *J Neurol*. June 2007;254(6):767–773.
39. Wilkins A. Cerebellar dysfunction in multiple sclerosis. *Front Neurol*. June 28, 2017;8:312. Available at: http://journal.frontiersin.org/article/10.3389/fneur.2017.00312/full.
40. Kalincik T, Buzzard K, Jokubaitis V, et al. Risk of relapse phenotype recurrence in multiple sclerosis. *Mult Scler*. 2014;20(11):1511-1522.
41. Kellor M, Frost J, Silberberg N, et al. Hand strength and dexterity. *Am J Occup Ther*. March 1971;25(2):77–83.
42. Hervault M, Balto JM, Hubbard EA, et al. Reliability, precision, and clinically important change of the Nine-Hole Peg Test in individuals with multiple sclerosis. *Int J Rehabil Res*. March 2017;40(1):91–93.
43. Yozbatiran N, Der-Yeghiaian L, Cramer SC. A Standardized Approach to Performing the Action Research Arm Test. *Neurorehabil Neural Repair*. January 2008;22(1):78–90.

44. Platz T, Pinkowski C, van Wijck F, et al. Reliability and validity of arm function assessment with standardized guidelines for the Fugl-Meyer Test, Action Research Arm Test and Box and Block Test: a multicentre study. *Clin Rehabil*. June 2005;19(4):404–411.
45. Carpinella I, Cattaneo D, Ferrarin M. Quantitative assessment of upper limb motor function in Multiple Sclerosis using an instrumented Action Research Arm Test. *J Neuroeng Rehabil*. 2014;11(1):67.
46. Marrie RA, Cutter GR, Tyry T, et al. Upper limb impairment is associated with use of assistive devices and unemployment in multiple sclerosis. *Mult Scler Relat Disord*. April 2017;13:87–92.
47. Forwell SJ, Zackowski KM. Team focus: occupational therapist. *Int J MS Care*. July 1, 2008;10(3):94–98.
48. Finlayson M, Garcia JD, Cho C. Occupational therapy service use among people aging with multiple sclerosis. *Am J Occup Ther*. June 2008;62(3):320–328.

27 Bladder and Bowel Dysfunction in Multiple Sclerosis

Courtenay K. Moore

KEY POINTS FOR CLINICIANS

- Bladder symptoms are very common among patients with multiple sclerosis (MS), with 50% to 80% reporting storage symptoms (urgency, frequency, urgency incontinence [UI]) and 30% to 50% reporting emptying issues.

- Neurogenic detrusor overactivity (NDO) is the most common cause of urgency, frequency, and UI.

- Detrusor underactivity (DUA), acontractility, and detrusor sphincter dyssynergia (DSD) are the most common causes of incomplete emptying.

- Fifty percent of MA patients will have both storage and emptying issues.

- There is no consensus on the evaluation and long-term management of MS patients. Therefore, the evaluation, workup, and follow-up should be tailored to each patient, assessing their risk factors for upper tract changes.

- First-line therapies for NDO include dietary and behavioral modification as well as pelvic floor physical therapy (PFPT).

- Second-line therapies for neurogenic overactive bladder (OAB) include anticholinergics and beta-3 agonists.

- Thirty percent of MS patients will require more invasive third- or fourth-line therapies.

- Bowel complaints are also common among MS patients, with 40% to 50% reporting chronic constipation and 29% to 51% fecal incontinence.

- Medications should be carefully screened as potential causes of bowel dysfunction.

- Constipation can be treated with fluid intake and dietary modifications, aggressive fiber supplementation, a regular time of evacuation, and over-the-counter medications.

- Fecal incontinence may be treated with dietary changes, over-the-counter medications to slow bowel motility, and sacral neuromodulation.

INTRODUCTION

MS is the most common progressive neurological disease affecting young men and women with an estimated worldwide prevalence of 2 to 2.5 million people (1). Both bladder and bowel dysfunction are highly prevalent among both men and women with MS. The 2005 North American Research Committee on Multiple Sclerosis (NARCOMS) survey collated responses from almost 10,000 patients with MS. Sixty-five percent of the responders experienced at least one moderate to severe urinary symptom (2). Urinary symptoms generally appear after a mean of 6 years and tend to increase in severity over time and with disease progression but can be the presenting symptom in 10% of patients (3). Tepavcevic and colleagues studied 93 patients with MS over a 6-year time frame, and demonstrated symptoms of bladder dysfunction in approximately 50% of men and women with MS on presentation and in 75% of men and women after 6 years of disease duration (4). Bowel complaints were also common, with constipation occurring in 53% to 54% of MS patients and fecal incontinence in 29% to 51% (5). Attention to bladder and bowel issues is an important part in managing patients with MS as both can have a profound impact on quality of life.

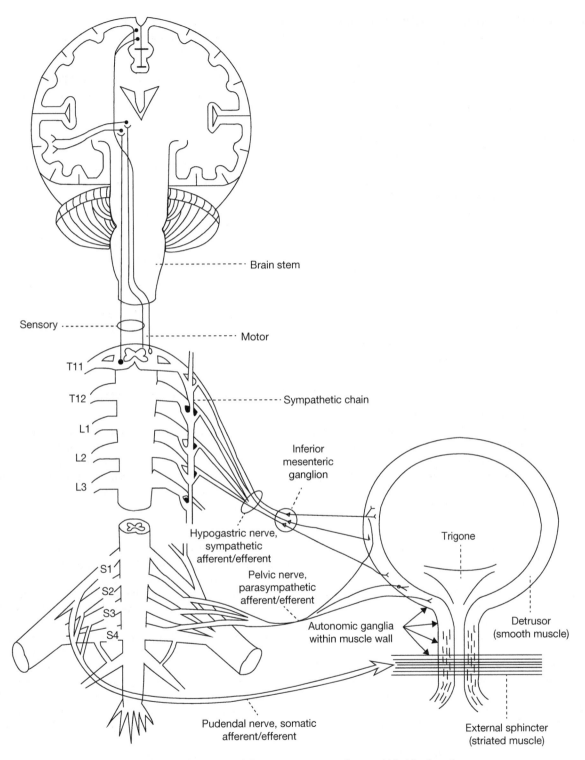

FIGURE 27.1 Diagram of the neuroanatomy of normal bladder function.

BLADDER AND BOWEL DYSFUNCTION IN MS

Pathophysiology and Symptoms

The neural pathways involved in micturition are organized as "on–off" circuits (Figure 27.1). Storage reflexes are controlled by sympathetic innervation during filling via the hypogastric nerve, which inhibits bladder contractions, and the pudendal nerve, which activates the external urinary sphincter while inhibiting parasympathetic innervation. As the bladder fills, increased visceral afferent neuron firing occurs, eventually resulting in activation of the parasympathetic system via the pelvic nerve and triggering a detrusor contraction and urethral relaxation via the pudendal nerve, thereby resulting in coordinated voiding (6).

Afferent sensation is relayed to the brain via the posterior and lateral white matter of the spinal cord, terminating in the pontine micturition center (PMC). As bladder filling continues, increased afferent neuron firing occurs, eventually resulting in the PMC triggering one of two responses: storage or voiding. With storage, the PMC then triggers further relaxation and storage of the bladder via activation of beta-receptors in the bladder and alpha-stretch receptors in the urethra, thereby relaxing the bladder and closing the urethra, via sympathetic control through the pudendal nerve. The conscious decision to void is controlled by the medial frontal cortex and the hypothalamus that modulate the activity of the periaqueductal area. Once the bladder reaches significant capacity, the PMC then triggers detrusor contraction and urethral relaxation, resulting in relaxation of the bladder outlet through the hypogastric nerve, via the parasympathetic nervous system, thereby resulting in urine flowing out of the bladder and urethra as the act of coordinated voiding (6).

Charil et al. mapped the lesion and disabilities on MRI on patients with relapsing and remitting MS and found a correlation between cervical spinal lesions below the PMC in the majority of patients with obstructive voiding symptoms and retention secondary to detrusor sphincter dyssynergia (DSD). Suprasacral lesions were associated with neurogenic detrusor overactivity (NDO), while sacral lesions corresponded with DUA and acontractility (7).

In MS patients, disruption of suprapontine circuitry removes the tonic sympathetic inhibitory control over the PMC and results in decreased bladder capacity and NDO. Lesions at the sacral level can result in DUA or contractility. Lesions between the PMC and sacral outlet can result in discoordination between the bladder and sphincter, resulting in DSD. Marrie et al. surveyed over 16,000 participants in the NARCOMS database and found that 80% of their respondents had complaints of bowel or bladder symptoms, often moderate to severe in nature, and 50% or more reported at least mild disability resulting from these symptoms (8). Bladder complaints among MS patients range from irritative voiding symptoms (urgency, frequency, UI) to incomplete emptying or retention.

According to various studies, OAB symptoms are most common with 31% to 85% of patients experiencing urinary frequency and urgency, 35% to 70% urge incontinence, 2% to 50% experiencing obstructive voiding symptoms, and 30% experiencing both irritative and obstructive symptoms.

Neurogenic bowel dysfunction (NBD), like neurogenic bladder, can cause storage, emptying or a combination of storage, and emptying issues. NBD is most commonly characterized by both constipation and fecal incontinence. Like the bladder, bowel dysfunction corresponds with the site of neurologic injury. Patients with supraconal upper motor lesions have hyperreflexic bowels with increased rectal and sigmoid compliance as well as increased sphincter tone resulting in stool retention and constipation (9). Patients with lower motor neuron lesions have areflexic bowels with loss of peristalsis resulting in slow stool propulsion, reduced rectal compliance, and lax anal tone (9).

Evaluation and Clinical Findings

Bladder and bowel function are integrally related to the patient's mental, cognitive, and functional status. The evaluation of patients with MS and elimination symptoms should include a detailed history, including prior treatments, a physical examination, assessing cognitive functional status, dexterity and any anatomical abnormalities and a fluid/bladders, and bowel diary (Tables 27.1 and 27.2).

Table 27.3 highlights potentially modifiable risk factors that can contribute to urinary incontinence and can be remembered using the DIAPPERS. In addition to a thorough history and physical examination a urinalysis should be performed at the initial visit. If the urinalysis is consistent with a urinary tract infection a urine culture should be sent. In accordance with American Urological Association Guidelines, a postvoid residual (PVR) should be obtained during the initial evaluation as part of a complete urodynamic. A PVR volume of less than 150 mL is considered normal.

A variety of screening questionnaires are available to assess urinary and pelvic floor complaints, including the urogenital distress inventory (UDI-6), and pelvic floor impact questionnaire (PFIQ) (10,11). The European Association of Urology recommends usage of the Qualiveen® (MAPI research trust), the only validated questionnaire to assess quality of life in patients with neurological disease (12).

Per American Urological Association, Urodynamic testing guidelines physicians should perform a complex cystometrogram (CMG), pressure flow analysis in patient's neurologic disease at risk for neurogenic bladder. When available, fluoroscopy and electromyography (EMG) should be used (13).

Litwiller et al. examined the urodynamic findings of 1,882 patients in 22 studies and found that 62% had NDO, 25% had DSD, 20% had DUA, and 10% had no significant urodynamic studies (UDS) findings (Table 27.4) (14).

TABLE 27.1 Possible Bladder Symptoms Experienced by Patients With MS

SYMPTOMS	DEFINITION
Urgency	The sudden strong desire to urinate that cannot be deferred
Frequency	A complaint by the patient that he or she voids too often
Urge incontinence	Involuntary urine leakage accompanied by an urgent desire to urinate
Nocturia	The complaint of needing to wake up one or more times a night to urinate
Urinary retention	A painful or nonpainful bladder that remains palpable or percussable after the patient has passed urine; may be associated with incontinence; generally a PVR volume of more than 150 mL
Hesitancy	Difficulty initiating a urine stream resulting in the delay in onset of voiding
Straining	Requiring additional muscular effort to initiate, maintain, or accelerate the urine stream

MS, multiple sclerosis; PVR, postvoid residual.

TABLE 27.2 Important Factors to Assess at the Time of Patient Interview Regarding Bladder Complaints

- Mental status/cognitive function
- Functional status (activities of daily living, walking, dexterity, transfer ability)
- Diet (caffeine, alcohol)
- Fluid intake habits (amount, does drink up until bedtime)
- Incontinence
- Recurrent UTIs
- PVR
- Urinary frequency and urgency symptoms
- Medications (type and timing)
- Other medical problems (CHF, PVD, DM)

CHF, congestive heart failure; DM, diabetes mellitus; PVD, peripheral vascular disease; PVR, postvoid residual; UTI, urinary tract infection.

TABLE 27.3 DIAPPERS: Potentially Treatable/Reversible Causes of Incontinence

Delirium: May be related to infection or metabolic disorder

Infection: Screen for infection with clean catch or straight-catheterized specimen, checking urinalysis, and culture and sensitivity when indicated

Atrophic vaginitis: Modifies vaginal pH and increases susceptibility to UTI; should be treated with transvaginal estrogen supplementation

Pharmaceuticals: Drugs that may cause urinary complaints including: (a) retention: alpha-agonists, opioids, anticholinergics; (b) incontinence: alpha blockers, muscle relaxants; and (c) urgency and frequency: diuretics, alcohol

Psychological: Assess for depression or cognitive impairment

Excess excretion: Causes of fluid accumulation in the body, including: peripheral edema, congestive heart failure, vascular disease, excessive oral fluid intake, diuretic usage

Restricted mobility: Difficulty ambulating to commode, problems with transfer, lack of assistance, distance to bathroom facilities, etc.

Stool impaction: Refer to gastroenterology if dietary modification and common oral fiber and laxatives are not sufficient

UTI, urinary tract infection.

TABLE 27.4 Common Findings on Urodynamic Testing and Associated Symptoms

URODYNAMIC FINDING	DEFINITION	ASSOCIATED SYMPTOMS
Detrusor overactivity without obstruction	Involuntary detrusor contractions during bladder filling with or without leakage	Urgency, frequency, urge incontinence, and nocturia
DSD	Detrusor contraction concurrent with an involuntary contraction of the urethral or periurethral striated muscle (may block urine outflow)	Urinary hesitancy, straining, or obstruction
Detrusor overactivity with outlet obstruction	Detrusor overactivity plus DSD (defined earlier). May occasionally obstruct urine flow altogether	Urinary urgency with hesitancy, straining, or obstruction
Detrusor overactivity with impaired contractility	Detrusor overactivity with reduced strength and/or duration of bladder contraction, resulting in prolonged bladder emptying and/or inability to completely empty in a timely fashion	Slow bladder emptying and/or urinary retention
Detrusor areflexia	Inability of the bladder to contract with routine filling at normal physiological volumes to elicit bladder emptying	Urinary retention

DSD, detrusor sphincter dyssynergia.

For patients with MS, the incidence of upper tract changes varies widely (0.8%–15%). At present, there are no consensus guidelines on upper tract imaging. Potential risk factors for upper tract changes include disease duration, advancing age, and pyramidal symptoms (15).

TREATMENT OF OAB/STORAGE SYMPTOMS

The goals of managing patients with neurogenic bladder are: to promote continence, preserve renal function, and improve the patients' quality of life (16). The NARCOMS study of 9,700 patients found that only 43% of participants with moderate-to-severe bladder symptoms had ever been evaluated by urology, and only 51% had received any anticholinergic medications for these symptoms (2).

The first-line therapies for NDO include behavioral/dietary modifications (Table 27.5), bladder training, and PFPT. Patients with idiopathic OAB generally experience a 40% improvement in their urinary complaints with lifestyle changes. However, these lifestyle modifications may not be as successful in patients with neurogenic conditions given cognitive impairment, high amplitude of the involuntary detrusor contractions or if the frontal cortex is involved, which would impair their ability to inhibit involuntary detrusor contractions.

However, several studies have shown PFPT to be beneficial in MS patients. De Ridder et al. conducted a prospective study of 30 women with MS and detrusor overactivity and found statistically significant improvement in pelvic floor muscle strength, functional bladder capacity, urinary frequency, and incontinence episodes (17). A larger randomized controlled study conducted by McClurg et al. showed that PFPT in combination with electrical stimulation reduced found combination therapy and was more effective in reducing incontinence episodes (85% vs. 47%, $p = .0028$) (18).

Pharmacotherapy is commonly utilized as a second-line therapy for neurogenic patients. Anticholinergics are the most commonly utilized medication, despite limited clinical data, and potential side effects including constipation, dry mouth, and mental status changes (Table 27.6). A 2009 Cochrane review assessing the efficacy, tolerability, and safety of these drugs in patients with MS patients. This review included five studies and found insufficient data to support any benefit of anticholinergics in the MS population (19). However, a large meta-analysis of 16 patients with NDO found more patients taking anticholinergics reported cure/improvement in urinary symptoms versus placebo (20). There were also significant improvements in urodynamic parameters including maximum cystometric capacity and lower detrusor pressure at highest contraction. There is a higher incidence of adverse events among patients taking anticholinergics; however, the anticholinergic drugs or different dosages assessed in this review was superior to another.

Mirabegron, a beta-3 agonist, the newest medication on the market for OAB has been shown to statistically reduce urinary frequency and incontinence episodes in patients with idiopathic OAB but not been studied in patients with NDO. While additional studies are needed to assess efficacy in MS patients, it may prove an attractive alternative given its more favorable side effect profile including no cognitive impairment, constipation, dry mouth, or impairment of bladder emptying.

Patients with OAB symptoms refractory to multiple medications and behavioral changes are candidates for more invasive therapies including: (a) percutaneous nerve stimulation (PTNS); (b) intradetrusor botulinum toxin injections; (c) sacral neuromodulation (SNM); (d) augmentation cystoplasty; and (e) urinary diversion.

TABLE 27.5   Behavioral Modifications for Urinary Symptoms in MS

FLUID TITRATION	PATIENTS ARE INSTRUCTED TO MODERATE DRINKING HABITS, FOCUSING ON NO MORE THAN 4–6 OUNCES OF FLUID PER HOUR
Reduce bladder irritant intake	Includes: Alcohol, caffeine, citrus juices, artificial sweeteners
Cut off oral fluids 2–3 hr before bedtime	Minimize the need for night time voiding and potential nocturia
Change medication timing	Do not take diuretics in evening; move bedtime medications 2–3 hr earlier
Scheduled voiding	Voiding by the clock to prevent bladder overfilling and potential incontinence episodes
Bladder retraining	Teaching patients who void too frequently methods to control urinary urge and extend time between voids
Kegel exercises	Teaching patients to improve voluntary control of pelvic floor muscles to control urinary urge and incontinence

MS, multiple sclerosis.

TABLE 27.6   Medications for the Treatment of Bladder Dysfunction

GENERIC NAME	BRAND NAME	ROUTE	DOSE	FREQUENCY
Anticholinergic medications for the treatment of OAB symptoms				
Fesoterodine	Toviaz	Oral	4 or 8 mg	Daily
Oxybutynin	Ditropan	Oral	5, 10, 15 mg	Up to three times a day
	Dirtropan XL	Oral	5, 10, 15 mg	Daily
	Oxytrol Patch	Topical	3.9 mg/d	One patch twice weekly
	Gelnique	Topical	10%	Daily
Solifenacin	Sanctura	Oral	20 mg	Twice a day
	Sanctura XR	Oral	60 mg	Daily
Darifenacin	Enablex	Oral	7.5, 15 mg	Daily
Tolterodine	Detrol	Oral	2, 4 mg	Twice a day
	Detrol LA	Oral	2, 4 mg	Daily
Alpha-adrenergic blockers for the treatment of impaired bladder emptying				
Tamsulosin	Flomax	Oral	0.4 mg	At bedtime
Alfuzosin	Uroxatral	Oral	10 mg	At bedtime
Doxazosin	Cardura	Oral	1, 2, 4, 8 mg	At bedtime
	Cardura XL	Oral	4, 8 mg	At bedtime
Silodosin	Rapaflo	Oral	4, 8 mg	At bedtime
Terazosin	Hytrin	Oral	1, 2, 5, 10 mg	At bedtime

OAB, overactive bladder.

PTNS uses intermittent stimulation to modulate the bladder reflex pathway via the tibial nerve. The posterior tibial nerve is a mixed sensory-motor nerve roots, and contains axons from L4-S3 nerve roots. Using either a needle or patch electrode, the electrical stimulation of these nerves by a needle evokes a central inhibition of the micturition reflex (16). Initial treatment consists of 12 thirty-minute weekly sessions. Most patients will require maintenance sessions based on return of symptoms typically at 2 to 4 months.

The efficacy of PTNS has been proven in several studies. In 2011, de Sèze and colleagues conducted a multicenter study of PTNS in 70 MS patients with refractory OAB symptoms (21). At 1 and 3 months, 82.6% and 83.3% patients, respectively reported improvement in OAB symptoms. Urgency, frequency, and incontinence episodes (all $p < .001$) were all significantly improved after both at 1 and 3 months. Twenty-six percent of subjects had no incontinence episodes at baseline and this increased to 45% after 1 month and to 47% of at 3 months.

In a recent prospective non-placebo-controlled trial of 83 MS patients with lower urinary tract symptoms (LUTS) refractory to medical therapy, 89% had a 50% or greater improvement in symptoms after initial treatment of PTNS (22). Treatment benefit was sustained for 2 years with a maintenance regimen of 3 weeks. At 2 years, there were significant decreases in daytime frequency and nocturia, as well as significant improvements in mean voided volume. At 2 years, urodynamic parameters including maximum cystometric capacity and volume at detrusor overacitvity increased while PVR and voiding pressure decreased.

Botulinum toxin A (Botox), abobotulinum toxin A (Dysport) acts by blocking the release of acetylcholine at the neuromuscular junction causing a reversible, temporary paralysis of the bladder muscle resulting in a decreased UI, and an increase in maximum cystometric capacity. Botulinum toxin A is currently the only U.S. Food and Drug Administration (FDA) approved botulinum toxin for the treatment of NDO. In two large multicenter, randomized, double-blind, placebo controlled phase 3 clinical trials of MS and spinal cord injury patients with NDO and with greater than 14 UI episodes refractory to anticholinergics were randomized to either 200 units, 300 units, or placebo (23,24). In both studies, 200 units of Botulinum toxin A statistically decreased UI episodes compared with placebo by −22 versus −13 at 6 weeks. Thirty-eight percent and 36% of patients were completely dry versus 7.6% of placebo. Patients who received 200 units of Botox also had statistically significant improvement in urodynamic parameters including increase in maximum cystometric capacity and a decrease in mean detrusor pressure at the first involuntary detrusor contraction. The median duration of effect was 42 weeks. The most common adverse events were urinary tract infection (UTI) (28%) and urinary retention (20%).

Denys et al. conducted a 3-year extension study and found that patients with NDO with a greater than or equal to 50% UI reduction after their first botulinum toxin A treatment continued to experience consistent improvements in UI and quality of life with subsequent treatments over the duration of 4 years, attesting to the continued efficacy of botulinum toxin A (25).

Sacral neuromodulation system (SNS) is a surgically implanted device FDA approved in 1997 for refractory OAB. The mechanism of action is not fully understood but theorized to stimulate sensory afferents which modulate the central nervous system (CNS) reflex pathway, inhibiting the ascending pathway of the micturition reflex and input to the PMC, preventing reflex micturition but not affecting volitional voiding (16). One important factor to consider when evaluating a patient for SNS is that MRIs of the spine are contraindicated, which is very relevant to the MS population.

While not FDA approved for NDO, the 2005 International Consultation on Incontinence recommended SNS for refractory NDO. There is limited data on SNS in MS patients. Minardi et al. performed a retrospective case series on 25 MS patients with neurogenic LUTS. Sixty percent of the patients went on to stage 2 implantation with a greater than 50% improvement in voiding symptoms (26).

In a meta-analysis by Kessler et al. looking at SNS for neurogenic LUT dysfunction for 26 independent studies with 357 patients found a pooled success rate was 68% for the test phase and 92% for permanent SNM, with a mean follow-up of 26 months. The pooled adverse event rate was 0% for the test phase and 24% for permanent SNS. When looking specifically at MS patients the success rate for the test phase and permanent SNS were 84% and 92%, respectively, suggesting SNS is effective for MS patients (27).

Chaabane et al. conducted a retrospective review of 62 patients (13 with MS) with neurogenic LUT dysfunction to assess the clinical and urodynamic effects of neuromodulation (28). Sixty-six percent had had more than 50% improvement in urodynamic parameters and bladder diary and went on to implantation. At a mean follow-up of 4.3 years, 75.7% of patients continued to report improvement. In these six cases, neuromodulation failed on average 12.0 ± 12.4 months after implantation. When specifically looking at patients with MS they found that only 50% had long-term success due to loss of efficacy. For patients with MS, the loss of efficacy followed a new relapse.

More invasive surgical options including urinary diversion and augmentation cystoplasty are options for patients who have failed the above therapies, who have a devastated urethra or a hostile bladder (impaired compliance or small capacity bladder). The goal of an augmentation cystoplasty is to surgically enlarge the bladder, restoring a low-pressure, continent, and compliant reservoir. This procedure is often performed using a segment of detubularized ileum.

Zachoval et al. reported the outcomes of augmentation ileocystoplasty performed in nine patients with MS. At 6 to 19 month follow-up, there was an increase in maximum mean detrusor capacity from 105 to 797 mL and a decrease in the maximum detrusor pressure from 53 cm H_2O to 30 cm H_2O (29). Elsewhere, in more varied but larger patient cohorts, the rates of continence 3 years after augmentation are high, as are the patient satisfaction rates. Therefore, augmentation ileocystoplasty is an effective surgical approach for patients with MS.

Contraindications to augmentation cystoplasty include inflammatory bowel disease, short gut syndrome, and inability to perform intermittent self-catheterization (ISC). In these patients, consideration should be given to a noncontinent urinary diversion.

TREATMENT OF INCOMPLETE EMPTYING/URINARY RETENTION

Up to 25% of patients with MS will experience urinary retention and require urinary catheterization of some form for voiding during the course of their disease (30). In MS patient DUA, impaired contractility and DSD are the most common reasons for incomplete emptying/urinary retention in patients with MS.

There is limited data on medical therapy for MS related incomplete emptying. Two small studies examined the effect of the alpha-blocker tamsulosin in MS patients with DSD. Kakizaki et al. reported an improvement in average and maximum flow rate but no statistically significant decrease in PVR (31). Similarly, Stankovich et al. found an increase in maximal flow rate but also a decrease in PVR (32).

Based on the small poor quality studies, in 2012, the National Clinical Guideline Center for the United Kingdom recommended against using alpha-blockers in patients with incomplete emptying secondary to neurologic disease (33).

Intermittent catheterization is the preferred method of bladder emptying in both men and women with adequate upper limb dexterity. Long-term use of indwelling catheters is complicated by chronic infection, leakage per urethra, urethral erosion, and potential long-term risk of malignancy. The UK MS treatment guidelines recommend use of a suprapubic tube rather than a urethral catheter for long-term drainage to reduce catheter-related complications including bacteriuria, recatheterization, and pain (33).

Botulimum toxin has been used in MS patients with DSD. de Sèze et al. conducted a double-blinded, placebo controlled trial injecting botulinum toxin into the external urinary sphincter in MS with DSD (34). There were no differences in mean postvoiding residual volume (PVR) between the placbo group (217 mL) and treatment (220 mL) (p = .45). A 2014 Cochrane Database Review and analysis concluded that transperineal botulinum toxin into the external sphincter improved voided urine volumes, but did not decrease PVR or decrease catheterization (35).

While SNS is FDA approved for idiopathic nonobstructive urinary retention, it has also been used in in neurogenic patients. Marinkovic and Gillen reported on 14 patients with MS who underwent SNS for urinary retention (36). Twelve patients went on to successful implantation. Preoperatively, self-catheterization volumes decreased from 308 mL compared to 50.5 mL (p < .001) at 4.3 years of follow-up. All 12 women went onto stage 2, voided successfully, and stopped self-catheterization. The reoperation rate was 17%, mainly for lead migration.

BOWEL DYSFUNCTION IN MS

Bowel symptoms are very common in patients with neurological conditions, and affect more than 50% of patients with MS. Both constipation and fecal incontinence are common, with constipation being more prevalent. A recent survey from the NARCOMS Patient Registry found that of the 502 participants, 39% reported constipation, 11% fecal incontinence, and 36% mixed constipation and incontinence (37). Bowel complaints can be the source of anxiety and social isolation, significantly affecting quality of life.

The pathophysiology of bowel dysfunction in MS varies with the site and severity of the neuralgic lesion. Sacral spinal cord lesions result in areflexic bowel, loss of peristalsis with increasing colonic transit time, and reduced rectal compliance and lax anal tone. Suprapontine lesions result in hyperreflexic bowels with increased rectal and sigmoid compliance as well as sphincter tone (2).

Evaluation and Clinical Findings

In 2010, the fourth International Consultation on Continence published an algorithm on the evaluation and managements of neurogenic bowel (38). The initial evaluation should include a detailed history including diet, medical conditions, past surgeries, and medications, which could affect bowel function (Tables 27.7 and 27.8). Physical examination should include abdominal, pelvic, and rectal examinations and sacral reflexes (voluntary anal sphincter contraction, deep perianal sensation, anal tone, anal and bulbocavernosus reflexes). Attention should be paid to rule out any abdominal masses, pelvic organ prolapse, hemorrhoids, and anal fissures. A rectal examination should be performed to assess the resting anal tone and external sphincter pressures. In addition, mental, cognitive, functional status (mobility, hand coordination), and environmental factors (toilet accessibility; assistive, care providers) should be assessed.

MS specific bowel questionnaires can be used including the Bowel Function Questionnaire for Persons with MS (BFQ-MS), a self-administered questionnaire consisting of 15 items pertaining to constipation, 13 items pertaining to fecal incontinence, and 20 items pertaining to both constipation and fecal incontinence. Several other validated questionnaires are available, including the Quality of Life Scoring Tool Relating to Bowel Management (QOL-BM), the Constipation Symptom Assessment Instrument (PAC-SYM), and the Brief Fecal Incontinence questionnaire (37).

It is recommended that any patient 50 or older undergo a fecal occult blood test yearly. Similar to neurogenic bladder, the primary aims of treatment neurogenic bowel are to achieve efficient bowel evaluation while avoiding fecal incontinence. Typical first-line therapies for the

TABLE 27.7 Screening Questions for Bowel Symptoms in Patients With MS

How are your bowel movements?

How many times do you move your bowels during a typical week?

What is the consistency of your bowel movements?

   If constipated: do you strain to pass stool?

      Do you have the sensation of incomplete emptying of the bowels?

Did you notice any changes in your bowel habits?

   If yes: what changes and for how long?

      What have you done to control the symptoms (behavioral changes, medications, etc.)?

Did you experience pain or discomfort when passing stool?

Did you have bowel accidents?

   If yes: did you leak stool or flatus?

      How much does it bother you?

      Do you need to wear protective garments?

      Are there any warning signs prior to an accident (urgency)?

      Did you do anything to make the problem better?

What does your diet consist of? (ask especially about fluid and fiber intake)

MS, multiple sclerosis.

TABLE 27.8 Medications That Can Precipitate or Exacerbate Bowel Dysfunction

Medications promoting constipation	Anticholinergics (fesoterodine, darifenacin, oxybutynin, solifenacin, tolterodine, trospium chloride)
	Antihypertensives (calcium channel blockers and central alpha agonists)
	Analgesics/narcotics (including nonsteroidal anti-inflammatory drugs, morphine, codeine)
	Antidepressants (selective serotonin reuptake inhibitors)
	Antipsychotics (chlorpromazine, clozapine, risperidone, olanzapine)
	Antihistamines (diphenhydramine, doxylamine, promethazine)
	Tricyclic antidepressants (amitriptyline, nortriptyline, imipramine, desipramine)
	Sedatives/tranquilizers (barbiturates, benzodiazepines, zolpidem)
	Antacids (aluminum and calcium compounds)
	Diuretics (triamterene, indapamide, hydrochlorothiazide)
	Iron supplements
Medications with diarrheal side effects	Antihypertensives (enalapril, metoprolol)
	Antiarrhythmics (quinidine)
	Antibiotics (penicillins, cephalosporins, carbapenems, antituberculosis agents, macrolides, sulfonamides, tetracyclines, quinolones)
	Antineoplastics (5-fluorouracil, capecitabine, irinotecan)
	Protease inhibitors (saquinavir, ritonavir, indinavir)
	Some diuretics (furosemide, indapamide, bumetanide)
	Antacids (magnesium hydroxide)
	Laxatives (bisacodyl, senna, lactulose, docusate, methylcellulose)

treatment of constipation include a high fiber diet, adequate fluid intake, and a timed bowel regimen. However, in a meta-analysis, Muller-Lissner found that dietary fiber was actually ineffective in improving colonic transit time in patients with chronic constipation, and might even induce symptoms of bloating or abdominal distension (39).

There are several types of medications that can be used to manage constipation if behavioral treatments fail (Table 27.9). Bulking agents work by increasing fecal mass to help stimulate peristalsis. It is important to ensure adequate hydration and fiber in the diet. Again, there is little data on their effectiveness in MS. Osmotic laxatives work by retaining fluid in the bowel. Stimulant laxatives work by increasing intestinal motility. Sodium dioctyl sulfosuccinate (sodium docusate) has properties of both a stimulant laxative and a stool softener. Unlike osmotic laxatives, stimulant laxatives are less likely to produce liquid stool and therefore fecal incontinence (40). Rectal stimulants are also useful can be given as an enema or suppository.

Several small studies have shown digital rectal stimulation and abdominal massages to be effective ways of stimulating bowel function (41).

Surgical interventions are indicated only in rare circumstances. These include the formation of a colostomy or an appendicostomy.

Treatment of Fecal Incontinence

In patients with fecal incontinence, dietary irritants (such as sugar substitutes, alcohol, and caffeine) should be eliminated as they cause stools to become looser (41). General antimotility drugs still remain the main treatment for fecal incontinence. The commonest of these are loperamide and codeine phosphate. However, care should be taken in evaluating whether the incontinence is actually

Treatment of Constipation

TABLE 27.9 Medications to Relieve Constipation

Bulking agents	Methylcellulose (Citrucel)
	Psyllium hydrophilic mucilloid (Metamucil)
	Polycarbophil (FiberCon)
	Guar gum (Benefiber)
	Malt soup extract (Maltsupex)
Stool softeners	Docusate (Colace, Surfak, Correctol, Dok)
Stimulant laxatives	Senna (Senokot, Ex-Lax, Senexon, Senna-Gen)
	Bisacodyl (Bisac-Evac, Biscolax, Dulcolax, Dacodyl, Fleet Bisacodyl Enema/Suppository)
	Castor oil
Osmotic laxatives	Lactulose (Constulose, Enulose, Generlac, Kristalose)
	Sorbitol
	Polyethylene glycol solution (Miralax)
	Glycerin suppository
Rectal stimulant	Suppository
	Enema

secondary to fecal overloading ("overflow incontinence") (40). Loperamide can be safely titrated according to the response. Bulking agents act by increasing stool mass and promoting fecal consistency, thereby decreasing diarrhea and improving the incontinence. Physical therapy (PT) with biofeedback may increase the strength of pelvic floor muscles and rectal sensory perception. Anal plugs can be used as a last resort in patients with refractory fecal incontinence. If these therapeutic measures fail, referral to a gastroenterologist is warranted. Surgical interventions include antegrade continence enemas, SNS, and, as a last resort, a colostomy.

CONCLUSION

Bladder and bowel symptoms are very common among MS patients and can significantly affect their quality of life. It is important that healthcare providers ask about both bowel and bladder complaints, as both can be treated and significantly improved with behavioral modifications, medical therapy, and, lastly, surgery.

KEY POINTS FOR PATIENTS AND FAMILIES

- Bladder and bowel issues are very common among patients with MS.
- Patients should discuss their bowel and bladder issues with their neurologists or primary care doctors, who can refer them to specialists if needed.
- There are many successful treatments for bladder and bowel dysfunction including physical therapy and mediation.
- Some patients may benefit from more invasive treatments if conservative measures fail.

REFERENCES

1. World Health Organization. Atlas: multiple sclerosis resources in the world. 2008. Available at: http://www.who.int/mental_health/neurology/ Atlas_MS_WEB.pdf.
2. Mahajan S, Patel P, Marrie R. The under treatment of overactive bladder symptoms in women with multiple sclerosis: an ancillary analysis of the NARCOMS Patient Registry. *J Urol.* 2010;183:1432–1437.
3. Mayo ME, Chetner MP. Lower urinary tract dysfunction in multiple sclerosis. *Urology.* January 1992;39(1):67–70.
4. Tepavcevic DK, Pekmezovic T, Stojsavljevic N, et al. Change in quality of life and predictors of change among patients with multiple sclerosis: a prospective cohort study. *Qual Life Res.* April 2014;23(3):1027–1037.
5. Crayton H, Heyman R, Rossman H. A multimodal approach to managing the symptoms of multiple sclerosis. *Neurology.* 2004;63(suppl 5):S12–S18.
6. Blaivas J, Holland NJ, Giesser B, et al. Multiple sclerosis bladder: studies and care. *Ann N Y Acad Sci.* 1984;436:328–346.
7. Charil A, Zijdenbos AP, Taylor J, et al. Statistical mapping analysis of lesion location and neurological disability in multiple sclerosis: application to 452 patient data sets.*Neuroimage.* July 2003;19(3):532–544.
8. Marrie R, Cutter G, Tyry T, et al. Disparities in the management of multiple sclerosis-related bladder symptoms. *Neurology.* 2007;68:1971–1978.
9. Martinez L, Neshatian L, Khavari R. Neurogenic bowel dysfunction in patients with neurogenic bladder. *Curr Bladder Dysfunct Rep.* December 2016;11(4):334–340.
10. Uebersax J, Wyman JF, Shumaker SA, et al. Short forms to assess life quality and symptom distress for urinary incontinence in women: the incontinence impact questionnaire and the urogenital distress inventory. *Neurourol Urodyn.* 1995;14:131–139.
11. Barber M, Kuchibhatla MN, Pieper CF, et al. Psychometric evaluation of 2 comprehensive condition-specific quality of life instruments for women with pelvic floor disorders. *Am J Obstet Gynecol.* 2001;185(6):1388–1395.
12. Phé V, Chartier-Kastler E, Panicker JN. Management of neurogenic bladder in patients with multiple sclerosis. *Nat Rev Urol.* May 2016;13(5):275–288.
13. Winters JC, Dmochowski RR, Goldman HB, et al. Urodynamic studies in adults: AUA/SUFU guideline. *J Urol.* December 2012;188(6 suppl):2464–2472.
14. Litwiller SE, Frohman EM, Zimmern PE. Multiple sclerosis and the urologist. *J Urol.* March 1999;161(3):743–757.
15. deSeze M, Ruffion A, Denys P, et al. The neurogenic bladder in multiple sclerosis: review of the literature and proposal of management guidelines. *Mult Scler.* 2007;13:915–928.
16. Sadiq A, Brucker BM. Management of neurogenic lower urinary tract dysfunction in multiple sclerosis patients. *Curr Urol Rep.* July 2015;16(7):44.
17. De Ridder D, Vermeulen C, Ketelaer P, et al. Pelvic floor rehabilitation in multiple sclerosis. *Acta Neurol Belg.* 1999;99:61–64.
18. McClurg D, Ashe RG, Lowe-Strong AS. Neuromuscular electrical stimulation and the treatment of lower urinary tract dysfunction in multiple sclerosis—a double-blind placebo-controlled, randomized clinical trial. *Neurourol Urodyn.* 2008;27:231–237.
19. Nicholas RS, Friede T, Hollis S, et al. Anticholinergics for urinary symptoms in multiple sclerosis. *Cochrane Database Syst Rev.* January 21, 2009;1:CD004193.
20. Madhuvrata P, Singh M, Hasafa Z, et al. Anticholinergic drugs for adult neurogenic detrusor overactivity: a systematic review and meta-analysis. *Eur Urol.* 2012;25;62(5):816–830.
21. de Sèze M, Raibaut P, Gallien P, et al. Transcutaneous posterior tibial nerve stimulation for treatment of overactive bladder syndrome in multiple sclerosis: a multicenter prospective study. *Neurourol Urodyn.* 2011;30:306–311.
22. Zecca C, Digesu GA, Robshaw P, et al. Maintenance percutaneous posterior nerve stimulation for refractory lower urinary tract symptoms in patients with multiple sclerosis: an open label, multicenter, prospective study. *J Urol.* 2014;191(3):697–702.
23. Cruz F, Herschorn S, Aliotta P, et al. Efficacy and safety of onabotulinum toxin A in patients with urinary incontinence due to neurogenic detrusor overactivity: a randomised, double-blind, placebo-controlled trial. *Eur Urol.* 2011;60(4):742–750.
24. Ginsberg D, Cruz F, Herschorn S, et al. Onabotulinum toxin A is effective in patients with urinary incontinence due to neurogenic detrusor activity regardless of concomitant anticholinergic use or neurologic etiology. *Adv Ther.* 2013;30(9):819–833.
25. Denys P, Dmochowski R, Aliotta P, et al. Positive outcomes with first onabotulinum toxin A treatment persist in the long term with repeat treatments in patients with neurogenic detrusor over activity. *BJU Int.* June 2017;119(6):926–932.
26. Minardi D, Muzzonigro G. Sacral neuromodulation in patients with multiple sclerosis. *World J Urol.* February 2012;30(1):123–128.
27. Kessler TM, La Framboise D, Trelle S, et al. Sacral neuromodulation for neurogenic lower urinary tract dysfunction: systematic review and meta-analysis. *Eur Urol.* December 2010;58(6):865–874.
28. Chaabane W, Guillotreau J, Castel-Lacanal E, et al. Sacral neuromodulation for treating neurogenic bladder dysfunction: clinical and urodynamic study. *Neurourol Urodyn.* April 2011;30(4):547–550.
29. Zachoval R, Pitha J, Medova E, et al. Augmentation cystoplasty in patients with multiple sclerosis. *Urol Int.* 2003;70(1):21–26.
30. Mahajan ST, Frasure HE, Marrie RA. The prevalence of urinary catheterization in women and men with multiple sclerosis. *J Spinal Cord Med.* November 2013;36(6):632–637.

31. Kakizaki H, Ameda K, Kobayashi S, et al. Urodynamic effects of alpha1-blocker tamsulosin on voiding dysfunction in patients with neurogenic bladder. *Int J Urol*. November 2003;10(11):576–581.

32. Stankovich EIu, Borisov VV, Demina TL. Tamsulosin in the treatment of detrusor-sphincter dyssynergia of the urinary bladder in patients with multiple sclerosis. *Urologiia*. July-August 2004;(4):48–51.

33. Stoffel JT. Chronic urinary retention in multiple sclerosis patients: physiology, systematic review of urodynamic data, and recommendations for care. *Urol Clin North Am*. August 2017;44(3):429–439.

34. de Sèze M, Petit H, Gallien P, et al. Botulinum a toxin and detrusor sphincter dyssynergia: a double-blind lidocaine-controlled study in 13 patients with spinal cord disease. *Eur Urol*. July 2002;42(1):56–62.

35. Utomo E, Groen J, Blok BF. Surgical management of functional bladder outlet obstruction in adults with neurogenic bladder dysfunction. *Cochrane Database Syst Rev*. May 24, 2014;(5):CD004927.

36. Marinkovic SP, Gillen LM. Sacral neuromodulation for multiple sclerosis patients with urinary retention and clean intermittent catheterization. *Int Urogynecol J*. February 2010;21(2):223–228.

37. Gulick E. Comparison of prevalance, related medical history, symptoms, and interventions regarding boweldysfunction in persons with multiple sclerosis. *J Neurosci Nurs*. 2010;42:E12–E23.

38. Abrams P, Andersson KE, Birder L, et al. Fourth international consultation on incontinence recommendations of the international scientific committee: evaluation and treatment of urinary incontinence, pelvic organ prolapse, and fecal incontinence. *Neurourol Urodyn*. 2010;29(1):213–240.

39. Muller-Lissner SA. Effect of wheat bran on weight of stool and gastrointestinal transit time: a meta analysis. *Br Med J (Clin Res Ed)*. 1988;296(6622):615–617.

40. DasGupta R, Fowler CJ. Bladder, bowel and sexual dysfunction in multiple sclerosis management strategies. *Drugs*. 2003;63(2):153–166.

41. Cotterill N, Madersbacher H, Wyndaele JJ, et al. Neurogenic bowel dysfunction: clinical management recommendations of the Neurologic Incontinence Committee of the Fifth International Consultation on Incontinence 2013. *Neurourol Urodyn*. June 22, 2017.

28 Sexual Dysfunction and Other Autonomic Disorders in Multiple Sclerosis

Samantha Domingo and Carolyn Fisher

KEY POINTS FOR CLINICIANS

- Autonomic dysfunction is common among individuals with multiple sclerosis (MS) and it involves both the sympathetic and parasympathetic branches of the autonomic nervous system.
- Autonomic dysfunction can lead to malfunction of urinary, cardiovascular, and thermoregulatory systems.
- Clinical symptoms associated with autonomic dysfunction in MS are heterogeneous.
- Autonomic dysfunction greatly influences the quality of life in patients with MS, and can significantly restrict activities of daily living.
- Autonomic dysfunction may be difficult to detect via traditional assessment methods.
- Sexual dysfunction is a common feature of MS.
- Sexual dysfunction causes in MS can stem from primary, secondary, and tertiary causes.

MS is associated with significant autonomic imbalance, with estimates that up to 90% of patients with MS have symptoms stemming from autonomic dysfunction (1). Autonomic dysfunction in MS is thought to be related to demyelinating plaques and axonal degeneration, which may disrupt critical pathways of the autonomic nervous system (ANS), including the brainstem, spinal cord, hypothalamus, and cerebral cortex (2–4). Autonomic dysfunction in MS involves both the sympathetic (SNS) and parasympathetic (PNS) branches of the ANS (1,5,6). Dysfunction of the SNS has been found to be a result of long-term clinical activity of MS (5). It has been postulated that, similar to other disease processes, chronic overactivation of the SNS could further contribute to the neurodegenerative process in progressive MS (7). Of note, SNS dysregulation may be more pronounced in patients who are in relapse (5) and progressive patients who are more severely disabled (7). PNS dysfunction, on the other hand, is closely related to disease progression and clinical disability (5,8).

Autonomic dysfunction can lead to malfunction of various body systems. Symptoms may manifest clinically as orthostatic intolerance, abnormal sweating, impaired thermoregulation, chronic fatigue, dysfunction of the pupillary reflexes, gastrointestinal symptoms, sleep disturbance, bladder or bowel dysfunction, and sexual dysfunction (SD). Autonomic dysfunction can greatly influence quality of life in patients with MS, and can significantly restrict activities

of daily living. Research has demonstrated that ANS imbalance correlates with duration of illness (1), disease progression (9), brain lesions (2), fatigue (10), inflammatory activity (7), and disability (2,5–7,11).

> *Autonomic dysfunction is frequent in MS and is thought to be directly related to lesions in specific areas of the central nervous system (CNS).*

SEXUAL DYSFUNCTION

SD, encompassing desire disorders, arousal disorders, orgasm disorders, and pain disorders, is among the myriad of symptoms of MS, with prevalence rates ranging from 40% to 80% in women and 50% to 90% in men (12–16). SD in MS can present early in the disease process (17). Some of the most common complaints in women include orgasmic dysfunction, loss of libido, inadequate vaginal lubrication, and genital numbness. For men, the most common presentation includes erectile dysfunction, loss of sexual confidence, orgasmic dysfunction, and genital numbness (16). Libido is typically associated with cerebral control, while arousal and response are related to spinal, autonomic reflexes (18,19).

Healthy sexual functioning relies on the intricate interplay of various systems including neurological, endocrine, vascular, and psychological; MS has a direct impact on one or more of these systems, heightening risk for the development of SD.

From a conceptual model, SD can be understood to have different levels of contributing factors that can be categorized into primary, secondary, and tertiary factors (20,21). Primary causes are those generally associated with cortex and spinal cord lesions and can include numbness, loss of libido, decreased lubrication, erectile dysfunction, and contributory medications. Secondary causes tend to stem from MS symptomatology including fatigue, spasticity, pain, bladder and bowel dysfunction, and cognitive difficulties. Tertiary causes are related to psychosocial factors including changes in social roles, mood disorders, demoralization, interpersonal difficulties, body image concerns, and fear of rejection, among others. Generally, individual cases will present with a combination of primary, secondary, and tertiary levels of contributing factors.

In terms of the pathophysiology of primary SD, it is understood that lesions in specific brain and spinal cord regions are associated with different presentations of SD in individuals with MS (22). For instance, erectile dysfunction, decreased vaginal lubrication, and changes in vaginal sensation were correlated with the T1-weighted images lesion load in the pons (23). Furthermore, a recent study examining the neuroanatomic correlates of female SD found that MS lesions in the occipital region had an impact on female sexual arousal; inadequate lubrication was associated with lesions in the left insular region, which typically contributes to the generation and mapping of visceral autonomic arousal states (24).

> *Sexual dysfunction in MS is related to primary (CNS lesions), secondary (other MS symptoms), and tertiary (psychosocial) factors.*

Assessment

Assessment of primary SD in MS poses several challenges, as there are very limited autonomic testing methodologies available (22). One study found that in individuals with MS and SD, there was more abnormal sympathetic skin response in the genitals than in the lower extremities, which could be indicative of subclinical autonomic dysfunction (25). More specific to erectile dysfunction, the recording of tumescence and rigidity during nocturnal erections can be utilized to identify primary or organic dysfunction (17).

In clinical settings, a comprehensive clinical interview can help to identify potential factors impacting SD symptoms. It is important to make note of potential side effects from medications and the impact of secondary MS symptoms (i.e., fatigue, urinary/bowel dysfunction, etc.). As such, there is evidence to support the relationship between SD and bladder dysfunction (26,27). In terms of tertiary symptoms, it is imperative to assess for depression in this population, as there is a strong association between depression severity and incidence of SD (28,29).

In addition to the standard clinical interview, there are validated tools designed to assess for SD in the MS population. The Multiple Sclerosis Sexuality and Intimacy Questionnaire 19 (MSISQ-19) is a 19-item self-report measure that addresses three dimensions of SD based on primary, secondary, and tertiary factors (30). The questionnaire, using a five-point Likert scale ranging in order of frequency of experience, assesses the level in which MS symptoms have interfered with the individual's sexual functioning in the previous 6 months. One of the advantages of utilizing this instrument is that it is the only one to date that is specifically designed for and validated in an MS population. Additionally, it only takes about 2 minutes to complete and patients are directed to discuss specific symptoms with their clinician if they score above a cutoff of 4 in terms of frequency. Finally, it is available for use in clinical and research settings at no cost. See Table 28.1 for a summary of assessment options.

Given the potential impact SD can have on quality of life, even when controlling for disability and other variables (15,31), it is paramount to incorporate screening and assessment into standard clinical practice. However, there are potential barriers that prevent practitioners from further inquiring into this area. Griswold (32) identified time limits with patients and feeling like the subject is outside the practitioner's role as the most common reasons why clinicians do not assess for SD in their daily practice. Frequently, patients do not volunteer concerns unless directly asked, but many are grateful when the subject is raised (33). Addressing potential barriers to assessment of SD is the key in facilitating adequate treatment. For instance, adequate training and practice in assessment can potentially increase the provider's comfort levels.

> *The topic of sexual dysfunction is frequently not brought up by both patients and clinicians during routine visits.*

TABLE 28.1 Assessment of Sexual Dysfunction in Multiple Sclerosis

- **Assess contributory medications (e.g., SSRIs)**
- **Conduct a comprehensive exam and history; identify contributing symptoms (e.g., fatigue)**
- **Evaluate concurrent perimenopause, menopause, and andropause status**
- **Obtain sexual history**
- **Incorporate screening tools such as the MSISQ-19**

MSISQ-19, Multiple Sclerosis Sexuality and Intimacy Questionnaire 19; SSRIs, selective serotonin reuptake inhibitors.

Treatment

Due to the complexity of the etiology of symptoms of SD in MS, treatment is likely to necessitate a multidisciplinary approach. Evidence-based SD treatment is an area of the literature that is still in its infancy, though there are a handful of studies examining pharmacological interventions in male and female patients with MS. There is modest evidence supporting the effectiveness of sildenafil in improving neurogenic erectile dysfunction in male patients with MS (34). In terms of female SD, sildenafil has demonstrated limited and inconsistent evidence in terms of therapeutic effectiveness (35,36). A pilot study by Lucio (37) incorporated pelvic floor training with electromyogram (EMG) biofeedback in female patients with MS and SD, and results showed improved vaginal tone, flexibility,

and reduced pain, but no improvement of desire, arousal, or orgasm. Interventions with a rehabilitation and counseling approach have shown more consistent and promising results (38,39). Despite limited research in this area, it is clear that treatment of SD is not unidimensional, and should incorporate a holistic approach which includes neurology, urology, nursing, social work, health psychology, and occupational and physical therapy (40). See Table 28.2 for a summary of interventions designed to target specific levels of SD.

The treatment of sexual dysfunction in MS is generally multimodal and multidisciplinary.

TABLE 28.2 Clinical Management of Sexual Dysfunction in Multiple Sclerosis

PRIMARY SEXUAL DYSFUNCTION	
SYMPTOM	**MANAGEMENT AND TREATMENT OPTIONS**
Decreased libido	CBT to address unhelpful beliefs about sexuality and sexual function; couples counseling; consider disease-modifying or symptomatic medications that could be contributing; body mapping exercises
Orgasmic dysfunction Premature/delayed ejaculation	Modify contributing medications if possible; focus on management of other symptoms; CBT may be considered
Decreased vaginal lubrication	Incorporate water-soluble lubricants prior to and during sexual activity and/or lubricants that contain menthol or other vasoactive agents to improve sensation; EMG biofeedback; pelvic floor training to stimulate arousal; hormonal therapy may be considered.
Erectile dysfunction	Consider use of PDE-5 inhibitors[a]; consider injectable medications such as prostaglandin.[b]
Genital numbness/ paresthesias	Genital sensation can be improved with more vigorous genital stimulation and use of vibrators; adequate management of paresthesias; CBT; couples counseling
SECONDARY SEXUAL DYSFUNCTION	
SYMPTOM	**MANAGEMENT AND TREATMENT OPTIONS**
Fatigue	Energy conservation strategies and planning for sexual activity; strategic napping; ambulation aids; pharmacologic treatment of fatigue
Bladder and bowel symptoms	Behavioral strategies (e.g., restricting fluid intake and planned bowel movements); self-catheterization before sexual activity; use of condoms for men to address urinary leakage; pharmacological interventions including the use of anticholinergic medications
Spasticity	Physical therapy focusing on range of motion exercises; consider taking antispasticity medication 30 min prior to sexual activity; explore alternative sexual positions to minimize discomfort or pain
Cognitive changes	Minimize nonsexual stimuli and maximize sensual and sexual stimuli to improve attention and concentration; consider cognitive rehabilitation
TERTIARY SEXUAL DYSFUNCTION	
SYMPTOM	**MANAGEMENT AND TREATMENT OPTIONS**
Depression	CBT; consider SNRIs such as venlafaxine, desvenlafaxine, or duloxetine due to fewer sexual side effects compared to SSRIs; consider adding bupropion to antidepressant regimen
Role reversal	If sexual partner is the primary caregiver, consider incorporating other family members to perform caregiving duties for the patient as to avoid "role conflict"; individual and/or couples counseling
Relationship issues	Couples counseling
Body image	CBT; couples counseling or sex therapy

[a]Sildenafil is the only medication that has been evaluated in clinical trials in men with MS.
[b]Prostaglandin and PDE-5 inhibitors contraindicated when patient is on nitrate-based cardiac medications, as they can lower blood pressure excessively.
CBT, cognitive behavioral therapy; EMG, electromyogram; PDE-5, phosphodiesterase type-5; SNRI, serotonin norepinephrine reuptake inhibitors; SSRI, selective serotonin reuptake inhibitors.

OTHER TYPES OF AUTONOMIC IMPAIRMENT IN MS

Cardiovascular Dysfunction

Estimates of the prevalence of cardiovascular autonomic dysfunction in patients with MS vary widely, from 10% to 55% (3,41,42). Cardiovascular abnormalities are likely due to injury of the cerebral pathways, which affect autonomic control of heart rate (43,44), and impairments are shown to involve both sympathetic and parasympathetic pathways (7,45).

Research consistently documents impaired heart rate variability (HRV) in patients with MS (7,8,43). Autonomic cardiovascular alterations, including impaired HRV, have been found to progress with severity and duration of MS (44,46,47). Specifically, cardiovascular autonomic dysfunction in patients with MS has been shown to correlate with midbrain lesion load (47), suggesting that with longer disease duration and more widespread plaques throughout the brain, impairment of cardiac autonomic balance may be increased (44). As such, autonomic cardiovascular testing may has been proposed as a surrogate marker for disease activity (2,7,48), particularly in light of research documenting that the relationship between autonomic dysfunction and MS disease duration may be independent of the presence of autonomic symptoms (7). Thus, assessment of cardiovascular autonomic function may be particularly useful to detect subclinical autonomic changes in MS (7,48). Standard cardiac autonomic tests include deep breathing test, Valsalva maneuver, blood pressure and heart rate responses to standing, and sustained handgrip.

> *Impaired heart rate variability has been consistently demonstrated in patients with MS.*

Orthostatic Intolerance

Orthostatic intolerance is one common manifestation of cardiovascular dysfunction. Orthostatic intolerance has been reported in up to 50% of patients with MS (49), and is thought to be a consequence of impaired sympathetic vasomotor control due to lesions in key parts of the brain (3,45). Notably, disability level is correlated with orthostatic intolerance (11). Manifestations of orthostatic dysfunction include syncope, dizziness, and postural orthostatic tachycardia syndrome (POTS). Orthostatic dizziness and syncope are common symptoms, and have been reported in up to 49% (41) and 55% (50) of patients with MS, respectively.

POTS is a form of orthostatic intolerance that has been commonly reported in patients with MS (11). Symptoms of POTS in patients with MS include fatigue, palpitations, orthostatic dizziness, and syncope, with the most commonly reported symptom being fatigue (50). The connection between POTS and MS may be attributed to demyelination of the brainstem and hemispheric lesions (50). POTS can exacerbate morbidity and disability already experienced in patients with MS, and lead to substantial limitation of daily activities and reduction in quality of life. Thus, POTS diagnosis and management are important considerations, and may result in improved quality of life in these patients.

> *Orthostatic dizziness, syncope, and POTS can be manifestations of orthostatic intolerance in patients with MS.*

Fatigue

Cardiovascular autonomic disturbance may also contribute to increased fatigue in patients with MS. Moreover, severity of autonomic dysfunction has been found to be more pronounced in patients who experience MS-related fatigue than those who do not, and the relationship between fatigue and autonomic dysfunction may be due, in part, to sympathetic vasomotor dysfunction (10).

Sleep Disturbance

Over 50% of patients with MS report sleep-related problems (51), which may be a result of dysautonomia in MS. Types of sleep disturbance may include difficulty initiating or sustaining sleep due to spasms or discomfort, snoring, and nocturia. Sleep disturbance may present clinically as insomnia, daytime fatigue, hypersomnolence, or depression (51). While sleep disturbance is common in patients with MS, it is often underdiagnosed and undertreated (see Chapter 22).

Impaired Thermoregulation

Patients with MS may experience abnormalities in body temperature regulation, although their prevalence has not been established. While the etiology of impaired thermoregulation in MS is multifactorial, areas of the SNS responsible for controlling thermoregulatory function are susceptible to demyelination, and this may contribute to increased sympathetic vasoconstriction in MS (52). The phenomenon of heat sensitivity is attributed to the detrimental effects of increased temperature on the conduction of action potentials along demyelinated axons. Abnormal thermoregulatory responses to heat stress, particularly decreased sweating, may further contribute to this problem (52). Notably, an estimated 60% to 80% of MS patients experience a temporary worsening of both physical and cognitive symptoms with heat exposure, which can greatly affect activities of daily living.

> *Impaired thermoregulatory responses may further contribute to heat sensitivity.*

PATIENT CASE A 44-year-old married female patient with relapsing–remitting MS (RRMS) presented to the clinic reporting decreased libido. She had been clinically stable while on fingolimod for about 8 months. However, she reported concerns about recent incidents of urinary and bowel incontinence. She endorsed increased stress and relationship concerns, which contributed to worsening of mood and increased anxiety symptoms. Since her last visit, there had been no other clinical changes, though she was concerned about incontinence issues, which had occurred twice in the past 3 months. Of note, presence of urinary tract infection had already been ruled out. Although otherwise clinically stable, this patient's worsening of mood and anxiety in relation to increased stress may have exacerbated autonomic dysregulation, which could potentially be impacting her bladder/bowel symptoms. In this case, management of the patient's symptoms included a referral urology to rule out medical etiology, and a referral to psychology to manage contributors of anxiety and mood. With the use of postvoiding residual by ultrasound, the urology referral revealed no concern of urinary retention. With the psychologist, the patient began cognitive behavioral therapy (CBT) to address mood and anxiety associated with relationship issues and bladder/bowel symptoms. CBT is a treatment modality that focuses on addressing beliefs and attitudes that may be interfering with the target behavior or symptom. For instance, the patient believed that she could not have a mutually satisfying sexual relationship with her husband if she had bladder or bowel control issues. Thus, this belief was challenged by way of evaluating the evidence supporting or debunking her belief, and the patient began identifying in therapy what intimacy meant for her. Behavioral strategies such as planning and scheduling bathroom breaks, voiding before sexual activity, and avoiding food and liquid intake a few hours prior to activity were discussed with the patient. Additionally, the patient underwent respiration and HRV biofeedback training as a way to learn to regulate autonomic functioning and enhance the parasympathetic response. Goals of autonomic regulation through biofeedback included reducing bladder and bowel incontinence, and further reducing anxiety associated with sexual activity. After four sessions, the patient demonstrated a reduction in anxiety and mood measures, improved relationship satisfaction, and decreased frequency of incontinence episodes.

KEY POINTS FOR PATIENTS AND FAMILIES

- Autonomic dysfunction is common in patients with MS, and can contribute to a wide variety of symptoms such as fatigue, dizziness with standing, abnormal bowel and bladder control, and SD.

- SD is a common feature of MS and can have an impact on mood and quality of life.

- There are many factors that can contribute to SD including unmanaged MS symptoms, depression, side effects from medications, issues with relationships and body image.

- In addition to adequate management of symptoms and medications contributing to SD, treatment of SD in MS can involve medications, counseling, or a combination of both.

REFERENCES

1. Gunal DI, Afsar N, Tanridag T, et al. Autonomic dysfunction in multiple sclerosis: correlation with disease-related parameters. *Eur Neurol*. 2002;48(1):1–5.
2. Acevedo AR, Nava C, Arriada N, et al. Cardiovascular dysfunction in multiple sclerosis. *Acta Neurol Scand*. 2000;101(2):85–88.
3. Vita G, Fazio MC, Milone S, et al. Cardiovascular autonomic dysfunction in multiple sclerosis is likely related to brainstem lesions. *J Neurol Sci*. 1993;120(1):82–86.
4. de Seze J, Stojkovic T, Gauvrit JY, et al. Autonomic dysfunction in multiple sclerosis: cervical spinal cord atrophy correlates. *J Neurol*. 2001;248(4):297–303.
5. Flachenecker P, Reiners K, Krauser M, et al. Autonomic dysfunction in multiple sclerosis is related to disease activity and progression of disability. *Mult Scler*. 2001;7(5):327–334.
6. Merkelbach S, Dillmann U, Kolmel C, et al. Cardiovascular autonomic dysregulation and fatigue in multiple sclerosis. *Mult Scler*. 2001;7(5):320–326.
7. Studer V, Rocchi C, Motta C, et al. Heart rate variability is differentially altered in multiple sclerosis: implications for acute, worsening and progressive disability. *Mult Scler J Exp Transl Clin*. 2017;3(2):1–11.
8. Monge-Argiles JA, Palacios-Ortega F, Vila-Sobrino JA, et al. Heart rate variability in multiple sclerosis during a stable phase. *Acta Neurol Scand*. 1998;97(2):86–92.
9. Merkelbach S, Haensch CA, Hemmer B, et al. Multiple sclerosis and the autonomic nervous system. *J Neurol*. 2006;253(suppl 1):I21–I25.
10. Flachenecker P, Rufer A, Bihler I, et al. Fatigue in MS is related to sympathetic vasomotor dysfunction. *Neurology*. 2003;61(6):851–853.
11. Adamec I, Bach I, Barusic AK, et al. Assessment of prevalence and pathological response to orthostatic provocation in patients with multiple sclerosis. *J Neurol Sci*. 2013;324(1-2):80–83.
12. Young CA, Tennant A, TONiC Study Group. Sexual functioning in multiple sclerosis: relationships with depression, fatigue and physical function. *Mult Scler*. 2016;23(9):1268–1275.
13. Zorzon M, Zivadinov R, Bosco A, et al. Sexual dysfunction in multiple sclerosis: a case-control study. I. frequency and comparison of groups. *Mult Scler*. 1999;5(6):418–427.

14. Zorzon M, Zivadinov R, Monti Bragadin L, et al. Sexual dysfunction in multiple sclerosis: a 2-year follow-up study. *J Neurol Sci.* 2001;187(1-2):1–5.

15. Tepavcevic DK, Kostic J, Basuroski ID, et al. The impact of sexual dysfunction on the quality of life measured by MSQoL-54 in patients with multiple sclerosis. *Mult Scler.* 2008;14(8):1131–1136.

16. Schairer LC, Foley FW, Zemon V, et al. The impact of sexual dysfunction on health-related quality of life in people with multiple sclerosis. *Mult Scler.* 2014;20(5):610–616.

17. Haensch CA, Jorg J. Autonomic dysfunction in multiple sclerosis. *J Neurol.* 2006;253(suppl 1):I3–I9.

18. Apostolidis AN, Fowler CJ. Evaluation and treatment of autonomic disorders of the urogenital system. *Semin Neurol.* 2003;23(4):443–452.

19. Lundberg PO, Brattberg A. Sexual dysfunction in selected neurologic disorders: hypothalamopituitary disorders, epilepsy, myelopathies, polyneuropathies, and sacral nerve lesions. *Semin Neurol.* 1992;12(2):115–119.

20. Foley FW, Iverson J. Sexuality and MS. In: Kalb RC, Scheinberg LC, eds. *MS and the Family.* New York, NY: Demos Publications; 1992:63–82.

21. Foley FW, Sanders A. Sexuality, multiple sclerosis, and women. *MS Management.* 1997;1(4):1–10.

22. Racosta JM, Kimpinski K, Morrow SA, et al. Autonomic dysfunction in multiple sclerosis. *Auton Neurosci.* 2015;193:1–6.

23. Zivadinov R, Zorzon M, Locatelli L, et al. Sexual dysfunction in multiple sclerosis: a MRI, neurophysiological and urodynamic study. *J Neurol Sci.* 2003;210(1-2):73–76.

24. Winder K, Linker RA, Seifert F, et al. Neuroanatomic correlates of female sexual dysfunction in multiple sclerosis. *Ann Neurol.* 2016;80(4):490–498.

25. Secil Y, Yetimalar Y, Gedizlioglu M, et al. Sexual dysfunction and sympathetic skin response recorded from the genital region in women with multiple sclerosis. *Mult Scler.* 2007;13(6):742–748.

26. Hulter BM, Lundberg PO. Sexual function in women with advanced multiple sclerosis. *J Neurol Neurosurg Psychiatry.* 1995;59(1):83–86.

27. Gruenwald I, Vardi Y, Gartman I, et al. Sexual dysfunction in females with multiple sclerosis: quantitative sensory testing. *Mult Scler.* 2007;13(1):95–105.

28. Gumus H, Akpinar Z, Yilmaz H. Effects of multiple sclerosis on female sexuality: a controlled study. *J Sex Med.* 2014;11(2):481–486.

29. Lew-Starowicz M, Rola R. Correlates of sexual function in male and female patients with multiple sclerosis. *J Sex Med.* 2014;11(9):2172–2180.

30. Sanders A, Foley FW, LaRocca NG, et al. The multiple sclerosis intimacy and sexuality questionnaire-19 (MSISQ-19). *Sex and Disabil.* 2000;18(1):3–26.

31. Nortvedt MW, Riise T, Frugard J, et al. Prevalence of bladder, bowel and sexual problems among multiple sclerosis patients two to five years after diagnosis. *Mult Scler.* 2007;13(1):106–112.

32. Griswold GA, Foley FW, Halper J, et al. Multiple sclerosis and sexuality: a survey of MS health professionals' comfort, training, and inquiry about sexual dysfunction. *Int J MS Care.* 2003;5(2):37–51.

33. Foley FW, Iverson J. Sexuality. In: *Multiple Sclerosis: A Guide for Families.* 3rd ed. New York, NY: Demos Medical Publishing; 2006:53–80.

34. Kratiras Z, Konstantinidis C, Thomas C, et al. P-01-015 efficacy of PDE-5 inhibitors in erectile dysfunction due to multiple sclerosis. *J Sex Med.* 2016;13(5):S145–S146.

35. Brown DA, Kyle JA, Ferrill MJ. Assessing the clinical efficacy of sildenafil for the treatment of female sexual dysfunction. *Ann Pharmacother.* 2009;43(7):1275–1285.

36. Dasgupta R, Wiseman OJ, Kanabar G, et al. Efficacy of sildenafil in the treatment of female sexual dysfunction due to multiple sclerosis. *J Urol.* 2004;171(3):1189–1193; discussion 1193.

37. Lucio A, D'ancona CA, Perissinotto MC, et al. Pelvic floor muscle training with and without electrical stimulation in the treatment of lower urinary tract symptoms in women with multiple sclerosis. *J Wound Ostomy Continence Nurs.* 2016;43(4):414–419.

38. Foley FW, LaRocca NG, Sanders AS, et al. Rehabilitation of intimacy and sexual dysfunction in couples with multiple sclerosis. *Mult Scler.* 2001;7(6):417–421.

39. Taylor B, Davis S. The extended PLISSIT model for addressing the sexual wellbeing of individuals with acquired disability or chronic illness. *Sex Disabil.* 2007;25(3):135–139.

40. Fletcher SG, Castro-Borrero W, Remington G, et al. Sexual dysfunction in patients with multiple sclerosis: a multidisciplinary approach to evaluation and management. *Nat Clin Pract Urol.* 2009;6(2):96–107.

41. Anema JR, Heijenbrok MW, Faes TJ, et al. Cardiovascular autonomic function in multiple sclerosis. *J Neurol Sci.* 1991;104(2):129–134.

42. Sterman AB, Coyle PK, Panasci DJ, et al. Disseminated abnormalities of cardiovascular autonomic functions in multiple sclerosis. *Neurology.* 1985;35(11):1665–1668.

43. Tombul T, Anlar O, Tuncer M, et al. Impaired heart rate variability as a marker of cardiovascular autonomic dysfunction in multiple sclerosis. *Acta Neurol Belg.* 2011;111(2):116–120.

44. Mahovic D, Lakusic N. Progressive impairment of autonomic control of heart rate in patients with multiple sclerosis. *Arch Med Res.* 2007;38(3):322–325.

45. Sanya EO, Tutaj M, Brown CM, et al. Abnormal heart rate and blood pressure responses to baroreflex stimulation in multiple sclerosis patients. *Clin Auton Res.* 2005;15(3):213–218.

46. Nasseri K, TenVoorde BJ, Ader HJ, et al. Longitudinal follow-up of cardiovascular reflex tests in multiple sclerosis. *J Neurol Sci.* 1998;155(1):50–54.

47. Saari A, Tolonen U, Paakko E, et al. Cardiovascular autonomic dysfunction correlates with brain MRI lesion load in MS. *Clin Neurophysiol.* 2004;115(6):1473–1478.

48. Nasseri K, Uitdehaag BM, van Walderveen MA, et al. Cardiovascular autonomic function in patients with relapsing remitting multiple sclerosis: a new surrogate marker of disease evolution? *Eur J Neurol.* 1999;6(1):29–33.

49. Flachenecker P, Wolf A, Krauser M, et al. Cardiovascular autonomic dysfunction in multiple sclerosis: correlation with orthostatic intolerance. *J Neurol.* 1999;246(7):578–586.

50. Kanjwal K, Karabin B, Kanjwal Y, et al. Autonomic dysfunction presenting as postural orthostatic tachycardia syndrome in patients with multiple sclerosis. *Int J Med Sci.* 2010;7:62–67.

51. Tachibana N, Howard RS, Hirsch NP, et al. Sleep problems in multiple sclerosis. *Eur Neurol.* 1994;34(6):320–323.

52. Davis SL, Wilson TE, White AT, et al. Thermoregulation in multiple sclerosis. *J Appl Physiol (1985).* 2010;109(5):1531–1537.

29 Spasticity Management in Multiple Sclerosis

Francois Bethoux and Mary Alissa Willis

KEY POINTS FOR CLINICIANS

- Spasticity, a component of the upper motor neuron syndrome, is a movement disorder characterized by a velocity-dependent increase in resistance to passive muscle stretch.

- Multiple sclerosis (MS) frequently causes spasticity, but the impact of spasticity in terms of discomfort and loss of function can be difficult to assess owing to other impairments (e.g., paresis, neuropathic pain, ataxia).

- Spasticity can help maintain function by compensating for loss of motor control (e.g., lower extremity extensor hypertonia facilitates standing).

- Spasticity treatment planning involves taking into account patient symptoms (e.g., muscle stiffness/tightness, muscle spasms) and examination findings (e.g., resistance to passive movement, range of motion limitations, observed spasms and clonus), and defining realistic goals.

- Muscle stretching and rehabilitation (physical/occupational therapy) must be considered when treating spasticity, alone or in combination with other treatments.

Spasticity is a movement disorder characterized by a velocity-dependent increase in resistance to passive muscle stretching related to increased tonic and phasic stretch reflexes (1). The presumed pathophysiological mechanism is a lack of descending inhibitory control on spinal cord neurons due to central nervous system (CNS) damage. Spasticity is a component of the upper motor neuron syndrome, which also includes weakness, loss of selective voluntary motor control, loss of dexterity, muscle spasms, synkinesis, and hyperreflexia.

The prevalence of spasticity in MS is high, with objective signs of spasticity noted in close to 60% of patients (2). Symptoms of spasticity were reported by 80% of responders in a survey from the North American Research Committee on MS (NARCOMS), with 35% of responders rating the symptoms as moderate or severe, and a predominant impact on the lower extremities (3). Spasticity severity was associated with worse disability, and was reported to interfere with many activities, particularly climbing stairs, walking, and sleeping. In this most recent survey, the majority of patients with spasticity reported that their symptoms were being addressed but less than half were satisfied with treatment of their spasticity.

EVALUATING SPASTICITY

Symptoms reported by the patient or a caregiver are essential in screening for spasticity (see Table 29.1). Beyond the basic symptoms, information should be sought about how spasticity impacts the patient's (and caregivers') activities and quality of life, asking for precise examples. For instance, painful spasms at night may disrupt sleep and cause increased fatigue the next day; stiffness in the hip adductors may interfere with hygiene and with the ability to perform intermittent catheterization; stiffness in the arms may interfere with the ability to get dressed, either independently or with the help of a caregiver. However, the description of symptoms can be misleading. For example, a patient may report that a limb is "stiff" because of difficulty voluntarily moving the affected limb, which is actually related to weakness without increase in tone. Paresthesias and neuropathic pain can be associated with a sensation of spasms, without involuntary muscle contraction on examination. Pain in MS is often multifactorial (neuropathic pain, musculoskeletal from abnormal posture and movement, pain from spasticity). A detailed interview, and the response to empirical symptomatic therapies, can help determine if the pain is likely to be primarily related to spasticity.

Examination is a key in confirming the presence of spasticity, assessing its severity, and identifying other pertinent neurological impairments (see Table 29.2). Dynamic phenomena ("spastic catch," abnormal movement patterns, spasms, clonus) are related to hyperexcitable reflexes, while static phenomena (decreased range of motion, fixed deformity) are related to changes in the rheological properties of musculoskeletal structures. In some patients, hypertonia is minimal at rest and becomes severe and bothersome with voluntary movement; therefore, spasticity should be assessed at rest (sitting or lying down) and with activity. Spasticity must be distinguished from other causes of abnormal muscle tone, particularly dystonia and extrapyramidal hypertonia (both more rarely encountered in MS). A complete neurological examination is warranted, as other impairments are likely to contribute to the patient's functional limitations.

> *Although screening for spasticity relies on patient-reported symptoms, the diagnosis must be confirmed by physical examination.*

Spasticity is most often evaluated by recording the signs and symptoms listed during a standard neurological examination. More standardized, quantitative clinician- or patient-reported measures are available to enhance outcome assessment (see Table 29.2). The Ashworth Scale, in its standard or modified versions, is widely used despite known limitations (4,5). Proper training is required to ensure inter and intrarelater reliability. Other measures of impairment and activity are important to consider, depending on the treatment goals (e.g., range of motion, muscle strength, pain, walking performance

TABLE 29.1 Symptoms and Signs Commonly Associated With Spasticity and the Upper Motor Neuron Syndrome

SYMPTOMS

Muscle stiffness or tightness
Difficulty performing voluntary movement
Clonus (sometimes described by patients as "shaking" or "tremor")
Muscle spasms
Pain (associated with spasms, stiffness, or passive movement)
Limb deformity
Difficulty attaining or maintaining adequate trunk and limb posture
Reported by caregivers: difficulty moving the limbs passively, difficult performing hygiene and care

CLINICAL FINDINGS

Velocity-dependent resistance to passive mobilization
"Clasp-knife" phenomenon (initial resistance to passive movement followed by sudden relaxation as the muscle continues to be stretched)
Abnormal limb or trunk posture, musculoskeletal deformity
Decreased passive range of motion
Hyperreflexia with or without clonus
Spastic cocontraction of agonist and antagonist muscles
Synergistic movement patterns
Flexor or extensor muscle spasms
Weakness
Loss of dexterity

TABLE 29.2 Outcome Measures for Spasticity Management

NAME	PURPOSE	MEASUREMENT SCALE AND COMMENTS
Clinical Measures		
Ashworth Scale (and modified versions)	To assess spasticity via resistance to passive movement	Applied to individual muscle groups; from 0 = no resistance to 4 = limb rigid in flexion or extension for each muscle or muscle group tested
Tardieu Scale	To assess spasticity via resistance to passive movement at three different speeds	R1: angle to first point of resistance during a fast stretch R2: angle to maximum range of motion during slow passive movement within physiological limits R2–R1 defines "dynamic tone"
Resistance to Passive Movement Scale	To assess spasticity via resistance to passive movement	Same rating scale as the Ashworth Scale, but examination and rating instructions are more standardized Predefined list of 26 passive movements to be tested Total score from 0 to 104
Patient Self-Report Measures		
Spasm Frequency Scale	To assess spasticity via spasm frequency	Ordinal scale from 0 = no spasm to 4 = more than 10 spontaneous spasms per hour
Spasticity Numeric Rating Scale	To assess the overall severity of spasticity	Ordinal scale from 0 = no spasticity, to 10 = worst possible spasticity
MS Spasticity Scale-88	To assess the impact of spasticity (how much patients are bothered by consequences of spasticity)	For each of 88 items, from 1 = not at all bothered, to 4 = extremely bothered Total score from 88 to 352

REPAS, Resistance to Passive Movement; SFS, Spasm Frequency Scale; NRS, Numeric Rating Scale; MSSS, MS Spasticity Scale tests, upper extremity function tests, generic quality of life measures).

MANAGEMENT OF SPASTICTY

While spasticity management does not alter MS disease activity, the use of disease therapies and treatment of spasticity-related symptoms are complementary in the overall management of patients with MS. The goals of spasticity management include

- Providing relief of symptoms
- Improving posture
- Improving function and/or ease of care (sometimes called "passive function")
- Preventing long-term complications (e.g., fixed contractures, decubiti)

Realistic goals should be discussed with patients and care providers early on.

A summary of treatment modalities is provided in Table 29.3. Muscle stretching must be a part of the treatment plan (except in rare cases where it is contraindicated). The National MS Society published booklets (*Stretching for People with MS: An illustrated manual*, and *Stretching with a Helper for People with MS: An illustrated manual*) available free of charge online or by mail to all people with MS (6). Greater improvement in patient reporting of spasticity was observed when stretching education was led by facilitators (7). Such studies of nonpharmacologic spasticity interventions are limited. Although the rationale for the use of rehabilitation in the management of spasticity is mostly empirical, skilled rehabilitation strategies should be considered, particularly when improvement of active function is sought.

TABLE 29.3 Summary of Treatment Modalities for Spasticity

TREATMENT	INDICATIONS	POTENTIAL ADVERSE EFFECTS/ COMMENTS
Rehabilitation/exercise (e.g., stretching, serial casting, splinting, orthotics, electrical stimulation, functional training)	Can be used across the spectrum of spasticity severity Should be considered in combination with all other treatment modalities	Tolerance to exercise and rehabilitation can be limited in MS
Oral medications (e.g., baclofen, tizanidine, dantrolene sodium, benzodiazepines)	Can be used across the spectrum of spasticity severity Starting at a low dose and titrating slowly is advised Medications can be combined, with close attention to cumulative side effects	Side effects include sedation, weakness, cognitive slowing, and liver toxicity for some medications
Cannabinoids (e.g., nabiximols)	Not approved in United States. Indicated in other countries for treatment-resistant moderate to severe MS-related spasticity. Dose should be individually titrated after positive response is observed during initial trial period	Side effects include dizziness, fatigue, and application site reactions
Local treatments (phenol/alcohol injections, BT injections)	To treat focal spasticity, or to address a focal problem related to diffuse spasticity Duration of effect: up to 36 mo with phenol, usually 3 mo with BT	Phenol/alcohol injections: local side effects (pain, chronic dysesthesia) BT injections: local side effects (pain, weakness, atrophy); systemic side effects (nausea, fatigue, respiratory infections, dysphagia, development of neutralizing antibodies, rare severe generalized side effects)
Neuromodulation (intrathecal baclofen therapy)	To treat severe diffuse spasticity refractory to oral medications and stretching A screening test should be performed to help with decision making and to refine expectation	Complications from surgery and anesthesia, wound dehiscence, pseudomeningocele, infection around the device, catheter malfunction, pump malfunction, baclofen withdrawal or overdose
Orthopedic surgery (tendon release, tendon transfer, osteotomy)	To address contractures and deformities resulting from spasticity These procedures are rarely used in MS	Complications include delayed healing and infection A period of immobilization is usually required It is important to optimize spasticity control before performing orthopedic surgery
Neurosurgery (neurotomy, selective dorsal rhizotomy)	To decrease spasticity by decreasing nerve input These procedures are rarely used in MS	Sensory loss, paresthesias, weakness

BT, botulinum toxin; MS, multiple sclerosis.

Management frequently involves a combination of complementary modalities to achieve the desired outcome. The MS Council for Clinical Practice Guidelines published evidence-based recommendations for the management of spasticity in MS and proposed a decision algorithm (8).

Oral antispasticity agents (Table 29.4) are widely used, although clinical trial evidence to support the efficacy of these medications in MS is limited (9). Some of

Stretching should be taught to all patients with spasticity or their caregivers, and should be performed daily.

these symptomatic medications are used off label. The MS Council guidelines and a European consensus statement (10)

TABLE 29.4   Oral Antispasticity Agents

MEDICATION	DOSE	ADVERSE EFFECTS	COMMENTS
Baclofen	Start: 5 to 10 mg/d Max: 80 mg/d in three to four divided doses per FDA recommendation, higher doses are used in practice as tolerated	Sedation, increased fatigue, confusion, dizziness, muscle weakness	Withdrawal: muscle stiffness, paresthesias, hallucinations, confusion, fever, seizures Overdose: hypotonia, respiratory depression, hypotension, coma Reduce dose in patients with impaired renal function
Tizanidine	Start: 2 to 4 mg/d Max: 36 mg/d in three to four divided doses	Sedation, dry mouth, dizziness, hypotension, elevated liver enzymes, hallucinations, muscle weakness	May potentiate effects of antihypertensive agents Reduce dose when given with fluoroquinolones (i.e., ciprofloxacin)
Benzodiazepines	Diazepam: Start: 2 mg qhs Max: 30 mg/d in three to four divided doses Clonazepam: Start: 0.5 mg qhs Max: 2 mg/d	CNS depression, muscle weakness	Withdrawal: anxiety, tremor, agitation, insomnia, seizures Overdose: respiratory depression, coma Often prescribed to relieve nocturnal spasms Frequently used to treat baclofen withdrawal
Gabapentin	Start: 100 to 300 mg/d Max: 3,600 mg/d in three to four divided doses	Nystagmus, diplopia, somnolence, ataxia, dizziness, peripheral edema, depression, and suicidal ideation	Secondary antispasticity agent Most useful in patients with paresthesias or neuropathic pain in addition to spasticity Reduce dose in patients with impaired renal function
Dantrolene sodium	Start: 25 mg/d Max: 400 mg/d in four divided doses	Sedation, GI symptoms, muscle weakness, hepatotoxicity	Potential for severe liver toxicity and the risk of weakness limit clinical use Fatal hepatitis in 0.3%. Follow liver function periodically Use lowest effective dose
Nabiximols	Titration for up to 14 d Should not exceed 12 sprays per day, with >15 min between sprays	Dizziness, fatigue, nausea, local reactions (pain, dysgeusia, ulceration).	Prescribed as second- or third-line agent, generally as combination therapy No withdrawal noted with therapy discontinuation
Levetiracetam	Start: 250 mg/d Max: 3,000 mg/d. Usually given twice daily	Sedation, confusion, nausea, depression, and suicidal ideation	Secondary antispasticity agent Was found to be effective on phasic signs of spasticity (spasms) but not on tonic signs of spasticity (resistance to passive movement) in a retrospective chart review of 12 MS patients Reduce dose in patients with impaired renal function
Clonidine	Start: 0.1 mg/d Max: 0.2 mg twice daily Transdermal patch is available	Bradycardia, hypotension, drowsiness, dry mouth, constipation, dizziness, pedal edema, depression	Secondary antispasticity agent Use with caution in patients with dysautonomia Avoid abrupt cessation because of possible rebound autonomic symptoms
Cyproheptadine	Start: 4 mg/d Max: 24 mg/d in three divided doses	Sedation, dry mouth, dizziness, weight gain	Cyproheptadine is used to alleviate the symptoms of baclofen withdrawal Reduce dose in patients with renal impairment

CNS, central nervous system; GI, gastrointestinal.

recommend baclofen and tizanidine as effective, first-line medications for spasticity. Monotherapy, in conjunction with stretching, is often at least partially effective for mild to moderate spasticity, although side effects can be a limiting factor, even with low doses. Dose escalation and combination of medications for severe spasticity are often limited by worsening sedation, increased weakness, or cognitive symptoms. Other considerations in choosing pharmacotherapy include cost, medication interactions, comorbidities, and patient's ability to follow instructions and to follow-up with the care provider. Antispasticity medications are usually started at a low dose and gradually titrated to limit side effects. Some of these medications should not be abruptly discontinued (e.g., baclofen). Table 29.4 summarizes the dosing and considerations for the most commonly used medications. It should be kept in mind that some other medications commonly used in MS can cause worsening of spasticity (e.g., interferon beta, selective serotonin re-uptake inhibitors [SSRIs]). Many other symptomatic medications may cause sedation or weakness (e.g., amitriptyline, anticholinergics for bladder management).

> *When prescribing oral medications for spasticity, slow dose titration is recommended to minimize side effects.*

There is growing interest in the use of cannabinoids to treat spasticity. Although not currently approved in the United States, an endocannabinoid modulator in the form of an oromucosal spray (Delta-9-tetrahydrocannabinol [THC]/cannabidiol [CBD], nabiximols) has been studied in several large clinical trials (11,12), and is approved in several European countries and Canada, to be used for treatment-resistant moderate to severe MS-related spasticity. Observational studies have reported a greater than 60% response rate (reduction in patient perception of spasticity) within 1 month of initiation of nabiximols. Dizziness and fatigue were the most common adverse effects noted in clinical trials and observational studies. Long-term safety—including effects on cognition and mood—with sustained use greater than 12 months remains unclear. (13)

Local treatments such as injection of anesthetic agents, chemical neurolysis, or botulinum toxin (BT) may facilitate stretching, improve comfort, and improve function by relaxing specific muscles or muscle groups. Owing to their transient effects, local anesthetics (lidocaine, etidocaine, bupivacaine) are sometimes used to evaluate the potential benefit of longer lasting procedures such as chemical neurolysis (e.g., phenol blocks) or chemodenervation (e.g., BT injections). Chemical neurolysis produces a much longer lasting (up to 36 months) nerve block by damaging nerve structures. Potential side effects include chronic dysesthesias.

Three formulations of BT-A (abobotulinum toxin A, onabotulinum toxin A, incobotulinum toxin A) and one formulation of BT-B (rimabotulinum toxin B) are available in the United States. Intramuscular BT injections are widely used to treat spasticity though only the forms of BT-A carry U.S. Food and Drug Administration (FDA) approval for spasticity (upper and lower limb for abobotulinum and onabotulinum toxin A; upper limb only for incobotulinum toxin A). The Therapeutics and Technology Assessment Subcommittee of the American Academy of Neurology concluded that BT is effective on upper and lower limb spasticity in reducing muscle tone and improving passive function (level A recommendation), and probably effective in improving active function (level B recommendation) in adults (14). BT is injected into a spastic muscle, preferably with electromyography (EMG), electrical stimulation, or ultrasound guidance, even though there is no definitive published evidence showing that guidance leads to improved outcomes (14).

There are few publications reporting on the efficacy and tolerability of BT therapy in MS, but data from other patient populations is consistent with clinical experience with MS patients. The therapeutic effect typically appears after 24 to 72 hours, peaks at 2 to 4 weeks, and usually lasts 10 weeks or more. Injections are typically repeated at 12 weeks. More frequent injections and use of high doses have been linked to the development of anti-BT antibodies with loss of clinical efficacy. It is estimated that BT diffuses approximately 30 mm around the injection site. Systemic side effects are uncommon, usually nonlife threatening (e.g., nausea, fatigue, dysphagia), and reversible, although severe complications (including generalized weakness, diplopia, severe dysphagia, urinary incontinence, respiratory compromise, in some cases leading to death) from spread of toxin effect have been reported. In addition, in recent trials of onabotulinum toxin A for upper extremity spasticity in the United States, more frequent respiratory infections were reported with active treatment compared to placebo. The BT preparations are not interchangeable. Attention must be given to dilution and dosing recommendations for each product.

> *Intramuscular injections of BT can help with focal spasticity, or when focal areas are targeted (e.g., difficulty opening the hand due to finger flexor spasticity, foot drop, hip adductor spasticity).*

Intrathecal baclofen (ITB) is approved by the FDA for the treatment of severe spasticity of spinal or cerebral origin refractory to oral antispasticity medications or when such medications are not tolerated. Administration of ITB reduces the incidence of CNS sedation compared to oral baclofen by allowing effective cerebrospinal fluid (CSF) concentrations to be achieved with much smaller doses of baclofen.

The medication is delivered directly into the intrathecal space via a programmable infusion system consisting of a battery-powered pump implanted subcutaneously in the lower abdominal wall and an intraspinal catheter (tip at the lower thoracic level usually) tunneled subcutaneously to the pump. The total daily dose and rate of administration of baclofen can be adjusted noninvasively via an external programming device. The benefits of ITB therapy in MS were reported in several publications (15–17). Potential complications were also well documented, and include complications from surgery, wound dehiscence, pseudomeningocele and CSF leak, infection, system malfunction, and baclofen withdrawal and overdose. In order to optimize outcomes, best practices should be followed (18). A bolus test injection (usually 25 to 100 mcg of ITB) should be performed in all patients (continuous infusion trials via an externalized intraspinal catheter are less commonly performed). It is critical that the patient and proxies understand their role in communicating with healthcare providers, the importance of routine follow-up visits for refills, the symptoms and signs of baclofen withdrawal and overdose, and instructions for emergency situations.

> *Intrathecal baclofen therapy is approved for severe spasticity refractory to first-line spasticity treatments. Thorough patient evaluation and education is warranted to optimize outcomes.*

OTHER CONSIDERATIONS

Spasticity increases with stress and noxious stimuli (e.g., pain, decubiti, urinary tract infection, and even ingrown toenail), and usually exhibits spontaneous fluctuations (typically increasing at night). Variations in ambient and core body temperature have been anecdotally reported to affect spasticity. For example, colder temperatures are often associated with increased spasticity.

It is important to remember that spasticity can also have beneficial consequences. For example, a patient may use extensor tone to stand and perform pivot transfers, which would otherwise be compromised by severe paraparesis. It is also believed that spasticity may decrease the risk of deep venous thrombosis and pressure ulcers by maintaining muscle tone in paralyzed muscles.

> *The role of spasticity in compensating for weakness must be taken into account when planning spasticity management.*

CONCLUSION

Spasticity is a common cause of discomfort and functional limitation in patients with MS. Successful spasticity management requires thorough assessments, a realistic treatment plan, and often multidisciplinary care. Key considerations before designing a spasticity management plan include

- Severity of resistance to passive movement
- Severity of spasms and clonus
- Pain with passive or active movement, or with spasms
- Dynamic versus resting spasticity
- Other neurological impairments (particularly weakness) that can impact function
- Degree of reliance on spasticity to perform critical functions (e.g., transfers)
- Complications related to spasticity (e.g., contractures, maceration, skin breakdown)
- Other factors contributing to spasticity (e.g., recurrent urinary tract infections)
- Patient's human and physical environment
- Patient/caregiver goals

PATIENT CASE

Ms. D, a 31-year-old right-handed mother of three young children, presents with left spastic hemiparesis in the context of relapsing-remitting multiple sclerosis (MS). She walks with no assistive device. Her main complaint is muscle spasms in the left toes, which are painful, and interfere with her ability to walk (she needs to stop and stretch her toes when the spasms occur). She also reports muscle stiffness in the left leg, and to a lesser degree in the left arm. On examination, there is left-sided weakness, mild in the left upper extremity (muscle testing four to 5/5), moderate in the left lower extremity (muscle testing three to 4/5). There is mild resistance to passive movement in the left upper and lower extremities, with the exception of the left ankle plantarflexors, where resistance to passive movement is severe (3/4 on the Modified Ashworth Scale) (5) with decreased range of motion in the left ankle/foot. Gait is hemiparetic with decreased left foot clearance due to foot drop and decreased active hip and knee flexion. Constant flexion of the toes upon standing and walking quickly becomes painful and forces the patient to rest. She walks 25 ft in 12 seconds.

(continued)

(continued)

Question: Does the patient need an intervention on her spasticity, and if so, what could be the main goals?

Answer: Based on the patient's complaints and examination findings, it appears that spasticity management could be beneficial, with the following broad goals: to reduce discomfort and pain associated with muscle spasms in the toes, and to facilitate walking. These goals should be discussed with the patient, along with the fact that weakness also contributes to the gait disturbance.

Question: Which first-line interventions can be offered?

Answer: The patient needs to start on a stretching regimen to improve or preserve range of motion in the left upper and lower extremities. She may benefit from wearing a left ankle-foot orthosis (AFO), and needs strengthening and gait training. To implement these interventions, a referral to physical therapy should be considered. It is also reasonable to discuss a symptomatic medication for spasticity (such as baclofen or tizanidine), starting with a low dose and with slow titration, as sedation and increased weakness could interfere with daytime activities.

Question: The patient attends several physical therapy sessions. She now stretches several times per day and exercises on a regular basis. She was unable to tolerate a left AFO because of her toe spasms. She started on baclofen, but could not increase the dose beyond 10 mg twice daily because of sedation. At that dose, her stiffness and spasms were not controlled so she discontinued the medication. Neurological examination is stable. The patient is frustrated because the spasms and pain in her toes prevent her from walking long distances and interfere with her ability to take care of her children. The physical therapist states that the patient is not able to fully perform the exercises because of her spasticity. Can other treatment options be offered?

Answer: Because the main problems related to spasticity are focal in the distal left lower extremity, it is reasonable to consider BT therapy Physical therapy should be continued after BT injections to allow further gait training.

Question: BT injections are administered in the left gastrocnemius, tibialis posterior, and toe flexor muscles. Toe spasms and pain "improved 85%" for 6 weeks, then gradually returned. She has been able to wear a left AFO, and does not catch her left foot as much. On examination, strength is stable; resistance to passive movement is improved in the ankle plantarflexors (from 3/4 to 2/4 on the Modified Ashworth Scale). Gait is improved with better left foot clearance. She walks 25 ft in 10 seconds (20% improvement). What is the next step?

Answer: The response from the first injection session is encouraging, but the duration of effect was relatively short, and there was only partial relief of toe spasms and pain. We recommend repeat BT injections with a higher dose, to continue with stretching and exercise, and to continue wearing the AFO. At this point, it is important to continue spasticity management, in the context of a chronic disease with high risk of worsening of disability over time.

PATIENT CASE

Ms. H. is a 37-year-old woman with primary progressive multiple sclerosis (MS). She was diagnosed with MS when leg stiffness and weakness failed to improve after cervical decompression and fusion. After a period of physical exertion, she develops low back pain, increased stiffness in the legs and spasms in the left leg. Her left knee is "locked up in a bent position." Examination shows spastic paraparesis, worse in the left leg than the right. Stiffness and spasms persist despite treatment with oral baclofen and tizanidine.

Question: Ms. H. describes symptoms of spasticity that limit function and produce significant discomfort despite maximally tolerated doses of two oral antispasticity agents. What modalities could be added to help reduce pain and possibly improve function?

(continued)

(continued)

Answer: She should start a stretching regimen to preserve and improve range of motion. A referral for physical therapy evaluation would also be appropriate. Injection of botulinum toxin (BT) in the left hamstrings (off label) may reduce spasms and when combined with physical therapy, improve the passive and active extension of the left knee.

Question: BT injections administered in the left hamstrings reduced pain by 50% and facilitated extension of the left knee. One month later, however, she develops severe extensor spasms in both legs, and her left knee is "locked up in an extended position." She complains of pain when she moves her legs, rated 8/10. On examination, there is severe resistance to passive movement in the legs, rated 3/4 on the Modified Ashworth Scale. Muscle testing is difficult to perform, but shows moderate diffuse weakness most severe at the hip flexors (3/5) and the tibialis anterior (3/5). She performs the timed 25 ft walk (T25FW) in 42 seconds using a rollator. She continues physical therapy and oral antispasticity agents. What other options should be considered?

Answer: Ms. H. now has severe diffuse spasticity with worsening pain and marginal ambulation. The examination does not reveal any obvious targets for local injections. Discussion of intrathecal baclofen (ITB) therapy is appropriate.

Question: A test injection of ITB 50 mcg is performed. The following pre- and postinjection measures are reported. Is the patient a good candidate for ITB therapy?

	PREINJECTION		POSTINJECTION	
Pain	8/10		2/10	
T25FW	42 s		25.6 s	
MANUAL MUSCLE TESTING*				
Hip flexors	4	2	3	2
Knee flexors	3	1	4	2
Knee extensors	3	3	3	4
Dorsiflexors	4	2	4	2
SPASTICITY (MODIFIED ASHWORTH SCALE)**				
Hip adductors	3	3	2	2
Knee flexors	3	3	1	3
Knee extensors	3	3	1	1
Plantarflexors	3	3	2	3

*Range 0 to 5, with higher scores indicating better strength.
**Range 0 to 4, with higher scores indicating more severe spasticity.

Answer: She chose to proceed with ITB pump surgery after the successful test injection. Following surgery, she experienced marked relief of spasticity, and after intensive rehabilitation her gait pattern improved. One year after pump placement, she reports that comfort and walking are significantly improved. She still has difficulty abducting the legs and discomfort on the inside of the thighs. Examination reveals mild to moderate spasticity in the legs with the exception of a Modified Ashworth Scale score of three in the hip adductors on both sides. She walks 25 ft in 17.6 seconds using a rollator and a left ankle-foot orthosis (AFO). Her gait has a scissoring appearance.

Question: This patient has overall good results with ITB therapy, physical therapy, and orthotics. Is there a role for other modalities in fine-tuning her spasticity management?

Answer: The dose of ITB was increased to address the residual spasticity in the hip adductors, but this caused increased leg weakness and difficulty walking, so was returned to the previous dose. BT injections were performed in the hip adductors bilaterally, which helped decrease pain, improve range of motion, and improve gait pattern. She continues to stretch and swim daily.

KEY POINTS FOR PATIENTS AND FAMILIES

- Many people with MS have spasticity, a type of muscle tightness that affects the control of movement.

- Other symptoms associated with spasticity include muscle spasms and a repetitive involuntary "shaking" called clonus, which often happens in the ankle.

- Spasticity does not equal weakness, though these often come together.

- Spasticity may cause discomfort and difficulty with usual activities.

- Treatment for spasticity begins with physical measures such as stretching and physical therapy.

- Certain medicines may reduce spasticity, although side effects may limit the ability to increase the dose.

- Botulinum toxin A is an injection treatment that is FDA-approved for the treatment of spasticity in the upper extremity (arm and hand) and in the lower extremity.

- Implanting a programmable pump under the skin to deliver baclofen in the spinal fluid may be useful for hard-to-treat severe spasticity.

REFERENCES

1. Lance J. Symposium synopsis. In: Feldman RG, Young RR, Koella WP, eds. *Spasticity: Disordered Motor Control*. Chicago, IL: Year Book Medical Publishers; 1980:485–494.
2. Matthews B. Symptoms and signs of multiple sclerosis. In: Compston A, Ebers G, Lassmann H, et al., eds. *Mc Alpine's Multiple Sclerosis*. London, UK: Churchill Livingstone; 1998.
3. Bethoux F, Marrie RA. A cross-sectional study of the impact of spasticity on daily activities in multiple sclerosis. *Patient*. 2016;9:537–546.
4. Ashworth B. Preliminary trial of carisoprodol in multiple sclerosis. *Practitioner*. 1964;192:540–542.
5. Bohannon R, Smith M. Inter-rater reliability of a modified Ashworth scale of muscle spasticity. *Phys Ther*. 1987;67:206–207.
6. Gibson B. *Stretching for People with MS: An Illustrated Manual*. New York, NY: National MS Society, 2016.
7. Hugos CL, Bourdette D, Chen Y, et al. A group-delivered °self-management program reduces spasticity in people with multiplesclerosis: a randomized, controlled pilot trial. *Mult Scler J Exp Transl Clin*. 2017;3:2055217317699993.
8. Multiple Sclerosis Council for Clinical Practice Guidelines. *Spasticity Management in Multiple Sclerosis*. Hackensack, NJ: Consortium of Multiple Sclerosis Centers; 2003.
9. Shakespeare D, Young C, Boggild M. Anti-spasticity agents for multiple sclerosis. *Cochrane Database Syst Rev*. 2009;4:CD001332.
10. Otero-Romero S, Sastre-Garriga J, Comi G, et al. Pharmacological management of spasticity in multiple sclerosis: systematic review and consensus paper. *Mult Scler*. 2016;22:1386–1396.
11. Zettl UK, Rommer P, Hipp P, et al. Evidence for the efficacy and effectiveness of THC-CBD oromucosal spray in symptom management of patients with spasticity due to multiple sclerosis. *Ther Adv Neurol Disord*. 2016;9:9–30.
12. Patti F, Messina S, Solaro C. Efficacy and safety of cannabinoid oromucosal spray for multiple sclerosis spasticity. *J Neurol Neurosurg Psychiatry*. 2016;87:944–951.
13. Koppel BS, Brust JC, Fife T, et al. Systematic review: efficacy and safety of medical marijuana in selected neurologic disorders: report of the Guideline Development Subcommittee of the American Academy of Neurology. *Neurology*. 2014;82(17):1556–1563.
14. Simpson DM, Hallet M, Ashman EJ, et al. Practice guideline update summary: botulinum neurotoxin for the treatment of blepharospasm, cervical dystonia, adult spasticity, and headache: report of the Guideline Development Subcommittee of the American Academy of Neurology. *Neurology*. 2016;86:1818-1826.
15. Stempien L, Tsai T. Intrathecal baclofen pump use for spasticity. *Am J Phys Med Rehab*. 2000;79:536–541.
16. Azouvi P, Mane M, Thiebaut J, et al. Intrathecal baclofen administration for control of severe spinal spasticity: functional improvement and long-term follow-up. *Arch Phys Med Rehab*. 1996;77:35–39.
17. Zahavi A, Geertzen JHB, Middel B, et al. Long term effect (more than five years) of intrathecal baclofen on impairment, disability, and quality of life in patients with severe spasticity of spinal origin. *J Neurol Neurosurg Psychiatry*. 2004;75:1553–1557.
18. Ridley B, Korth Rawlins P. Intrathecal baclofen therapy: ten steps towards best practice. *J Neurosci Nursing*. 2006;38:72–82.

Multiple Sclerosis and Mobility

Francois Bethoux, Jacob J. Sosnoff, and Keith McKee

KEY POINTS FOR CLINICIANS

- Walking and balance impairment are frequent consequences of multiple sclerosis (MS), affecting up to 75% of persons with MS over the course of the disease.
- Gait and balance abnormalities may occur early in the disease, even before a clinical disturbance can be identified on examination.
- Impaired walking and balance have a profound impact on an individual's ability to function and quality of life.
- Neurological impairments and comorbidities both contribute to walking and balance impairment, sometimes making it difficult to identify specific targets for intervention.
- A variety of tools are available to assess walking and balance in patients with MS. A combination of functional tests and questionnaires is usually recommended for identification and monitoring purposes.
- There is a growing body of evidence showing the effects of rehabilitation/exercise, medications, and assistive devices on walking and balance in MS.

Mobility is a complex construct which can be defined as "moving by changing body position or location or by transferring from one place to another, by carrying, moving, or manipulating objects, by walking, running, or climbing, and by using various forms of transportation" (1). In this chapter, we focus on walking and balance, which represent two major elements of mobility.

WHAT CAUSES MOBILITY LIMITATIONS IN MULTIPLE SCLEROSIS?

There are multiple causes to balance and walking limitations in multiple sclerosis (MS). The primary etiology is the damage caused to the central nervous system (CNS) by the disease process. Among neurological impairments, abnormal motor control (paresis, spasticity, and ataxia) in the lower extremities is the most obvious offender. Indeed, studies have reported a correlation between balance impairment, muscle weakness (2), and spasticity (3), as well as between walking limitations and muscle weakness (4) or spasticity (5). Often, other impairments contribute to the problem, such as loss of sensation in the lower extremities, slowed spinal somatosensory conduction (6), motor and sensory loss in the upper extremities (impacts gait pattern

and interferes with the ability to use assistive devices), visual disturbance, cognitive impairment, and fatigue.

The impact of cognitive impairment is demonstrated through the common deterioration in walking performance while performing a cognitive task, in MS patients more so than in healthy controls (7). Dual-tasking also leads to deterioration of spatiotemporal parameters of gait (8), even at the early stage of the disease (9). These observations suggest that MS patients with gait disturbance may benefit from consciously "focusing on their legs" to preserve their ability to maintain their balance while walking and to avoid falling.

The relationship between balance, walking performance, and fatigue is complex. A few investigations report that experimentally induced fatigue negatively impacts postural control (10), and there are limited reports that fatigue is related to balance. Even though some studies report a correlation between self-reported fatigue and altered gait parameters (11) or walking performance (12), others failed to demonstrate a significant change in walking performance on timed tests over the course of the day, despite a worsening in self-reported fatigue (13). A recent literature review and meta-analysis showed a moderate correlation between perceived fatigue and motor fatigability, but the authors point out that these represent distinct constructs (14).

The role of comorbidities in balance and walking impairment should not be overlooked. With aging, patients with MS may develop the same musculoskeletal disorders as the general population (osteoarthritis, back pain, and osteoporosis). Moreover, MS can indirectly increase the risk of musculoskeletal comorbidities. For example, an abnormal gait pattern may cause early osteoarthritis of the lower extremities and low back pain because of abnormal body mechanics and osteoporosis may develop as a consequence of decreased ambulation. Addressing these problems may result in significant improvement of mobility, even if neurological impairments remain unchanged. Conversely, addressing abnormal gait patterns early is important in limiting the risk of musculoskeletal complications. Other comorbidities may also have an impact. Marrie et al. analyzed data on 8,983 individuals with MS in the North American Research Committee on Multiple Sclerosis Registry and found that the presence of cardiovascular comorbidities increased the risk of ambulatory disability (15). Even depression, a frequent comorbidity in MS, may impact ambulation by decreasing a patient's motivation to walk and to exercise.

> *Cognitive impairment and comorbidities should be assessed when managing ambulation and balance impairment.*

> *It is important to address gait deviations early, to limit the risk of long-term musculoskeletal complications which may further affect mobility.*

MOBILITY AND FALLS

The issue of imbalance and falls cannot be overlooked in a discussion about mobility and MS. The incidence of falls is high in MS. An international sample of over 500 individuals with MS reported that 56% suffered at least one fall whereas 37% had greater than two falls over a 3-month period (16). Other studies suggest that falls are present in individuals with limited mobility (17). Many risk factors for falling have been identified, including a higher level of disability, impaired mobility, imbalance, cognitive impairment, bladder dysfunction, and fear of falling (18). The use of an assistive device is associated with an increased risk of falling, but this likely is simply a marker of increased disability, which is a known risk factor for falling, rather than a direct effect of assistive devices (19). The main concern related to falls is the occurrence of injuries, particularly fractures (20,21), which are more frequent in patients with a higher level of disability,

but may also occur early in the disease course (22). Since decreased mobility is also associated with an increased risk of osteoporosis, it is essential to perform bone density testing and initiate interventions to reduce fall risk in patients who report falls or are at high risk of falling.

> *Patients with MS and mobility limitations should be asked systematically about falls.*

BALANCE IMPAIRMENT IN MS

The ability to maintain an upright posture, even when standing still, is dependent on complex interplay of three major sensory systems (somatosensory, visual, and vestibular) and appropriate motor commands. If function is altered in any of these processes, then impairments in balance also referred to as postural control are observed. Given the dispersed neural damage in individuals with MS, it is not surprising that approximately 80% of MS patients have balance impairment (23,24). Impaired balance in MS is characterized by increased amount of postural sway during quiet stance, decreased responses to postural perturbation (6), and reduced stability boundary (10) and tends to correlate with disability level (3). As previously stated, balance impairment is frequently implicated in falls in the MS community (25).

Given the commonality of balance impairment in MS, numerous approaches ranging from self-report (e.g., patient-reported outcomes) to laboratory-based biomechanical analyses to quantify standing balance have been validated (Table 30.1). It is recommended that a combination of both objective and subjective measures of balance should be utilized to fully characterize balance since they reflect different aspects of balance (26). Perhaps the most common patient report outcome measure is the Activities-specific Balance Confidence Scale (27). This self-report measure has individuals indicate their confidence in completing everyday balance tasks without losing their balance. This questionnaire could be completed prior to the office visit and the total score can be followed over time. Some items refer to cold weather conditions (icy sidewalks) and may not be relevant in all locales.

Performance tests of balance control allow for the characterization of impairment. The Romberg Test assesses changes in postural sway with eyes open and eyes closed. It is used to determine proprioceptive contributions to static standing balance and recently has been validated in a large MS sample (28).

Balance rating scales such as the Berg Balance Scale (BBS) or Mini-Balance evaluation systems test (Mini-BEST) can be used in a rehabilitation setting. Both scales rate an

TABLE 30.1   Tools for Balance Assessment in MS

ASSESSMENT TOOL	PURPOSE	DESCRIPTION
Interview	Screen for balance limitations and obtain pertinent history	Presence and severity of limitations Pertinent neurological symptoms and comorbidities Safety issues (falls) Interventions tried in the past and results
Physical examination	Assess impairments and observe gait	Neurological impairments (e.g., weakness, spasticity, sensory loss, ataxia, visual loss, cognitive impairment) Other contributing impairments (e.g., musculoskeletal problems) Describe gait pattern (includes effort needed to walk, need for assistive device, safety issues)
Balance performance tests	Quantify balance performance via direct observation	Romberg Test: Observed postural sway with eyes open vs. eyes closed
Rating scales of balance	Rate balance performance via direct observation	BBS: 14 common balance tasks; Mini-Balance Evaluation Systems Test: 14-item balance scale that measures dynamic balance specifically anticipatory transitions, postural responses, and sensory orientation.
Self-report questionnaires	Assess the patient's perception of balance limitations	Activities-specific Balance Confidence scale (assesses confidence participant can complete activity of daily living without losing balance) Falls Efficacy Scale: The fall efficacy scale is designed to assess the degree of perceived efficacy, i.e., self-confidence of the individual at avoiding a fall during 10 activities of daily living. The score ranges from 10 to 100.
Quantitative balance control	Quantify various components of gait	Posturography, accelerometry, inertial sensors

BBS, Berg Balance Scale; MS, multiple sclerosis.

individual's ability to complete a series of balance tasks. The BBS requires individuals to maintain positions of varying difficulty and perform specific tasks such as standing and sitting unsupported, and turning to look over shoulders. The mini-BEST test incorporates tasks of anticipatory transitions, postural responses to perturbations and sensory orientation. Although both measures are valid in patients with MS (29), it has been suggested that Mini-BEST may be more suitable for individuals with limited disability.

Quantification of balance impairment via biomechanical analysis utilizing motion capture, force platforms (e.g., posturography), or inertial sensors is performed in research settings. Although costly, these systems appear to more sensitive to balance deficits in preclinical impairment (30). Additionally, these systems tend to be predictive of future falls more so than clinical assessments (31). A potential barrier to the clinical utility of these biomechanical analyses is the lack of consensus of the most appropriate parameters to utilize.

REHABILITATION AND EXERCISE FOR BALANCE IMPAIRMENT IN MS

There is a body of evidence supporting the use of various interventions to improve balance in individuals with MS (25,32,33) (Table 30.2).

Rehabilitation and exercise should be considered as first-line interventions when aiming to improve balance, and carried out concomitantly with other interventions. There is evidence that endurance and resistance training can improve balance in individuals with MS (25,32). The benefits seem to be greatest when the exercises include standing positions and much less so when completed seated. Maximal improvements in balance result from approaches that challenge balance and functional movements (25). Interventions targeting an individual's unique balance impairment tend to have the most benefit (33). The use of exergaming as a balance rehabilitation approach has shown preliminary promise (34).

The optimal amount of rehabilitation or exercise to improve balance in individuals with MS is not clear. It has been suggested that a higher volume of exercise results in greater improvements in balance (25). In general, it is recommended that exercises need to be challenging to the individual.

It is important to note that the vast majority of evidence concerning rehabilitation and exercise effects on balance in MS has been based on data from mild to moderately disabled individuals. Caution should be taken when generalizing the positive impact of rehabilitation on balance in severely disabled individuals. There is some pilot data suggesting that seated balance control is modifiable in individuals who are not ambulatory (35).

TABLE 30.2 Interventions to Improve Balance

Exercise	Aerobic exercise	Exercise regimen needs to be adjusted as the patient's functional capacity changes.
	Resistance training	Resistance training performed in standing positions has greater benefit to balance
	Aquatic exercise	
	Walking exercise (with appropriate assistive devices and orthoses for safety)	Involving family members or care partners, or involvement in group exercise sessions, may improve adherence as well as safety and quality of exercise.
	Balance exercise	Improvement of balance performance was demonstrated after exercise programs— specifically focusing on balance.
Rehabilitation	Training in motor and sensory strategies	A referral to neurologic physical therapy should be systematically considered when balance is impaired.
		Physical therapy can and should be used in combination with other interventions to optimize outcomes.
		Published evidence showing the efficacy of rehabilitation interventions on balance is limited.
		Improvement of balance performance was demonstrated with focused balance training.
		Periodic reevaluation is needed.

MS AND AMBULATION

Clinicians involved in the care of patients with MS are well aware that MS frequently affects ambulation. Indeed, the tests and scales most commonly used to monitor the disease course involve some aspect of walking, including walking speed in the Timed 25 Foot Walk (T25FW), walking distance and use of an assistive device in the Expanded Disability Status Scale (EDSS). Walking limitations are one of the most visible consequences of the disease. Only recently have more detailed data on the prevalence and impact of walking limitations in MS become available. An estimated 75% of persons with MS (PwMS) experience a limitation of their ability to walk or of their mobility over the course of the disease (36,37). In a survey among over 1,000 PwMS, 41% reported having difficulty walking (38).

Several publications demonstrate the importance of walking limitations, and their profound impact on the lives of PwMS. Lower limb function was ranked first among 12 bodily functions within a population of 162 PwMS, whether the duration of their disease was under 5 years or over 15 years (39). Abnormal gait parameters are correlated with patient-reported ability to perform activities of daily living (40). Walking limitations have been linked to unemployment (41). However, in the large survey mentioned earlier, 39% of PwMS stated that they rarely or never discussed this problem with their physician, suggesting that walking limitations are not always addressed in the healthcare setting (38).

Assessing Ambulation

In order to address walking limitations, it is helpful for healthcare professionals to identify the problem and assess its severity. A variety of measures are available, although only some have been fully validated in MS (Table 30.3) (42).

Simple questions such as "How is your walking?" are a great way to start the conversation, but are usually not enough to determine the extent of the problem and develop a treatment plan. Specific information should be sought about the amount of walking actually performed (e.g., "Do you walk every day?," "Do you walk outside your home?," "How far can you walk without stopping?"), including the use of assistive devices or other support, and safety indicators ("Do you ever fall?," "When was the last time you fell?," "Did you sustain any injuries from falling?"). Validated questionnaires, such as the MS Walking Scale-12 (MSWS-12), are now available to gather patient feedback about walking performance in daily activities in a standardized manner (43). These questionnaires can be filled in by the patient before an office visit; the responses to each item facilitate the interview, and the total score can be monitored over time. Since healthcare providers rarely observe patients walking in their own home environment, self-report measures are a useful complement to clinical tests performed in the office.

> *Validated questionnaires such as the MS Walking Scale-12 (MSWS-12) provide information that can guide the assessment of ambulation limitations.*

Clinical examination allows the characterization of a gait abnormality and provides information on the underlying impairments: neurological impairments such as paresis, spasticity, cerebellar ataxia, sensory loss, and other contributing impairments such as osteoarthrosis of lower extremity joints or other musculoskeletal problems. Gaining an understanding of the causal factors is essential in designing an appropriate treatment plan.

Walking tests performed in the clinic or gait laboratory allow the provider to gather quantitative information about walking performance and gait disturbance. Among timed

TABLE 30.3 Assessment Tools for Ambulation in MS

ASSESSMENT TOOL	PURPOSE	DESCRIPTION
Interview	Screen for ambulation limitations and obtain pertinent history	Presence and severity of limitations Pertinent neurological symptoms and comorbidities Safety issues (falls) Interventions tried in the past and results
Physical examination	Assess impairments and observe gait	Neurological impairments (e.g., weakness, spasticity, sensory loss, ataxia, visual loss, cognitive impairment) Other contributing impairments (e.g., musculoskeletal problems) Describe gait pattern (includes effort needed to walk, need for assistive device, safety issues)
Walking performance tests	Quantify walking performance via direct observation	Timed tests on short distance (e.g., T25FW, 10-m walk, timed up and go) Timed tests on long distance (e.g., 2-min walk, 6-min walk) Tests of walking distance (e.g., walking distance from EDSS) Six Spot Step Test (walking as quickly as possible along a rectangular field while kicking five cylinder blocks out of their marked circles)
Rating scales of walking	Rate walking performance via direct observation	Ambulation Index (combination of need for assistive device and time to walk 25 ft) Dynamic Gait Index (rates the degree of impairment on various maneuvers that involve walking and balance) Rivermead Visual Gait Assessment (quantification of gait disturbance rates deviations from normal postures and movements while walking)
Self-report questionnaires	Assess the patient's perception of walking limitations	MSWS-12 (assesses how MS affected various aspects of walking in the past 2 wk) Patient-Determined Disease Steps (assesses the level of walking limitations) Rivermead Mobility Index (assesses various aspects of mobility, including walking)
Instrumented measurement of walking in daily life	Quantify walking in daily life via a device worn by the patient	Pedometry Accelerometry GPS
Quantitative gait analysis	Quantify various components of gait	Spatiotemporal parameters of gait Kinetics of gait Kinematics of gait Energy expenditure

EDSS, Expanded Disability Status Scale; GPS, global positioning system; MS, multiple sclerosis; MSWS-12, MS Walking Scale-12; T25FW, timed 25 foot walk.

walking tests, the T25FW (44), a test of maximum (but safe) walking speed on a short distance, is the most frequently used in clinical and research settings. The T25FW is both easy to administer and validated and a 20% change in performance is thought to be clinically significant (45). The 2-minute walk (2MW) and the 6-minute walk (6MW) (46) are considered as measures of walking endurance, but are not as often administered, mostly because of feasibility issues (administration time, need for a long hallway, and in some patients need for recovery time). In addition to providing a number that can be monitored over time, these tests give an opportunity for the clinician to observe the patient's gait pattern.

> *The timed 25 foot walk (T25FW) is the most commonly used test of walking performance in MS, but longer walking tests can provide information on walking endurance.*

Ambulation rating scales are generally used in a rehabilitation setting and allow the provider to attribute scores to observed gait deviations, including the use of assistive devices. The Dynamic Gait Index assesses performance on eight walking tasks designed to challenge the patient's dynamic balance (e.g., walking with horizontal or vertical head movements), and is correlated with reported falls (47).

Quantification of gait disturbance via gait analysis is traditionally performed in research settings and in some clinical centers, as a full gait analysis system is costly, requires a large space and specialized staff to run the tests and to interpret the data, and testing is time consuming. Less cumbersome, more affordable, and more user-friendly systems allow the measurement of spatiotemporal parameters of gait in the clinic (48). Abnormalities of gait pattern in MS have been described in several publications (Table 30.4) and can be detected early in the disease, before a gait disturbance is noted on examination (49). The energetic cost of walking (measured with the rate of oxygen consumption) is increased in patients with MS compared to healthy controls.

More recently, pedometers, accelerometers, and, less frequently, global positioning systems (GPS), have been used in research studies to measure walking and activity in the patient's own environment. Although these devices may provide a more accurate picture of ambulation in daily activities, the clinical significance and psychometric properties (validity, reliability, and sensitivity to change) of the results, usually expressed in step counts or activity counts, have not been fully determined. Published data to date suggest that step counts and activity counts are reduced in those with MS compared to healthy subjects, and that the reduction is greater when the level of walking disability is greater, as it would be expected (50).

TABLE 30.4 Common Gait Abnormalities in MS

- Decreased walking speed
- Decreased (in some cases increased) cadence
- Decreased step and stride length
- Increased step width
- Increased double support time
- Decreased swing phase
- Increased step variability

MS, multiple sclerosis.

Improving Ambulation

There is a growing body of evidence supporting the use of various interventions to improve ambulation in MS (Table 30.5).

REHABILITATION AND EXERCISE

Rehabilitation and exercise should be considered as the first-line interventions when trying to improve ambulation, and carried out concomitantly with other interventions. Routine exercise is encouraged in MS, alone or in a group, at home or in a gym, on a regular basis. Exercise was shown to have a beneficial effect on aerobic capacity, walking speed, walking endurance, and functional performance in MS (51,52), in addition to improving fatigue, mood, and health-related quality of life (53). Many MS patients have difficulty initiating an exercise routine on their own; therefore, a referral to a physical therapist (preferably with experience in MS) to develop an individualized home exercise program is often helpful. Gait rehabilitation is a more thorough and intense training performed by a physical therapist and usually includes

TABLE 30.5 Interventions to Improve Ambulation

TYPE OF INTERVENTION	DESCRIPTION	COMMENTS
Exercise	Stretching (with assistance if needed) Aerobic exercise Resistance training Aquatic exercise Walking exercise (with appropriate assistive devices and orthoses for safety)	Exercise program often needs to be initiated under the guidance of a physical therapist. Exercise regimen needs to be adjusted as the patient's functional capacity changes. Involving family members or care partners, or involvement in group exercise sessions, may improve adherence as well as safety and quality of exercise. Improvement of walking performance was demonstrated after exercise programs.
Rehabilitation	Stretching performed by physical therapist Exercise supervised by physical therapist Traditional gait and balance training Training to the use of assistive devices and orthoses Periodic reevaluation is needed Training to home exercise program Technology-assisted gait training 　BWSTT 　FES-assisted BWSTT or cycling 　Robotic-assisted BWSTT	A referral to neurologic physical therapy should be systematically considered when ambulation is impaired. Physical therapy can and should be used in combination with other interventions to optimize outcomes. Published evidence showing the efficacy of rehabilitation interventions on walking is limited. Improvement of walking performance was demonstrated with traditional gait training. Robot-assisted BWSTT may not be superior to traditional gait training, based on one publication. Periodic reevaluation is needed.
Assistive devices and orthoses	Unilateral support: 　Cane, crutch, walking stick Bilateral support: 　Bilateral canes or crutches 　Walker: standard, two-wheel, four-wheel (with hand brakes, basket, and seat) Foot FlexR, Foot Up, Dictus Band AFO 　Plastic, solid, or articulated ankle 　Usually custom-molded as opposed to off-the-shelf carbon fiber KAFO KO HFAD FES devices for foot drop	There is limited evidence showing the efficacy of assistive devices and orthoses in MS. An uncontrolled pilot study of the HFAD showed significant improvement of walking performance and leg strength at 8 and 12 wk.

(continued)

TABLE 30.5 Interventions to Improve Ambulation (*continued*)

TYPE OF INTERVENTION	DESCRIPTION	COMMENTS

Medications	DMTs (to help prevent worsening of walking limitations due to disease activity)
	Dalfampridine (approved to improve walking in patients with MS, based on improvement of walking speed in phase 3 clinical trials)
	Symptomatic medications:
	  For spasticity (see Chapter 29)
	  For pain (see Chapter 25)
	  For other symptoms as indicated
	Treatments for comorbidities (e.g., cardiovascular, respiratory, musculoskeletal)
		Slowing of disability progression was demonstrated with some DMTs.
		The efficacy of dalfampridine was established using the T25FW with a responder analysis, and more recently with the 6-MW test.
		The effects of symptomatic medications and treatments for comorbidities on ambulation in MS are rarely assessed.

Surgical treatments	Orthopedic surgery
	  For musculoskeletal injuries related to falls
	  For contractures and limb deformity (e.g., tendon release, osteotomy) related to spasticity
	  For severe osteoarthritis or other musculoskeletal comorbidity
	Neurosurgical interventions for spasticity
	ITB therapy
	Selective dorsal rhizotomy
	Tibial nerve neurotomy
		Decision making is often difficult, because of a lack of evidence to guide decision making, and because of uncertainty regarding the functional results of surgical interventions.
		ITB therapy is approved for the treatment of severe spasticity refractory to oral medication in a variety of conditions including MS. Published data suggest that ambulation can be preserved in carefully selected ambulatory MS patients treated with ITB.

6-MW, 6 minute walk; AFO, ankle foot orthosis; BWSTT, body weight supported treadmill training; DMT, disease-modifying therapy; FES, functional electrical stimulation; HFAD, hip flexion assist device; ITB, intrathecal baclofen; KAFO, knee ankle foot orthosis; KO, knee orthosis; MS, multiple sclerosis; T25FW, timed 25 foot walk.

stretching and range of motion exercises, strengthening exercises, and task-specific training (e.g., gait and balance training, training to climb stairs). Published evidence shows a small but significant improvement of walking performance after physical therapy (54). In addition, physical therapists help determine the need for assistive devices and orthoses, and train patients to use them properly and safely. Body weight supported treadmill training (BWSTT) was shown to be effective at improving walking performance in MS (55) and can be performed with the help of one or two physical therapists to move the legs or with the assistance of a robotic device. However, this training may not be more effective than traditional gait training (56).

> *Rehabilitation and exercise are the first line of treatment for ambulation limitations in MS.*

ASSISTIVE DEVICES AND ORTHOSES

Assistive devices include canes, crutches, and walkers, all of which are routinely recommended when MS compromises gait efficiency and/or gait safety. These devices are meant to improve the efficiency of gait, to decrease the musculoskeletal stress due to gait deviations, and to decrease the risk of falling. Despite extensive empirical experience, there is very little published evidence on the efficacy of these assistive devices. Although these devices are prescribed by a physician, it is strongly recommended to involve a physical therapist for evaluation and training, as mentioned earlier. Ankle foot orthoses (AFOs) are commonly used to correct foot drop, but their effect on gait may be limited and needs to be better studied (57). Heavier orthoses such as knee ankle foot orthoses (KAFO) can be helpful in controlling hyperextension of the knee, but are often too heavy for routine use.

> *Assistive devices should be considered to improve the efficiency and safety of walking, and to preserve mobility in nonambulatory patients.*

Recently, "active" devices promoting active movement (instead of immobilizing a limb segment) have become available. For example, functional electrical stimulation (FES) devices using peroneal nerve stimulation can trigger active dorsiflexion to correct foot drop during specific portions of the gait cycle. These FES devices consist of a cuff worn on the proximal lower leg containing the electrodes, and a mechanism (heel switch or tilt sensor) to trigger the stimulation at the appropriate time in the gait cycle (i.e., from the time the foot is lifted off the floor to the time it makes contact with the floor again). Although FES devices for foot drop have received extensive publicity, published evidence in MS is scarce and sometimes contradictory (58,59). Also, the hip flexion assist device (HFAD), which consists of two elastic bands attached proximally to a waist belt and distally to the shoe, significantly improved walking performance in a pilot study on 21 MS patients (60).

In patients who walk only in their home ("household ambulators"), and in those who lose the ability to ambulate altogether, mobility can be preserved by using a wheelchair. Power mobility devices (i.e., power wheelchairs and scooters) are considered when upper extremity function is impaired. It is essential to customize these devices to the abilities and needs of the patient, and to their environment. For example, custom seating may be needed in patients with poor trunk control, and the size of the wheelchair should be compatible with the space available within the home. This requires a thorough evaluation by qualified rehabilitation professionals.

MEDICATIONS

Dalfampridine (also called fampridine in other parts of the world), an extended-release formulation of 4-aminopyridine, was approved in the United States and other countries as a symptomatic medication to improve walking in patients with MS, based on improved walking speed (on T25FW testing) in two phase 3 placebo-controlled clinical trials (61,62). Dalfampridine is prescribed at the dose of 10 mg twice daily (12 hours apart). A lower dose (5 mg twice daily) was shown to be ineffective (63). Higher doses showed no added efficacy, but caused an increased frequency of serious adverse events (particularly seizures) in a phase 2 dose-ranging study. The risk of seizures is a significant concern, and patients should be educated to take the medication as prescribed. Common side effects include urinary tract infections, insomnia, dizziness, headache, nausea, and paresthesias. Anaphylactic reactions temporally related to dalfampridine dosing have been reported in the postmarketing experience. Since this medication is excreted predominantly in the urine, estimated creatinine clearance should be known before initiating treatment and monitored at least annually, and it should be used with caution in individuals older than 50 years owing to more common occurrence of mild renal impairment in this subgroup of patients. Dalfampridine is contraindicated in patients with a history of seizure or with moderate or severe renal impairment (creatinine clearance of 50 mL/min or less).

In practice, dalfampridine can be considered in any MS patient with walking limitations, as no predictors of response to treatment (such as MS course or baseline disability level) were identified in clinical trials. The percentage of dalfampridine responders (based on sustained improvement of walking speed on the T25FW) is expected to be comprised between 35% and 45% based on data from the phase 3 clinical trials, and the benefit was generally seen between 2 and 4 weeks after treatment initiation (61,62). It is therefore important to measure walking speed at baseline, and after a trial period of up to 8 weeks. Perceived improvement of walking is also an important outcome; in the clinical trials, treatment responders exhibited a significant improvement on the MSWS-12, compared to nonresponders. There is no evidence to suggest that successful treatment with dalfampridine changes the need for mobility devices (such as a cane or a walker); therefore, it is important to agree on realistic expectations with the patient. Patient education should also include potential safety issues, such as noncompliance with dosing (particularly trying to make up for missed doses or reducing the time between doses), and the fact that the tablets should not be crushed or cut in order to preserve the pharmacokinetic properties of the extended release formulation. Prescribing dalfampridine does not preclude a referral to physical therapy or the prescription of assistive devices. If these interventions have not already been implemented, it is desirable to initiate them either before starting the medication (allows to evaluate the specific effects of each intervention) or concomitantly with treatment initiation.

> *Dalfampridine is approved by the Food and Drug Administration (FDA) to improve walking in patients with MS, based on an improvement in walking speed in clinical trials.*

Other medications can contribute directly or indirectly to improve or preserve walking. Medications targeting symptoms that interfere with walking, such as spasticity (see Chapter 29) and pain, may enhance walking performance, although the functional effects of these drugs are rarely tested, or the functional tests used are not consistent (64).

It is worth noting that some medications may cause worsening of gait disturbance and imbalance because of side effects such as somnolence, dizziness, or weakness. Therefore, in the presence of an abrupt deterioration of walking performance, it is important to review a current medication list, along with other potential factors such as MS exacerbation or progression, infection, or other acute illness.

SURGICAL TREATMENTS

Two types of surgical treatments can be contemplated to improve ambulation in MS: neurosurgical interventions to control spasticity and orthopedic surgery.

Among neurosurgical interventions for spasticity, intrathecal baclofen (ITB) therapy is the most common. Two case series in MS patients showed that ambulation is usually preserved after the implantation of a baclofen pump (65,66), but improvement of gait pattern has not been demonstrated. Although selective dorsal rhizotomy or tibial nerve neurotomy are sometimes used in MS on the basis of their effects on gait in patients with cerebral palsy and stroke, there is no published evidence in MS to our knowledge.

Musculoskeletal comorbidity has been shown to impact the level of disability in MS (see Chapter 35). Conversely, gait deviations from neurological impairments cause stress on the musculoskeletal system; severe spasticity can cause contractures and limb deformity; and falls can cause fractures, sprains, and other musculoskeletal injuries. It is therefore important to recognize and treat musculoskeletal problems in the presence of MS. Unfortunately, there is little evidence to guide clinical decision making, especially when surgery is considered. Even if MS does not contraindicate surgery, the functional results are less predictable than in the general population, and prolonged rehabilitation is often needed. Disease management and spasticity control should be optimized before elective musculoskeletal surgery. One publication recommended the use of prophylactic corticosteroids at the time of surgery (67), but this remains controversial owing to a possible negative effect of corticosteroids on healing and infectious risk and the lack of evidence that surgery or anesthesia increases the risk of MS exacerbation (68).

> *Although surgery is not contraindicated in MS, the use of surgical treatments to improve ambulation requires careful patient selection and intensive rehabilitation.*

CONCLUSION

Preserving mobility can be an uphill battle in MS, involving the patient, family, personal care providers, and healthcare providers. Considering the physical, psychological, and socioeconomic consequences of loss of mobility, it is essential to identify, understand, and address walking and balance impairment as early as possible, often starting with simple and safe interventions such as exercise, physical therapy, symptomatic medications, and the use of assistive devices. Ambulation and balance should be monitored periodically in the comprehensive management of MS, using validated performance tests and questionnaires. Further research is needed to better understand the pathophysiology of mobility impairments, to validate outcome measures for mobility, and to further test the efficacy and safety of various interventions (and combination of interventions) in subgroups of patients.

KEY POINTS FOR PATIENTS AND FAMILIES

- MS frequently causes issues with walking and balance, which in turn restrict mobility.

- Walking and balance can be affected early in the disease course, and impact daily activities and quality of life. Therefore, it is important to bring difficulties with walking and balance to the attention of your healthcare provider.

- Walking and balance can be assessed through performance tests and questionnaires, and technological innovations have made it easier to measure walking and balance in a person's own environment.

- Exercise and rehabilitation play a key role in helping maintain or improve walking and balance. Exercises can be adapted to a person's abilities, often with input from a physical therapist.

- Medications, braces, and assistive devices can also help make walking and balance tasks safer and easier.

REFERENCES

1. World Health Organization. International Classification of Functioning, Disability, and Health. Available at http://apps.who.int/classifications/icfbrowser/. Accessed August 22, 2017.
2. Chung LH, Remelius JG, Van Emmerik RE, et al. Leg power asymmetry and postural control in women with multiple sclerosis. *Med Sci Sports Exerc.* 2008;40(10):1717-1724.
3. Sosnoff JJ, Shin S, Motl RW. Multiple sclerosis and postural control: the role of spasticity. *Arch Phys Med Rehabil.* 2010;91(1):93-99.
4. Thoumie P, Lamotte D, Cantalloube S, et al. Motor determinants of gait in 100 ambulatory patients with multiple sclerosis. *Mult Scler.* 2005;11:485-491.
5. Sosnoff JJ, Gappmaier E, Frame A, et al. Influence of spasticity on mobility and balance in persons with multiple sclerosis. *J Neurol Phys Ther.* 2011;35:129-132.
6. Cameron MH, Horak FB, Herndon RR, et al. Imbalance in multiple sclerosis: a result of slowed spinal somatosensory conduction. *Somatosens Mot Res.* 2008;25(2):113-122.
7. Wajda DA, Sosnoff JJ. Cognitive-motor interference in multiple sclerosis: a systematic review of evidence, correlates, and consequences. *Biomed Res Int.* 2015;2015:720856.
8. Hamilton F, Rochester L, Paul L, et al. Walking and talking: an investigation of cognitive-motor dual tasking in multiple sclerosis. *Mult Scler.* 2009;15:1215-1227.
9. Kalron A, Dvir Z, Achiron A. Walking while talking: difficulties incurred during the initial stages of multiple sclerosis disease process. *Gait Posture.* 2010;32:332-335.
10. Van Emmerik RE, Remelius JG, Johnson MB, et al. Postural control in women with multiple sclerosis: effects of task, vision and sympto-matic fatigue. *Gait Posture.* October 2010;32(4):608-614.
11. Huisinga JM, Filipi ML, Schmid KK, et al. Is there a relationship between fatigue questionnaires and gait mechanisms in persons with multiple sclerosis? *Arch Phys Med Rehabil.* 2011;92:1594-1601.
12. Karpatkin H, Cohen ET, Rzetelny A, et al. Effects of intermittent versus continuous walking on distance walked and fatigue in persons with multiple sclerosis: a randomized crossover trial. *J Neurol Phys Ther.* 2015;39:172-178.
13. Feys P, Gijbels D, Romberg A, et al. Effect of time of day on walking capacity and self-reported fatigue in persons with MS: a multicenter trial. *Mult Scler.* 2012;18(3):351-357.
14. Loy BD, Taylor RL, Fling BW, et al. Relationship between perceived fatigue and performance fatigability in people with multiple sclerosis: a systematic review and meta-analysis. *J Psychosom Res.* September 2017;100:1-7. doi:10.1016/j.jpsychores.2017.06.017.
15. Marrie RA, Rudick R, Horwitz R, et al. Vascular comorbidity is associated with more rapid disability progression in multiple sclerosis. *Neurology.* 2010;74:1041-1047.
16. Nilsagård Y, Gunn H, Freeman J, et al. Falls in people with MS—an individual data meta-analysis from studies from Australia,

Sweden, United Kingdom and the United States. *Mult Scler.* 2015;21(1):92-100.

17. Kasser SL, Jacobs JV, Foley JT, et al. A prospective evaluation of balance, gait, and strength to predict falling in women with multiple sclerosis. *Arch Phys Med Rehabil.* 2011;92:1840-1846.

18. Sosnoff JJ, Socie MJ, Boes MK, et al. Mobility, balance and falls in persons with multiple sclerosis. *PLOS ONE.* 2011;6(11):e28021.

19. Coote S, Finlayson M, Sosnoff JJ. Level of mobility limitations and falls status in persons with multiple sclerosis. *Arch Phys Med Rehabil.* 2014;95(5):862-866.

20. Cameron MH, Poel AJ, Haselkorn JK, et al. Falls requiring medical attention among veterans with multiple sclerosis: a cohort study. *J Rehabil Res Dev.* 2011;48:13-20.

21. Peterson EW, Cho CC, von Koch L, et al. Injurious falls among middle aged and older adults with multiple sclerosis. *Arch Phys Med Rehabil.* 2008;89:1031-1037.

22. Moen SM, Celius EG, Nordsletten L, et al. Fractures and falls in patients with newly diagnosed clinically isolated syndrome and multiple sclerosis. *Acta Neurol Scand Suppl.* 2011;191:79-82.

23. Karst GM, Venema DM, Roehrs TG, et al. Center of pressure measures during standing tasks in minimally impaired persons with multiple sclerosis. *J Neurol Phys Ther.* 2005;29(4):170-180.

24. Cameron MH, Lord S. Postural control in multiple sclerosis: implications for fall prevention. *Curr Neurol Neurosci Rep.* 2010;10(5):407-412.

25. Gunn H, Markevics S, Haas B, et al. Systematic review: the effectiveness of interventions to reduce falls and improve balance in adults with multiple sclerosis. *Arch Phys Med Rehabil.* 2015;96(10):1898-1912.

26. Cameron MH, Huisinga J. Objective and subjective measures reflect different aspects of balance in multiple sclerosis. *J Rehabil Res Dev.* 2013;50(10):1401-1410.

27. Powell LE, Myers AM. The Activities-specific Balance Confidence (ABC) Scale. *J Gerontol A Biol Sci Med Sci.* 1995;50A(1):M28-M34.

28. Kalron A. The Romberg ratio in people with multiple sclerosis. *Gait Posture.* 2017;54:209-213.

29. Williams KL, Low Choy NL, Brauer SG. Are changes in gait and balance across the disease step rating scale in multiple sclerosis statistically significant and clinically meaningful? *Arch Phys Med Rehabil.* September 2016;97(9):1502-1508.

30. Solomon AJ, Jacobs JV, Lomond KV, et al. Detection of postural sway abnormalities by wireless inertial sensors in minimally disabled patients with multiple sclerosis: a case-control study. *J Neuroeng Rehabil.* 2015;12:74.

31. Prosperini L, Fortuna D, Giannì C, et al. The diagnostic accuracy of static posturography in predicting accidental falls in people with multiple sclerosis. *Neurorehabil Neural Repair.* 2013;27:45-52.

32. Sosnoff JJ, Sung J. Reducing falls and improving mobility in multiple sclerosis. *Expert Rev Neurother.* 2015;15(6):655-666.

33. Paltamaa J, Sjögren T, Peurala SH, et al. Effects of physiotherapy interventions on balance in multiple sclerosis: a systematic review and meta-analysis of randomized controlled trials. *J Rehabil Med.* 2012;44(10):811-823.

34. Taylor MJ, Griffin M. The use of gaming technology for rehabilitation in people with multiple sclerosis. *Mult Scler.* 2015;21(4):355-371.

35. Rice LA, Isaacs Z, Ousley CO, et al (in press). Investigation of the Feasibility of an Intervention to Manage Fall Risk Among Wheeled Mobility Device Users With Multiple Sclerosis. *Int J MS Care.*

36. Swingler RJ, Compston DA. The morbidity of multiple sclerosis. *Q J Med.* 1992;83:325-337.

37. Hobart JC, Lamping DL, Fitzpatrick R, et al. The Multiple Sclerosis Impact Scale (MSIS-29): a new patient-based outcome measure. *Brain.* 2001;124:962-973.

38. La Rocca N. Impact of walking impairment in multiple sclerosis: perspectives of patients and care partners. *Patient.* 2011;4:189-201.

39. Heesen C, Böhm J, Reich C, et al. Patient perception of bodily functions in multiple sclerosis: gait and visual function are the most valuable. *Mult Scler.* 2008;14:988-991.

40. Paltamaa J, Sarasoja T, Leskinen E, et al. Measures of physical functioning predict self-reported performance in self-care, mobility, and domestic life in ambulatory persons with multiple sclerosis. *Arch Phys Med Rehabil.* 2007;88:1649-1657.

41. Edgley K, Sullivan MJ, Dehoux E. A survey of multiple sclerosis: II. Determinants of employment status. *Can J Rehabil.* 1991;4:127-132.

42. Bethoux F, Bennett S. Evaluating walking in patients with multiple sclerosis: which assessment tools are useful in clinical practice? *Int J MS Care.* 2011;13(1):4-14.

43. Hobart JC, Riazi A, Lamping DL, et al. Measuring the impact of MS on walking ability: the 12-item MS Walking Scale (MSWS-12). *Neurology.* 2003;60:31-36.

44. Rudick RA, Cutter G, Reingold S. The multiple sclerosis functional composite; a new clinical outcome measure for multiple sclerosis trials. *Mult Scler.* 2002;8:359-365.

45. Kragt JJ, van der Linden FA, Nielsen JM, et al. Clinical impact of 20% worsening on Timed 25-foot Walk and 9-hole Peg Test in multiple sclerosis. *Mult Scler.* 2006;12:594-598.

46. Goldman M, Marrie RA, Cohen JA. Evaluation of the six-minute walk in multiple sclerosis subjects and healthy controls. *Mult Scler.* 2007;14:383-390.

47. Cattaneo D, Regola A, Meotti M. Validity of six balance disorders scales in persons with multiple sclerosis. *Disabil Rehabil.* 2006;28:789-795.

48. Givon U, Zeilig G, Achiron A. Gait analysis in multiple sclerosis: characterization of temporal-spatial parameters using GAITRite functional ambulation system. *Gait Posture.* 2009;29:138-142.

49. Martin CL, Phillips BA, Kilpatrick TJ, et al. Gait and balance impairment in early multiple sclerosis in the absence of clinical disability. *Mult Scler.* 2006;12:620-628.

50. Gijbels D, Alders G, Van Hoof E, et al. Predicting habitual walking performance in multiple sclerosis: relevance of capacity and self-report measures. *Mult Scler.* 2010;16:618-626.

51. Rampello A, Franceschini M, Piepoli M, et al. Effect of aerobic training on walking capacity and maximal exercise tolerance in patients with multiple sclerosis: a randomized crossover controlled study. *Phys Ther.* 2007;87(5):545-559.

52. Dalgas U, Stenager E, Jakobsen J, et al. Resistance training improves muscle strength and functional capacity in multiple sclerosis. *Neurology.* 2009;73(18):1478-1484.

53. Dalgas U, Stenager E, Jakobsen J, et al. Fatigue, mood and quality of life improve in MS patients after progressive resistance training. *Mult Scler.* 2010;16:480-490.

54. Learmonth YC, Ensari I, Motl RW. Physiotherapy and walking outcomes in adults with multiple sclerosis: systematic review and meta-analysis. *Phys Ther Rev.* 2016;21:160-172.

55. Pilutti LA, Lelli DA, Paulseth JE, et al. Effects of 12 weeks of supported treadmill training on functional ability and quality of life in progressive multiple sclerosis: a pilot study. *Arch Phys Med Rehabil.* 2011;92:31-36.

56. Xie X, Sun H, Zeng Q, et al. Do patients with multiple sclerosis derive more benefit from Robot-assisted gait training compared with conventional walking therapy on motor function? A meta-analysis. *Front Neurol.* June 13, 2017;8:260. doi:10.3389/fneur.2017.00260. eCollection 2017.

57. Sheffler LR, Hennessey MT, Knutson JS, et al. Functional effect of an ankle foot orthosis on gait in multiple sclerosis: a pilot study. *Am J Phys Med Rehabil.* 2008;87(1):26-32.

58. Barrett CL, Mann GE, Taylor PN, et al. A randomized trial to investigate the effects of functional electrical stimulation and therapeutic exercise on walking performance for people with multiple sclerosis. *Mult Scler.* 2009;15(4):493-504.

59. Paul L, Rafferty D, Young S, et al. The effect of functional electrical stimulation on the physiological cost of gait in people with multiple sclerosis. *Mult Scler.* 2008;14(7):954-961.

60. Sutliff M, Naft J, Stough D, et al. Efficacy and safety of a hip flexion assist orthosis in ambulatory multiple sclerosis patients. *Arch Phys Med Rehabil.* 2008;89(8):1611-1617.

61. Goodman AD, Brown TR, Krupp LB, et al. Sustained-release oral fampridine in multiple sclerosis: a randomised, double-blind, controlled trial. *Lancet.* 2009;373:732-738.

62. Goodman AD, Brown TR, Edwards KR, et al. A phase 3 trial of extended release oral dalfampridine in multiple sclerosis. *Ann Neurol.* 2010;68:494-502.

63. Yapundich R, Applebee A, Bethoux F, et al. Evaluation of dalfampridine extended release 5 and 10 mg in multiple sclerosis: a randomized controlled trial. *Int J MS Care.* 2015;17(3):138-145.

64. Shakespeare D, Young C, Boggild M. Anti-spasticity agents for multiple sclerosis. *Cochrane Database of Syst Rev.* 2003;4:CD001332.

65. Sadiq SA, Wang GC. Long-term intrathecal baclofen therapy in ambulatory patients with spasticity. *J Neurol.* 2006;253:563-569.

66. Bethoux F, Stough D, Sutliff M. Treatment of severe spasticity with intrathecal baclofen therapy in ambulatory multiple sclerosis patients: 6-month follow-up. *Arch Phys Med Rehab.* 2004;84:A10.

67. Dickerman RD, Schneider SJ, Stevens QE, et al. Prophylaxis to avert exacerbation/relapse of multiple sclerosis in affected patients undergoing surgery. *J Neurosurg Sci.* 2004;48:135-137.

68. D'hooghe MB, Nagels G, Bissay V, et al. Modifiable factors influencing relapses and disability in multiple sclerosis. *Mult Scler.* 2010;16(7):773-785.

31 General Health and Wellness in Multiple Sclerosis

Mary R. Rensel, Brandon P. Moss, and Carrie M. Hersh

KEY POINTS FOR CLINICIANS

- Multiple sclerosis (MS) patients need to have a primary care provider, yet access to primary care is compromised by a variety of barriers.
- Preventive medicine is important in all stages of MS to lessen the risk of comorbidities and subsequent worsening of neurologic disability.
- Comorbidities increase the risk of physical disability in MS, decrease quality of life, and worsen MS outcomes.
- Lifestyle strategies may affect long-term outcomes in MS patients.
- Encourage regular exercise, smoking cessation, and good nutrition for health promotion and to decrease the risk of comorbidities in MS patients.
- Smoking cessation may lessen long-term disability in MS patients.
- MS patients should be systematically screened and treated for vitamin D deficiency.
- Consider mind–body therapies such as meditation and yoga to help MS symptoms.

OVERVIEW

Patients with MS need routine treatment and monitoring by a neurologist with experience in MS. In addition, we now know that age-appropriate health screens, vascular risk management, and management of other health conditions are equally important, but are not routinely addressed by neurologists. There is increasing evidence that other medical and mental health conditions such as hypertension, hypercholesterolemia, and depression may influence the level of disability from MS (see Chapter 35). Therefore, other healthcare providers are needed, particularly a primary care provider (PCP), to help comanage patients living with MS for optimal care.

In addition to conventional medicine, there is growing public and scientific interest in incorporating lifestyle strategies to optimize MS care as part of an integrative model of medicine. Many of these interventions are rooted in a global approach to health and wellness. Recommended wellness interventions are summarized in Table 31.1.

Comorbidities and adverse lifestyle factors negatively affect the clinical phenotype of the disease, time to diagnosis, disability progression, and health-related quality of life. MS patients will need a cane earlier if they have a single physical comorbidity and even earlier with multiple comorbidities (1). Lifestyle factors shown to have a positive impact on physical disability in MS include adequate social support; emotional health; and healthy behaviors including exercise, smoking cessation, obesity management, and prevention of vascular comorbidities (1–3).

COMMON PRIMARY CARE ISSUES IN MS PATIENTS

There are primary care issues that are common in MS patients, such as osteoporosis, vitamin D deficiency, depression, fatigue, and sleep disorders. Osteoporosis in MS patients may be related to the use of steroids due to limited ambulation (4), or perhaps related to the disease itself. Vitamin D deficiency is common in MS patients and common in higher latitudes. There is some evidence that vitamin D deficiency may play a role in triggering MS, or even in promoting disease activity once a person has been diagnosed with MS (5). This is not certain at present, but is another important reason to maintain recommended vitamin D levels (see section on vitamin D for more detailed information). Managing vascular risk factors or comorbidities (hypertension, cholesterol, obesity, diabetes, and smoking) is important for cardiovascular health, but recent data show that risk factor modification may also be important in limiting MS disease severity including physical disability (6,7).

TABLE 31.1 Principal Recommendations for Wellness Interventions in MS

Diet	• Eat a Mediterranean low-salt, low-saturated fat diet consistent with USDA guidelines.
Vitamin D Supplementation	• Maintain a minimum 25(OH)D level of 30 ng/mL consistent with Endocrine Society guidelines. • Vitamin D3 supplementation is preferred over vitamin D2. • Although there is no established treatment approach, supplementation with 1,000 IU of vitamin D3 for levels between 20 and 30 ng/mL and 2,000 IU of vitamin D3 for levels <20 ng/mL is one general treatment approach.
Exercise	• Follow the minimum recommendations for exercise according to the US NCHPAD guidelines: • 20–60 min sessions of moderate intensity aerobic training 3–4 d/wk • 10–15 min sessions of strength training 2–3 d/wk • 10–15 min sessions of stretching exercises daily
Tobacco Smoking Cessation	• A combination program incorporating behavioral and pharmacologic interventions for smoking cessation can be beneficial. • Behavioral interventions: written materials containing advice on quitting, multisession group therapy, individual counseling sessions • Pharmacologic interventions: NRT, varenicline, bupropion, cystine, nortriptyline
Screening for Psychiatric Comorbidities and Referral to Mental Health Services	• Use a validated screening tool for depression regularly in clinical practice (two-item screen, BDI, CES-D, CMDI, HADS, PHQ-9). • Follow general practice guidelines for the treatment of depression, bipolar disorder, and anxiety. • There is no evidence supporting the use of one psychotropic medication over another in the MS population.
Preventative care	• See primary care provider at a minimum annually.

25(OH)D3, 25-hydroxyvitamin D3; BDI, Beck Depression Inventory; CES-D, Center for Epidemiologic Studies Depression Scale; CMDI, Chicago Multiscale Depression Inventory; HADS, Hospital Anxiety and Depression Scale; IU, international units; MS, multiple sclerosis; NCHPAD, National Center on Health, Physical Activity and Disability; NRT, nicotine replacement therapy; PHQ-9, Patient Health Questionnaire-9; USDA: United States Department of Agriculture.

Depression, fatigue, and sleep disorders are very common in MS patients and are addressed separately in this text.

The prevalence of smoking in MS patients is similar to the general population. In addition to commonly known health risks, smokers have an increased risk of developing autoimmune conditions including MS, as well as have higher levels of disability in the context of MS (8). Smoking cessation has been associated with decreased rate of disability in MS (9). MS patients should be referred to a smoking cessation program in their community and prescribed pharmaceutical products, as this combination of treatments dramatically increases the success rates (10).

The prevalence of alcoholism in MS patients is also similar to the general population. Patients should discuss their alcohol intake in detail with their care team. Excess alcohol should be avoided since it may adversely affect several body systems including the neurologic system, and if there is alcohol dependency or abuse, it should be aggressively addressed. Alcohol intake should be limited or altogether avoided with various medications commonly prescribed for the management of MS, including interferons, antiepileptic medications, and benzodiazepines.

Patients with MS are faced with various barriers to accessing primary care. First, it may be difficult for MS patients to travel to nonaccessible facilities because of physical limitations. Second, some MS patients require frequent visits for management of complex issues either related or unrelated to their disease, and additional healthcare visits for preventive services may seem burdensome from a

practical and financial standpoint. Third, the symptoms of MS affect directly or indirectly many body systems (e.g., urological, musculoskeletal); therefore, patients with MS may contact their neurology team first for help. Yet, owing to the many general health issues with relevance to MS, it is imperative that patients routinely visit with a PCP to perform preventive care as well as to treat known conditions. It is also the role of the neurology team to encourage regular visits with a PCP, smoking cessation, mental health screening, social connectedness, and healthy behaviors to help promote general wellness and lessen the risk of comorbidities.

> It is imperative that MS patients routinely visit with a primary care provider to perform preventive care as well as to treat known medical conditions.

HEALTH PROMOTION

Health promotion includes setting goals and establishing health-enhancing behaviors, such as regular exercise, good nutrition, and stress management. In individuals with MS, health promotion has been shown to improve employment, physical conditioning and strength, quality of life, and even to lessen the severity of MS (11–13). Specific health-promoting behaviors are discussed in detail in the following section. However, in the setting of MS, initiating and maintaining healthy behaviors often requires individualized guidance from a multidisciplinary team. For example, there is good evidence showing that regular exercise is important in MS; therefore, we encourage specific planning for exercise programming in the MS population. Because of barriers such as physical impairment, fatigue, and cognitive limitations, MS patients can benefit from having access to physical therapy (PT) and occupational therapy (OT) to help map out a home exercise plan, improve strength and balance, and to enrich activities of daily living. MS patients should also have access to mental health professionals as part of their care team to help with stress management, emotional health, goal setting, motivation to change behaviors, and the management of coexisting psychiatric disorders.

As health practitioners, we want to give our patients all the opportunities and tools to facilitate health promotion. Health promoting tools include individualized education, shared medical appointments, community programs, and a plethora of electronic resources (e.g., applications [apps] for smart phones and information accessible on the Internet). Smart phone apps and wearables can help the patient obtain health information, set personal goals, and track healthy behaviors and wellness indicators (14,15). The Internet is another vast source of information and guidance on healthcare information and has enhanced the opportunities for patients to be more engaged and active in coping with and managing their disease. Information, guidance, and sometimes support can be obtained online from various sources, including healthcare providers, patient support organizations, general medical information sites, and other MS patients through chat rooms and forums. While the Internet makes information seeking easy, one must be reminded that it is not a neutral technology, and the contents can be biased (e.g., by commercial interests or personal opinions) or lack evidence-based medicine to support their claims (16). Eighty percent of patients looking for information online will find what they are looking for and the common users of the Internet are patients with long-standing illness (17). It is the healthcare providers' role to point the patients to a variety of resources with accurate information on healthy lifestyle education.

> *Encourage multiple sclerosis (MS) patients to set goals and promote healthy behaviours:*
>
> 1. *Follow a healthy diet*
> 2. *Perform regular exercise*
> 3. *Engage in regular visits with the primary care provider (PCP) to prevent and manage comorbidities*
> 4. *Promote smoking cessation*
> 5. *Moderate alcohol intake*
> 6. *Manage stress*
> 7. *Correct vitamin D deficiency*
> 8. *Connect with the community (e.g., volunteer)*
> 9. *Enhance self-advocacy*

GENERAL HEALTH AND WELLNESS IN MS

Wellness is a lifelong, personalized process through which people make informed choices about their lifestyle behaviors and activities across multiple interrelated dimensions in order to lead their best lives. While all patients with MS should seek optimal health and wellness practices, each person's disease state and underlying comorbidities present individual challenges to meeting these goals.

Exercise in MS

MS patients typically report a sedentary lifestyle, which can be associated with their level of disability, severity of symptoms, or lack of knowledge on the importance of exercise for MS. A growing body of evidence shows that exercise can be helpful and is safe for patients with MS. Fatigue, physical and emotional health, and quality of life have been shown to be positively affected by various types of exercise, including aerobic training (18), resistance training (19), and yoga (20). Therefore, regular aerobic activity should be encouraged in MS patients. Most patients can either exercise on their own or with the help of PT/OT specialists help to improve physical functioning and to develop an appropriate home exercise program. Some patients with more advanced disability and cognitive impairment may require closer individualized care.

Emerging evidence suggests further potential benefits of exercise in MS. Studies have reported an increase in brain-derived neurotropic factors (BDNF) and insulin-like growth factor (IGF) with aerobic activity, suggesting the potential enhancement of neuronal repair and brain plasticity with exercise (21). Other studies have shown that a higher level of cardiopulmonary fitness was associated with faster physical performance and greater brain activation on defined tasks, providing evidence that exercise may help cognition (22).

RECOMMENDATIONS FOR EXERCISE

Based on the evidence discussed earlier, routine exercise is important in MS and should be encouraged. Yet, MS patients often cannot tolerate the intensity and frequency of training recommended in healthy adults. The U.S. National Center on Health, Physical Activity and Disability Guidelines for patients with MS recommend 20 to 60 minute sessions of moderate intensity aerobic training at least 3 to 4 d/wk and 10 to 15 minute sessions of strength training 2 to

3 d/wk (23). They also include daily stretching exercises for at least 10 to 15 minutes. These guidelines caution patients to closely monitor heart rate and blood pressure regularly if they have dysautonomia, and patients should maintain a cool environment to avoid heat sensitivity.

The effects of exercise in MS patients include:

1. *Lessening MS symptoms such as fatigue*
2. *Decreasing risk of vascular comorbidities*
3. *Increasing conditioning and strength*
4. *Improving quality of life—both physical and emotional*
5. *Possibly promoting nerve repair*

Vitamin D and MS

An increasing number of studies support a positive role for vitamin D in MS. Low sunlight and ultraviolet (UV) radiation exposure, as well as low vitamin D levels and intake, are inversely correlated with the risk of developing MS (5). Lower vitamin D levels have been associated with an increase in MRI activity (24) and an increase in risk of relapse (25). These studies may explain the findings that MS relapses are typically in the Fall and Spring when vitamin D levels reach their nadir. There have been pediatric MS studies showing that low vitamin D levels increased the risk of relapses in clinically isolated syndrome (CIS) (26).

Multiple phase I and II randomized controlled trials (RCTs) have now been conducted to assess the safety and utility of vitamin D supplementation (27–32). None of these studies were powered for clinical outcome measures, and only one of these studies (29) was powered for an MRI measure of disease activity. This one-year, randomized, double-blind, placebo-controlled trial evaluated 20,000 international units (IU) of vitamin D3 as an add-on therapy to interferon (IFN) beta-1b. Total T2 lesion volume was the primary endpoint. Median change in T2 lesion volume was 287 mm^3 in the placebo group compared to 83 mm^3 in the treatment group, but the difference did not meet statistical significance (p = .105). The total number of gadolinium-enhancing lesions, a secondary endpoint, decreased significantly in both groups (p = .002), but this change was significantly higher in the vitamin D group (p = .004) with a change in the median number of lesions from 0.6 to 0.1 in the treatment arm. Several ongoing RCTs are investigating the utility of vitamin D as adjunctive therapy to disease-modifying therapies (DMTs) and may help provide a more definitive answer regarding the impact of vitamin D on disease activity and worsening of disability in MS (33–35).

In summary, vitamin D appears to play a role in the risk of developing MS and in the activity of the disease. Yet, the majority of MS patients are deficient in vitamin D. The recommended dose of calcium for the adult population is 1,200 mg/d, and the recommended vitamin D dose is at least 600 mg/d. Additional doses of vitamin D$_3$ may be needed, depending on the serum level of vitamin D 25-OH. Dosing of vitamin D3 can range from 2,000 to 4,000 IU daily or higher with the target being near 60 ng/mL. Depending on the individual, one could also encourage regular exposure to the sun, for example, 10 minutes daily or 30 minutes a few times per week, with the use of sunscreen for more extended periods in the sun. However, patients should first be counselled to discuss potential risks of sunlight expsosure with their healthcare provider.

MS patients should be treated with at least 1,000 international units (IU) of vitamin D$_3$ daily, adjusted according to the vitamin D 25-OH blood level. Maintain vitamin D$_{25}$ OH levels near 60 ng/mL, and assess at least annually.

Osteoporosis and MS

Patients with MS have multiple risk factors for osteoporosis: impaired gait, sedentary lifestyle, and the use of steroids (4). It has been shown that MS patients have a high risk of osteoporosis even with a normal gait (36). Daily long-term steroid use has been associated with an increased risk of osteoporosis; yet, pulse steroids given every few months have not been associated with bone degradation (37). Bone loss can be prevented by proper nutrition, limited alcohol intake (37), weight-bearing exercise as able (38), and calcium and vitamin D supplementation. Recently, calcium supplementation has been associated with possible cardiovascular events; therefore, patients need to discuss risk and benefits with their primary care physician (39). We are not aware of published guidelines on the prevention and management of osteoporosis specific to MS. Testing for osteoporosis and supplementation with calcium and vitamin D should be considered in MS patients with a history of fracture, gait impairment, low vitamin D levels, and/or frequent steroid usage (38). Considering the increasing complexity of the management of bone health, referral to the patient's PCP is advisable.

Healthy nutrition, smoking cessation, decreased alcohol intake, and regular exercise with weight bearing promote bone health.

Smoking and MS

Smoking has general negative health effects and has additionally been shown to have direct links to MS disease activity. Cigarette smoke contains thousands of compounds, many of which have direct toxicity to oligodendroglia and neurons, or influence immune function. People who have ever smoked or who have passively been exposed to tobacco smoke during their lifetime are at higher risk of MS compared to those who have never smoked. Smoking has also been associated with a delay in the diagnosis of MS, worse disease progression, increased likelihood of having active MS on MRI, decreased quality of life, and increased risk of bone fracture (9). There is not as much information on vapor cigarettes and their effects on MS. MS patients should be educated regarding the deleterious effects of smoking and should be advised to quit.

Smoking is common in individuals with MS. One factor that may increase the likelihood of smoking and create a challenge for smoking cessation in MS is mental health issues. In a recent population-based prevalence study, it was reported that smoking rates differ between those with no history of mental health concerns (22.5%), those with some mental health concerns reported in their life time (34.8%), and those with mental health concerns in the past month (41.0%) (40). These numbers suggest that persons with mental health concerns in the general population are approximately twice as likely to smoke as compared to those without mental health concerns. At the same time, it is estimated that up to 54% of individuals with MS may be diagnosed with major depressive disorder, up to 13% with a bipolar disorder, up to 35% with an anxiety disorder, 22% with an adjustment disorder, and 3% with a psychotic disorder (see Chapter 20).

There is evidence supporting that adequate treatment of depression and anxiety can help smokers quit (41). Referral to a mental health provider can help in several ways including addressing co-occurring mental health concerns, increasing motivation and self-efficacy, identifying goals based on stage of change, applying behavioral principles such as self-monitoring and identifying trigger situations, and relapse prevention. The Centers for Disease Control (CDC) has issued recommendations for interventions to promote smoking cessation (42).

Smoking cessation recommendations as per CDC (43) are the following:

1. Brief encouragement and assistance by a doctor
2. Individual, group, or telephone counseling
3. Behavioral therapies
4. Treatments that include person to person contact and more intensity
5. Programs to deliver treatments using mobile phones

6. Medications to aid smoking cessation have been found to be effective; nicotine replacement, buproprion SR, and varenuicline tartrate
7. Counseling and medication are both effective; using them together is more effective than either therapy alone

Obesity and MS

The rates of obesity are higher in the MS population compared to the general population (44). Further, a higher body mass index (BMI) was found in patients who were married, male, employed, and had other comorbidities such as diabetes or arthritis. One study found that 60% of MS patients were overweight, which was associated with an increase in physical disability levels; even individuals with a mild level of disability had a higher risk of being overweight (45). Importantly, obesity is associated with hypertension, hypercholesterolemia, and type 2 diabetes, and these conditions are individually associated with an increased risk of MS-related physical disability. Additionally, obesity has been found to be common in the pediatric population with MS (46). It is the role of the MS care provider to encourage a PCP, as part of their healthcare team, to engage in preventive medicine practices, including nutritional education.

Emotional Health and MS (see Chapter 20)

As mentioned earlier, psychological issues are common among MS patients. The strongest predictors of depression in MS include modifiable factors such as fatigue impact, low mobility, resiliency, self-esteem, self-efficacy, and coping style. Psychological diagnosis and treatments as well as wellness programming may lessen the risk and/or consequences of depression in MS patients (47). Stress is also common due to the chronic unpredictable nature of MS. Given the under-recognition and under-treatment of psychiatric comorbidities in MS, regular screening is indicated with validated screening tests, where they exist. There is no evidence for any one treatment strategy over another in the MS population, so management of psychiatric comorbidities should follow general practice guidelines. Several studies, including one RCT, also suggest a potential role for stress management in MS, and stress management strategies can be offered to patients who are interested (48).

INTEGRATIVE MEDICINE AND MS

Integrative medicine (IM) combines treatments from conventional medicine and complementary medicine for which there is some high-quality evidence of safety and effectiveness (49).

MS Patients and IM

Nearly 60% of MS patients have tried IM, and the rate has increased over the last decade (50) with the advent of popularized health and wellness approaches. The types of IM modalities that have been reported to be used by MS patients include reflexology, massage therapy, yoga, meditation, diet, omega-3 fatty acid supplements, acupuncture, Reiki, tai chi, and vitamins and supplements (51). MS patients tend to use IM due to several reasons: dissatisfaction with conventional medicine, wanting more control over their disease management, enhancement of their sense of well-being, and MS symptom relief. MS patients with a longer course of MS, higher educational levels, female sex, and high level of fatigue tend to use IM more than others (52).

Nutritional Issues in Relation to MS

At this time, there is no direct evidence of a nutritional aetiology related to the development of MS. Nonetheless, there are studies linking high intake of saturated fats, calories, salt, and animal products with an increased risk of MS (53,54). Conversely, a plant-based diet with high fish intake, low salt, and lowered saturated fat has been associated with lessening the risk of MS (55). Polyunsaturated fatty acids are thought to encourage a healthy immune system. Linolenic acid was tested in the 1960s as a possible treatment for MS, and the results were mixed (56).

A low salt Mediterranean diet has been recommended. The type of fat in the Mediterranean diet has a higher omega 3:6 ratio. Omega-3 fatty acids are found in various sources: flaxseed, soy, soybean oil, canola oil, walnuts, fish, and fish oils. There are some findings suggesting that fish oils are well tolerated with DMTs for MS although they did not consistently influence the relapse rate of MS (57). A healthy diet with fewer sugars and processed foods may increase the energy level of MS patients. MS patients have high rates of constipation, so patients should be educated on the need to eat three regular meals, eat high-fiber meals, have adequate water intake, and eat fruits and vegetables regularly.

While there is no convincing evidence in support of a particular diet in MS, a plant-based, anti-inflammatory, nutritional regimen appears to be the most strongly indicated for optimal health. The 2015 to 2020 Dietary Guidelines from the U.S. Department of Agriculture include general dietary approaches with the goal of optimizing health and minimizing chronic diseases (58). Such recommendations include: a variety of vegetables, whole fruits, grains (at least half of which should be whole grains), fat-free or low-fat dairy products (including milk, yogurt, cheese, and fortified soy beverages), a variety of proteins (including seafood, lean meats and poultry, eggs, legumes, nuts, seeds, and soy products), high-fiber foods, and oils. The guidelines limit added sugars, processed foods, salt intake to less than 2,300 mg/d, total fat in the diet to 20% to 35% of calories, saturated fat intake less than 10% of calories, and trans fats.

The daily fluid intake recommendations may need to be adjusted according to the daily caffeine intake, medical conditions, and activity level. Nutritional therapy consultation can help to educate the patient on a healthy diet. There have been multiple studies looking at isolated nutritional supplement to help the MS patient, and to date no particular consistent positive findings occurred when patients added an isolated supplement of vitamin E, vitamin C, fish oils, evening primrose oil, or vitamin A (Table 31.2). To promote wellness, we have issued the following suggestions for our MS patients:

1. Follow a low-salt Mediterranean diet, low-fat diet while avoiding high intake of saturated fats.
2. Eat vegetables for at least two meals per day, five to seven servings a day. Serving size varies, low starch vegetables serving size is ½ cup cooked or one cup raw vegetables as a serving. It is important to eat a variety of colorful vegetables.
3. Eat three to five servings daily of a colorful variety of fruits.
4. Eat proteins daily. Proteins include meat, poultry, fish, eggs, beans, and nuts. *Limit meat to* 4 to 6 times a month.
5. Increase intake of whole grains in your cereals, breads, and pastas.
6. Eliminate simple carbohydrates such as white flour and white sugar.
7. At this time there is no known necessity to avoid gluten to help treat MS.
8. Fish may be helpful for the immune system; tuna or salmon have high levels of omega-3 oils.
9. Follow the ChooseMyPlate.gov recommendations on the balance of food products and portion sizes on your plate. Choose more vegetables and proteins than grains or fruit on your plate.
10. Maintain a healthy weight.
11. Limit salt intake.

TABLE 31.2 Outcomes of Studies of IM Interventions in MS Patients

POSITIVE FINDINGS	NEGATIVE FINDINGS
Fish oil	Antioxidant vitamins
St. John's wort	Ginkgo
Omega-3 fatty acids	Vitamin C
Coenzyme Q10	Vitamin E
Cannabis	Vitamin B_{12}
Low dose naltrexone	Ginseng
Meditation	Vitamin A
Therapeutic touch	Prolonged fasting
Aerobic exercise	Inosine
Reflexology	Bee venom
Music therapy	
Yoga	

IM, integrative medicine; MS, multiple sclerosis.

Supplements and MS

There is no known combination of supplements that helps to treat MS. That being said, there are multiple trials of over-the-counter products to help MS symptoms or disease management. The goal of supplementation is to promote a healthy immune system. MS patients may want to avoid immune system stimulating supplements such as Echinacea, oral garlic tabs, zinc, Astralagus, Cat's claw, maitake mushroom, mistletoe, and stinging nettle. There is a theoretical risk of stimulating the immune system in an MS patient thereby worsening the disease. As stated earlier, studies of fish oils as a therapy for MS have yielded mixed results. Evening primrose or flaxseed oil will increase the daily intake of omega-3 which may help the immune system although at this time there is no conclusive evidence to this effect. There are clinical trials from years ago showing that Linoleic acid can help relapses and possibly disability progression in two of three clinical trials (56). Vitamin B complex and Coenzyme Q10 tablets may help improve fatigue in MS. Urinary tract infections (UTI) are common in MS patients and can lead to worsening of MS symptoms. Vitamin C and cranberry tablets may help protect against UTIs. The potential benefits of vitamin D supplementation were discussed earlier.

> *Supplements to consider in MS include: multivitamin daily, vitamin D, calcium, B Complex vitamins, coenzyme Q10, vitamin C, and cranberry. "Immune boosters" should be avoided.*

Mind–Body Therapies and Healing Touch in MS

There are various mind–body therapies available to our patients; yet, there have been few controlled trials that demonstrate their efficacy in MS. Mind–body therapies include meditation, yoga, biofeedback, and acupuncture. There is level 3 evidence that MS patients can benefit from mind–body therapies including meditation (59). Meditation, including Qigong, tai chi, and walking meditation were shown to help MS patients with quality of life, depression, pain, and fatigue (60–62). Yoga can be helpful for MS patients with various levels of disability and it may help with fatigue (20). Music therapy has been shown to help MS patients with depression and gait disorder. Acupuncture is a component of traditional Chinese medicine. Although up to 20% of MS patients have tried acupuncture (63), clinical trials with acupuncture are too limited to provide definitive information regarding MS symptoms. There are studies of acupuncture helping spinal cord injury pain (64). There are reports of mind–body therapies helping particular symptoms of MS. One such study is with biofeedback improving refractory bowel symptoms (65). Self-hypnosis was compared to progressive muscle relaxation for MS pain; it showed self-hypnosis helped pain intensity and interference (66).

There is another practice called *Healing Touch* that is a hands-mediated therapy where a practitioner lays hands near or on the body to direct healing energy. Healing Touch has potential clinical effectiveness in improving health-related quality of life in chronic disease management. Healing Touch is generally safe, with no serious adverse effects having been reported (67). There are various types of Healing Touch, and some have been studied in clinical trials in MS patients. Reflexology is an alternative medicine technique involving activating pressure points with the hands on various parts of the body. There is a study showing reflexology helping MS symptoms: motor, sensory, and bladder symptoms (68). There are other studies showing that sham massage and reflexology both help MS symptoms equally; therefore, this is another practice that needs further research in MS (69). Reiki is an ancient Japanese healing method that involves "laying on the hands." It has been reported to help stress, depression, and pain in various other medical conditions (70). There are multiple systematic reviews of controlled trials of Reiki and this was not found to be effective in various outcomes including pain and anxiety in various settings, including diabetic peripheral neuropathy (PN) and fibromyalgia pain (71). There is inconclusive evidence of Reiki's effectiveness in MS (63).

Healing Touch practices can be a potential source of help for our patients with little potential of side effects or harm. There are generally many community-based options for learning these techniques that are readily accessible at a low cost to the patient.

SUMMARY

Despite well-known barriers, education on wellness, preventive medical care, and lifestyle optimization is extremely important for people with MS, and strong efforts should be made to ensure it is provided. These healthy lifestyle practices, including diet, physical activity, weight control, stress reduction, and tobacco discontinuation, are aimed at lowering the risk of developing chronic diseases and serve as an adjunct treatment for those chronic diseases already present. Comorbidities worsen long-term outcomes in MS patients; therefore, early and persistent healthy lifestyle practices in MS may effect long-lasting changes in the level of disability. More research is needed to determine how these active healthy practices can enhance long-term outcomes in MS patients. Altogether, the integration of lifestyle management with conventional medicine provides a multidimensional treatment approach to optimize overall health in individuals with MS. The impact of comorbidity prevention and/or treatment and lifestyle strategies deserves further investigation using larger studies across multiple regions to evaluate the impact of these interventions on disease-related outcomes on a more global scale.

KEY POINTS FOR PATIENTS AND FAMILIES

- See a primary care provider regularly to prevent and/or treat other conditions that can affect the level of physical disability of MS.

- Exercise regularly, seek a referral to physical and occupational therapy to help with MS symptoms, and to set up and maintain a home exercise program.

- Healthy nutrition is important; see a nutritionist if you need help starting or modifying your food plan.

- Take supplementary vitamin D and calcium; keep vitamin D level at 50 ng/mL or higher.

- Maintain a healthy weight.

- Stop smoking.

- Moderate alcohol intake.

- Consider mind–body therapies like meditation to help with feeling better.

- Optimal screening, diagnosis, and management of psychological and/or psychiatric issues like stress, depression, and anxiety.

SUGGESTED WEBSITES FOR PATIENTS WITH MS

National MS Society: www.NMSS.org

Mellen Center: my.clevelandclinic.org/multiple_sclerosis_center/default.aspx

FDA: www.fda.gov

NIH: information on current and past clinical trials in MS: nih.gov

NCCAM The National Center for Complementary and Alternative Medicine: nccam.nih.gov/health/decisions/practitioner.htm

REFERENCES

1. Marrie RA, Rudick R, Horwitz R, et al. Vascular comorbidity is associated with more rapid disability progression in multiple sclerosis. *Neurology*. 2010;74(13):1041–1047.
2. Mohr DC, Goodkin DE, Bacchetti P, et al. Psychological stress and the subsequent appearance of new brain MRI lesions in MS. *Neurology*. 2000;55(1):55–61.
3. Marrie RA, Horwitz RI, Cutter G, et al. Association between comorbidity and clinical characteristics of MS. *Acta Neurol Scand*. 2011;124(2):135–141.
4. Hearn AP, Silber E. Osteoporosis in multiple sclerosis. *Mult Scler*. 2010;16(9):1031–1043.
5. Wingerchuk DM. Supplementing our understanding of vitamin D and multiple sclerosis. *Neurology*. 2010;74(23):1846–1847.
6. Marrie RA, Horwitz R, Cutter G, et al. Comorbidity delays diagnosis and increases disability at diagnosis in MS. *Neurology*. 2009;72(2):117–124.
7. Sundstrom P, Nystrom L. Smoking worsens the prognosis in multiple sclerosis. *Mult Scler*. 2008;14(8):1031–1035.
8. Healy BC, Ali EN, Guttmann CR, et al. Smoking and disease progression in multiple sclerosis. *Arch Neurol*. 2009;66(7):858–864.
9. Manouchehrinia A, Tench CR, Maxted J, et al. Tobacco smoking and disability progression in multiple sclerosis: United Kingdom cohort study. *Brain*. 2013;136(pt 7):2298–2304.
10. West R, Raw M, McNeill A, et al. Health-care interventions to promote and assist tobacco cessation: a review of efficacy, effectiveness and affordability for use in national guideline development. *Addiction*. 2015;110(9):1388–1403.
11. Watt D, Verma S, Flynn L. Wellness programs: a review of the evidence. *CMAJ*. 1998;158(2):224–230.
12. Stuifbergen AK, Becker H, Blozis S, et al. A randomized clinical trial of a wellness intervention for women with multiple sclerosis. *Arch Phys Med Rehabil*. 2003;84(4):467–476.
13. Ennis M, Thain J, Boggild M, et al. A randomized controlled trial of a health promotion education programme for people with multiple sclerosis. *Clin Rehabil*. 2006;20(9):783–792.
14. Yousef A, Jonzzon S, Suleiman L, et al. Biosensing in multiple sclerosis. *Expert Rev Med Devices*. 2017;14(11):901–912.
15. Sasaki JE, Sandroff B, Bamman M, et al. Motion sensors in multiple sclerosis: narrative review and update of applications. *Expert Rev Med Devices*. 2017;14(11):891–900.
16. Korp P. Health on the Internet: implications for health promotion. *Health Educ Res*. 2006;21(1):78–86.
17. Rogers MA, Lemmen K, Kramer R, et al. Internet-delivered health interventions that work: systematic review of meta-analyses and evaluation of website availability. *J Med Internet Res*. 2017;19(3):e90.
18. Petajan JH, Gappmaier E, White AT, et al. Impact of aerobic training on fitness and quality of life in multiple sclerosis. *Ann Neurol*. 1996;39(4):432–441.
19. Dalgas U, Stenager E, Jakobsen J, et al. Fatigue, mood and quality of life improve in MS patients after progressive resistance training. *Mult Scler*. 2010;16(4):480–490.
20. Oken BS, Kishiyama S, Zajdel D, et al. Randomized controlled trial of yoga and exercise in multiple sclerosis. *Neurology*. 2004;62(11):2058–2064.

21. Gold SM, Schulz KH, Hartmann S, et al. Basal serum levels and reactivity of nerve growth factor and brain-derived neurotrophic factor to standardized acute exercise in multiple sclerosis and controls. *J Neuroimmunol*. 2003;138(1-2):99–105.

22. Prakash RS, Snook EM, Erickson KI, et al. Cardiorespiratory fitness: a predictor of cortical plasticity in multiple sclerosis. *Neuroimage*. 2007;34(3):1238–1244.

23. Rimmer JH, Vanderbom KA, Graham ID. A New Framework and Practice Center for Adapting, Translating, and Scaling Evidence-Based Health/Wellness Programs for People With Disabilities. *J Neurol Phys Ther*. April 2016;40(2):107–114. doi: 10.1097/NPT.0000000000000124. PMID: 26945430.

24. Loken-Amsrud KI, Holmoy T, Bakke SJ, et al. Vitamin D and disease activity in multiple sclerosis before and during interferon-beta treatment. *Neurology*. 2012;79(3):267–273.

25. Runia TF, Hop WC, de Rijke YB, et al. Lower serum vitamin D levels are associated with a higher relapse risk in multiple sclerosis. *Neurology*. 2012;79(3):261–266.

26. Mowry EM, Krupp LB, Milazzo M, et al. Vitamin D status is associated with relapse rate in pediatric-onset multiple sclerosis. *Ann Neurol*. 2010;67(5):618–624.

27. Burton JM, Kimball S, Vieth R, et al. A phase I/II dose-escalation trial of vitamin D3 and calcium in multiple sclerosis. *Neurology*. 2010;74(23):1852–1859.

28. Kampman MT, Steffensen LH, Mellgren SI, et al. Effect of vitamin D3 supplementation on relapses, disease progression, and measures of function in persons with multiple sclerosis: exploratory outcomes from a double-blind randomised controlled trial. *Mult Scler*. 2012;18(8):1144–1151.

29. Soilu-Hanninen M, Aivo J, Lindstrom BM, et al. A randomised, double blind, placebo controlled trial with vitamin D3 as an add on treatment to interferon beta-1b in patients with multiple sclerosis. *J Neurol Neurosurg Psychiatry*. 2012;83(5):565–571.

30. Sotirchos ES, Bhargava P, Eckstein C, et al. Safety and immunologic effects of high- vs low-dose cholecalciferol in multiple sclerosis. *Neurology*. 2016;86(4):382–390.

31. Stein MS, Liu Y, Gray OM, et al. A randomized trial of high-dose vitamin D2 in relapsing-remitting multiple sclerosis. *Neurology*. 2011;77(17):1611–1618.

32. Wingerchuk DM, Lesaux J, Rice GP, et al. A pilot study of oral calcitriol (1,25-dihydroxyvitamin D3) for relapsing-remitting multiple sclerosis. *J Neurol Neurosurg Psychiatry*. 2005;76(9):1294–1296.

33. Smolders J, Hupperts R, Barkhof F, et al. Efficacy of vitamin D3 as add-on therapy in patients with relapsing-remitting multiple sclerosis receiving subcutaneous interferon beta-1a: a Phase II, multicenter, double-blind, randomized, placebo-controlled trial. *J Neurol Sci*. 2011;311(1-2):44–49.

34. Dorr J, Ohlraun S, Skarabis H, et al. Efficacy of vitamin D supplementation in multiple sclerosis (EVIDIMS Trial): study protocol for a randomized controlled trial. *Trials*. 2012;13:15.

35. Bhargava P, Cassard S, Steele SU, et al. The vitamin D to ameliorate multiple sclerosis (VIDAMS) trial: study design for a multicenter, randomized, double-blind controlled trial of vitamin D in multiple sclerosis. *Contemp Clin Trials*. 2014;39(2):288–293.

36. Simonsen CS, Celius EG, Brunborg C, et al. Bone mineral density in patients with multiple sclerosis, hereditary ataxia or hereditary spastic paraplegia after at least 10 years of disease—a case control study. *BMC neurology*. 2016;16(1):252.

37. Jang HD, Hong JY, Han K, et al. Relationship between bone mineral density and alcohol intake: a nationwide health survey analysis of postmenopausal women. *PLOS ONE*. 2017;12(6):e0180132.

38. Zikan V. Bone health in patients with multiple sclerosis. *J Osteoporos*. 2011;2011:596294.

39. Tankeu AT, Ndip Agbor V, Noubiap JJ. Calcium supplementation and cardiovascular risk: a rising concern. *J Clin Hypertens (Greenwich)*. 2017;19(6):640–646.

40. Strine TW, Mokdad AH, Balluz LS, et al. Depression and anxiety in the United States: findings from the 2006 Behavioral Risk Factor Surveillance System. *Psychiatr Serv*. 2008;59(12):1383–1390.

41. Keyser-Marcus L, Vassileva J, Stewart K, et al. Impulsivity and cue reactivity in smokers with comorbid depression and anxiety: possible implications for smoking cessation treatment strategies. *Am J Drug Alcohol Abuse*. 2017;43(4):432–441.

42. Maciosek MV, LaFrance AB, Dehmer SP, et al. Health benefits and cost-effectiveness of brief clinician tobacco counseling for youth and adults. *Ann Fam Med*. 2017;15(1):37–47.

43. Smoking and Tobacco Use. https://www.cdc.gov/tobacco/data_statistics/fact_sheets/cessation/quitting/index.htm

44. Marrie RA, Horwitz RI. Emerging effects of comorbidities on multiple sclerosis. *Lancet Neurol*. 2010;9(8):820–828.

45. Khurana SR, Bamer AM, Turner AP, et al. The prevalence of overweight and obesity in veterans with multiple sclerosis. *Am J Phys Med Rehabil*. 2009;88(2):83–91.

46. Yeh E, Ramanathan M, Weinstock-Guttman B. Obesity as a risk factor in pediatric demyelinating disorders. *Neurology*. 2011;76(9):A131.

47. Berzins SA, Bulloch AG, Burton JM, et al. Determinants and incidence of depression in multiple sclerosis: a prospective cohort study. *J Psychosom Res*. 2017;99:169–176.

48. Artemiadis AK, Vervainioti AA, Alexopoulos EC, et al. Stress management and multiple sclerosis: a randomized controlled trial. *Arch Clin Neuropsychol*. 2012;27(4):406–416.

49. Complementary, Alternative, or Integrative Health: What's In a Name? https://nccih.nih.gov/sites/nccam.nih.gov/files/Whats_In_A_Name_06-16-2016.pdf

50. Berkman CS, Pignotti MG, Cavallo PF, et al. Use of alternative treatments by people with multiple sclerosis. *Neurorehabil Neural Repair*. 1999;13(4):243–254.

51. Bowling AC. Complementary and alternative medicine in multiple sclerosis. *Continuum (Minneap Minn)*. 2010;16(5 Multiple Sclerosis):78–89.

52. Marrie RA, Hadjimichael O, Vollmer T. Predictors of alternative medicine use by multiple sclerosis patients. *Mult Scler*. 2003;9(5):461–466.

53. Farez MF, Fiol MP, Gaitan MI, et al. Sodium intake is associated with increased disease activity in multiple sclerosis. *J Neurol Neurosurg Psychiatry*. 2015;86(1):26–31.

54. Ghadirian P, Jain M, Ducic S, et al. Nutritional factors in the aetiology of multiple sclerosis: a case-control study in Montreal, Canada. *Int J Epidemiol*. 1998;27(5):845–852.

55. Alter M, Yamoor M, Harshe M. Multiple sclerosis and nutrition. *Arch Neurol*. 1974;31(4):267–272.

56. Dworkin RH, Bates D, Millar JH, et al. Linoleic acid and multiple sclerosis: a reanalysis of three double-blind trials. *Neurology*. 1984;34(11):1441–1445.

57. Bates D, Cartlidge NE, French JM, et al. A double-blind controlled trial of long chain n-3 polyunsaturated fatty acids in the treatment of multiple sclerosis. *J Neurol Neurosurg Psychiatry*. 1989;52(1):18–22.

58. U.S. Department of Health and Human Services and U.S. Department of Agriculture. *2015–2020 Dietary Guidelines for Americans*. 8th ed.; 2015. Available at: http://health.gov/dietaryguidelines/2015/guidelines/.

59. Tavee J, Stone L. Healing the mind: meditation and multiple sclerosis. *Neurology*. 2010;75(13):1130–1131.

60. Grossman P, Kappos L, Gensicke H, et al. MS quality of life, depression, and fatigue improve after mindfulness training: a randomized trial. *Neurology*. 2010;75(13):1141–1149.

61. Tavee J, Rensel M, Planchon SM, et al. Effects of meditation on pain and quality of life in multiple sclerosis and peripheral neuropathy: a pilot study. *Int J MS Care*. 2011;13(4):163–168.

62. Wahbeh H, Elsas SM, Oken BS. Mind-body interventions: applications in neurology. *Neurology*. 2008;70(24):2321–2328.

63. Schwartz CE, Laitin E, Brotman S, et al. Utilization of unconventional treatments by persons with MS: is it alternative or complementary? *Neurology*. 1999;52(3):626–629.

64. Nayak S, Shiflett SC, Schoenberger NE, et al. Is acupuncture effective in treating chronic pain after spinal cord injury? *Arch Phys Med Rehabil*. 2001;82(11):1578–1586.

65. Preziosi G, Raptis DA, Storrie J, et al. Bowel biofeedback treatment in patients with multiple sclerosis and bowel symptoms. *Dis Colon Rectum*. 2011;54(9):1114–1121.

66. Jensen MP, Barber J, Romano JM, et al. A comparison of self-hypnosis versus progressive muscle relaxation in patients with multiple sclerosis and chronic pain. *Int J Clin Exp Hypn*. 2009;57(2):198–221.

67. Anderson JG, Taylor AG. Effects of healing touch in clinical practice: a systematic review of randomized clinical trials. *J Holist Nurs*. 2011;29(3):221–228.

68. Siev-Ner I, Gamus D, Lerner-Geva L, et al. Reflexology treatment relieves symptoms of multiple sclerosis: a randomized controlled study. *Mult Scler*. 2003;9(4):356–361.

69. Hughes CM, Smyth S, Lowe-Strong AS. Reflexology for the treatment of pain in people with multiple sclerosis: a double-blind randomised sham-controlled clinical trial. *Mult Scler*. 2009;15(11):1329–1338.

70. Vitale A. An integrative review of Reiki touch therapy research. *Holist Nurs Pract*. 2007;21(4):167–179; quiz 180-161.

71. Lee MS, Pittler MH, Ernst E. Effects of reiki in clinical practice: a systematic review of randomised clinical trials. *Int J Clin Pract*. 2008;62(6):947–954.

32

Complementary and Alternative Medicine: Practical Considerations

Allen C. Bowling

KEY POINTS FOR CLINICIANS

- Conventional healthcare providers may not discuss complementary and alternative medicine (CAM) therapies with their patients even though the majority of multiple sclerosis (MS) patients use some form of CAM and these CAM therapies exhibit a wide range of risk–benefit profiles.

- CAM therapies that are low risk and possibly therapeutic and thus might be worth consideration by some MS patients include acupuncture, cooling, cranberry, ginkgo biloba, mindfulness, low-dose naltrexone, tai chi, vitamin B_{12}, vitamin D, and yoga.

- CAM therapies that are less worthy of consideration because they are low risk but have unknown efficacy in MS include fish oil, the Swank diet, and gluten-restricted diets.

- CAM therapies that should be approached with caution or avoided owing to lack of efficacy, uncertain efficacy, or potential risks include antioxidants, bee venom therapy, Chinese herbal medicine, echinacea (and other "immune-stimulating" supplements), and cannabis.

- Clinicians who provide objective information about CAM therapies to their patients may provide a valuable role in informed decision making about CAM and may thereby facilitate the appropriate use of CAM. Likewise, clinicians who do not discuss CAM issues may silently endorse CAM and indirectly perpetuate the misuse of CAM in patients who are under their care.

The use of unconventional medicine, also known as CAM is popular among MS patients yet may not be openly discussed at clinic visits. In the general population, CAM is used by 30% to 50%, whereas among those with MS it is used by 50% to 75% (1–3). Conventional healthcare providers may not address CAM with their MS patients for a variety of reasons, including limited time and limited CAM knowledge or experience. The remarkable advances in disease-modifying therapies over the past several years have greatly improved treatment options, but the increased complexity of decision making and monitoring associated with some of these therapies may make it even more challenging for clinicians to interact with MS patients about CAM issues. This chapter is aimed at providing busy clinicians with an easy-to-use, concise guide to CAM therapies they are likely to encounter in practice. There are several key points that provide context for the wide range of CAM therapies. Specific CAM therapies that are discussed in this chapter are shown in Table 32.1. More detailed,

comprehensive, and critical reviews of MS-relevant CAM therapies may be found elsewhere (1–3).

TABLE 32.1 MS-Relevant CAM Therapies

Acupuncture, Chinese herbal medicine, and traditional Chinese medicine	Ginkgo biloba
	"Gluten sensitivity"
Antioxidants	Low-dose naltrexone
Bee venom therapy	
Cannabis	Mindfulness
Cooling therapy	
Cranberry	Tai chi
Echinacea and other "immune-stimulating" supplements	Vitamin B_{12}
Fish oil and the Swank diet	Vitamin D
	Yoga

CAM, complementary and alternative medicine; MS, multiple sclerosis.

DEFINITIONS AND CLASSIFICATION SCHEMES

In the CAM field, there are a variety of terms. The broadest term, *unconventional medicine*, is often defined as therapies that are not typically taught in medical schools or generally available in hospitals. The way in which these unconventional therapies are used is the basis for *complementary and alternative medicine (CAM)*: *complementary* indicates that the unconventional therapies are used in conjunction with conventional medicine, whereas *alternative* indicates that they are used instead of conventional medicine. The National Institutes of Health (NIH) has developed a classification scheme that divides CAM therapies into seven different categories (Table 32.2) (1,2).

CAM Therapies

ACUPUNCTURE, CHINESE HERBAL MEDICINE, AND TRADITIONAL CHINESE MEDICINE

Acupuncture is the most widely known and, among MS patients, perhaps most widely practiced component of the ancient, multimodal healing method known as traditional Chinese medicine (TCM). Other components of TCM include herbs, nutrition, tai chi, exercise, stress reduction, and massage (1,2). Studies of MS and acupuncture are extremely limited (4). Studies in other conditions indicate that acupuncture is effective for pain, nausea, and vomiting (1,2). There are no well-conducted studies of Chinese herbal medicine in MS. In terms of safety, acupuncture is generally well tolerated. In contrast, Chinese herbal medicine, which is often provided in conjunction with acupuncture, poses theoretical risks. Many of the commonly used herbs (including Asian ginseng, astragalus, and maitake and reishi mushrooms) may activate immune cells and could thereby worsen MS or antagonize the effects of MS disease-modifying medications (1,2).

If patients are using acupuncture, be sure to directly ask whether they are receiving Chinese herbal medicine along with acupuncture.

TABLE 32.2 National Institutes of Health Classification of CAM

Natural Products
Vitamin and mineral supplements, herbs
Manipulative and Body-Based Practices
Chiropractic manipulation, massage
Mind and Body Medicine
Meditation, yoga, guided imagery
Movement Therapies
Feldenkrais, pilates
Traditional Healing
Native American medicine
Energy Medicine
Healing touch, Reiki, magnet therapy
Whole Medical Systems
Naturopathy, traditional Chinese medicine, Ayurveda

CAM, complementary and alternative medicine.

Acupuncture is generally safe and may alleviate pain. In contrast, for disease-modifying effects or symptomatic relief in MS, Chinese herbal medicine is of unknown efficacy and carries theoretical risks.

ANTIOXIDANTS

Various antioxidant supplements are touted for MS. There is theoretical evidence that by inhibiting free radical-induced damage antioxidants could decrease myelin and axonal injury. In addition, studies in the animal model of MS indicate that antioxidants are therapeutic. However, several antioxidants "activate" immune cells and thus could worsen MS or antagonize the effects of disease-modifying medications. Clinical trials of antioxidants in MS are limited and inconclusive. Some of these trials have not been powered adequately (5,6).

Common antioxidants include coenzyme Q10, selenium, and vitamins A, C, and E.

There is a theoretical basis and animal model evidence to suggest that antioxidants could be therapeutic in MS, but antioxidants also carry theoretical risks in MS and there are not any MS clinical trials that provide definitive evidence of safety and efficacy.

BEE VENOM THERAPY

Bee venom therapy (BVT) involves the use of bee stings for possible medical benefits. There is a long history of BVT use in MS (2). However, studies of BVT in MS are limited. In the most rigorous clinical trial to date, BVT in 26 patients with relapsing–remitting and secondary-progressive MS did not produce therapeutic effects on multiple outcome measures, including relapse rate, disability, MRI activity, quality of life, and fatigue (7). Another study of nine progressive MS patients did not find any therapeutic effects—four of the nine patients were withdrawn due to neurological worsening during the study (8). BVT is generally safe, but anaphylactic reactions occur rarely. Also, periorbital bee stings, which are sometimes claimed to treat optic neuritis, may actually cause optic neuritis and should be avoided (1,2).

In MS, BVT has not been shown to produce any clear therapeutic effects and it may rarely cause serious side effects.

CANNABIS

Cannabis, also referred to as marijuana, contains tetrahydrocannabinol (THC) and other compounds known as cannabinoids (CBs). CBs have a wide range of biochemical effects that could, in theory, exert symptomatic and disease-modifying effects in MS. However, clinical trials of CBs in MS have produced variable results. Some, but not all, studies have shown improvement in pain and patient-reported spasticity ("subjective spasticity") (1–3,9). In the largest and most rigorous study in MS, CBs produced subjective, but not objective, evidence for relief of spasticity and pain (10). A CB oromucosal spray (Sativex) is licensed for use outside the United States.

Sativex has produced variable results in clinical trials evaluating multiple MS symptoms, including pain, spasticity, bladder dysfunction, and sleeping difficulties (11,12). Cannabis use has been associated with multiple adverse effects, including addiction, cognitive dysfunction, psychosis, anxiety, depression, suicide, stroke, cardiac ischemia, sedation, nausea, vomiting, impaired driving, seizures, incoordination, and poor pregnancy outcomes (2,13,14). In the United States, cannabis use is illegal at the federal level, but many states have legalized "medical marijuana" for those with MS and multiple other conditions (2,13,14).

> *In states in which "medical marijuana" is legal for use in MS, patients may mistakenly assume that as it is legal, cannabis has been proven to be safe and effective in MS.*

Clinical trials of cannabis use in MS have generally produced positive results for pain and subjective spasticity. Cannabis may produce significant side effects, and its use is illegal in many states and countries.

COOLING THERAPY

The aim of cooling therapy is to make therapeutic use of the long-recognized temperature sensitivity that occurs in MS. It is known that MS symptoms frequently worsen with body warming and may improve with cooling. Various cooling strategies have been developed (2). Simple methods include drinking cold beverages, avoiding exposure to warm environments, and staying in air-conditioned areas. More sophisticated approaches utilize specially designed cooling garments. MS clinical trials of variable quality have reported improvement in multiple symptoms with cooling (2,15,16). The most rigorous study, which was randomized, blinded, and controlled, found objective improvement in walking and visual function and subjective improvement in cognition, strength, and fatigue (16). Cooling is generally safe. The garments may be awkward to use. Cooling may provoke neurological worsening in the small fraction of MS patients who, paradoxically, are cold-sensitive (2).

> *Cooling is a simple strategy that may be underutilized in the MS community.*

Cooling is a simple, inexpensive approach that has little risk and multiple potential symptomatic benefits.

CRANBERRY

Cranberry is relevant to MS because MS-induced urinary retention increases the risk of urinary tract infections (UTIs) and the fruit of the cranberry plant may prevent UTIs. Some, but not all, clinical trials of cranberry indicate that it may prevent UTIs (2,13,17). Importantly, cranberry is not effective for treating UTIs. Although cranberry is generally well tolerated, chronic use may increase the risk of kidney stones and cranberry use has rarely been associated with bleeding and prolongation of the international normalized ratio (INR) in those on warfarin (13). Cranberry may be taken in the form of tablets, capsules, or juice.

> *Cranberry's likely mechanism of action—inhibition of bacterial adhesion to uroepithelium—is different from the mechanism of action of any conventional UTI medication.*

Cranberry is usually well tolerated and may prevent UTIs. It should not be used to treat UTIs.

ECHINACEA AND OTHER "IMMUNE-STIMULATING" SUPPLEMENTS

It is claimed erroneously in some lay publications that, as MS is an immune condition, MS patients should take "immune-stimulating" supplements such as echinacea. Lists of various supplements that are known to activate T cells and macrophages are then provided and recommended for MS patients. This information is incorrect, and the recommendations are potentially dangerous. These supplements could actually worsen MS or antagonize the effects of disease-modifying medications. Based on animal models or in vitro studies, multiple herbs, vitamins, and minerals are associated with T cell or macrophage activation (Table 32.3) (1,2,13).

There is no evidence that "immune-stimulating" supplements provide any therapeutic effects in MS. In fact, owing to theoretical risks, these supplements should actually be avoided or used with caution.

FISH OIL AND THE SWANK DIET

For decades, it has been hypothesized that polyunsaturated fatty acids (PUFAs), such as fish oil, may have disease-modifying effects in MS. Fatty acids exist in saturated and polyunsaturated forms. PUFAs include omega-3 and omega-6 fatty acids. Fish oil contains omega-3 fatty acids (2,18,19).

TABLE 32.3 Herbs, Vitamins, and Minerals With Possible "Immune-Stimulating" Effects

Alfalfa	Melatonin
Antioxidants	Maitake mushroom
Ashwagandha (*Withania somnifera*)	Mistletoe
Asian ginseng	Shiitake mushroom
Astragalus	Siberian ginseng
Cat's claw	Stinging nettle
Echinacea	Zinc
Garlic	

In the 1940s, a dietary approach known as the "Swank diet" was developed. This diet was low in saturated fat and high in PUFAs. It was claimed to have disease-modifying effects in MS, but the studies of this diet are inconclusive because they were not randomized, controlled, or blinded (18,19).

There have been several clinical trials of omega-3 fatty acid supplementation in MS. These studies have been inconclusive (18,19). One large, controlled, randomized, double-blind trial of fish oil supplements did not report statistically significant effects, but there was a trend that favored the treatment group ($p < .07$) (20). A more recent rigorous, MRI-based study of fish oil as monotherapy or as combination therapy with interferon beta-1a did not find an effect of fish oil on its primary outcome measure of MRI activity or on multiple secondary outcome measures, including relapse rate, disability progression, fatigue, and quality of life (21). Since this trial was relatively small ($n = 92$) and of short–moderate duration (6 months for monotherapy, 18 months for combination therapy), it may not have been long enough and may have lacked statistical power to be absolutely definitive. However, there were no clear "trends" that favored fish oil for the multiple outcome measures. Fish oil is usually well tolerated. The clinical trials of fish oil in MS have not indicated any significant safety issues or antagonism of interferon effects. The Food and Drug Administration (FDA) classifies fish oil as "generally regarded as safe" ("GRAS"). Fish oil may have mild anticoagulant effects. Also, PUFAs, especially in high doses, may produce vitamin E deficiency and thus supplementation with modest doses of vitamin E (100 international units [IU] daily) may be reasonable (2,17,21).

> *Fish oil (and other dietary approaches) should not be used instead of conventional disease-modifying medications.*

Fish oil is generally well tolerated. However, clinical trials of fish oil in MS have been inconclusive. Similarly, the clinical trial of the Swank diet has significant flaws and is inconclusive.

GINKGO BILOBA

Ginkgo biloba has been used for centuries as a herbal therapy. It contains chemical constituents with a wide range of potential pharmacological activities, including anti-inflammatory and antioxidant effects. Through these actions, ginkgo could, in theory, exert symptom-relieving and disease-modifying actions in MS. One large study of ginkgo found that it was *not* effective for treating MS attacks. Limited MS clinical trials for possible symptomatic effects found improvement in fatigue but not cognitive dysfunction (3,22,23). Ginkgo is usually well tolerated, but there are some potential drug interactions and side effects. It may rarely cause seizures and produce anticoagulant effects. Mild side effects include headaches, rashes, dizziness, nausea, vomiting, and diarrhea (1,13).

> *Ginkgo should probably be avoided in those with seizures and those who are undergoing surgery, have coagulopathies, or take antiplatelet or anticoagulant medications.*

Limited clinical trials suggest that ginkgo improves fatigue but is ineffective for cognitive dysfunction and MS attacks. Ginkgo has limited side effects.

"GLUTEN SENSITIVITY"

Over the past several years, there has been a dramatic increase in interest in "gluten sensitivity," which has been paralleled by an increase in the availability of gluten-free foods. "Celiac disease," also known as "celiac sprue" and "gluten-sensitive enteropathy," is a well characterized form of gluten sensitivity that affects about 1% of the general population. This condition may cause significant malabsorption and is diagnosed on the basis of symptoms, antibody testing, and small-bowel biopsy. It is treated with a gluten-free diet (2,24,25).

It has been proposed that there is a milder and much more common variant of celiac disease that is known by several terms, including "gluten sensitivity," "non-celiac gluten sensitivity," and "celiac lite." With this condition, it is claimed that gluten may cause intestinal symptoms (diarrhea, abdominal pain, bloating) as well as extraintestinal symptoms (headache, lethargy, ataxia). It is also claimed that chronic neurological symptoms may be provoked in MS patients who have "gluten sensitivity." At this time, "gluten sensitivity" is difficult to diagnose or study as there are not any established diagnostic criteria. This condition has not been studied specifically in the MS population. It is a fairly benign experiment to limit or eliminate gluten from the diet of MS patients who believe they may have this condition, but this may be laborious and expensive. Also, this "casual" self-treatment approach may delay diagnosis and lead to inappropriate or inadequate management and treatment in those who actually have celiac disease (2,24–27).

"Gluten sensitivity" is a poorly defined condition that has not been fully characterized in MS or in the general population. Diagnostic testing for celiac disease should be considered in those who have significant gastrointestinal symptoms that are provoked by gluten.

LOW-DOSE NALTREXONE

Treatment with low doses of oral naltrexone, an opiate antagonist used for opiate and alcohol addiction, has been claimed to be therapeutic for many medical conditions, including MS. It is claimed that in MS, low-dose naltrexone (LDN) relieves symptoms and also modifies the disease course by decreasing the attack rate and slowing disability progression.

Much of the lay writing about LDN is based on anecdotal reports (2). Three clinical trials of LDN in MS have produced mixed results. One study in primary progressive MS reported improved spasticity, worsened pain, and no effect on other outcome measures, including fatigue, depression, and quality of life (28). Two other studies used similar clinical trial designs to evaluate LDN in relapsing and progressive forms of MS. One of these studies found improvement in pain and mental health (29), while the other did not report any therapeutic effects (30). Based on available evidence, LDN appears to be generally well tolerated. In one of the clinical trials, one patient with progressive MS experienced neurological worsening. In patients who are treated with opiates, LDN could provoke withdrawal.

> *LDN should probably be avoided in patients who are treated with opiates.*

LDN appears to be generally well tolerated. Therapeutic effects have been inconsistent in the studies of LDN in MS.

MINDFULNESS

Mindfulness refers to the psychological quality of bringing one's complete attention to the present moment in a nonjudgmental way. Training people to use this approach has been studied especially for the relief of stress and anxiety in an approach known as "Mindfulness Based Stress Reduction." Mindfulness approaches have also been studied in many other medical and psychological conditions (2). In MS, several mindfulness clinical trials of variable quality have reported improvement in multiple symptoms, including anxiety, depression, fatigue, balance, pain, and overall quality of life (31). Mindfulness is usually well tolerated. This approach should be taught by those who are able to recognize serious psychological or psychiatric issues for which mindfulness is not appropriate. In some cases, meditation and other relaxation methods may cause spasms and produce anxiety ("relaxation-induced anxiety"), fear of losing control, and disturbing thoughts (2).

> *Although mindfulness has undergone extensive clinical study over the past 30 years, it may be unfamiliar to many conventional health providers.*

Mindfulness is a low-risk approach that may relieve anxiety and multiple other MS-associated symptoms.

TAI CHI

Tai chi is an ancient healing approach. Like acupuncture, tai chi is a component of the multimodal healing method of TCM. There are multiple clinical trials of tai chi in MS, but these are of variable quality. The most consistent benefits in these studies have been with balance and quality of life. Other reported therapeutic effects include flexibility, lower extremity strength, gait, and pain (32,33). Tai chi is generally well tolerated. It may cause strained muscles and joints. Modified forms of tai chi are available for those with disabilities (2).

Tai chi is a generally safe therapy that has been reported as a low-risk therapy that has produced improvement in multiple MS symptoms in limited clinical trial testing.

VITAMIN B$_{12}$

Lay publications sometimes claim that vitamin B$_{12}$ supplements produce therapeutic effects in MS. There is no strong clinical evidence to support such an approach. Several studies indicate that there is a small fraction of MS patients who have vitamin B$_{12}$ deficiency. MS patients who are vitamin B$_{12}$-deficient should be supplemented. Vitamin B$_{12}$ supplements are generally well tolerated. Rarely, these supplements may cause rashes, diarrhea, and itching (1,2,13).

> *Since vitamin B$_{12}$ deficiency may mimic MS and a subgroup of MS patients are vitamin B$_{12}$-deficient, MS patients should have a vitamin B$_{12}$ level determined at least once.*

Vitamin B$_{12}$ supplements are generally safe. Supplementation with vitamin B$_{12}$ is only indicated in those with vitamin B$_{12}$ deficiency.

VITAMIN D

Vitamin D has many potential effects on MS. It has been known for years that MS patients are at risk for developing osteopenia and osteoporosis, and vitamin D is important for maintaining bone density. In addition to these effects on bones, studies over the past decade have raised the possibility that, through immune-regulating effects, vitamin D might have disease-modifying (and preventive) actions in MS, and, possibly by improving leg function and gait stability, vitamin D could improve neurological function in MS (2,34).

Observational studies have shown that low blood levels and low intake of vitamin D are associated with a higher risk for developing MS. Low blood levels are also associated with a higher risk of converting from clinically isolated syndrome (CIS) to MS and with a higher risk for attacks, MRI activity, and disability progression in those with MS. Interventional studies of vitamin D in MS have been published but these are of variable quality and have reported mixed results to date. High-quality intervention studies are needed (35).

Vitamin D is usually well tolerated. The recommended daily amount (RDA) is 600 to 800 IU. The daily tolerable upper intake level (UL) is 4,000 IU daily. High doses may cause nausea, vomiting, fatigue, hypertension, and renal damage. Emerging evidence indicates that high doses (>4,000 IU daily) or high blood levels (>55 ng/mL) of vitamin D could *increase* the risk of fractures, falls, cardiovascular disease, all-cause mortality, and some cancers, including pancreatic (1,2,13,36,37).

In reasonable doses, vitamin D is generally safe. Limited studies indicate that vitamin D could have preventive, disease-modifying, and symptomatic effects in MS. Further studies are needed in this area. Vitamin D supplementation should be considered in MS patients with low vitamin D levels.

YOGA

Yoga is a component of Ayurveda, an ancient healing approach developed in India. Although yoga is widely used in some MS communities, it has undergone limited clinical trial investigation in MS. Multiple symptoms have been reported to be improved with yoga in MS trials. The most consistent symptomatic benefit has been with fatigue and mood (38,39). Yoga is generally well tolerated and may be modified for those with disabilities (2).

Yoga is a generally well-tolerated approach that may improve fatigue and multiple other symptoms in MS.

CONCLUSION

CAM use is common among MS patients, yet CAM may not be discussed with MS patients in some healthcare settings. Conventional healthcare providers may provide a valuable role in the care and education of their MS patients by providing guidance about CAM use. It may be especially helpful to provide general information about CAM and also specific, MS-relevant information about the risks and benefits of CAM therapies.

KEY POINTS FOR PATIENTS AND FAMILIES

- When trying to decide about using some form of CAM, discuss this with a healthcare provider. The risks and benefits of the CAM therapy should be obtained and reviewed before making a decision.

- If no objective information is available about a CAM therapy, it should be approached with caution.

- Vitamins, minerals, and herbs should be used with caution as they, like drugs, have the potential to worsen medical conditions or interact with other medications. There is limited information about the safety and effectiveness of dietary supplements in MS and when used in combination with MS medications.

- There are *no* CAM approaches that have been proven to be disease modifying and there are *many* conventional medications that have been proven to have this effect. CAM approaches should be used in conjunction with disease-modifying therapy rather than as an alternative.

- Information about CAM and MS is ever-changing. As a result, it is important to have ongoing discussions with a healthcare provider about CAM therapies that are being used or are being considered.

REFERENCES

1. Bowling AC. Complementary and alternative medicine and multiple sclerosis. *Neurol Clin.* 2011;29:465–480.
2. Bowling AC. *Optimal Health and Multiple Sclerosis: A Guide to Integrating Lifestyle, Alternative, and Conventional Medicine.* New York, NY: Springer Publishing; 2014.
3. Yadav V, Bever C, Bowen J, et al. Summary of evidence-based guideline: complementary and alternative medicine in multiple sclerosis: report of the guideline development subcommittee of the American Academy of Neurology. *Neurology.* 2014;82:1–10.
4. Karpatkin HI, Napolione D, Siminovich-Blok B. Acupuncture and multiple sclerosis: a review of the evidence. *Evid Based Compl Altern Med.* 2014;972935. doi:10.1155/2014/972935.
5. Plemel JR, Juzwik CA, Benson CA, et al. Over-the-counter antioxidant therapies for use in multiple sclerosis: a systematic review. *Mult Scler.* 2015;21:1485–1495.
6. Carvalho AN, Firuzi O, Gama MJ, et al. Oxidative stress and antioxidants in neurological diseases: is there still hope? *Curr Drug Targets.* 2017;18:705–718.
7. Wesselius T, Heersema DJ, Mostert JP, et al. A randomized crossover study of bee sting therapy for multiple sclerosis. *Neurology.* 2005;65:1764–1768.
8. Castro HJ, Mendez-Inocencio JI, Omidvar B, et al. A phase I study of the safety of honeybee venom extract as a possible treatment for patients with progressive forms of multiple sclerosis. *Allergy Asthma Proc.* 2005;26:470–476.
9. Koppel BS, Brust JCM, Fife T, et al. Systematic review: efficacy and safety of medical marijuana in selected disorders: report of the guideline development subcommittee of the American Academy of Neurology. *Neurology.* 2014;82:1556–1563.
10. Zajicek J, Fox P, Sanders H, et al. Cannabinoids for treatment of spasticity and other symptoms related to multiple sclerosis (CAMS study): multicentre randomised placebo-controlled trial. *Lancet.* 2003;362:1517–1526.
11. Zajicek J, Sanders HP, Wright DE, et al. Cannabinoids in multiple sclerosis (CAMS) study: safety and efficacy data for 12 months follow-up. *J Neurol Neurosurg Psychiatry.* 2005;76:1664–1669.
12. Barnes MP. Sativex: clinical efficacy and tolerability in the treatment of symptoms of multiple sclerosis and neuropathic pain. *Exp Opin Pharmacother.* 2006;7:607–615.

13. Jellin JM, Gregory PJ, Batz F, et al. *Pharmacist's Letter/Prescriber's Letter Natural Medicines Comprehensive Database*, 8th ed. Stockton, CA: Therapeutic Research Faculty; 2017.

14. National Academies of Sciences, Engineering, and Medicine. *The Health Effects of Cannabis and Cannabinoids: The Current State of Evidence and Recommendations for Research.* Washington, DC: The National Academies Press; 2017.

15. Meyer-Heim A, Rothmaier M, Weder M, et al. Advanced lightweight cooling-garment technology: functional improvements in thermosensitive patients with multiple sclerosis. *Mult Scler.* 2007;13:232–237.

16. NASA/MS Cooling Study Group. A randomized controlled study of the acute and chronic effects of cooling therapy for MS. *Neurology.* 2003;60:1955–1960.

17. Juthani-Mehta M, Van Ness PH, Bianco L, et al. Effect of cranberry capsules on bacteriuria plus pyuria among older women in nursing homes: a randomized controlled clinical trial. *J Amer Med Assoc.* 2016;316:1879–1887.

18. Stewart TM, Bowling AC. Polyunsaturated fatty acid supplementation in MS. *Int MS J.* 2005;12:88–93.

19. Mehta LR, Dworkin RH, Schwid SR. Polyunsaturated fatty acids and their potential therapeutic role in multiple sclerosis. *Nature Clin Pract Neurol.* 2009;5:82–92.

20. Bates D, Cartlidge N, French J, et al. A double-blind controlled trial of long chain n-3 polyunsaturated fatty acids in the treatment of multiple sclerosis. *J Neurol Neurosurg Psychiatry.* 1989;52:18–22.

21. Torkildsen O, Wergelend S, Bakke S, et al. Omega-3 fatty acid treatment in multiple sclerosis (OFAMS study). *Arch Neurol.* 2012;69(8):1044–1051. doi:10.101/archneurol.2012.283.

22. Lovera J, Bagert B, Smoot K, et al. Ginkgo biloba for the improvement of cognitive performance in multiple sclerosis: a randomized, placebo-controlled trial. *Mult Scler.* 2007;13:376–385.

23. Johnson SK, Diamond BJ, Rausch S, et al. The effect of Ginkgo biloba on functional measure in multiple sclerosis: a pilot randomized controlled trial. *Explore (NY).* 2006;2:19–24.

24. Troncone R, Jabri B. Coeliac disease and gluten sensitivity. *J Intern Med.* 2011;269:582–590.

25. Sapone A, Bai JC, Ciacci C, et al. Spectrum of gluten-related disorders: consensus on new nomenclature and classification. *BMC Med.* 2012;10:13.

26. DiSabatino A, Corazza GR. Nonceliac gluten sensitivity: sense or sensibility? *Ann Intern Med.* 2012;156:309–311.

27. Hadjivassiliou M, Sanders DS, Grünewald RA, et al. Gluten sensitivity: from gut to brain. *Lancet Neurol.* 2010;9:318–330.

28. Gironi M, Martinelli-Boneschi F, Sacerdote P, et al. A pilot trial of low-dose naltrexone in primary progressive multiple sclerosis. *Mult Scler.* 2008;14:1076–1083.

29. Cree BA, Kornyeyeva E, Goodin DS. Pilot trial of low-dose naltrexone and quality of life in multiple sclerosis. *Ann Neurol.* 2010;68:145–150.

30. Sharafaddinzadeh N, Moghtaderi A, Kashipazha D, et al. The effect of low-dose naltrexone on quality of life of patients with multiple sclerosis: a randomized placebo-controlled trial. *Mult Scler.* 2010;16:964–969.

31. Simpson R, Booth J, Lawrence M, et al. Mindfulness based interventions in multiple sclerosis—a systematic review. *BMC Neurol.* 2014;14:15.

32. Zou L, Wang H, Xiao Z, et al. Tai chi for health benefits in patients with multiple sclerosis: a systematic review. *PLOS ONE.* 2017;12(2):e0170212.doi:10.1371/journal.pone.0170212.

33. Mills M, Allen J. Mindfulness of movement as a coping strategy in multiple sclerosis. A pilot study. *Gen Hosp Psychiatry.* 2000;22:425–431.

34. Pierrot-Deseilligny C, Souberbielle JC. Vitamin D and multiple sclerosis: an update. *Mult Scler Relat Disord.* 2017;14:35–45.

35. Mowry E. Vitamin D insufficiency and supplementation in MS: findings from clinical studies. *Int J MS Care.* 2015;17(suppl 2):9–16.

36. Bowling AC. Integrating vitamin D into the overall therapeutic strategy for MS. *Int J MS Care.* 2015;17(suppl 2):17–21.

37. Ross AC, Taylor CL, Yaktine AL, et al., eds. *Dietary Reference Intakes for Calcium and Vitamin D.* Washington, DC: The National Academies Press; 2010.

38. Oken BS, Kishiyama S, Zajdel D, et al. Randomized controlled trial of yoga and exercise in multiple sclerosis. *Neurology.* 2004;62:2058–2064.

39. Cramer H, Lauche R, Azizi H, et al. Yoga for multiple sclerosis: a systematic review and meta-analysis. *PLOS ONE* 2014;9(11):e112414. doi:10.371/journal.pone.0112414.

33

Pediatric Multiple Sclerosis

Amy T. Waldman

KEY POINTS FOR CLINICIANS

- Pediatric and adult multiple sclerosis (MS) have similar clinical symptoms.

- The presence of encephalopathy and a polysymptomatic presentation with diffuse central nervous system (CNS) involvement is more suggestive of acute disseminated encephalomyelitis (ADEM).

- For children presenting with transient neurological symptoms, such as paresthesias, the diagnosis of MS may not be recognized by a pediatrician or other healthcare professional, especially if the symptoms self-resolve, the neurological examination is normal, or limited imaging is performed. Therefore, a high index of suspicion for pediatric MS is required.

- In children with clinical symptoms consistent with MS (vision changes, paresthesias, weakness, balance, and gait difficulties), the MRI criteria for dissemination in space and dissemination in time proposed by the 2017 revisions to the McDonald Criteria are applicable to children, especially those older than 11 years.

- Children with MS have more frequent relapses early in the disease course and a greater T2 lesion volume at disease onset than adults; however, they generally have a slower progression to disability.

- Primary progressive MS is exceedingly rare in children and should prompt consideration of alternative diagnoses such as metabolic, mitochondrial, or neurodegenerative disorders (including leukodystrophies).

- In pediatric MS, relapse management is similar to adult MS, typically beginning with methylprednisolone, 20 to 30 mg/kg/d (maximum of 1,000 mg) for 3 to 5 days.

- Adult dosing of disease-modifying therapy (interferon beta and glatiramer acetate) is generally prescribed, although interferons should be titrated up to the full dose to minimize potential side effects.

- Pediatric MS clinical trials are helping to understand the efficacy, safety, and tolerability of MS therapies in pediatric patients.

- While disability can be minimal in pediatric MS, cognitive evaluation is a key aspect of care.

Pediatric MS was first described in 1922. Thirty-six years later, one of the first retrospective studies on pediatric MS, which enrolled 40 children with MS between 1920 and 1952, concluded that children and adults with MS have similar clinical profiles including symptoms and physical and laboratory (cerebral spinal fluid [CSF]) findings. Shortly thereafter, pediatric MS was recognized by the first expert panel organized to establish a definition of clinically definite MS. In 1961, Dr. George Schumacher and colleagues permitted the inclusion of children (older than 10 years) in their clinical description of the disease (1).

Although pediatric MS has been recognized for almost a century, dedicated pediatric MS centers, facilitated by national collaborative programs, have been established mostly over the past decade. Pediatric MS research has also grown substantially. Although many similarities exist between pediatric- and adult-onset MS, there are notable differences, too. Such differences, which have raised questions about the impact of age, genetic susceptibility, and environmental exposures on the developing immune system, will hopefully lead to a greater understanding of the pathophysiology of the disease. This chapter highlights these unique issues relevant to the diagnosis and prognosis for MS in our youngest patients.

DEFINITIONS OF ACQUIRED DEMYELINATING SYNDROMES IN CHILDREN

Perhaps the greatest challenge in diagnosing MS in children is the growing recognition of the spectrum of demyelinating and neuroinflammatory conditions affecting the brain and spinal cord. In 2007, the International Pediatric MS Study Group proposed working definitions to allow for greater consistency in the diagnosis of ADEM, pediatric MS, and other acquired demyelinating syndromes in childhood (2). By creating a uniform language, the group hoped for more accurate diagnostic and prognostic data. These definitions were updated in 2013 (see Table 31.1), and additional phenotypes (see Table 33.2) have been further characterized since the 2013 revisions.

As in adults, pediatric MS is a chronic disease defined by neurological events separated in time and space affecting any age (including those younger than 10 years). The consensus definitions allow for the diagnosis of MS using MRI scans to confirm dissemination in time and space. The 2017 McDonald Criteria are applicable to children (see Diagnosis and MRI section in this chapter) (3). Ninety-five percent of children have relapsing–remitting MS (4); secondary progression rarely occurs during childhood or adolescence. Primary progressive MS is exceedingly rare in children; therefore, a progressive clinical course in a child should prompt consideration of genetic, metabolic, mitochondrial, neoplastic, and other disorders.

TABLE 33.1 International Pediatric MS Study Group Definitions

ACQUIRED DEMYELINATING SYNDROMES	PROPOSED CONSENSUS DEFINITIONS	COMMENTS
ADEM (monophasic)	• A first polyfocal clinical CNS event with presumed inflammatory cause • Encephalopathy that cannot be explained by fever is present • MRI typically shows diffuse, poorly demarcated, large, >1–2 cm lesions involving predominantly the cerebral white matter; T1 hypointense white matter lesions are rare; deep gray matter lesions (e.g., thalamus or basal ganglia) can be present • No new symptoms, signs, or MRI findings after 3 mo following the incident ADEM	• Encephalopathy is defined as an alternation in consciousness (e.g., stupor, lethargy) or behavioral change unexplained by fever, systemic illness, or postictal symptoms • A single clinical event of ADEM can evolve over a period of 3 mo, with fluctuations in clinical symptoms and severity • MRI findings alone are insufficient for the diagnosis of ADEM • Documentation of a prior infection and isolation of an infectious agent are not required for diagnosis
Multiphasic ADEM	• New event of ADEM 3 m or more after the initial event that can be associated with new or reemergence of prior clinical and MRI findings	• The new event must meet the clinical criteria for ADEM, including the presence of encephalopathy. Serial MRIs of patients with multiphasic ADEM, obtained following resolution of the second demyelinating event, should ultimately show a complete or partial resolution in the MRI lesions, in contrast to serial MRI findings in patients with MS that typically demonstrate ongoing accrual of asymptomatic lesions
Neuromyelitis optica (IPMSSG definitions published in 2013)	• Must have optic neuritis and acute myelitis as major criteria • Must have at least two of three supportive criteria: (a) contiguous spinal MRI lesion extending over three or more segments, (b) brain MRI not meeting diagnostic criteria for MS, or (c) anti-aquaporin-4 IgG seropositive status	• Brain lesions, located in the hypothalamus, brain stem, or diffuse cerebral white matter, have been described in children who have typical features of NMO • NMO should be considered in the differential diagnosis of children with ADEM due to overlapping clinical features (e.g., diffuse cerebral lesions and contiguous spinal cord MRI lesions) • These criteria were published before NMO Spectrum Disorder was further classified by the presence or absence of NMO-IgG antibodies (5)

(continued)

TABLE 33.1   International Pediatric MS Study Group Definitions (*continued*)

ACQUIRED DEMYELINATING SYNDROMES	PROPOSED CONSENSUS DEFINITIONS	COMMENTS
CIS	• A first monofocal or multifocal CNS demyelinating event; encephalopathy is absent, unless due to fever	• The term CIS is applied to the first clinical demyelinating event (i.e., isolated in time) that does not meet the criteria for another syndrome • Examples include isolated optic neuritis, transverse myelitis, and brainstem syndromes • The study group elected to define CIS as multifocal if the clinical features could be attributed to more than one CNS site and monofocal if the clinical symptoms could be attributed to a single CNS lesion. These distinctions are based solely on clinical findings. The term multifocal cannot be applied to a clinically monofocal presentation in which the MRI shows multiple asymptomatic lesions
Pediatric MS	Any of the following: • Two or more nonencephalopathic CNS clinical events separated by more than 30 d, involving more than one area of the CNS • One nonencephalopathic episode typical of MS which is associated with MRI findings consistent with 2010 Revised McDonald criteria for DIS and in which a follow-up MRI shows at least one new enhancing or nonenhancing lesion consistent with DIT MS criteria • One ADEM attack followed by a nonencephalopathic clinical event, 3 or more months after symptom onset, that is associated with new MRI lesions that fulfill 2010 Revised McDonal DIS criteria • A first, single, acute event that does not meet criteria for ADEM and whose MRI findings are consistent with the 2010 Revised McDonald criteria for DIS and DIT (applies only to children ≥12 y old)	• The DIS criteria have less predictive value in younger children, thus caution must be used in applying these criteria to confirm an MS diagnosis in children younger than 12 y

ADEM, acute disseminated encephalomyelitis; CIS, clinically isolated syndrome; CNS, central nervous system; CSF, cerebrospinal fluid; DIS, dissemination in space; DIT, dissemination in time; FLAIR, fluid attenuated inversion recovery; IgG, immunoglobulin G; NMO, neuromyelitis optica; NMOSD, neuromyelitis optica spectrum disorder; MS, multiple sclerosis.
Source: Krupp LB, Tardieu M, Amato MP, et al. International Pediatric Multiple Sclerosis Study Group criteria for pediatric multiple sclerosis and immune-mediated central nervous system demyelinating disorders: revisions to the 2007 definitions. *Mult Scler*. 2013;19:1261–1267.

INCIDENCE OF PEDIATRIC MS

Approximately 3% to 5% of adults with MS experience their first attack prior to 18 years of age (6). The incidence of pediatric MS in the United States is 0.5 per 100,000 children, or 379 new cases each year according to a study performed using a large health maintenance organization database in southern California (7). The same study estimated the incidence of all demyelinating diseases (including ADEM, optic neuritis, and transverse myelitis) to be 1.6 per 100,000, or 1,246 new cases per year (7). In comparison, a prospective national Canadian study reported an incidence of an initial demyelinating syndrome of 0.9 per 100,000 children (8). Another prospective national study determined the incidence of pediatric MS (<16 years) in Germany to be 0.3 per 100,000 children (9). The variation between studies may reflect different methodologies or may be due to

different environmental and genetic factors. For example, age, race, ethnicity, and residence may alter susceptibility for pediatric MS.

> *Three percent of MS patients experience their first symptom in childhood.*

DEMOGRAPHICS

The risk of pediatric MS increases with age. Multiple studies have shown an increased risk in pediatric MS after 10 to 11 years of age (9–11) (see section on Risk of MS after a first demyelinating event), whereas ADEM commonly occurs between 3 and 8 years of age (12–14).

TABLE 33.2 Additional Pediatric Disorders

ACQUIRED DEMYELINATING SYNDROMES	PROPOSED CONSENSUS DEFINITIONS	COMMENTS
ADEM followed by recurrent optic neuritis	All of the following are present: • Initial presentation fulfills criteria for ADEM • ON diagnosed after ADEM with objective evidence of loss of visual function • The ON occurs after a symptom-free interval of 4 wk and not as part of the ADEM or recurrent ADEM • Diagnostic criteria for pediatric MS are not fulfilled • Oligoclonal bands are not detected in the CSF (a pleocytosis may be present) • MRI reveals typical brain or spinal cord T2 lesions consistent with ADEM initially; however, subsequent imaging shows resolution or near-complete resolution of lesions and new brain or spinal cord lesions do not appear during the ON attacks	• Initial clinical features and imaging are typical of ADEM; however, with time, there is resolution of clinical symptoms, examination findings, and MRI abnormalities extrinsic to the optic nerves. Attacks of only recurrent optic neuritis occur

Chronic relapsing inflammatory optic neuropathy	• Optic neuritis and at least one relapse
	• Objective evidence for loss of visual function
	• Response to immunosuppressive treatment and relapse on withdrawal or dose reduction of immunosuppressive treatment
	  – NMO-IgG seronegative
	  – MRI confirms contrast enhancement of the acutely inflamed optic nerves
		• In this disorder, recurrent attacks isolated to the optic nerves occur without any other CNS involvement

ADEM, acute disseminated encephalomyelitis; CNS, central nervous system; CSF, cerebral spinal fluid; MS, multiple sclerosis; NMO-IgG, neuromyelitis optica immunoglobulin G; ON, optic neuritis.
Source: Krupp LB, Tardieu M, Amato MP, et al. International Pediatric Multiple Sclerosis Study Group criteria for pediatric multiple sclerosis and immune-mediated central nervous system demyelinating disorders: revisions to the 2007 definitions. *Mult Scler*. 2013;19:1261–1267; Huppke P, Rostasy K, Karenfort M, et al. Acute disseminated encephalomyelitis followed by recurrent or monophasic optic neuritis in pediatric patients. *Mult Scler*. 2013;19(7):941–946; Petzold A, Plant GT. Chronic relapsing inflammatory optic neuropathy: a systematic review of 122 cases reported. *J Neurol*. 2013;261(1):17–26. (15,16).

Although younger children are more likely to present with ADEM and older children have monofocal or multi-focal clinically isolated syndromes (Table 33.1), there are exceptions, and the proposed International Pediatric MS Study Group criteria, not age, should be used to diagnose acquired demyelinating syndromes in children.

> *The risk of pediatric MS increases after 11 years of age.*

Overall, the proportion of males and females presenting with demyelinating diseases is approximately equal; however, the female:male ratio is approximately 2:1 in pediatric MS whereas there is perhaps a male predominance in ADEM (12,13).

Many pediatric studies have demonstrated a lower proportion of white/Caucasian race among pediatric-onset MS compared to adult-onset disease (6,15–17). Although referral bias may influence the proportion of minorities at some centers, there is growing evidence to suggest that the risk of MS is increased in African American and Asian children as well as those with a Hispanic background. The influence of race and ethnicity on disease severity is addressed later in the chapter (see section on Relapses).

The difference in demographics between children and adults with MS may be due to differences in susceptibility among different races and ethnicities in children or may reflect more diverse populations living in areas of higher MS risk. In fact, a Canadian study demonstrated a higher proportion of patients with Caribbean, Asian, or Middle Eastern ancestry than the adult MS population from the same area, suggesting that risk of MS may be determined in part by disease risk in the place of residence during childhood, in addition to ancestry (17).

OTHER RISK FACTORS

Environmental risk factors for MS have been the subject of much research. As noted earlier, the place of residence during childhood influences the risk of MS. The prevalence of

MS increases proportionate to distance from the equator, perhaps owing to decreased sun exposure. Lower serum levels of vitamin D increase the risk of pediatric and adult MS (10,18) and have been linked to an increased relapse rate in pediatric MS (see subsequent section on Relapses) (19). Large-scale retrospective analyses have also shown an increased risk for MS in children of mothers with lower levels of exposure to ultraviolet (UV) radiation in the first trimester of pregnancy (20).

Other factors contributing to adult MS also have been investigated in children. The *HLA-DRB1*1501/1503* allele linked to increased susceptibility in adult MS has been shown to confer similarly increased risk upon pediatric patients of European ancestry presenting with acquired demyelinating syndromes (21). A remote Epstein–Barr virus (EBV) infection is also associated with an increased risk of MS. The presence of antibodies against EBV nuclear antigen along with the presence of the *HLA-DRB1*1501* allele markedly increases MS risk in adults (22). However, a genetic–environmental interaction has not been shown in children. Rather, the *HLA-DRB1*15* genotype, remote EBV infection, and vitamin D insufficiency (defined as <75 nmol/L which corresponds to 30 ng/mL) are independent risk factors for pediatric MS (10). Absence of these three risk factors is associated with a low risk of MS (5%) (10). In a national prospective study of children with acquired demyelinating syndromes, approximately 57% of the children with all the three factors have been diagnosed with MS (10). Higher body mass index is also a risk factor for pediatric MS (23).

Although the *HLA-DRB1* allele and Epstein–Barr nuclear antigen-1 seropositivity are independent risk factors, the *HLA-DRB1* allele may be implicated in the role of herpes simplex virus (HSV) in MS. One study showed that HSV played a protective role against MS in children with the *HLA-DRB1* allele, and that the risk of MS was increased in those with HSV who did not have the allele (23). The same study demonstrated a decreased risk of MS in children previously exposed to cytomegalovirus (CMV) (23).

A French study linked parental smoking at home to increased risk (adjusted relative risk [RR] = 2.12) of pediatric-onset MS as compared to controls. The investigators also found that the risk was higher still with longer duration of exposure in children older than 10 years (RR = 2.49) (24). Though several studies pointed to a possible relationship between Hepatitis B vaccination and subsequent development of pediatric MS, more stringent analyses have found vaccination to have no effect on risk (25).

> *The presence of the HLA-DRB1 allele, remote EBV infection, vitamin D deficiency, and parental smoking increase the risk of pediatric MS.*

CLINICAL FEATURES

Signs and Symptoms

The clinical symptoms in pediatric MS are very similar to adult-onset disease. CNS demyelination may result in visual disturbances, sensory manifestations, weakness or spasticity, balance difficulties, gait abnormalities, or bowel and bladder dysfunction localizing to the brain or spinal cord. Lhermitte's sign and Uhthoff's phenomenon also occur in children.

One of the most common presenting symptoms of MS in both children and adults is optic neuritis, characterized by decreased visual acuity, red color desaturation, and visual field deficits. Compared to adults, children are more likely to have bilateral involvement, especially children younger than 10 years. Children often present with significant vision loss (visual acuities of 20/200 or worse); however, the visual recovery is favorable as most achieve a visual acuity of 20/40 or better (26,27). Many of the children in these studies received intravenous corticosteroids, which may have helped improve outcome (see section on Relapses). Children with bilateral optic neuritis are not at higher risk for MS compared to those presenting with unilateral optic neuritis. Rather, risk of MS after optic neuritis increases with age at presentation, regardless of whether the child has unilateral or bilateral disease. The presence of asymptomatic MRI lesions outside the visual system markedly increases the risk of MS (11) (see Figure 33.1 and section on risk of MS after a first demyelinating event).

Optic neuritis is also a presenting symptom of neuromyelitis optica spectrum disorder (NMOSD) (see section on Differential Diagnosis). Bilateral or chiasm involvement at any age should prompt the clinician to consider further evaluation for NMOSD.

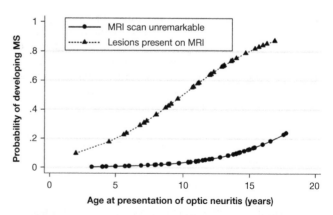

FIGURE 33.1 Probability of developing MS after optic neuritis according to age at presentation and MRI findings (defined as ≥1 lesion on T2-weighted imaging outside of the visual system) in children.

MS, multiple sclerosis.

Source: Waldman AT, Stull LB, Galetta SL, et al. Pediatric optic neuritis and risk of multiple sclerosis: meta-analysis of observational studies. *J AAPOS.* 2011;15:441–446.

Bilateral optic neuritis is more common than unilateral optic neuritis in children younger than 10 years.

Laboratory Studies

CEREBROSPINAL FLUID

A lumbar puncture is routinely recommended for all children presenting with demyelinating disease, although some physicians are less inclined to order a spinal tap for isolated optic neuritis (28). Only about 70% of physicians routinely obtain CSF studies in isolated optic neuritis (28).

Oligoclonal bands are present in about 60% of children with MS and are more common in children older than 11 years.

The presence of oligoclonal bands (OCB) in the CSF is not as high in children with MS as seen in adults: approximately 60% of children with MS have OCB (10) compared to 85% of adults with MS (29) (see Chapter 9). Once again, age is a key factor as younger children (younger than 11 years) are more likely to have an elevated CSF white blood cell (WBC) count with a higher number of polynuclear cells (neutrophils), although a lymphocytic predominance is present in all ages (30). In the same study, OCBs were present in 63% of older children (11 years of age or older) but in only 43% of younger children with MS. Similarly, an elevated immunoglobulin G (IgG) index was seen in 68% of older children versus 35% of younger children. In adults, the presence of OCB during a first demyelinating event increases the risk of having a second clinical attack within a year (31,32). Although children with a positive IgG profile and the absence of neutrophils in the CSF had shorter times to their second attack in one study, further confirmation is needed to determine whether the CSF profile is associated with the risk and timing of subsequent attacks (30).

OTHER LABORATORY INVESTIGATIONS

The evaluation of a child with any demyelinating disease should include a complete blood count, erythrocyte sedimentation rate, and antinuclear antibody (33). In addition, a basic metabolic panel, angiotensin-converting enzyme, C-reactive protein, thyroid stimulating hormone, B_{12} level, and folate are typically ordered by a majority of physicians to exclude mimics of CNS demyelination (28). A serum vitamin D_{25} (OH) level is commonly obtained, as vitamin D deficiency may increase susceptibility to MS and influence relapse rate. Further laboratory studies are often selected on the basis of the clinical phenotype, such as serum neuromyelitis optica (NMO) IgG antibody testing in a patient

presenting with optic nerve and spinal cord symptoms or a metabolic workup or lysosomal enzymes in a child with a history of developmental regression.

Myelin oligodendrocyte glycoprotein (MOG), located on the outer portion of the myelin sheath, has been explored in the past as a potential target or marker of demyelination. However, the detection of antibodies to MOG using enzyme-linked immunosorbent assay (ELISA) and Western blot was inconsistent (34). Recent advancement in cell-based assays has enabled more accurate detection of antibodies to MOG. In children with acute demyelinating syndromes, the presence of MOG antibodies is predictive of a non-MS phenotype (i.e., the child does not fulfill the International Pediatric MS Study Group definition for MS) in two separate longitudinal studies of several months duration (34,35). Antibodies to MOG are more frequently present in acute demyelinating syndromes involving (a) younger children, (b) those with an ADEM phenotype (with encephalopathy and polyfocal disease), (c) those with elevated CSF cell counts, and (d) children in whom OCBs are absent (35,36). The combination of MOG antibody and oligoclonal band results is further informative in determining the likelihood of an MS diagnosis. In a cohort of 65 children with a first acquired demyelinating syndrome, children who were positive for OCB and negative for antibodies to MOG ($N = 14$) were more likely to have MS (79% MS, 21% non-MS), whereas none of the 15 patients with positive MOG antibodies and absent OCB fulfilled criteria for MS (34). The spectrum of MOG-associated disease is broad, with clinical features of ADEM, ON, transverse myelitis, and NMO. Additional studies have shown that MOG antibodies are rare in patients who have antibodies to aquaporin-4 (37). The presence of MOG antibodies is not indicative of a monophasic disorder as relapses do occur and are more likely if high titers of MOG antibodies are present (35). Of note, the detection of MOG antibodies has recently become available as a clinical test in the United States. More data are needed to interpret the diagnostic, treatment, and prognostic implications of a positive (or negative) MOG test.

MRI

MRI of the brain and/or spinal cord is the standard of investigation for children with suspected demyelinating disease. As in adults, T2/fluid attenuated inversion recovery (FLAIR) hyperintensities are found in children with MS throughout the supra- and infratentorial brain and spinal cord. In order of decreasing frequency, brain lesions can be found in the deep white matter, juxtacortical white matter, periventricular white matter, corpus callosum, internal capsule, cortical gray matter, deep gray nuclei, brain stem, and cerebellum (34). Most lesions in children measure less than 1 cm axially (and 1.5 cm longitudinally). However, larger lesions are also common in pediatric MS, as 65% of a pediatric MS cohort had at least one lesion measuring more than 2 cm (34).

Brain lesion volumes were compared between children with clinically isolated syndromes (CISs) and adults with MS. At the time of a first demyelinating event, children have similar supratentorial lesion volumes but increased infratentorial lesion volumes compared to adults with established MS (35). Comparing the first MRI scan of the brain between children and adults, another study also demonstrated an increased number of T2 lesions (>3 mm^2), large T2 lesions (>1 cm), posterior fossa lesions, and gadolinium-enhancing lesions in children compared to adults (36). With follow-up imaging, the same study also showed that children had more new T2 hyperintensities and more gadolinium-enhancing lesions compared to adults (36).

The MRI scan in prepubertal children (younger than 11 years) presents additional challenges. While the number of T2 lesions on the initial MRI scan is similar between children under 11 years and 11 years or older, younger children have fewer discrete ovoid lesions and more large lesions (>1 cm) (37). Additional trends in the younger group included fewer enhancing lesions and more deep gray matter involvement. On follow-up imaging, a reduction in the number of T2 hyperintensities was observed in the prepubertal group with MS. ADEM is often diagnosed in these patients because of their age and MRI appearance (see the section on Differential Diagnosis) but patients with ADEM should first and foremost meet clinical criteria as defined by the International Pediatric MS Study Group (Table 33.1).

Diagnosis

As in adults, pediatric MS is diagnosed after two events, separated in time and space. The 2010 and 2017 revisions to the McDonald Criteria specifically addressed the application of these criteria to the pediatric population. The McDonald Criteria were designed and validated in adults presenting with a CIS. The MRI portion of the McDonald Criteria regarding dissemination in time and space are appropriate for children with CIS, especially those older than 11 years.

> *The 2010 McDonald Criteria can be used to demonstrate dissemination in time and space, especially in children older than 11 years.*

Differential Diagnosis

Clinicians must take care to exclude a number of other conditions that may present with CNS involvement, including other acquired demyelinating disorders (ADEM, NMOSD, transverse myelitis, and fulminant demyelinating diseases) as well as metabolic, infectious, vascular, genetic, neoplastic, mitochondrial, and systemic inflammatory disorders.

According to the International Pediatric MS Study Group definitions, a first demyelinating event in childhood meets the criteria for ADEM if encephalopathy is present and the child has a multifocal/polysymptomatic presentation. In the absence of one or both of these criteria, the child has a CIS, which can be monofocal or multifocal based on the clinical symptoms. For example, optic neuritis with asymptomatic brain lesions at the time of the initial presentation is considered a monofocal CIS.

One of the biggest diagnostic challenges is differentiating between ADEM and a first attack of MS. ADEM is clinically distinguished if encephalopathy and multifocal deficits are present (see Table 33.1); however, exceptions occur. Some neurologists have questioned the inclusion of encephalopathy for a diagnosis of ADEM. As stated by the International Pediatric MS Study Group, the inclusion of encephalopathy improves specificity for ADEM.

> *ADEM is characterized by encephalopathy and multifocal deficits.*

MRI has also been used to differentiate ADEM from MS. ADEM is typically associated with multiple large asymmetric lesions in the white matter and deep gray nuclei; the brain stem, cerebellum, and spinal cord may also be affected. The following criteria can be used with a sensitivity of 81% and specificity of 95% to distinguish a first attack of MS from ADEM. At the time of an initial demyelinating event, the diagnosis of MS is likely if two of the following are present: (a) two or more periventricular lesions, (b) the presence of black holes (enhancing or nonenhancing), or (c) the absence of a diffuse bilateral lesion pattern.

> *Using MRI to differentiate between ADEM and MS, the presence of two of the following favors a diagnosis of MS: (a) two or more periventricular lesions, (b) the presence of one or more T1 hypointensities, or (c) the absence of a diffuse bilateral lesion pattern.*

Traditionally, ADEM is considered a monophasic illness; however, relapses do occur in ADEM. A relapse within 3 months of the initial event or one that occurs within 1 month of the withdrawal of steroids is not considered a new attack but rather part of the original event. However, relapses occurring more than 3 months after the initial event and more than 1 month after steroids may be diagnosed as multiphasic ADEM, whether the same CNS site or new CNS sites are affected (see Table 33.1).

Encephalopathy must also be present for a diagnosis of multiphasic ADEM.

The revised definitions by the International Pediatric MS Study Group acknowledged that a child who has a relapse after ADEM could be confirmed to have pediatric-onset MS if the following criteria are met: (a) the relapse does not include encephalopathy, (b) the relapse occurs more than 3 months after the first attack meeting the criteria for ADEM, and (c) new MRI findings occur that meet 2010 McDonald criteria for dissemination in space (2).

A rare entity has been described called "ADEM followed by recurrent or monophasic optic neuritis in pediatric patients" (15). As the name implies, children meet criteria for ADEM initially, but ultimately relapses are limited to the optic nerves. This entity is different from MS by the lack of subsequent CNS involvement extrinsic to the optic nerves. The diagnostic criteria are included in Table 33.2.

In 2013, the International Pediatric MS Study Group also proposed the following definition for NMO: the presence of both optic neuritis and myelitis as well as either a longitudinally extensive lesion (measuring three vertebral segments or more) on an MRI of the spinal cord or NMO-IgG antibody positivity (2). An MRI of the brain may also reveal lesions, especially in the deep gray matter or brain stem. Large, diffuse subcortical white matter lesions can also occur (37). Subsequently, criteria for NMOSD were proposed, notably with stratification by NMO-IgG antibody positivity (5). These criteria, described in Chapter 38, are often used in children, although more information is needed on the prevalence of NMO-IgG positivity. Some patients with symptoms similar to NMOSD but with negative NMO-IgG testing have been found to have anti-MOG antibodies (34,37).

Aside from demyelinating diseases, there are a number of other disorders that mimic CNS demyelination. The differential diagnosis is similar to adults (as discussed in Chapter 10). Especially relevant to the pediatric population, metabolic diseases, or leukodystrophies should be considered in some children. Children with these diseases often have a progressive decline without clear relapses. Such a clinical presentation is unlikely to be primary progressive MS, which is extremely rare in children. Other organ involvement (eye, skin, liver, heart, etc.) should prompt consideration for genetic leukoencephalopathies. Also, bilateral deep gray matter involvement is common in ADEM or even NMOSD but can also be present in other conditions, such as metabolic disorders, toxic encephalopathies, or hypoxic–ischemic injury.

Risk of MS After a First Demyelinating Event

MRI is a useful tool in predicting the risk of MS after a CIS. In children with a normal MRI of the brain at the time of their initial event, the risk of developing MS is approximately 2% (Figure 33.2) (10). Accordingly, while a normal brain MRI is prognostically favorable, it does not exclude the possibility of a relapse (recurrent optic neuritis without brain lesions or recurrent transverse myelitis) (10). For those children with T2/FLAIR hyperintensities in the brain at the time of their first attack, the risk of MS is increased if nonenhancing T1 hypointense lesions and/or one or more periventricular lesion(s) are present. This risk is further increased with persistent T1 lesions on serial images (38).

> *At the time of a first demyelinating event, the presence of one or more T1 hypointense lesion(s) and/or one or more periventricular lesion(s) is associated with an increased risk of MS.*

As noted previously, the risk of MS increases with age. In children (younger than 18 years) with optic neuritis, the risk of MS increases by 32% for every 1 year increase in age over 2 years, after adjusting for the presence or absence of asymptomatic brain lesions on MRI (see Figure 33.1) (11). Another study also examined the relation between age and MRI lesions and their influence on MS risk after a first demyelinating event (including ADEM, transverse myelitis, etc.). After stratifying by the presence of T2 lesions on MRI, the risk is further defined by the age, which doubles in children over 11.85 years (10) (see Figure 33.2).

Relapses

Similar to adults, a relapse is typically defined by the presence of symptoms localizing to the CNS that persist for at least 24 hours and are not related to a fever or illness (39). The onset of symptoms should be separated from the onset of a previous attack by at least 30 days. The clinical presentation of MS attacks in children resembles that seen in adults, though attacks are often more severe (defined as a visual acuity of 20/200 or worse or an Expanded Disability Status Scale [EDSS] score of 3.0 or higher). Investigators at one center categorized roughly one-half of pediatric attacks as severe, with only 10% to 17% of adult exacerbations filling the same criteria. They also found more attacks in pediatric patients involve the brain stem/cerebellum and cerebral hemispheres (39).

> *A higher relapse rate is seen in children compared to adults. Low serum 25OH vitamin D levels and nonwhite race are also associated with a higher relapse rate.*

Three specific factors have been associated with a greater relapse rate: younger age at onset, lower serum vitamin D levels, and nonwhite race. Compared to adults, children have a significantly higher annualized relapse rate, which was demonstrated repeatedly with multiple statistical models and methodologies (40). A retrospective study

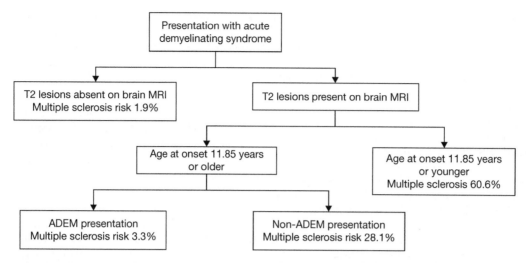

FIGURE 33.2 MS risk stratification algorithm for children presenting with an acute demyelinating syndrome. This classification scheme predicts the diagnosis in children presenting with an acute demyelinating syndrome with 83.7% accuracy.

MS, multiple sclerosis.

Source: Banwell B, Bar-Or A, Arnold DL, et al. Clinical, environmental, and genetic determinants of multiple sclerosis in children with acute demyelination: a prospective national cohort study. *Lancet Neurol.* 2011;10:436–445.

observed a correlation between serum 25-hydroxyvitamin D3 level, adjusted for time of year, and relapse rate (19). The same study also demonstrated an increased relapse rate in Hispanic children (19), a finding that concurs with another study's conclusion that Hispanic children are more likely to experience breakthrough disease with first-line disease-modifying therapy (DMT) (15). African American patients also had more relapses than white patients in a Detroit cohort (16). Pediatric patients seem to recover more completely from exacerbations. One study found that 66% of children with severe initial demyelinating events recovered fully, as opposed to 46% of adults from the same center. Incomplete recovery from one event predicted the same in later relapses (39). Moreover, the rate of disability progression in children increases with each relapse in the first 2 years (41).

> *Pediatric MS attacks are generally treated with intravenous methylprednisolone at 20 to 30 mg/kg/d for 3 to 5 days, and 50% of physicians prescribe an oral prednisone taper.*

Pediatric MS attacks are managed similarly to adults. Intravenous corticosteroids are used as a first-line therapy, although an expert panel agreed that not every flare requires treatment (28). Rather, the clinical presentation with respect to the severity of the attack influences the decision to treat. Although adults are often treated with 1 g/d of intravenous methylprednisolone, children generally receive 20 to 30 mg/kg of body weight per day (maximum of 1 g/d) for 3 to 5 days, with 50% of the panel routinely using a subsequent oral steroid taper (28). For patients who do not improve with methylprednisolone, intravenous immunoglobulin and plasmapheresis have also been used to treat acute attacks in children; however, the expert panel did not reach a consensus with respect to the definition of treatment failure or protocol for initiation of a second-line acute relapse treatment.

MANAGEMENT

The management of pediatric MS is a complex undertaking, driven by the child's clinical course and often requiring the participation of a multidisciplinary team including neurologists, neuro-ophthalmologists, neuropsychologists, urologists, physiatrists, physical and occupational therapists, school nurses, and teachers. Education of patient, family (both parents and siblings), caregivers, and school as to the nature of the disease and its management should be thorough and ongoing to ensure that each child receives the best care possible. Frequent evaluations, such as clinical examinations every 3 months, and regular MRI scans (every 3–6 months) for the first year may be necessary to assess for disease progression, assess for medication compliance/adherence and side effects, and counsel the family.

Generally, treatment of pediatric MS closely resembles that of adult MS—clinicians commonly recommend long-term use of DMT and management of more severe attacks with corticosteroids (see earlier section on Relapses). Although they are not Food and Drug Administration (FDA)-approved for children younger than 18 years, interferon beta-1a and beta-1b and glatiramer acetate have similar safety and efficacy as in adults and should be initiated in children with established MS and those identified as high risk (i.e., CIS with asymptomatic brain lesions). Interferons should be initiated at lower doses and titrated up to adult dosing to decrease side effects (such as flu-like symptoms) (42). Otherwise, the dosing is not weight based or reduced owing to age alone. Neutralizing antibodies to interferons are infrequently seen in children (43). A dual-placebo-controlled 215-patient trial of oral fingolimod compared with intramuscular interferon-beta-1 found that fingolimod reduced annualized relapse rate by 82% over interferon, with similar benefits on MRI measures of MS disease activity (44). Safety and tolerability were quite good. Fingolimod is now FDA-approved for relapsing-remitting MS in children (ages 10 years and older). Data on long-term safety has not been established.

> *Although they are not Food and Drug Administration (FDA)-approved for children, interferon beta and glatiramer acetate should be initiated in children with MS and clinically isolated syndrome (CIS; at high risk for MS).*

The International Pediatric MS Study Group has defined inadequate treatment response in pediatric MS (which applies only to those patients who have been treated with full-dose therapy for a minimum of 6 months and have been fully compliant during this time) as (a) an increase or no reduction in relapse rate, or new T2 or contrast enhancing lesions on MRI from pretreatment period, or (b) ≥ two confirmed relapses (clinical or MRI relapses) within a 12-month period or less (45). Multiple treatments have been proposed, such as switching DMT or adding corticosteroids, intravenous immunoglobulin, or plasma exchange at regular intervals (45). Natalizumab has been used in selected children with MS who have failed first-line therapy (45,46). Although children are generally thought to have lower exposure rates to John Cunningham (JC) virus (47,48), the risk of progressive multifocal leukoencephalopathy (PML) in the pediatric population has not been defined and remains a concern. Rituximab is not approved by the FDA for the treatment of MS; however, it is often used in pediatric MS and other neuroinflammatory diseases (49,50) due to its efficacy in reducing new clinical attacks and MRI lesions in adults (51). Dosing regimens and schedules vary. Although the risk of PML is believed to be less for rituximab compared to natalizumab, there have been cases of PML with rituximab use in other disease populations, although usually in combination with other immune-modulating therapies. Of note, there is a risk of hypogammaglobulinemia with rituximab. Oral therapies, such as immunosuppressive agents, such as cyclophosphamide, azathioprine, and mycophenolate, have also been used in children failing first-line therapy. The use of mitoxantrone in children is discouraged by the International Pediatric MS Study Group due to its risk profile (cardiotoxicity and risk of leukemia [45]).

As in adult MS, other therapies may be required for disabling symptoms. Physical, occupational, and speech therapy may be offered, as needed. Spasticity may require baclofen or dantrolene. Benzodiazepines and botulinum toxin may also be used but do not have FDA indications for spasticity in children. The commonly used medications for fatigue in adults (amantadine and modafinil) do not have FDA indications for MS fatigue in children but are frequently used in pediatrics. Oxybutynin and hyoscyamine have pediatric indications for neurogenic bladder; hyoscyamine can also be used for neurogenic bowel. Tolterodine does not have FDA approval for pediatric dosing but is used in children. Gabapentin and pregabalin have been tried for neuropathic pain (although they are also off-label for pediatrics). Antidepressants may be required for some children; however, given the FDA boxed-warnings on the use of antidepressants in children, these medications are often best initiated and titrated by a psychiatrist. Although many of the symptomatic medications are not specifically approved by the FDA for MS-related symptoms (particularly in children), many have been studied in children with other etiologies (such as cerebral palsy, traumatic brain injury, etc.), and dosing is often extrapolated from such studies or adult data.

PROGNOSIS

A major goal of MS therapy is to slow the progression of physical and cognitive disability. Generally, pediatric-onset MS patients maintain lower EDSS scores for a longer period of time after disease onset as compared to adult-onset patients. In a longitudinal study, the interval between onset and conversion to secondary progressive MS and irreversible disability was about 10 years longer in pediatric-onset patients. However, conversion occurred when childhood-onset patients were approximately 10 years younger than their adult counterparts (41).

Cognitive decline may occur both more frequently and at an accelerated rate in pediatric patients, perhaps owing to the effects of demyelination on brains that have not yet reached the final stages of maturation. In a group of 63 Italian children, a neuropsychological test battery classified 31% as cognitively impaired, with 15 found to have an IQ score of under 90; follow-up 2 years later placed 70% of the same cohort in the cognitive impairment group (48,49). Pediatric MS patients scored lowest on tests at both sessions involving verbal comprehension, complex attention, and memory. The authors found that a younger age at onset correlated with cognitive impairment at the first assessment, whereas older age and higher educational level at initial testing correlated with cognitive impairment at the time of follow-up. Other studies with smaller cohorts have similarly found cognitive impairment in approximately one third of children with MS. Commonly affected functions include attention and processing speed as well as verbal abilities. Younger age of onset and/or longer disease length predicted impairment in several independent studies (50,51), indicating a need for close surveillance and/or early interventions in these cases.

> MS progresses more slowly in children; however, children reach irreversible disability at younger ages compared to adults.

CONCLUSION

In general, pediatric and adult MS share similar clinical symptoms, CSF profiles, and lesion characteristics on MRI scans. Similar diagnostic criteria are used in pediatric and adult MS. The mechanisms influencing the age of onset are poorly understood. Genetic and environmental risk factors are currently being studied in both groups, and exposure to viruses in the pediatric years may influence the biological onset of disease. Although similarities exist between pediatric- and adult-onset MS, there are a number of differences between the groups. Children have higher relapse rates and greater T2 lesion volumes yet slower progression of disability. Hypotheses for this paradox have included greater edema with less myelin damage or better remyelination and repair (36,39). The unique characteristics that may influence the disease progression in children is the subject of considerable pediatric MS research. Moreover, pediatric clinical trials of DMTs are elucidating effective MS therapies for our youngest patients.

PATIENT CASE   A 5-year-old presents to the ED with a 1-day history of horizontal diplopia. He would squint to focus or close one eye. He was noted to veer to the side while walking down the hallway causing him to walk into walls. There was no recent fever, illness, or vaccination. He was not fatigued, altered, or confused.

Question: What evaluation is needed?

Answer: The child should be evaluated by a neurologist and a neuro-ophthalmologist. The differential diagnosis for a sudden, acquired focal neurologic deficit is broad and includes neuroinflammatory, vascular, and oncologic diseases. The examination was notable for a right sixth nerve palsy, right-sided dysmetria, and ataxia.

An MRI of the brain, C-, and T-spine, without and with gadolinium, should be obtained. In children, when neuroinflammatory disease is being considered, the sedation needs of the child often factor into the initial decision to image only the brain or the brain, C-, and T-spine. Laboratory studies should include an antinuclear antibody profile and angiotensin-converting enzyme for rheumatologic mimics of neuroinflammation. Epstein–Barr virus (EBV) serology, and vitamin D 25(OH) are also typically obtained as risk factors for MS. A lumbar puncture should be performed and assessed for white and red blood cell counts, protein, glucose, culture, and oligoclonal bands (OCBs).

The MRI revealed a large irregular lesion seen as an increased T2 signal involving the right side of the pons and right brachium pontis. The signal abnormality extended to the surface of the brain stem at the origin of the right sixth cranial nerve, but also affected the pons in the area of the nucleus for the sixth cranial nerve. On postcontrast imaging, there was contrast enhancement of this lesion. There were also foci of T2 prolongation noted within the white matter of the genu of the corpus callosum left of midline, right frontal lobe white matter, splenium of the corpus callosum on the left, left frontal lobe periventricular white matter, right posterior temporal white matter, and left parietal white matter. There was enhancement of the two left medial parietal and deep left frontal lesions adjacent to the frontal horn and slightly more superior.

The spinal tap revealed four white blood cells and zero red blood cells. The cerebral spinal fluid (CSF) glucose was 50 with a protein of 15. OCBs were present with seven bands in the CSF that were not present in the serum. The remainder of the laboratory tests were notable for evidence of a prior EBV infection and low-normal vitamin D 25-OH (32 ng/mL).

Question: What is the diagnosis?

Answer: The diagnosis is monofocal clinically isolated syndrome as the child presented with symptoms localizing to an infratentorial lesion. The classification of monofocal versus multifocal is based on the clinical symptoms, not the MRI lesion distribution. The presence of additional lesions extrinsic to the

(continued)

(continued)

symptomatic lesion raises concern that this is a first attack of multiple sclerosis (MS). The sensitivity and specificity of the McDonald criteria to confirm MS at the incident attack are decreased in younger children; thus, caution is recommended in applying these criteria to confirm dissemination in time and space at a first attack in children younger than 12 years.

Question: What do you do now?

Answer: It is reasonable to treat the patient at this point with a course of high-dose corticosteroids (i.e. intra-venous methylprednisolone 20-30 mg/kg/d, maximum of 1 g/day, for 3-5 days). Some physicians will follow intravenous methylprednisolone by a prednisone taper, typically lasting 2 weeks. Information about the side effects of corticosteroids and expectation of treatment response should be reviewed with the family.

He steadily improved with the administration of steroids.

Question: What do you do now?

Answer: Repeat imaging should be obtained 3 months after the initial attack. The presence of at least one new enhancing or nonenhancing lesion in the patient would confirm the diagnosis of MS. A second attack in a distinct region of the brain would also confirm the diagnosis of MS. For this patient, a follow-up scan revealed new T2 hyperintense lesions in the periventricular white matter and the diagnosis of MS was confirmed.

Question: What do you do now?

Answer: The family was offered treatment with interferon-beta or glatiramer acetate. Physicians should be aware that not all manufacturers of these drugs offer injection training in pediatric patients.

PATIENT CASE   A 14-year-old female presents to the ED after waking up in the morning with blurry vision in the left eye. She complained of pain behind her left eye. Her examination was notable for a left relative afferent pupillary defect, visual acuity of 20/200 in the left eye, blurred disc margin in the left eye, and decreased color vision on the left using Ishihara color plates.

Question: What evaluation is needed?

Answer: The child should be assessed by a neurologist and neuro-ophthalmologist to determine the extent of the central nervous system (CNS) involvement. An MRI of the brain without and with gadolinium is the standard of care to evaluate for asymptomatic lesions outside the visual system. As noted in the previous case, laboratory studies (including antibodies to neuromyelitis optica [NMO]-immunoglobulin G [IgG]) and a lumbar puncture may be obtained. An MRI of the C- and T-spine may be necessary, especially if the neurological examination is abnormal to assess for clinically silent lesions.

Formal neuro-ophthalmological examination confirmed the earlier findings. No clinical abnormalities were appreciated in the right eye. The remainder of the neurological examination was normal. MRI of the brain revealed a T2/fluid attenuated inversion recovery (FLAIR) hyperintensity in the left optic nerve. Three additional T2/FLAIR hyperintensities were seen in the periventricular region, and one discrete lesion was present in the juxtacortical white matter. None of the lesions enhanced after the administration of gadolinium. She was seronegative for NMO-IgG.

Question: What is the diagnosis?

Answer: The diagnosis is unilateral optic neuritis, or, in this case, a monofocal clinically isolated syndrome (CIS). While the presence of lesions in the periventricular and juxtacortical white matter does meet McDonald Criteria for dissemination in space, she has not demonstrated dissemination in time (which requires the presence of enhancing and nonenhancing lesions simultaneously to diagnosis dissemination in time on a single MRI scan).

(continued)

(continued)

Question: What do you do now?

Answer: It is reasonable to treat her at this point with a course of high-dose corticosteroids due to her severe visual impairment (i.e. intravenous methylprednisolone 20-30 mg/kg/d, maximum 1g/d, for 3-5 days, followed by a prednisone taper if desired). It should be noted, however, that the use of corticosteroids for optic neuritis is a topic of ongoing research to determine whether it affects the visual or neurologic outcomes. Information about the side effects of corticosteroids and expected treatment response should be addressed. She will also require regular neurological examinations and repeat MRI scans to assess for disease progression.

Question: What is her risk for MS?

Answer: She is considered at high risk for MS given her age and the presence of asymptomatic T2/FLAIR hyperintensities in the brain. She should be offered disease-modifying therapy (DMT; interferon beta or glatiramer acetate) even though she does not meet diagnostic criteria for MS.

Question: How should DMT be initiated?

Answer: The physician should present the family with all of the current first-line therapies (interferon beta-1a and 1b and glatiramer acetate) with a review of the differences in route, frequency, and side effects for each medication. In general, the dosing is similar for children and adults, although the interferons should all be titrated upward to decrease side effects. Not all children and families accept initiation of DMT at the first attack and the advantages and disadvantages should be thoroughly reviewed.

Question: What is the long-term prognosis for pediatric MS?

Answer: While many children have more frequent relapses early in the disease course, some children have slower disease progression. Children should be encouraged to fully participate in their usual activities. Frequent neurological examinations and serial imaging are important to monitor disease progression.

KEY POINTS FOR PATIENTS AND FAMILIES

- MS affects children as well as adults; however, the course of the illness and symptoms are different in each person, regardless of age.
- Children with MS should see a neurologist regularly and repeat MRI scans even when they feel well.
- Goals of treatment include controlling acute inflammation, reducing the frequency of relapses and accrual of new MRI lesions, slowing physical and cognitive decline, and maximizing quality of life for the affected child.
- Children should be encouraged to participate in activities they enjoy, and regular exercise is encouraged.
- Children may require an individualized education plan through their school if they have difficulties with coursework or miss school because of medical appointments or hospitalizations.

REFERENCES

1. Poser CM, Brinar VV. Diagnostic criteria for multiple sclerosis: an historical review. *Clin Neurol Neurosurg.* 2004;106:147–158.
2. Krupp LB, Tardieu M, Amato MP, et al. International Pediatric Multiple Sclerosis Study Group criteria for pediatric multiple sclerosis and immune-mediated central nervous system demyelinating disorders: revisions to the 2007 defintions. *Mult Scler.* 2013;19:1261–1267.
3. Thompson AJ, Banwell BL, Barkhof F, et al. Diagnosis of multiple sclerosis: 2017 revisions of the McDonald criteria. *Lancet Neurol.* 2018;17:162–173.
4. Polman CH, Reingold SC, Banwell B, et al. Diagnostic criteria for multiple sclerosis: 2010 revisions to the McDonald criteria. *Ann Neurol.* 2011;69:292–302.
5. Wingerchuk DM, Banwell B, Bennett JL, et al. International consensus diagnostic criteria for neuromyelitis optica spectrum disorders. *Neurology.* 2015;85:177–189.

6. Chitnis T, Glanz B, Jaffin S, et al. Demographics of pediatric-onset multiple sclerosis in an MS center population from the northeastern United States. *Mult Scler.* 2009;15:627–631.

7. Langer-Gould A, Zhang JL, Chung J, et al. Incidence of acquired CNS demyelinating syndromes in a multiethnic cohort of children. *Neurology.* 2011;77:1143–1148.

8. Banwell B, Kennedy J, Sadovnick D, et al. Incidence of acquired demyelination of the CNS in Canadian children. *Neurology.* 2009;72:232–239.

9. Pohl D, Hennemuth I, von Kries R, et al. Paediatric multiple sclerosis and acute disseminated encephalomyelitis in Germany: results of a nationwide survey. *Eur J Pediatr.* 2007;166:405–412.

10. Banwell B, Bar-Or A, Arnold DL, et al. Clinical, environmental, and genetic determinants of multiple sclerosis in children with acute demyelination: a prospective national cohort study. *Lancet Neurol.* 2011;10:436–445.

11. Waldman AT, Stull LB, Galetta SL, et al. Pediatric optic neuritis and risk of multiple sclerosis: meta-analysis of observational studies. *J AAPOS.* 2011;15:441–446.

12. Tenembaum S, Chamoles N, Fejerman N. Acute disseminated encephalomyelitis: a long-term follow-up study of 84 pediatric patients. *Neurology.* 2002;59:1224–1231.

13. Tenembaum S, Chitnis T, Ness J, et al. Acute disseminated encephalomyelitis. *Neurology.* 2007;68:S23–S36.

14. Dale RC, de Sousa C, Chong WK, et al. Acute disseminated encephalomyelitis, multiphasic disseminated encephalomyelitis and multiple sclerosis in children. *Brain.* 2000;123(pt 12):2407–2422.

15. Huppke P, Rostasy K, Karenfort M, et al. Acute disseminated encephalomyelitis followed by recurrent or monophasic optic neuritis in pediatric patients. *Mult Scler.* 2013;19(7):941–946.

16. Petzold A, Plant GT. Chronic relapsing inflammatory optic neuropathy: a systematic review of 122 cases reported. *J Neurol.* 2013;261(1):17–26.

17. Kennedy J, O'Connor P, Sadovnick AD, et al. Age at onset of multiple sclerosis may be influenced by place of residence during childhood rather than ancestry. *Neuroepidemiology.* 2006;26:162–167.

18. Munger KL, Levin LI, Hollis BW, et al. Serum 25-hydroxyvitamin D levels and risk of multiple sclerosis. *JAMA.* 2006;296:2832–2838.

19. Mowry EM, Krupp LB, Milazzo M, et al. Vitamin D status is associated with relapse rate in pediatric-onset multiple sclerosis. *Ann Neurol.* 2010;67:618–624.

20. Staples J, Ponsonby AL, Lim L. Low maternal exposure to ultraviolet radiation in pregnancy, month of birth, and risk of multiple sclerosis in offspring: longitudinal analysis. *BMJ.* 2010;340:c1640.

21. Disanto G, Magalhaes S, Handel AE, et al. HLA-DRB1 confers increased risk of pediatric-onset MS in children with acquired demyelination. *Neurology.* 2011;76:781–786.

22. De Jager PL, Simon KC, Munger KL, et al. Integrating risk factors: HLA-DRB1*1501 and Epstein-Barr virus in multiple sclerosis. *Neurology.* 2008;70:1113–1118.

23. Gianfrancesco MA, Stridh P, Rhead B, et al. Evidence for a causal relationship between low vitamin D, high BMI, and pediatric-onset MS. *Neurology.* 2017;88:1623–1629.

24. Mikaeloff Y, Caridade G, Tardieu M, et al. Parental smoking at home and the risk of childhood-onset multiple sclerosis in children. *Brain.* 2007;130:2589–2595.

25. Mikaeloff Y, Caridade G, Rossier M, et al. Hepatitis B vaccination and the risk of childhood-onset multiple sclerosis. *Arch Pediatr Adolesc Med.* 2007;161:1176–1182.

26. Bonhomme GR, Waldman AT, Balcer LJ, et al. Pediatric optic neuritis: brain MRI abnormalities and risk of multiple sclerosis. *Neurology.* 2009;72:881–885.

27. Taimur M, Healy BC, Benson LA. Factors associated with recovery from acute optic neuritis in patients with multiple sclerosis. *Neurology.* 2014;82:2173–2179.

28. Waldman AT, Gorman MP, Rensel MR, et al. Management of pediatric central nervous system demyelinating disorders: Consensus of United States neurologists. *J Child Neurol.* 2011;26:675–682.

29. Chitnis T, Bar-Or A. Pediatric MS: biological presentation and research update. In: Chabas D, Waubant EL, eds. *Demyelinating Disorders of the Central Nervous System in Childhood.* New York, NY: Cambridge University Press; 2011.

30. Chabas D, Ness J, Belman A, et al. Younger children with MS have a distinct CSF inflammatory profile at disease onset. *Neurology.* 2010;74:399–405.

31. Bosca I, Magraner MJ, Coret F, et al. The risk of relapse after a clinically isolated syndrome is related to the pattern of oligoclonal bands. *J Neuroimmunol.* 2010;226:143–146.

32. Tintore M, Rovira A, Brieva L, et al. Isolated demyelinating syndromes: comparison of CSF oligoclonal bands and different MR imaging criteria to predict conversion to CDMS. *Mult Scler.* 2001;7:359–363.

33. Hahn JS, Pohl D, Rensel M, et al. Differential diagnosis and evaluation in pediatric multiple sclerosis. *Neurology.* 2007;68:S13–S22.

34. Hacohen Y, Absoud M, Deiva K, et al. Myelin oligodendrocyte glycoprotein antibodies are associated with a non-MS course in children. *Neurol Neuroimmunol Neuroinflamm.* 2015;2:e81.

35. Hennes EM, Baumann M, Schanda, K, et al. Prognostic relevance of MOG antibodies in children with an acquired demyelinating syndrome. *Neurology.* 2017;89:900–908.

36. Fernandez-Carbonell C, Vargas-Lowy D, Musallam A, et al. Clinical and MRI phenotype of children with MOG antibodies. *Mult Scler.* 2016;22(2):174–184

37. Jarius S, Ruprecht K, Kleiter I, et al. MOG-IgG in NMO and related disorders: a multicenter study of 50 patients. Part 1: Frequency, syndrome specificity, influence of disease activity, long-term course, associated with AQP4-IgG, and origin. *J Neuroinflammation.* 2016;13:279.

38. Verhey LH, Branson HM, Shroff MM, et al. MRI parameters for prediction of multiple sclerosis diagnosis in children with acute CNS demyelination: a prospective national cohort study. *Lancet Neurol.* 2011;10:1065–1073.

39. Fay AJ, Mowry EM, Strober J, et al. Relapse severity and recovery in early pediatric multiple sclerosis. *Mult Scler.* 2012;18(7):1008–1012.

40. Gorman MP, Healy BC, Polgar-Turcsanyi M, et al. Increased relapse rate in pediatric-onset compared with adult-onset multiple sclerosis. *Arch Neurol.* 2009;66:54–59.

41. Renoux C, Vukusic S, Mikaeloff Y, et al. Natural history of multiple sclerosis with childhood onset. *N Engl J Med.* 2007;356:2603–2613.

42. Banwell B, Reder AT, Krupp L, et al. Safety and tolerability of interferon beta-1b in pediatric multiple sclerosis. *Neurology.* 2006;66:472–476.

43. Kuntz NL, Chabas D, Weinstock-Guttman B, et al. Treatment of multiple sclerosis in children and adolescents. *Expert Opin Pharmacother.* 2010;11:505–520.

44. Chitnis T et al. PARADIGMS: a randomised double-blind study of fingolimod versus interferon ß-1a in paediatric multiple sclerosis. Late breaking news oral presentation presented at: the 7th Joint ECTRIMS-ACTRIMS meeting on October 28, 2017; Paris, France.

45. Chitnis T, Tenembaum S, Banwell B, et al. Consensus statement: evaluation of new and existing therapeutics for pediatric multiple sclerosis. *Mult Scler.* 2012;18:116.

46. Ghezzi A, Pozzilli C, Grimaldi LM, et al. Safety and efficacy of natalizumab in children with multiple sclerosis. *Neurology.* 2010;75:912–917.

47. Kean JM, Rao S, Wang M, et al. Seroepidemiology of human polyomaviruses. *PLOS Path.* 2009;5:e1000363.

48. Knowles WA, Pipkin P, Andrews N, et al. Population-based study of antibody to the human polyomaviruses BKV and JCV and the simian polyomavirus SV40. *J Med Virol.* 2003;71:115–123.

49. Tzaribachev N, Koetter I, Kuemmerle-Deschner JB, et al. Rituximab for the treatment of refractory pediatric autoimmune diseases: a case series. *Cases J.* 2009;2:6609.

50. Dale RC, Brilot F, Duffy LV, et al. Utility and safety of rituximab in pediatric autoimmune and inflammatory CNS disease. *Neurology.* 2014;83:142–150.

51. Hauser SL, Waubant E, Arnold DL, et al. B-cell depletion with rituximab in relapsing-remitting multiple sclerosis. *N Eng J Med.* 2008;358:676–688.

34

Women's Issues

Megan E. Esch, Bridgette Jeanne Billioux, and Ellen M. Mowry

KEY POINTS FOR CLINICIANS

- Multiple sclerosis (MS) is more prevalent in women, and the female-to-male ratios of incident and prevalent MS seem to be increasing.
- Multiple factors likely contribute to the sex differences seen in MS, including genetic, hormonal, and immune factors.
- Sex hormones have effects in the immune system and seem to play a role in MS.
- Contraception is an important consideration in women of childbearing age on disease-modifying therapies (DMTs); both hormonal and nonhormonal contraception are reasonable options, though both have associated risks and challenges in the woman with MS.
- The age at onset of menarche may be associated with risk of developing MS.
- The premenstrual period is sometimes associated with worsened MS symptoms and may be associated with an increased rate of relapse.
- Sexual dysfunction is a common, but often overlooked, concern in women with MS.
- MS has no effect in and of itself on fertility, although some medications used in the treatment of MS may affect fertility.
- Although it does not affect the overall disease course, pregnancy itself is associated with a decreased rate of relapse, particularly in the third trimester, while there is a rebound increase in the rate of relapse in the first few months postpartum.
- Many medications used to treat MS are contraindicated during pregnancy and should be reviewed if a woman becomes or decides to become pregnant.
- Relapses during pregnancy are often treated with intravenous (IV) steroids, although steroids are ideally avoided during the first trimester.
- Postpartum risk of relapse may be decreased with prophylactic intravenous immunoglobulin (IVIG) given intrapartum and postpartum, or postpartum alone.
- Breastfeeding may be associated with a lower risk of relapse postpartum, but studies are conflicting.
- Many MS medications, including DMTs, are contraindicated during breastfeeding and should be reviewed if a patient decides to breastfeed.
- Menopause may be associated with worsened symptoms and progression.
- MS patients are at a higher risk for osteoporosis and osteopenia after menopause.

MS, like many other autoimmune diseases, is well known to be more prevalent in women, particularly those of childbearing age, than men. Many factors, including the neuroendocrine axis and its effects on immunological function, may contribute to these predilections. Given the evidence for hormonal effects on MS, many female hormonal factors have been evaluated for their effect on MS, including the onset of puberty, the menstrual cycle, oral contraceptive pills (OCP), pregnancy, breastfeeding, and menopause.

Pregnancy in MS is a very important topic in the management of the disease, both due to the fact that women of childbearing age are disproportionately affected by the disease, but also because of the many management issues that arise when a person with MS desires to become pregnant. During pregnancy, hormone levels change, impacting the MS relapse rate. Preventing relapses and managing flares and other symptoms can be challenging, as many medications typically used in MS patients are contraindicated during pregnancy. In addition, young women with MS are often concerned about the effects of pregnancy on disease progression; other concerns include the likelihood of passing on MS to offspring and whether, in light of its associated disabilities, MS impacts the ability to become pregnant or to have a safe delivery. This chapter aims to address the many issues pertinent to the management of MS in women.

SEX DIFFERENCES AND HORMONAL INFLUENCE ON MS

MS is well known to have a higher incidence and prevalence in women, with a prevalence approaching 3:1 in comparison to men, and some evidence suggests that this ratio has increased over the past few decades (1). The most common form of MS, the relapsing–remitting type (relapsing-remitting MS [RRMS]), has a largely female predominance; primary progressive MS tends to affect males and females equally, with a possible slight male preponderance (2). Men with MS tend to acquire disability more rapidly compared to women among those with an MS onset between the ages of 16 and 49 years but not when onset occurred at age 50 years or more (3); they also tend to incur more cognitive disability than women, although this latter result may have been confounded by disease duration or other factors for which statistical analyses did not account (4). MS also tends to affect women at a slightly younger age than men, with a median difference in onset of 2 to 3 years (5). Data regarding sex differences in the use of DMTs are conflicting. In general, the effect of DMTs on the rate of clinical relapses does not differ between sexes (6,7). Interferons (IFNs) in particular do not seem to have an overall gender effect in RRMS (8,9); however, at least one study has demonstrated a later onset of relapse in men treated with IFN compared to women. However, there is a higher risk of disability progression (10). One study of patients with primary progressive MS suggested that men treated with glatiramer acetate had lower rates of progression compared to untreated men; this effect was not seen in women (11). There are likely multiple factors underlying these differences between men and women with MS, including genetic, hormonal, and immune factors.

There is a disproportionate occurrence of MS in women, which may be further increasing.

There are interesting sex differences in the immune system, which likely play a role in the phenotypic differences of MS in men compared to women. Females tend to show a stronger immune response than males; they have higher baseline immunoglobulin levels and CD4+ T cells than males. Females also have a more sustained immunological response to antigenic challenges (12). In general, autoimmune diseases are much more common in women than men. Interestingly, many of these autoimmune diseases also seem to be affected by hormonal changes, as seen in menstrual cycle fluctuations, pregnancy, and menopause (6). There are some specific sex differences in the immune systems of patients with MS; for example, women have a greater T-cell response to myelin proteolipid protein, as well as a comparatively increased cytokine secretion in response to lymphocyte stimulation with myelin proteins, than men (13).

Hormonal factors likely play an important role in MS in general. An overwhelming majority of patients are diagnosed between 15 and 50 years of age. On average, MS typically begins early in the third decade, with less than 1% of MS patients experiencing symptoms prior to onset of puberty. Also, the risk of developing MS declines beyond onset of menopause; these correlations between MS onset and age suggest a role for hormonal factors in MS (6). Sex hormones, including estrogens, progestins, and androgens, have multiple effects on the nervous system and also act as immunomodulators. Specifically, sex hormones have a significant influence on T-helper (Th) lymphocytes. In brief, Th lymphocytes are classified into two types: Th1 (proinflammatory) and Th2 (anti-inflammatory) cell types on the basis of their secretion of different cytokines. Th1 cells secrete proinflammatory interleukin (IL)-1, IL-2, IL-12, tumor necrosis factor alpha (TNF alpha), and IFN gamma, whereas Th2 cells secrete anti-inflammatory IL-4, IL-5, IL-6, and IL-10 (14). Estrogen affects levels of these cytokines, largely dependent on the concentration of hormone. With higher concentrations of estrogen (as in pregnancy), TNF alpha levels are decreased and IL-10 levels are increased; conversely, with lower levels of estrogen, TNF alpha levels are increased. Estrogen also stimulates humoral immunity and Th2 cellular function, and it inhibits natural killer cell activity and T suppressor cell activity. Progesterone decreases IL-1 and IFN gamma, and stimulates IL-4, acting as a relative immunosuppressant (15). These hormones act synergistically, as well. Testosterone, like progesterone, tends to act as an immunosuppressant (16).

Although these are incompletely understood, there seem to be multiple genetic and epigenetic factors associated with the effect of sex differences in MS. Several studies of half-sib, avuncular pairs, and extended family pedigrees suggest a maternal parent of origin effect in MS, in which individuals related through the maternal line are more likely to be affected than individuals related through the paternal line (17). There is also a well-known association of MS with *HLA-DRB1*1501*, which is a specific human leukocyte antigen (HLA) class II allele of the major histocompatibility complex; this association appears stronger in women compared to men (13). Polymorphisms in apolipoprotein E (APOE) and CD95 genes have been associated in some studies with disease severity in women with MS. Also, a relationship has been reported between MS and polymorphisms in the estrogen receptor gene (16).

SEX HORMONES AND OCPs IN MS

As noted earlier, estrogens and progesterones shift the immune response from a Th1 to a Th2 pattern and downregulate proinflammatory cytokines, which would theoretically have a protective role in MS. In animal studies using the MS mouse model, experimental allergic encephalomyelitis, administration of estrogen tends to lessen the severity of disease, and oophorectomy worsens disease (18). Given these findings in animal models, studies have been conducted with exogenous estrogens in female MS patients.

Estriol is an estrogen unique to pregnancy, and its concentrations are highest during the third trimester of pregnancy, that is, when MS relapse rates are lowest. Administration of estriol in nonpregnant females with MS has been associated with a reduction in inflammatory cytokines (IFN-gamma), a decrease in MRI activity, and improved clinical outcomes in women with MS (19,20). Voskuhl et al. recently published results of a phase 2 trial evaluating the effects of estriol in combination with glatiramer acetate (GA) on reduction in annualized relapse rate (ARR). Estriol plus GA demonstrated modestly reduced ARR at 24 months, with 0.25 relapses per year (95% CI: 0.17–0.37) in the group on combination therapy compared to 0.37 relapses per year (95% CI: 0.25–0.53) in GA alone, with an adjusted rate of relapse of 0.63; this corresponded to a *p*-value of .077. The investigators also demonstrated an effect on cortical gray matter loss, but did not demonstrate significant change in number of enhancing or T2 lesions, nor whole brain volume (20). The small study sample size limited the power of the result, and phase 3 trials may be warranted to more definitively evaluate the impact of the combination of therapies.

In addition to estriol's singular association with pregnancy, it is also unique in its receptor-binding affinity compared to other estrogens. Its weak binding properties to both the alpha and the beta estrogen receptor subunits have been thought to play a role in its reduced association with gynecological malignancies, cardiovascular risk, and endometrial proliferation compared to other estrogens (21–24). At least one study demonstrated increased rates of abnormal menstrual bleeding, enlarged uterine fibroids, and increased risk of thrombotic events (19) in females treated with estriol, though larger studies failed to reproduce all but abnormal menses as significant side effects (20).

> *Oral contraceptive pills are safe to use in MS patients, although one must consider the risk of deep vein thrombosis (DVT), particularly in patients with limited mobility.*

Oral contraceptives and their potential effects on MS have also been studied. The data are limited and the results are conflicting. Some studies suggest that there may be a lower incidence of MS in OCP users, whereas others did not show any significant difference between OCP users and nonusers (25,26). In 2016, the US Medical Eligibility Criteria for Contraceptive Use was modified to include evidence-based recommendations regarding contraceptive use in MS patients. The recommendations were based on a published review of literature, which is overall lacking for all forms of contraceptive use in MS, including oral contraceptives. In general, OCP use is not contraindicated in patients with MS, but caution must be exercised when prescribing these for MS patients with limited mobility due to the increased risk of clotting and thromboembolic events conferred by OCP use. Additionally, progesterone derivatives may incur higher risk of changes in bone mineral density, which in turn increases risk of osteopenia and osteoporosis (27). Increased risk of osteopenia with progesterone exposure is an important consideration in MS patients who may have increased lifetime exposure to corticosteroids.

Nonoral hormonal contraception and nonhormonal contraception are also options for the MS patient wishing to avoid pregnancy. Permanent or semipermanent forms of contraception (e.g., intrauterine devices and implants) may be a preferred mechanism for preventing pregnancies in patients on particularly teratogenic DMTs given their increased efficacy, reliability, and ease of use. Barrier devices and vaginal rings are also reasonable considerations, although concerns regarding difficulties with fine motor control, vaginal stenosis, and spasticity of the lower extremities may cause functional limitations in use of these methods. It is important for the provider to counsel patients on the most effective forms of contraception depending on the patients' current intentions to become pregnant, the current DMT, and any functional constraints that may affect proper use of contraception.

PUBERTY, MENSTRUAL CYCLE, AND MS

Given that less than 1% of MS diagnoses are made in prepubescent females, and the known influence of sex hormones on the pathophysiology of MS, assessing pubertal influences on MS is indicated. The data are, for the most part, conflicting, likely in part due to small sample sizes, which have made it difficult to draw reasonable conclusions regarding age of menarche and the development of MS. Two small cohort studies demonstrated no association between age of onset of menarche and risk of development of MS (28,29). However, Ramagopalan et al. conducted a large cohort study, inclusive of 5,493 MS patients of both sexes. They demonstrated a younger age of onset of puberty was significantly associated with increased overall risk of acquiring MS in females, but not males (30). These findings were corroborated in a smaller Danish study (31). A separate small cohort of patients demonstrated that earlier age of menarche is associated with earlier onset of first MS symptoms (32), but the correlation of timing of first MS symptoms was not demonstrated in Ramagopalan's study. Although it needs to be replicated, it is interesting to note that one small study demonstrated that menarche status may also influence the rate of relapses in pediatric MS; girls in the 6 months preceding and following menarche incur the highest risk of relapses in the pediatric population (33).

Beyond puberty, many female MS patients report fluctuations in their symptoms corresponding to changes in their menstrual cycle. These symptoms may include fatigue, myalgias, depression, decreased endurance, worsened spasticity, weakness, incoordination, and abnormalities in gait, sensation, vision, or sphincter function (16,34). Although data on the relationship between the menstrual cycle and MS exacerbations are limited, one questionnaire-based study suggested a higher rate of MS exacerbations occurring in the premenstrual period compared to the rest of the menstrual cycle in a group of premenopausal women with MS (35). Worsening of symptoms and exacerbations during the premenstrual period may be explained by the relative drop in estrogen and progesterone, leading to a Th1/Th2 shift (35).

FERTILITY IN MS

MS does not appear to have any direct effect on fertility (5), although one Swedish study suggested that the frequency of infertile women might be higher in the MS population than in the general population (36). An Italian study in postmenopausal women demonstrated that females with MS were significantly more likely to be childless compared to their healthy counterparts, but this was not associated with fertility status (37). Factors that may influence MS patients' decisions regarding motherhood include lack of a stable relationship, the influence of perceived disability on parenting, and concerns about MS transmission to offspring (36,37).

Although MS itself does not seem to affect fertility, some medications for MS may have effects on fertility. Pregnancy may be avoided or postponed because of DMT. Specifically, mitoxantrone has been found to cause significantly protracted or even irreversible amenorrhea after prolonged use (38). Cyclophosphamide exerts a toxic effect on the ovaries and reduces ovarian reserve. Cyclophosphamide also frequently leads to amenorrhea with definitive amenorrhea in up to 33% of female patients

receiving pulse dosing for treatment of progressive MS (36). However, mitoxantrone and cyclophosphamide are not commonly used in the treatment of MS.

> *MS has no direct effect on fertility, but the desire to start a family may be influenced by various personal or psychosocial issues that should be considered when counseling patients.*

SEXUAL DYSFUNCTION

Not to be overlooked in this population is the increased frequency of sexual dysfunction (SD) compared to healthy populations. SD is present in as many as 80% of females with MS, but very few women discuss sexual concerns with their treating physicians (39). The presence of SD is noted as soon as 2 to 5 years after diagnosis of MS, presumably when many affected women might otherwise be planning families (40). SD may be related to white matter lesions themselves, which cause decreased lubrication and genital sensation, bladder control problems, or difficulty with orgasm. In addition to the physical manifestations of SD, common complaints of SD in women include fatigue, low libido or arousal, and the psychosocial impacts of body image and self-esteem (39,41,42). One large cohort study demonstrated a significantly more negative association of SD on mental, as opposed to physical, aspects of health-related quality of life (43). Psychosocial factors associated with SD are considerable in MS patients; these include lower education level, residence in less-populated or rural communities, positive depression screening index, and negative assessment of relationship status (39,42). The influence of SD on the desire to start a family is not certain, but this is worth considering in counseling patients who may be seeking family planning advice. In addition to the possible role of SD in family planning, identifying SD as a role in overall quality of life is important for all females with MS.

> *SD is common, but underreported in women with MS. The impact of SD on mental health quality of life is significant, and warrants discussion between physician and patient.*

PREGNANCY IN MS

After the decision to conceive has been made, the course of pregnancy may be a concern to the MS patient. The concern of whether or not pregnancy affects the overall course of MS has been debated widely for years. In the past, MS patients were advised against pregnancy owing to concerns that it worsens disease prognosis. However, in more recent years it has been found that pregnancy does not seem to have a detrimental effect on the overall disease course. Some studies have suggested that pregnancy may even have a positive effect on MS prognosis, including decreasing the rate of progression to irreversible disability and time to transition to progressive forms of MS (44–48). One recent large, retrospective study suggested that pregnancy has no long-term effect on the course of disease but may be associated with more rapid progression to secondary progressive MS (49), which further clouds the picture of the long-term effects of pregnancy on the disease course of MS.

> In general, pregnancy does not have a detrimental effect on the overall disease course, though there is suggestion it may be associated with more rapid progression to secondary progressive MS.

While it is unclear how pregnancy affects the long-term course of MS, it is well established that pregnancy affects the course of MS in the short term. Pregnancy is associated with a decrease in disease activity, particularly in the third trimester, with a rebound increase in risk of relapse in the first few months postpartum (50). The Pregnancy in Multiple Sclerosis Study (PRIMS), a multicenter European prospective observational study, found that there was a slight reduction in relapse rate during the first two trimesters, and a substantial reduction during the third trimester, with an ARR of 0.2 relapses/y during the third trimester compared to 0.7 prior to pregnancy. Postdelivery, there was an increase in ARR to 1.2 over the first 3 months postpartum, after which the ARR returned to the rate prior to pregnancy (51). This phenomenon is likely related to the relative immunosuppressive state during pregnancy produced by increases in estrogen, progesterone, and glucocorticoids, and other factors leading to a shift toward anti-inflammatory Th2 responses. Although pregnancy is thought to be protective against MS exacerbations, some underlying MS symptoms may worsen during pregnancy, including fatigue, spasticity, bowel and bladder dysfunction, and difficulty with mobility or ambulation (16). Following the landmark PRIMS results, multiple international studies were completed that replicated the intra- and postpartum ARR trends demonstrated in PRIMS (52,53).

> Pregnancy is associated with a decrease in disease activity, particularly in the third trimester, with a rebound increase in disease activity postpartum.

The results of PRIMS prompted investigation into the predictors of postpartum relapse. Follow-up studies demonstrated that prepregnancy relapse rate, intrapartum relapse rate, and prepregnancy severity of disability each predicted increased postpartum relapse rate (54,55). Use of DMT at any point during the 2 years preconception demonstrated a protective effect toward early postpartum relapse. Importantly, time to conception after cessation of DMT at any point within the 2-year period prior to conception did not affect postpartum relapse rate (55).

MS patients may also have concerns about the potential safety of pregnancy for both themselves and fetal development. In general, MS patients show no increase in fetal malformations, spontaneous abortions, risk of preeclampsia, preterm delivery, caesarean delivery, or gestational diabetes compared to the general population (50,56). Women with MS do not seem to have an increase in complications during pregnancy compared to women without MS (57). One recent Turkish study demonstrated that urinary tract infection (UTI) was significantly increased in a pregnant MS cohort compared to controls, and that 1-minute Apgar scores were significantly lower in neonates born to women with MS; Apgar scores in this group improved at 5 minutes and were comparable to neonates born to healthy women (56).

Information about genetics is also important to discuss with MS patients who are interested in becoming pregnant. While the risk of developing MS in the general population is about 0.2%, the risk increases to 3% to 5% in a child with a parent affected by MS, which is a 15- to 25-fold increase. This risk increases further to 30.5% in the event that both parents are affected by MS (16). Studies evaluating whether MS transmission is greater, depending on which parent is affected, have produced conflicting results (58–60).

DMTs in Pregnancy

The continuation or discontinuation of DMT both during pregnancy and postpartum are important considerations. Pregnancy is known to reduce the risk of relapse of patients with MS; however, it does not eliminate the risk. Traditionally, MS patients are counseled to stop DMTs before trying to conceive, although clinicians should review the potential risks and benefits of continuing DMTs on a case-by-case basis (61). The recommended time between stopping a therapy and attempting pregnancy varies by medication and by practitioner. It may be helpful for patients to meet with their obstetrician for help with pregnancy timing and planning so as to minimize the length of time off DMTs. While some of the older DMTs have been studied more extensively, less is known about the safety of the newer therapies during pregnancy, although the literature is expanding.

> In general, patients are advised to discontinue disease-modifying therapy prior to conception.

In general, the information known about IFN beta and GA is relatively reassuring. The large molecular size of IFN beta may prevent transportation across the placental barrier. Although studies regarding IFN in human pregnancy are limited, animal studies of IFN administration in pregnancy demonstrated higher risk of spontaneous abortion when the medication was dosed late in pregnancy and at 2 to 40 times the recommended human dosing. In humans, there was some early evidence of decreased birth weight in babies exposed to IFN in utero, and a possible slight increase in rate of spontaneous abortion in women taking IFN during pregnancy (62). However, recent data published from two large IFN registries showed similar rates of birth defects and spontaneous abortion in pregnancies exposed to IFN in the first trimester of pregnancy compared to nondrug exposed pregnancies (63,64). There is ultimately no clear evidence of teratogenicity with use of IFNs (62,65). Due to the animal data and early data suggesting possible association with increased spontaneous abortion and fetal malformations, IFN remains a Food and Drug Administration (FDA) category C drug.

GA has not been shown to cause birth defects in animal studies. Previously, there was a suggestion that there may be an increased risk of spontaneous abortion with its use (66). However, a review of studies that include nearly 500 pregnancy exposures to glatiramer demonstrated there is no increased risk to the fetus exposed to GA in early pregnancy (67). Two large-cohort studies of pregnant women exposed to GA demonstrated no increased risk of spontaneous abortion or fetal abnormalities in drug-exposed fetuses (68,69). GA is the only available DMT for MS that has been classified as a category B drug by the FDA.

Oral therapies for MS, including fingolimod, dimethyl fumarate, and teriflunomide are relatively new. Fingolimod has demonstrated embryolethality and teratogenicity in animal studies, at weight-based doses less than weight-based human equivalents. Malformations included persistent truncus arteriosus and ventral septal defects (70,71). The largest human registry available included 66 reported pregnancies exposed to fingolimod. The outcomes suggest there is an increased risk of spontaneous abortion and fetal abnormalities that may be attributed to the intended target of fingolimod; sphingosine-1-phosphate receptors are known to play a role in vascular formation during embryogenesis (72). Based on the pharmacologic profile, it is recommended patients intending to conceive discontinue the use of fingolimod at least 2 months prior to conception to ensure complete metabolism and excretion of drug (70).

In animal studies, dimethyl fumarate (DMF) demonstrates an increased risk of fetal toxicity and embryolethality, including delayed ossification, delayed sex maturation, low birth weight, and neurodevelopmental abnormalities. Plasma concentrations of the active metabolite monomethyl fumarate at toxic doses were as high as 16 times the plasma concentration of humans receiving the recommended daily dose but reached toxic effect in some animals at plasma concentrations lower than those of humans on the recommended daily dose (68). Some of the fetal abnormalities seen in animals may be related to decreased maternal food consumption leading to low fetal birth weight. Preliminary postmarketing clinical data do not suggest increased risk of spontaneous abortion or fetal abnormalities in early pregnancy exposure to DMF; however, the available fetal animal data should give pause to clinicians treating patients of childbearing potential with DMF, particularly in women whom a reliable form of contraception is not in use (73). Although there are no published recommendations regarding the period of time a woman should wait to conceive following discontinuation of DMF, it is known that the drug is not detected in blood after 24 hours of last dose (74).

Among the newer oral therapies, teriflunomide is currently the only FDA-approved pregnancy category X therapy available for treatment of MS (75). Preclinical studies demonstrated embryolethality and teratogenicity at plasma concentrations lower than recommended human doses (76). Data are available regarding teriflunomide in 70 human pregnancies, which have demonstrated no increased risk of spontaneous abortion or embryo–fetal developmental abnormalities (77). Of note, teriflunomide can be found in the semen of men treated with teriflunomide; male-to-female transfer of teriflunomide via semen may result in very low detectable levels of teriflunomide in female partners. If females taking teriflunomide desire to conceive, they should undergo a cholestyramine or activated charcoal elimination protocol prior to attempting pregnancy; similarly, men undergoing treatment desiring children with their female partners should also undergo elimination (76). Likewise, if a woman becomes pregnant while exposed to teriflunomide, the same elimination procedure should be implemented to minimize risk to the developing fetus (76).

The monoclonal antibodies are of increased interest in the treatment of MS due to their efficacy, and ease of administration. Of the monoclonal antibodies, natalizumab has been available for use in MS the longest, and there is more clinical safety available for the drug than its newer counterparts. Preclinical trials of natalizumab demonstrated variable teratogenicity; at supratherapeutic doses in animal models, there is evidence of increased spontaneous abortion, anemia, thrombocytopenia, and thymic atrophy (78). The largest registry of pregnant women exposed to natalizumab within 3 months prior to conception through the end of pregnancy has reported the outcomes of 355 pregnancies. The data did not suggest any evidence of drug effect on fetal malformation; the rate of spontaneous abortions in women exposed to natalizumab was similar to the rate of spontaneous abortion in the general population (79). A smaller study of 102 pregnancies exposed to natalizumab was compared to both disease matched and healthy controls. No differences in fetal outcomes existed when exposed pregnancies were compared to disease-matched controls; however, there was an increased risk of spontaneous abortion and lower birth weight in both natalizumab-exposed pregnancies and disease-matched controls compared to healthy controls. The authors note that the rate of spontaneous abortion in the healthy control group was actually lower than the general population, which may have contributed to these findings (80). One small case series of 13 pregnancies looked at natalizumab exposure during the third trimester of pregnancy. This series did demonstrate reversible and non–life-threatening anemia and thrombocytopenia in neonates. Natalizumab was detectable in the umbilical cord blood at the time of delivery in tested samples and as long as 6 months after delivery (81). Notably, the population of women exposed to natalizumab in the third trimester had experienced severely refractory MS: some experienced severe relapses in the setting of withdrawal of natalizumab prior to pregnancy, and others steroid-refractory relapses during the course of pregnancy, which required continuation of natalizumab throughout pregnancy, or the reinitiation of therapy in late pregnancy, highlighting the real-world difficulties of making therapy decisions with women with more aggressive MS who desire to conceive.

Alemtuzumab demonstrates increased risk of secondary autoimmunity, particularly thyroid-associated diseases and immune thrombocytopenia. Animal studies of alemtuzumab exposure demonstrated increased rate of spontaneous abortion and lymphocytopenia (82). There are no human studies of alemtuzumab in significant numbers of pregnancies available for review, though early studies suggest there is no increased risk of preterm birth, spontaneous abortion, or fetal abnormalities compared to the general population (83). Given the risk of secondary autoimmunity and concern for neonatal thyrotoxicosis and lymphocytopenia, it is recommended that women wait for at least 4 months after alemtuzumab infusion before attempting to conceive (82).

Animal studies of supratherapeutic doses of the rituximab, and its humanized analogue ocrelizumab, infused during organogenesis demonstrated decreased populations of B cells in offspring. Levels of B cells returned to normal at about 6 months of age (84). Renal toxicity and bacterial infections due to immunosuppression were seen in the offspring of animal mothers treated with ocrelizumab (85). Outcomes of one study of rituximab use for a variety of indications in 153 pregnant women demonstrated an increased risk of preterm birth and spontaneous abortion compared to the general population. The most common neonatal abnormality demonstrated was hematologic disorders, which were transient and non–life threatening in all but one case; there was no evidence of increased teratogenicity due to drug effect (86). These outcomes should be viewed cautiously, as some autoimmune conditions treated with rituximab are associated with early miscarriage, and the data may not directly apply to rituximab use in MS cohorts. No human pregnancy studies specifically regarding rituximab or ocrelizumab use in MS cohorts has been completed. Prescriber information of ocrelizumab currently suggests that patients wait 6 months after infusion to begin attempting conception given the presence of detectable serum drug levels at 6 months (85).

Current DMTs and their respective FDA pregnancy categories are provided in Table 34.1.

Treatment of Exacerbations During Pregnancy

In the event of MS relapse during pregnancy, short doses of high-dose corticosteroids can be used, much as in non-pregnant patients. Corticosteroids are known to cross the placenta; however, most of the prednisolone and hydrocortisone that cross to the placenta are converted to less active metabolites by placental syncytiotrophoblasts (61). Methylprednisolone is typically the preferred agent of treatment, with a 3- to 5-day course being the most common course of treatment with or without a subsequent, short prednisone taper (5,61). While short-term therapy with glucocorticoids is generally considered safe in pregnant women, there have been some adverse effects described. Studies have reported a possible mild increase in orofacial abnormalities in fetuses exposed to prednisone in the first trimester; hence, high doses of prednisone ideally should be avoided in the first trimester, when palate formation is occurring (87). Otherwise, short courses of prednisone and other corticosteroids can be safely tolerated in the second and third trimesters. On the other hand, prolonged tapering courses of corticosteroids are associated with an increased risk of gestational diabetes, hypertension, sodium retention, edema, and premature rupture of membranes, and should hence be avoided during pregnancy (66).

> *Short courses of high-dose steroids may be used to treat MS relapses in pregnant women.*

Symptomatic Treatment During Pregnancy

Many medications used in the symptomatic treatment of MS (i.e., spasticity or urinary dysfunction) are contraindicated during pregnancy (5). For a listing of commonly used symptomatic medications in MS and their pregnancy classifications, please refer to Table 34.2.

> *Many symptomatic therapies are contraindicated during pregnancy.*

Delivery in MS

Women with MS do not experience increased obstetrical or neonatal complications compared to unaffected women (61). Neither general nor spinal anesthesia is contraindicated in MS, as neither has a particular effect on the disease. Decisions regarding labor and delivery procedures should hence be based entirely on obstetrical

TABLE 34.1 MS Therapies and FDA Pregnancy Categories

DRUG	U.S. FDA PREGNANCY CATEGORY	COMMENT
Dexamethasone	C	Avoid during first trimester
Methylprednisolone	C	Avoid during first trimester
Interferon beta	C	Possible increase in spontaneous abortions
Glatiramer acetate	B	Possible decrease in birth weight
Natalizumab	C	Possible risk of hematologic abnormalities during third trimester
Fingolimod	C	Possible increase in spontaneous abortions; possible risk of cardiovascular abnormalities
Alemtuzumab	C	
Rituximab	C	Possible risk of hematologic abnormalities
Ocrelizumab	C	Increased risk of infections and renal toxicity in animals
Teriflunomide	X	Fetal malformation and embryo–fetal death in animals
Methotrexate	X	Craniofacial and limb defects, CNS abnormalities, miscarriage
Cyclophosphamide	D	Impaired fetal growth, malformations of skeleton, palate, limbs, and eyes
Azathioprine	D	
Cyclosporine A	C	
Mitoxantrone	D	
Intravenous immunoglobulin	C	Probably safe

Class A: Adequate, well-controlled studies in pregnant women have not shown an increased risk of fetal abnormalities to the fetus in any trimester of pregnancy.

Class B: Animal studies have revealed no evidence of harm to the fetus. However, there are no adequate and well-controlled studies in women. Or animal studies have shown an adverse effect, but adequate and well-controlled studies in pregnant women have failed to demonstrate a risk to the fetus in any trimester.

Class C: Animal studies have shown an adverse effect and there are no adequate and well-controlled studies in pregnant women, or no animal studies and no adequate and well-controlled studies in pregnant women.

Class D: Adequate well-controlled or observational studies in pregnant women showed a risk to the fetus. However, benefits of therapy may outweigh the potential risks. For example, the drug may be acceptable if needed in a life-threatening situation or serious disease for which safer drugs cannot be substituted.

Class X: Adequate well-controlled or observational studies in animals or pregnant women have demonstrated positive evidence of fetal abnormalities or risks. The use of the product is contraindicated in women who are or may become pregnant.

CNS, central nervous system; FDA, Food and Drug Administration; MS, multiple sclerosis.

Source: Adapted from Ferrero S, Pretta S, Ragni N. Multiple sclerosis: management issues during pregnancy. *Eur J Obstet Gynecol Reprod Biol*. 2004;115:3–9; Coyle PK, Johnson K, Pardo L, et al. Pregnancy outcomes in patients with multiple sclerosis treated with glatiramer acetate (Copaxone 1). In: *Proceedings of the 55th Annual Meeting of the American Academy of Neurology*. Honolulu, HI; March 29–April 5, 2003. *Neurology*. 2003;60(5)(suppl 1). A60 [abstract].

evaluation. Although there is no particular increase in the rate of complications in MS patients during delivery, there may be some potential differences from the general population which should be considered. Some MS patients have some degree of pelvic floor weakness, as well as spasticity and fatigue, which can hamper an efficient abdomen–pelvic push; this may lead to requiring more assistance during delivery. In MS patients with diaphragmatic insufficiency, there may be an increased risk of respiratory failure intra- or postpartum, possibly leading to a need for prolonged monitoring. In addition, MS patients on chronic corticosteroid therapy may be at an increased risk of acute adrenocortical failure postpartum and should be closely monitored for such (5).

> *In general, delivery is no more complicated in MS patients than in the general population.*

Postpartum Relapse and Prevention

While pregnancy confers some protection from MS relapses, there is a higher risk of relapse in the postpartum period. It is generally recommended that patients who were on DMTs prior to pregnancy resume DMTs immediately postpartum, unless they plan on breastfeeding. One retrospective study of 893 pregnancies demonstrated that higher preconception and midpregnancy ARRs as well as greater preconception disability score are risks for relapse in the first 3 months postpartum, while use of DMT for any duration prior to conception protects against relapse during the same time period (50). The best prevention for postpartum relapse, then, is to prevent preconception relapses by selection of an effective DMT for the patient.

Few studies have considered the use of nontraditional DMTs in preventing postpartum relapses. A prophylactic 3- to 5-day course of high-dose steroids may provide up to 4 weeks of protection from relapse and can be used postpartum; steroids are also not contraindicated during

TABLE 34.2 Symptomatic MS Treatments and FDA Pregnancy Categories

CATEGORY	DRUGS FOR SYMPTOMATIC TREATMENT
Class B	Oxybutynin
	Cyclobenzaprine
	Tamsulosin
Class C	Baclofen
	Carbamazepine
	Darifenacin
	Dantrolene
	Tizanidine
	Gabapentin
	Dalfampridine
	Amantadine
	Most selective serotonin reuptake inhibitors[a]
	Serotonin–norepinephrine reuptake inhibitors
	Bupropion
	Tolterodine
	Solifenacin
	Trospium
Class D	Most benzodiazepines
	Phenytoin

FDA, Food and Drug Administration; MS, multiple sclerosis.
[a]Some research associates use of citalopram, fluoxetine, and sertraline with persistent pulmonary hypertension of the newborn (PPHN) when taken during the last half of pregnancy (88). Paroxetine is considered "less safe" given a small increased risk of cardiovascular abnormalities in one study (89).
Source: Adapted from Ghezzi A, Zaffaroni M. Female-specific issues in multiple sclerosis. *Expert Rev Neurother.* 2008;8(6):969-977; *Micromedex® Healthcare Series* [intranet database]. Version 5.1. Greenwood Village, CO: Thomson Reuters (Healthcare) Inc. Accessed November 8, 2012. (90)

breastfeeding, although they should be used cautiously, as there have been rare cases of orofacial malformations and adrenal suppression in neonates when high-dose corticosteroids are given late term (61,91,92). Intravenous immunoglobulin (IVIG) may also be considered to prevent relapse in the postpartum period; in one study, IVIG was found to reduce the relapse rate by 33% (93). In a study by Achiron et al., IVIG was studied both intrapartum as well as postpartum as prophylaxis against postpartum relapses. Both groups had significantly lower rates of relapse, with the intrapartum IVIG group having a slightly lower rate of relapse compared to the postpartum group (94). IVIG is also considered to be safe in breastfeeding women (66). One study looked at the role of estradiol and progestin in the immediate postpartum period in preventing relapses. The study was stopped early due to slow recruitment, but interim analysis did not demonstrate significant difference in relapses between exposure to hormone and controls (95,96).

> *Unless breastfeeding, DMTs should generally be restarted postpartum.*

BREASTFEEDING IN MS

The effect of breastfeeding on MS is somewhat controversial. Breastfeeding has been shown to dampen the proinflammatory response in MS by returning the IFN gamma-producing CD4+ T cells to normal levels (61). Further, exclusive breastfeeding decreases postpartum relapses with an associated decrease in proinflammatory TNF-alpha-producing CD4+ T cells (97–99). Early studies evaluating the effect of breastfeeding on the clinical course of MS showed conflicting data; these studies demonstrated either no significant difference in relapse rate between patients who breastfed or bottle-fed, or minimal benefit with breastfeeding (5). More recently, a small prospective cohort of 32 postpartum women with MS found that women who breastfed exclusively for the first 2 months postpartum were approximately 5 times less likely to have an MS relapse during the first-year postpartum when compared to women who did not breastfeed or who supplemented formula with breastfeeding (97). A larger prospective study of about 300 women by Portaccio et al., however, found no difference in relapse rate profiles between women who breastfed and those who did not after adjusting for covariates, although the distinction of exclusive breastfeeding was not made in this study (100). While there may be a relative decrease in relapse rates in the first 6 months postpartum in women who breastfeed, this seems to be more prominent in women who breastfeed exclusively. Caution in this interpretation is needed, however, as women who exclusively breastfeed may have less severe disease at baseline, enabling their ability to breastfeed without supplementation in the postpartum period (101). Further, the benefit to mothers with MS of exclusive breastfeeding may decline or be lost when supplemental feeds are initiated (99). In general, there seems to be no significant effect on overall disease progression or evolution in MS patients who have breastfed (5), and decisions about breastfeeding should probably be driven by the mother's personal choice.

In patients who want to breastfeed, caution must be taken when prescribing medications, as many medications used in MS treatment may be excreted in breast milk. While steroids are known to be transferred to breast milk, infant exposure to corticosteroids from breast milk is thought to be minimal (5). Nevertheless, overuse of corticosteroids during breastfeeding is not recommended, as they can potentially suppress infant growth. Based on pharmacologic profile, high doses of corticosteroids are associated with more exposure to the breastfeeding infant. Recommendations for discarding breast milk following steroid ingestion depend on the dose and choice of glucocorticoid; discussion with the medical provider is necessary to determine the need for discarding breast milk (102,103). IVIG is generally thought to be safe during lactation (57). Mitoxantrone, cyclosporine A, cyclophosphamide, and azathioprine should not be used in lactating women, as these agents are secreted in the breast milk.

One small study demonstrated that IFN beta is secreted into human breast milk in concentrations less than 0.006%, and no infants exposed to breast milk in IFN-exposed mothers were affected. However, it is generally not recommended in lactating women (67,104). There are insufficient data on GA and breastfeeding at this time (5). Neither IFN nor GA is orally absorbed, and the molecular weight of both drugs likely prevents their transfer from mother to baby via breast milk. Fingolimod and teriflunomide are excreted in the breast milk of rats; however, it is unknown if the medications are excreted in human milk, and they are generally not recommended in breastfeeding woman. There are not significant data regarding the excretion of DMF in human breast milk. Natalizumab is present in human breast milk; however, this drug is not orally bioavailable. Rituximab and ocrelizumab are excreted in animal milk, but data are unavailable in humans. Their oral bioavailability of both rituximab and ocrelizumab has not been established.

Given the limited data in all DMTs regarding the transfer of DMTs through human breast milk, the potential risks associated with exposing infants to these medications are mostly unknown. Thus, DMTs are generally not recommended in breastfeeding patients. A discussion with the patient regarding the benefits of early breastfeeding versus the risk of postpregnancy relapse is warranted.

> *Breastfeeding may be associated with a decreased relapse rate in the first year postpartum, but this effect seems to be more evident in women who breastfeed exclusively.*

> *IVIG is safe to use during breastfeeding. Steroids can be used with caution during lactation. DMTs and immunosuppressants are generally contraindicated during breastfeeding.*

IMAGING IN PREGNANT AND BREASTFEEDING WOMEN

When concerned for relapse during pregnancy or postpartum, the clinician may be inclined to acquire MRI. A large retrospective Canadian review of exposure to MRI in the first trimester of pregnancy demonstrated no increased risk of stillbirth, neonatal death, or congenital abnormalities in compared to nonexposed pregnancies. The same study demonstrated no increased risk of congenital anomalies in fetuses exposed to gadolinium-based contrast at any time during pregnancy.

Gadolinium-based contrast agents in exposed fetuses did demonstrate slight increased risk of broad spectrum rheumatologic and inflammatory disorders, and increased risk of stillbirths (105). The most recent American College of Radiology guidelines recommend caution when administering gadolinium-based contrast agents during pregnancy, unless a significant benefit outweighs risk of fetal exposure (106). The FDA currently considers gadolinium-based contrast agents pregnancy category class C.

Gadolinium-based contrast agents are excreted into the breast milk in minute fractions. Serum clearance of gadolinium in renally intact patients occurs within the first 24 hours of administration. It is estimated that less than 0.0004% of mother's gadolinium dose is systemically exposed to the infant after transfer of contrast agent to breast milk through the infant's GI tract (107,108). Although potential and theoretical concerns may exist when exposing infants to any agent, there have been no reports of complications due to breastfeeding infants exposed to gadolinium. The American College of Radiology guidelines consider it safe to breastfeed after exposure gadolinium (106).

> *Gadolinium-based contrast agents provide negligible exposure to breastfeeding infants. It is considered safe to continue breastfeeding after administration of IV gadolinium.*

MENOPAUSE IN MS

There is a relative dearth of information on MS and menopause. There is some evidence that menopause may correlate with the onset of progressive worsening disease. In one early study, prior to use of modern DMTs, 54% of postmenopausal patients reported worsening of their MS disability and progressive symptomatology (109). A more recent study demonstrated that the onset of menopause marks a modest but statistically significant worsening of clinician-rated disability on the Expanded Disability Scale Score (EDSS); this finding is independent of age of onset of menopause and controlled for DMT use (110). In the same cohort, patient-reported outcomes of their functional change did not reflect a worsening despite that their objective clinical findings did.

In addition to interest regarding postmenopausal changes in MS itself, one must be aware of the variety of hormone-related symptoms associated with menopause that may mimic MS features. Bowel and bladder dysfunction, frequent hot flashes, cognitive slowing, and sleep changes are features of menopause that become more prominent perimenopausally, and may either mimic or exacerbate baseline symptoms in the MS patient. Physiologic issues, such as osteoporosis and osteopenia, are especially relevant to women with MS, as those who have been treated with high doses of steroids and who have impaired mobility are at an even higher risk of osteoporosis. Bone density scanning should hence be considered in postmenopausal patients. Weight-bearing exercises should also be recommended to all MS patients, unless a contraindication exists. In addition, calcium and vitamin D supplements may be beneficial (11).

Postmenopausal hormone replacement therapy (HRT) has demonstrated variable impact on disability outcomes. A Swedish registry observed that the majority of postmenopausal patients experienced no self-reported change in their MS symptoms while on HRT (111). On the contrary, a small cohort of postmenopausal MS patients on HRT did demonstrate a statistically significant improvement in self-reported quality of life compared to patients not on HRT; however, it is noted that the HRT group also had a statistically shorter duration of disease (112). Nevertheless, existing data regarding the impact of hormonal exposure on the inflammatory nature of MS, warrants further investigation in various hormonal stages of life, from prepuberty to postmenopause.

> *Postmenopausal patients are at a higher risk of osteoporosis or osteopenia. Menopause may be associated with modestly worsened clinical disability, although this may be related to menopause itself. Data are inconclusive regarding the effect of HRT on quality of life in postmenopausal patients with MS.*

KEY POINTS FOR PATIENTS AND FAMILIES

- Pregnancy is not contraindicated in patients with MS.
- Notify your care provider if you become pregnant, or plan on becoming pregnant, as some medications used in the treatment of MS may not be safe for use during pregnancy.
- Pregnancy reduces the risk of MS flare, especially in the third trimester.
- Most doctors recommend patients discontinue their DMTs during or prior to pregnancy.
- If you are at a particularly high risk of relapse, your care provider may recommend continuing your DMT prior to, and possibly during, pregnancy.
- If a relapse occurs during pregnancy, a short course of high-dose steroids may be used for management.
- Risk of complications during pregnancy and delivery in MS is the same as the general population.
- General and spinal anesthesia are safe in MS patients during delivery.
- Notify your care provider if you plan on breastfeeding, as some medications used for MS may be secreted in the breast milk and should not be taken if you plan on breastfeeding.

REFERENCES

1. Sellner J, Kraus J, Awad A, et al. The increasing incidence and prevalence of female multiple sclerosis—a critical analysis of potential environmental factors. *Autoimmun Rev.* 2011;10(8):495–502.
2. Thompson AJ, Polman CH, Miller DH, et al. Primary progressive multiple sclerosis. *Brain.* 1997;120:1085–1096.
3. Tremlett H, Devonshire V. Is late-onset multiple sclerosis associated with a worse outcome? *Neurology.* 2006;67:954–959.
4. Savettieri G, Messina D, Andreoli V, et al. Gender-related effect of clinical and genetic variables on the cognitive impairment in multiple sclerosis. *J Neurol.* 2004;251:1208–1214.
5. Ghezzi A, Zaffaroni M. Female-specific issues in multiple sclerosis. *Expert Rev Neurother.* 2008;8(6):969–977.
6. Coyle PK. Gender issues. *Neural Clin.* 2005;23:39–60.
7. Li R, Sun X, Shu Y, et al. Sex differences in outcomes of disease-modifying treatments for multiple sclerosis: a systematic review. *Mult Scler Relat Disord.* February 2017;12:23–28.
8. Rudick RA, Kappos L, Kinkel R, et al. Gender effects on intramuscular interferon beta-1a in relapsing-remitting multiple sclerosis: analysis of 1406 patients. *Mult Scler.* 2011;17:353–360.
9. Magyari M, Koch-Henriksen N, Laursen B, et al. Gender effects on treatment response to interferon-beta in multiple sclerosis. *Acta Neurol Scand.* 2014;130:374–379.
10. Trojano M, Pellegrini F, Paolicelli D, et al. Post-marketing of disease modifying drugs in multiple sclerosis: an exploratory analysis of gender effect in interferon beta treatment. *J Neurol Sci.* 2009;286:109–113.

11. Wolinsky JS, Narayana PA, O'Connor P, et al. Glatiramer acetate in primary progressive multiple sclerosis: results of a multinational, multicenter, double-blind, placebo-controlled trial. *Ann Neurol.* 2007;61:14–24.
12. Whitacre C. Sex differences in autoimmune disease. *Nat Immunol.* 2001;2:777–780.
13. Greer J, McCombe P. Role of gender in multiple sclerosis: clinical effect and potential molecular mechanisms. *J Neuroimmunol.* 2011;234(5):7–18.
14. Sharrief K. Cytokines in multiple sclerosis: pro-inflammation or pro-remyelination? *Mult Scler.* 1998;4:169–173.
15. Gilmore W, Weiner LP, Correale J. Effect of estradiol on cytokine secretion by proteolipid protein-specific T cell clones isolated from multiple sclerosis patients and normal control subjects. *J Immunol.* 1997;158:446–451.
16. Schwendimann R, Alekseeva N. Gender issues in multiple sclerosis. *Int Rev Neurobiol.* 2007;79:377–392.
17. Ramagopalan S, Knight J, Ebers G. Multiple sclerosis and the major histocompatibility complex. *Curr Opin Neurol.* 2009;22(3):219–225.
18. Jansson L, Olsson T, Holmdahl R. Estrogen induces a potent suppression of experimental autoimmune encephalomyelitis and collagen-induced arthritis in mice. *J Neuroimmunol.* 1994;53:203–207.
19. Sicotte NL, Live SM, Klutch R, et al. Treatment of multiple sclerosis with the pregnancy hormone estriol. *Ann Neurol.* 2002;52:421–428.
20. Voskuhl R, Wang H, Wu TC, et al. Estriol combined with glatiramer acetate for women with relapsing-remitting multiple sclerosis: a randomised, placebo-controlled, phase 2 trial. *Lancet Neurol.* 2016;15:35–46.
21. Eckler K. Are all estrogens created equal? *Menopause.* 2004;11:7–8.
22. Enmark E, Gustafsson JA. Oestrogen receptors—an overview. *J Intern Med.* 1999;246:133–138.
23. Lemon HM. Oestriol and prevention of breast cancer. *Lancet.* 1973;1:546–547.
24. Hutchinson M. Oestrogen therapy for multiple sclerosis: not the way forward. *Int MS J.* 2003;10(3):98.
25. Alonso A, Jick SS, Olek MJ, et al. Recent use of oral contraceptives and the risk of multiple sclerosis. *Arch Neurol.* 2005;62:1362–1365.
26. Thorogood M, Hannaford PC. The influence of oral contraceptives on the risk of multiple sclerosis. *Br J Obstet Gynaecol.* 1998;105:1296–1299.
27. Houtchens MK, Zapata LB, Curtis KM, et al. Contraception for women with multiple sclerosis: guidance for healthcare providers. *Mult Scler.* 2017;23(6):757–764.
28. Antonovsky A, Leibowitz U, Smith HA, et al. Epidemiologic study of multiple sclerosis in Israel. I. An overall review of methods and findings. *Arch Neurol.* 1965;13:183–193.
29. Gustavsen MW, Page CM, Moen SM, et al. Environmental exposures and the risk of multiple sclerosis investigated in a Norwegian case-control study. *BMC Neurol.* 2014;14:196.
30. Ramagopalan SV, Valdar W, Criscuoli M, et al. Age of puberty and the risk of multiple sclerosis: a population based study. *Eur J Neurol.* 2009;16:342–347.
31. Nielsen N, Harpsøe M, Simonsen J, et al. Age at menarche and risk of multiple sclerosis: a prospective cohort study based on the Danish national birth cohort. *Am J Epidemiol.* March 2017; 185(8):712–719.
32. Sloka JS, Pryse-Phillips WE, Stefanelli M. The relation between menarche and the age of first symptoms in a multiple sclerosis cohort. *Mult Scler.* 2006;12(3):333–339.
33. Lulu S, Graves J, Waubant E. Menarche increases relapse risk in pediatric multiple sclerosis. *Mult Scler.* 2016;22(2):193–200.
34. Wilson S, Donnan P, Swingrem R, et al. A serial observational study on hormonal influences in MS symptoms. *Mult Scler.* 2004;SS188–SS189.
35. Zordrager A, DeKeyser J. The premenstrual period and exacerbations in multiple sclerosis. *Eur Neurol.* 2002;48:204–206.
36. Cavalla P, Rovei V, Masera S, et al. Fertility in patients with multiple sclerosis: current knowledge and future perspectives. *Neurol Sci.* 2006;27:231–239.
37. Ferraro D, Simone AM, Adani G, et al. Definitive childlessness in women with multiple sclerosis: a multicenter study. *Neurol Sci.* 2017;38(8):1–7. doi:10.1007/s10072-017-2999-1.
38. Cohen BA, Mikol DD. Mitoxantrone treatment of multiple sclerosis: safety considerations. *Neurology.* 2004;63(suppl 6):S28-S32.
39. Lew-Starowicz M, Rola R. Prevalence of sexual dysfunctions among women with multiple sclerosis. *Sex Disabil.* 2013;31:141–153.
40. Nortvedt MW, Riise T, Frugård J, et al. Prevalence of bladder, bowel and sexual problems among multiple sclerosis patients two to five years after diagnosis. *Mult Scler.* January 2007;13(1):106–112.
41. Foley FW. Assessment and treatment of sexual dysfunction in multiple sclerosis. In: Giesser, BS, ed. *Primer on Multiple Sclerosis.* 2nd ed. Los Angeles, CA: Oxford University Press; 2016.
42. Bartnik P, Wielgos A, Kacperczyk J, et al. Sexual dysfunction in female patients with relapsing-remitting multiple sclerosis. *Brain Behav.* 2017;7:e00699.
43. Schairer LC, Foley FW, Zemon V, et al. The impact of sexual dysfunction on health-related quality of life in people with multiple sclerosis. *Mult Scler.* April 2014;20(5):610–616.
44. Stenager E, Stenager EN, Jensen K. Effect of pregnancy on the prognosis for multiple sclerosis, a 5-year follow-up and investigation. *Acta Neurol Scand.* 1994;90:305–308.
45. Dwosh E, Guimond C, Duquette P, et al. The interaction of MS and pregnancy: a critical review. *Int MS J.* 2003;10:38–42.
46. Runmarker B, Andersen O. Pregnancy is associated with a lower risk of onset and a better prognosis in multiple sclerosis. *Brain.* 1995;118(pt 1):253–261.
47. Masera S, Cavalla P, Prosperini L, et al. Pariety is associated with longer time to reach irreversible disability milestones in women with multiple sclerosis. *Mult Scler.* 2015;21(10):1291–1297.
48. D'Hooghe MB, Nagels G, Uitdehaag BM. Long-term effects of childbirth in MS. *J Neurol Neurosorg Psychiatry.* 2010;81(1):38–41.
49. Karp I, Manganas A, Sylvestre MP, et al. Does pregnancy alter the long-term course of multiple sclerosis? *Ann Epidemiol.* 2014;24:504–508.
50. Caon C. Pregnancy in MS. In: Olek MJ, ed. *Multiple Sclerosis.* Totowa, NJ: Humana; 2005:145–159.
51. Confavreux C, Hutchinson M, Hours MM, et al. Rate of pregnancy related relapse in multiple sclerosis. *N Engl J Med.* 1998;339(5):285–291.
52. Salemi G, Callari G, Gammino M, et al. The relapse rate of multiple sclerosis changes during pregnancy: a cohort study. *Acta Neurol Scand.* 2004;110(1):23–26.
53. Fragoso YD, Finkelsztejn A, Comini-Frota ER, et al. Pregnancy and multiple sclerosis: the initial results from a Brazilian database. *Arq Neuropsiquiatr.* 2009;67(3A):657–660.
54. Vukusic S, Hutchinson M, Hours M, et al. Pregnancy and multiple sclerosis (the PRIMS study): clinical predictors of post-partum relapse. *Brain.* 2004;127(pt 6):1353–1360.
55. Hughes SE, Spelman T, Gray OM, et al. Predictors and dynamics of postpartum relapses in women with multiple sclerosis. *Mult Scler.* 2014;20(6):739–746.
56. Yalcin SE, Yalcin Y, Yavuz A, et al. Maternal and perinatal outcomes in pregnancies with multiple sclerosis: a case-control study. *J Perin Med.* 2016;45(4):455–460.
57. Ferrero S, Pretta S, Ragni N. Multiple sclerosis: management issues during pregnancy. *Eur J Obstet Gynecol Reprod Biol.* 2004;115:3–9.
58. Hupperts R, Broadley S, Mander A, et al. Patterns of disease in concordant parent-child pairs with multiple sclerosis. *Neurology.* 2001;57:290–295.
59. Kantarci OH, Barcellos LF, Atkinson EJ, et al. Men transmit MS more often to their children vs. women: the Carter effect. *Neurology.* 2006;67:305–310.
60. Herrera BM, Ramagopalan SV, Orton S, et al. Parental transmission of MS in a population-based Canadian cohort. *Neurology.* 2007;69:1208–1212.
61. Tsui A, Lee M. Multiple sclerosis and pregnancy. *Curr Opin Obstet Gynecol.* 2011;23:435–439.

62. Sandberg-Wolheim M, Frank D, Goodwin TM, et al. Pregnancy outcomes during treatment with interferon β-1a in patients with multiple sclerosis. *Neurology*. 2005;65(6):802–806.

63. Sandberg-Wollheim M, Alteri E, Moraga MS, et al. Pregnancy outcomes in multiple sclerosis following subcutaneous interferon beta-1a therapy. *Mult Scler*. 2011;17(4):423–430.

64. Coyle PK, Sinclair SM, Scheuerle AE, et al. Final results from the Betaseron (interferon β-1b) pregnancy registry: a prospective observational study of birth defects and pregnancy-related adverse events. *BMJ Open*. 2014;4:e004536.

65. Boskovic R, Wide R, Wolpin J, et al. The reproductive effects of β interferon therapy in pregnancy: a longitudinal cohort. *Neurology*. 2005;65(6):807–811.

66. Ferrero S, Esposito F, Pretta S, et al. Fetal risks related to the treatment of multiple sclerosis during pregnancy and breastfeeding. *Expert Rev Neurother*. 2006;6(12):1823–1831.

67. Fragoso Y. Glatiramer acetate to treat multiple sclerosis during pregnancy and lactation: a safety evaluation. *Expert Opin Drug Saf*. 2014;13(12):1743–1748.

68. Coyle PK, Johnson K, Pardo L, et al. Pregnancy outcomes in patients with multiple sclerosis treated with glatiramer acetate (Copaxone 1). In: *Proceedings of the 55th Annual Meeting of the American Academy of Neurology*. Honolulu, Hawaii; March 29–April 5, 2003. *Neurology*. 2003;60(5)(suppl 1). A60 [abstract].

69. Herbstritt SA, Glatiramer acetate during early pregnancy: a prospective cohort study. *Mult Scler*. 2016;22(6):810–816.

70. GILENYA (fingolimod) capsules, for oral use. Full Prescribing Information. Available at: https://www.pharma.us.novartis.com/sites/www.pharma.us.novartis.com/files/gilenya.pdf. Revised February 2016. Accessed July 9, 2017.

71. Gilenya-Product Information as approved by the CHMP on 19 April 2012, pending endorsement by the European Commission. Available at: http://www.ema.europa.eu/docs/en_GB/document_library/Other/2012/04/WC500125687.pdf. Accessed July 9, 2017.

72. Karlsson G, Francis G, Koren G, et al. Pregnancy outcomes in the clinical development program of fingolimod in multiple sclerosis. *Neurology*. 2014;82(8):674–680.

73. Gold R, Phillips JT, Havrdova E, et al. Delayed-release dimethyl fumarate and pregnancy: preclinical studies and pregnancy outcomes from clinical trials and postmarketing experience. *Neurol Ther*. 2015;4:93–104.

74. TECFIDERA (dimethyl fumarate) delayed-release capsules, for oral use. Available at: https://www.tecfidera.com/content/dam/commercial/multiple-sclerosis/tecfidera/pat/en_us/pdf/full-prescribing-info.pdf. Revised January 2017. Accessed July 10, 2017.

75. https://www.accessdata.fda.gov/drugsatfda_docs/label/2012/202992s000lbl.pdf. Accessed November 24, 2012.

76. AUBAGIO (teriflunomide) tablets, for oral use: highlights of prescribing information. Available at: http://products.sanofi.us/aubagio/aubagio.pdf. Revised November 2016. Accessed July 11, 2017.

77. Kieseier B, Benamor M. Pregnancy outcomes following maternal and paternal exposure to teriflunomide during treatment for relapsing–remitting multiple sclerosis. *Neurol Ther*. 2014;3:133–138.

78. TYSABRI (natalizumab) injection, for intravenous use: Highlights of Prescribing Information. Available at: https://www.tysabri.com/content/dam/commercial/multiple-sclerosis/tysabri/pat/en_us/pdfs/tysabri_prescribing_information.pdf. Revised May 2016. Accessed July 11, 2017.

79. Friend S, Richman S, Bloomgren G, et al. Evaluation of pregnancy outcomes from the Tysabri® (natalizumab) pregnancy exposure registry: a global, observational, follow-up study. *BMC Neurol*. 2016;16:150.

80. Ebrahimi N, Herbstritt S, Gold R, et al. Pregnancy and fetal outcomes following natalizumab exposure in pregnancy. A prospective, controlled observational study. *Mult Scler*. 2015;21(2):198–205.

81. Haghikia A. Natalizumab use during the third trimester of pregnancy. *JAMA Neurol*. 2014;71(7):891–895.

82. CAMPATH (alemtuzumab) injection for intravenous use: highlights of prescribing information. Available at: http://www.campath.com/pdfs/2014-09-Campath_US_PI.pdf. Revised 2014. Accessed July 12, 2017.

83. Oh J, Achiron A, Chambers C, et al. Pregnancy outcomes in patients with RRMS who received Alemtuzumab in the clinical development program (S24.008). Abstract presented at: American Academy of Neurology Annual Meeting; April 15–21, 2016; Vancouver, British Columbia. *Neurology*. April 5, 2016;86(suppl 16):S24.008.

84. RITUXAN (rituximab) injection, for intravenous use: highlights of prescribing information. Available at: https://www.gene.com/download/pdf/rituxan_prescribing.pdf. Revised April 2016. Accessed July 13, 2017.

85. OCREVUS (ocrelizumab) injection, for intravenous use: highlights of prescribing information. Available at: https://www.accessdata.fda.gov/drugsatfda_docs/label/2017/761053lbl.pdf. Revised March 2017. Accessed July 13, 2017.

86. Chakravarty E, Murray ER, Kelman A, et al. Pregnancy outcomes after maternal exposure to rituximab. *Blood*. 2011;117:1499–1506.

87. Park-Wyllie L, Mazzotta P, Pastuszak A, et al. Birth defects after maternal exposure to corticosteroids: prospective cohort study and meta-analysis of epidemiological studies. *Teratology*. 2000;62:385–392.

88. Nonacs R. *SSRIs and PPHN: A Review of the Data* [Internet]. Boston, MA: Massachusetts General Hospital, Center for Women's Mental Health; November 10, 2009. Available at: http://www.womensmentalhealth.org/posts/ssris-and-pphn-a-review-of-the-data/

89. Wurst KE, Poole C, Ephross SA, et al. First trimester paroxetine use and the prevalence of congenital, specifically cardiac, defects: a meta-analysis of epidemiological studies. *Birth Defects Res A Clin Mol Teratol*. 2010;88:159.

90. Micromedex® Healthcare Series [intranet database]. Version 5.1. Greenwood Village, CO: Thomson Reuters (Healthcare) Inc. Available at: http://www.micromedexsolutions.com/micromedex2/librarian. Accessed November 8, 2012.

91. Beitans Beitins IZ, Bayard F, Ances IG, et al. The transplacental passage of prednisone and prednisolone in pregnancy near term. *J Pediatr*. 1972;81:936–945.

92. Homar V, Grosek S, Battelino T. High-dose methylprednisolone in a pregnant woman with Crohn's disease and adrenal suppression in her newborn. *Neonatology*. 2008;94:306–309.

93. Haas J. High dose IVIG in the postpartum period for prevention of exacerbation of MS. *Mult Scler*. 2000;6(suppl 2):S18–S20.

94. Achiron A, Kischner I, Dolev M, et al. Effect of intravenous immunoglobulin treatment on pregnancy and postpartum-related relapses in multiple sclerosis. *J Neurol*. 2004;251(9):1133–1137.

95. Vukusic S, Ionescu I, El-Etr M, et al. The prevention of postpartum relapses with progestin and estradiol in multiple sclerosis (POPART'MUS) trial: rationale, objectives and state of advancement. *J Neurol Sci*. 2009;286:114–118.

96. Vukusic S, Ionescu I, El-Etr M. Post partum progestin and estriol in multiple sclerosis. 28th Congress of the European Committee for Treatment and Research in Multiple Sclerosis (ECTRIMS). Abstract 143. Presented October 12, 2012.

97. Langer-Gould A, Huang S, Gupta R, et al. Exclusive breastfeeding and the risk of postpartum relapses in women in multiple sclerosis. *Arch Neurol*. 2009;66(8):958–963.

98. Langer-Gould A, Gupta R, Huang S, et al., Interferon- gamma-producing T cells, pregnancy, and postpartum relapses of multiple sclerosis. *Arch. Neurol*. 2010;67:51–57.

99. Hellwig K, Kuge M, Gold R, et al. When supplemental infant feedings begin, postpartum multiple sclerosis relapses return. *Neurology*. 2012;78:P06.186.

100. Portaccio E, Ghezzi A, Hakiki B, et al. Breastfeeding is not related to postpartum relapses in multiple sclerosis. *Neurology*. 2011;77(2):145–150.

101. Langer-Gould A, Beaber B. Effects of pregnancy and breast-feeding on the multiple sclerosis disease course. *Clin Immunol.* 2013;149:244–250.
102. Ost L, Wettrell G, Björkhem I, et al. Prednisolone excretion in human milk. *J Pediatr.* 1985;106(6):1008.
103. Cooper S, Felkins K, Baker T, et al. Transfer of methylprednisolone into breast milk in a mother with multiple sclerosis. *J Hum Lact.* May 31, 2015;31(2):237–239.
104. Hale TW, Siddiqui AA, Baker TE. Transfer of interferon B-1a into human breastmilk. *Breastfeed Med.* 2012;7(2):123–125.
105. Ray JG, Vermeulen MJ, Bharatha A, et al. Association between MRI exposure during pregnancy and fetal and childhood outcomes. *JAMA.* 2016;316(9):952–961.
106. ACR Manual on Contrast Media. Version 10.3. 98. Administration of contrast media to pregnant or potentially pregnant patients. Available at: https://www.acr.org/-/media/ACR/Files/Clinical-Resources/Contrast_Media.pdf. Revised June 15, 2017. Accessed July 31, 2017.
107. Rofsky NM, Weinreb JC, Litt AW. Quantitative analysis of gadopentate diglumine excreted in breast milk. *J Magn Reson Imaging.* 1993;3:131–132.
108. Kubik-Huch RA, Gottstein Alame NM, Frenzel T, et al. Gadopentetate diglumine excretion into human breast milk during lactation. *Radiology.* 2000;216:555–558.
109. Smith R, Studd JW. A pilot study of the effect upon multiple sclerosis of the menopause, hormone replacement therapy and the menstrual cycle. *J R Soc Med.* 1992;85(10):612–613.
110. Bove R, Healy B, Musallam A, et al. Exploration of changes in disability after menopause in a longitudinal multiple sclerosis cohort. *Mult Scler.* June 2016;22(7):935–943.
111. Holmqvist P, Wallberg M, Hammar M, et al. Symptoms of multiple sclerosis in women in relation to sex steroid exposure. *Maturitas.* 2006;54:149–153.
112. Bove R, White CC, Fitzgerald KC, et al. Hormone therapy use and physical quality of life in postmenopausal women with multiple sclerosis. *Neurology.* October 4, 2016;87(14):1457–1463.

35 Multiple Sclerosis and Associated Comorbidities

Yuval Karmon, Caila B. Vaughn, Shumita Roy, Svetlana Primma Eckert, and Bianca Weinstock-Guttman

---

KEY POINTS FOR CLINICIANS

- The most commonly reported comorbidities in multiple sclerosis (MS) are depression, anxiety, hypertension, hyperlipidemia, and chronic lung disease.
- Several studies have shown an increased rate of vascular comorbidities in MS patients.
- Presence of vascular comorbidities may delay MS diagnosis and hasten disability progression.
- Smoking has been reported to adversely affect the risk for MS disease progression.
- A less favorable lipid profile (high low-density lipoprotein [LDL]-C) has been shown to be associated with a worse MS outcome.
- Hypothyroidism is one of the most common autoimmune comorbidities in MS patients and should always be screened for and addressed, especially in interferon-treated patients, as it can affect fatigue, cognitive functions, and mood, as well as general well-being.
- Higher reported rates of mood disorders (including depression) and sleep disorders (insomnia, obstructive sleep apnea, and restless leg syndrome) were reported in MS patients.
- Late onset MS can be ascertained in patients older than 50 years, and is characterized by a lower rate of relapsing disease, usually presenting with a primary progressive course, or an earlier conversion to a secondary progressive course.

COMORBIDITIES IN MULTIPLE SCLEROSIS

Comorbidity in general refers to the cumulative burden of illnesses other than the disease of main interest (1). Comorbidities are not limited to a specific disease or population, and as expected their extent and frequency increase with age, adding to the morbidity associated with the primary condition (1). MS is a chronic disease that affects the central nervous system (CNS), and is considered the second most common cause of disability among young adults after trauma (2). Comorbid health behaviors and lifestyle factors, such as smoking, alcohol intake, and limited physical activity, can substantially affect the risk and outcomes of chronic diseases in general, and of MS in particular.

Overview

Over the last few years, several studies underscoring the high prevalence and importance of comorbidities were reported. It was found that the most commonly reported comorbidities in MS were depression, anxiety, hypertension, hyperlipidemia, and chronic lung disease (3). Interestingly, most of them were commonly present at the time of MS diagnosis.

Various comorbidities as well as smoking have been found to be associated with diagnostic delays (4), lower adherence to treatment, increased disability progression (5), increased hospitalization and healthcare utilization (6), and, most importantly, lower health-related quality of life (morbidity) and higher mortality (7,8).

Timely recognition of comorbid conditions in clinical practice is the most desirable goal, and the aim of this chapter is to increase the awareness for medical comorbid health conditions in patients with MS.

Most comorbidities can be managed with medications or lifestyle changes.

Mental Comorbidities

As mentioned earlier, depression and anxiety were found to be of the most common comorbidities in MS patients and frequently are the most difficult to address. Their impact on quality of life is considerable. Depression in MS patients has a lifetime prevalence of 50%, whereas anxiety has a lifetime prevalence of 36%. These comorbidities are discussed in detail in Chapter 20.

Vascular Comorbidities

The clinical heterogeneity observed among MS patients may stem from different factors including underlying comorbidities. A study (n = 8,983) in the North American Research Committee on Multiple Sclerosis (NARCOMS) registry evaluated the association between disability in MS and the presence of several vascular risk factors (9). Participants who reported more than one vascular comorbidity (diabetes, hypertension, heart disease, hypercholesterolemia, and peripheral vascular disease) at the time of diagnosis had a higher risk of ambulatory disability, and the risk increased with the number of vascular conditions reported (hazard ratio [HR]/condition for early gait disability 1.51; 95% confidence interval [CI]: 1.41–1.61). Vascular comorbidities at any point during the disease course also raised the risk of ambulatory disability (adjusted HR for unilateral walking assistance 1.54; CI: 1.44–1.65). This study suggests that outcome in MS might be affected by vascular comorbidities developed at the time of MS symptom onset, or later during the disease course.

In another publication on the same patient sample, the presence of obesity, smoking, and physical or mental comorbidities was associated with a significant delay in diagnosing MS (for up to 11 years from the time of symptom onset) (5). This effect persisted even after accounting for demographic and clinical characteristics. These results were further confirmed in a recent Danish study where preexisting comorbidities including cerebrovascular, cardiovascular, lung, and cancer comorbidities increased the risk for diagnostic delays of MS with odds ratios (OR) for delaying the diagnosis as high as 4.04 in patients with cardiovascular comorbidities. The authors also showed increased mortality in MS patients with psychiatric, cerebrovascular, cardiovascular, lung, diabetes, and cancer comorbidities as well (8). Possible explanations include the presence of a preexisting disease that can mask the symptoms of MS, and new symptoms being mistakenly attributed to the preexisting condition. Additionally, for both cardiovascular disease (CVD) and lung disease, adverse health behaviors, such as

smoking and other injurious lifestyle behaviors, may entail disregard for new symptoms, potentially causing hesitancy to seeking medical advice (8). The existing burden of illness could also negatively affect the MS outcomes in general.

Further analysis showed that vascular, musculoskeletal, and psychiatric comorbidities, and obesity were associated with more severe disability at the time of MS diagnosis. After adjustment, the OR for moderate disability compared with mild disability at diagnosis was 1.51 (CI: 1.12–2.05) in participants with a vascular comorbidity and 1.38 (CI: 1.02–1.87) in those with obesity (5). These findings were recently replicated in a population-based cohort (8). A potential approach to slowing MS progression may require a more aggressive management of vascular and other comorbidities, including behavioral changes (e.g., dietary intervention, active exercise programs, and smoking cessation).

Two nationwide Danish studies evaluating mortality among MS patients reported that patients with MS had a 30% higher risk of death due to CVD, including cerebrovascular disease, compared with the age-matched general population (10,11), while a 6% higher risk of death due to CVD (excluding stroke) was observed in a study from South Wales (12). Another Danish study (13) showed that the risk of CVD among MS patients is still low, yet higher than in the general population, particularly in the short-term correcting for age. The risk of myocardial infarction (MI) was 0.2% among patients with MS (adjusted infusion-related reactions [IRR] = 1.84; 95% CI: 1.28–2.65, compared with population cohort members), whereas the 1-year risk of stroke was 0.3% (adjusted IRR = 1.96; 95% CI: 1.42–2.71), and the IRR for heart failure was 1.92 (95% CI: 1.27–2.90). A possible explanation may be that increased prevalence of CVD is often associated with reduced mobility and ability to exercise, as recently shown in a large cohort of MS patients (14,15).

Hyperlipidemia

The retrospective analysis of NARCOMS registry participants mentioned earlier reported that dyslipidemia was associated with an increased risk for disability progression in MS (5,9). In a previously published study, our group showed that fasting serum lipid profile evaluated in a group of 492 MS patients (age: 47.1 ± 10.8 years; disease duration: 12.8 ± 10.1 years) followed for approximately 2 years (2.2 ± 1.0 years) correlated with disability and MRI outcomes (quantitative MRI findings at baseline were available for 210 patients). Expanded Disability Status Scale (EDSS) worsening was associated with higher baseline LDL (p = .006) and total cholesterol (p = .001) levels, with trends for higher triglyceride levels (p = .025); high-density lipoprotein (HDL) was not associated with clinical disease status. A similar pattern was found for MS Severity Score (MSSS) worsening (p = .008 for total cholesterol). However, higher HDL levels (p < .001) were associated with lower contrast-enhancing lesion volume. Higher total cholesterol was associated with a trend for lower brain parenchymal fraction (p = .033) (16). Increased total cholesterol was also found to be associated with increases in the number of contrast-enhancing lesions on brain MRI in clinically isolated syndrome (CIS) patients following a first clinical demyelinating event (17).

Dyslipidemia can potentiate inflammatory processes at the vascular endothelium, possibly leading to the induction of adhesion molecules and the recruitment of monocytes (18–20). Associations between dyslipidemia and increased inflammation are well established in conditions such as atherosclerosis, CVD, metabolic syndrome, and obesity (21). Similarly, in the context of other autoimmune diseases, a strong association between dyslipidemia and CVD was shown in systemic lupus erythematosus (SLE) (22) and an increased cardiovascular risk and dyslipidemia have been reported in rheumatoid arthritis (23) as well. HDL and LDL also modulate the function and survival of pancreatic beta cells in type 2 diabetes mellitus (24). Neuromyelitis optica patients were reported to have significantly higher serum cholesterol triglycerides but lower LDL compared to healthy controls (25). Therefore, a direct influence of hyperlipidemia on the inflammatory and/or neurodegenerative processes in MS (in addition to the known increased risk for cardiovascular pathology) is possible.

Smoking

Smoking was shown to be associated with an increased risk to develop MS (26). More recently, the relation of smoking to disease progression was also evaluated, the results being still contradictory (27,28). One study, which included 780 MS patients who had never smoked, 428 ex-smokers, and 257 who currently smoked, found that current smokers (OR 2.42, 95% CI: 1.09–5.35) and ex-smokers (1.91, 1.02–3.58) were more likely to present with primary progressive MS (PPMS) than with relapsing–remitting MS (RRMS). Potential confounders (comorbid obesity or vascular risk factors) were unfortunately not assessed in this study (29).

Several studies also suggest that smoking is associated with an increased risk of disability progression in patients with MS. In a study using information from the General Practice Research Database (30), smokers with RRMS were three times more likely to develop secondary progressive MS (SPMS) than were nonsmokers, whereas only 20 of 179 patients who were never-smokers or ever-smokers had a progressive course. In another study of individuals with newly diagnosed MS ($n = 122$), the proportion of patients who developed SPMS after a median follow-up time of 6 years was 72% for ever-smokers who began smoking before the age of 15 years, 40% for ever-smokers who began smoking after the age of 15 years, but only 26% for those who had never smoked (31). Another study followed 129 patients with a CIS who were at high risk of developing MS on the basis of findings from MRI and cerebrospinal fluid (CSF) examination. After 3 years, 75% of smokers developed MS compared with only 51% of nonsmokers (HR 1.8, 95% CI: 1.2–2.8). In two studies including the one from our

group (27,29), smoking was associated with an increased number of gadolinium-enhancing lesions, increased T2-weighted lesion volume, and greater brain atrophy (27). Neither study included a control group of smokers without MS to assess whether smoking has additive or multiplicative effects on brain imaging measures, such as brain volume.

Antiphospholipid Antibodies

Although antiphospholipid antibody syndrome (APLS) was first described in the context of connective tissue diseases such as SLE, it was soon recognized that the condition can exist as an isolated syndrome. Primary APLS (PAPLS) is an autoimmune disorder characterized by recurrent thrombosis, miscarriages, and thrombocytopenia in the presence of antiphospholipid antibodies (APLA) and persistently positive (+) anticardiolipin or lupus anticoagulant (LA) tests. It has been established that APLAs are heterogeneous and bind to various antigenic targets (32). Some studies reported a higher prevalence of various APLAs in MS as compared to other neurological disorders (33). When MRIs of MS patients were compared to those of PAPLS patients (34), they showed significantly higher T2 and T1 lesion volumes. The same study also demonstrated that APLA+ RRMS and SPMS patients showed significantly higher T2 lesion volume, lower gray matter fraction (GMF), and lower normal-appearing gray matter magnetization transfer ratio (MTR) when compared to APLA− patients (35). It is possible that APLA mediates heterogeneous cerebral pathology that needs to be further investigated. A recent study from our group suggests that prospectively followed APLA+ RRMS patients treated with interferon beta (IFNb)-1a developed more severe MRI and clinical disease activity (relapses and sustained disability progression) as compared with APLA− RRMS patients treated with IFNb-1a (36), although a decreased effect of IFN cannot be ruled out.

Recently, it was suggested that some phospholipids actually serve as natural anti-inflammatory compounds. Several autoantibodies in MS were found to target a phosphate group in phosphatidylserine and oxidized phosphatidylcholine derivatives (Table 35.1) (38). The presence of certain APLAs, therefore, might be a marker for an ongoing systemic underlying inflammatory process. On the other hand, administration of those phospholipids might also become an optional MS therapy in the future.

Other Autoimmune Comorbidities

Several studies investigating the prevalence of other autoimmune comorbidities in MS compared with the general population showed conflicting results (41,46,47), often related to differences in study design (48). Although the targeted autoimmune diseases were found more frequently in MS patients compared to the general population, their absolute frequency is low; therefore, their presence is unlikely to have a substantial effect on MS at the population level, but may have an impact at the individual level (Table 35.1).

TABLE 35.1 Evidence Supporting the Role of Comorbidities in MS

COMORBIDITY OR RISK FACTOR	REFERENCES	FINDINGS
CV comorbidity	(5,9,37) (NARCOMS registry) (5,9,37) (10–13)	A higher risk to develop ambulatory disability with the presence of more vascular risk factors Median time to disability shortens with presence of vascular risk factors (12.8 vs. 18.8 y) Risk of CV death is higher than in general population
Smoking	(26) (27–31) (27,29)	Is associated with increased risk to develop MS Its association with MS progression is controversial Was associated with more brain atrophy, Gad-positive lesions, and T2-weighted lesion volume
Hyperlipidemia	(5,9,37) (16) (16) (16)	Retrospective analysis of NARCOMS registry: dyslipidemia was associated with an increased risk for disability progression in MS Fasting serum lipid profile evaluated in 492 patients correlated with disability and MRI outcomes EDSS worsening was associated with higher baseline LDL and total cholesterol Higher HDL levels were associated with lower contrast-enhancing lesion volume
APLA	(35) (36) (38)	APLA+ RRMS/SPMS had higher T2 lesion volume, lower GMF, and lower normal-appearing gray matter MTR when compared to APLA– patients APLA+ RRMS patients treated with IFN beta-1a developed more severe MRI and clinical disease activity (relapses, and sustained disability progression) as compared with APLA– RRMS patients treated with IFN beta-1a Administration of phosphatidylserine and oxidized phosphatidylcholine derivatives ameliorated EAE by suppressing activation and inducing apoptosis of autoreactive T cells
Autoimmune comorbidities	(100,101) (39,40) (41–43) (44,45)	Inflammatory bowel disease—questionable association (conflicting results) Varying rates for rheumatoid arthritis in MS (0.9%–4.4%) Hypothyroidism rates are considered to be high in MS male and female patients (up to 9%)

APLA+, antiphospholipid antibodies positive; APLA–, antiphospholipid antibodies negative; CV, cardiovascular; EAE, experimental autoimmune encephalomyelitis; EDSS, Expanded Disability Status Scale; GMF, gray matter fraction; HDL, high-density lipoprotein; IFN, interferon; LDL, low-density lipoprotein; MS, multiple sclerosis; MTR, magnetization transfer ratio; NARCOMS, North American Research Committee on Multiple Sclerosis; RRMS, remitting–relapsing MS; SPMS, secondary progressive MS.

In the New York State Multiple Sclerosis Consortium (NYSMSC) study (42) (n = 3,019), 0.8% of patients with MS had comorbid SLE, and an even higher rate of SLE was observed in MS patients' relatives (1.8%). Varying frequencies were also reported for rheumatoid arthritis (RA) (41–43) (0.9%–4.4%). Data from the NYSMSC revealed a much higher rate of RA, 9.8% in first-degree relatives of MS patients compared with the patients themselves (2%) (42). Thyroid dysfunction was also reported to be more frequent than expected in MS patients, with frequencies of up to 9% in both males and females (47). This rate was actually found to be significantly higher than a control group only for male MS patients in particular (control group rates: male 1.9%, female 9.2%). Two other studies (44,45) using a control or reference group identified an increased risk. Therefore, MS patients should be screened for thyroid dysfunction (often related to autoimmune thyroiditis), as it could affect energy level, fatigue, mood, and cognitive functions significantly, and proper management should be initiated, since it is easily treatable.

Disease-modifying therapies approved for MS can be also associated with secondary development of autoimmune diseases (see Chapters 13 and 14). IFNb therapy has been reported to induce antithyroid antibodies and to precipitate thyroid clinical disease in patients with preexisting antibodies (49,50). Okanoue and colleagues have suggested that IFNb can induce autoimmune disorders including autoimmune thyroiditis, hemolytic anemia, thrombocytopenia, SLE, rheumatoid arthritis, and psoriasis. However, these autoimmune diseases (except for autoimmune thyroiditis) are in general rare events among IFNb therapy users, and may develop at a higher frequency in MS patients in general, as previously mentioned (51). There are also rare reported cases of IFNb-associated SLE in the literature and subacute cutaneous lupus has been previously reported (52). Crispin and Diaz-Jouanen described a case of a woman who developed SLE while on continuous therapy with IFNb-1a for 3 years (53). Occasional cases of myasthenia gravis following IFNb therapy have also been described (54). Treatment with glatiramer acetate (GA) was also reported to be associated with autoimmune diseases such as Crohn's disease, myasthenia gravis, and arthritis (55–58).

New challenges are also envisioned as novel immunologically active agents were incorporated into the MS therapeutic arsenal. An increased risk for autoimmune diseases was observed in patients treated with alemtuzumab (Lemtrada®), a very potent treatment for RRMS. Thyroid disease was seen most frequently, in approximately 40% of treated patients (59), and individual risk was shown to be modified by smoking and family history of autoimmune diseases, which should be incorporated into the patient counseling process prior to treatment initiation (60).

Other Comorbidities

Physical comorbidities other than autoimmune diseases seem to be common in patients with MS as well. Comorbidities reported in the large NARCOMS registry sample, besides the ones already mentioned, included arthritis (16%, excluding RA), irritable bowel syndrome (13%), and chronic lung disease (13%) (61). This list includes three of the five leading causes of disability in the general population (hypertension, lung disease, arthritis, back or spine problems, and heart disease) (62). In the parallel self-report from the nationally representative Canadian Community Health Survey (63), 302 respondents with MS reported comorbidities that included back problems (35%), nonfood allergies (29%), arthritis (26%), hypertension (17%), and migraine (14%). All these comorbidities have to be assessed, differentiated from MS-related deficits and symptoms, and treated appropriately. Data from several studies have indicated that sleep disorders and related disorders are more common in patients with MS than in the general population (64). In a large cohort of U.S. veterans with MS (n = 16,074), 940 (6%) had sleep disorders compared with 3% of veterans without MS. Sleep disturbance was defined as the presence of at least one abnormal diagnostic polysomnogram or sleep disorder identified during study period (65). Restless legs syndrome (RLS) was also reported with a frequency ranging from 13.3% to 37.5% depending on the cohort studied (66,67). In most of these studies, RLS occurred substantially more often in individuals with MS than in the general population. A screening questionnaire-based study of a large MS population from Northern California showed that a startling proportion of the patients with underlying sleep disorders including obstructive sleep apnea, insomnia, and RLS are underdiagnosed. In this study, out of 2,375 patients who completed questionnaires and met inclusion criteria, 898 (37.8%) screened positive for obstructive sleep apnea, 746 (31.6%) for moderate to severe insomnia, and 866 (36.8%) for RLS in contrast to only 4%, 11%, and 12% of the cohort reporting being diagnosed by a healthcare provider with obstructive sleep apnea, insomnia, and RLS, respectively (68). Obesity was found to be as prevalent in MS patients as in the general population (50%) (69) which could potentially contribute to the development of sleep disorders as well, such as obstructive sleep apnea.

Comorbidities and Therapeutic Decisions

Comorbidities can affect the treatment of MS, including the selection of whether to initiate treatment, the specific choice of treatment, and its subsequent effectiveness. Severe,

uncontrolled depression, for example, is a contraindication for the use of IFNb (70). Many clinical trials in patients with MS exclude individuals with severe comorbidities or substance abuse disorders, and therefore may not reflect "real-life" results (71). Consequently, the safety, tolerability, and effectiveness of most drugs are not known in such patients. Depression is seen in higher frequency among MS patients and is also recognized for affecting compliance and adherence to disease-modifying therapy (72) and therefore needs to be frequently screened for. Some medications may be contraindicated in patients with certain comorbidities as well. Concurrent ischemic heart disease or hypertension, as well as the use of certain medications (e.g., beta- or calcium channel blockers) were found to be associated with a higher risk for developing heart rhythm problems with fingolimod, requiring close monitoring for 24 hours in a hospital setting following the first dose, compared to the usual 6-hour outpatient monitoring for patients without known vascular comorbidities (73). Previous history of a seizure disorder is usually a contraindication for treatment with 4-aminopyridine (dalfampridine, Ampyra®), which is indicated to improve walking in patients with MS (74).

Finally, the most proactive way to address some of the mentioned comorbidities is to prevent them. Potentially modifiable lifestyle risk factors, such as smoking, alcohol overuse, physical inactivity, obesity, and malnutrition, which are associated with some common comorbidities (including hypertension, diabetes, hyperlipidemia, ischemic heart disease, and chronic lung disease) should be screened for with appropriate support for interventions and counselling at patient visits.

Evidence suggests that comorbidities might:

- *Delay the time between MS symptom onset and diagnosis*
- *Affect the clinical phenotype/severity of MS at presentation*
- *Affect disability progression and health-related quality of life*
- *Have significant effects on treatment decisions*

AGING AND MS

The most recently estimated prevalence of MS in the United States is approximately 1,000,000 (75), and about one-half of individuals with MS are older than 55 years. Most neurologists are hesitant to diagnose MS in elderly patients. In fact, previous diagnostic criteria excluded the diagnosis of MS on the basis of age alone (76). However, population-based studies have shown that the prevalence of late onset MS (>50 years) is not rare, ranging between 4.6% and 9.4% of all cases of MS (77). It is also very likely that patients presenting with a diagnosis after age 50 represent a heterogeneous mixture of patients with true late-onset MS and those with unrecognized symptoms earlier in life. Of those with MS, about 90% will have a life expectancy similar to their counterparts. This also means that the majority of patients will live with the disease at least 20 years if diagnosed in their late 50s. Few studies have been conducted to evaluate the effects of aging on MS disease course.

A distinction should be made between two main groups: those who age with MS while diagnosed at an earlier age, as opposed to the group of patients who are being diagnosed with MS at an older age (late onset MS).

Aging With MS

In a study using hospital discharge notes, older adults with MS experienced more infectious complications, such as pneumonia, urinary tract infection, sepsis, or cellulitis, as compared with their non-MS counterparts who were more likely to have diagnoses of MI, congestive heart failure, stroke, angina, diabetes, and lung disease (78). At the same time, aging individuals with MS have an increased risk for vascular comorbidities as previously mentioned.

In the last two decades, it has become evident that the underlying MS pathology involves, in addition to the well-known inflammatory process, a significant neurodegenerative component that is primarily responsible for the irreversible neurological clinical progression. This neurodegenerative process probably starts at the very early stages of the disease, but is more prominent in later stages of the disease. Brain parenchymal atrophy, as measured by MRI, represents the best surrogate marker for assessing the associated ongoing neurodegenerative processes in MS, and is considered the best predictor for disability progression (79). In particular, the thalamus and basal ganglia have been implicated in the process of "central" atrophy. Thalamic atrophy has been reported early on, even in children diagnosed with MS (80), CIS (81), and adult phenotypes of MS, including RRMS, SPMS, and PPMS. The thalamic volume increases in typically developing children (82) and decreases in healthy adults (83). It is important to account for the late development and natural aging changes of the thalamus when interpreting the findings in MS, particularly when MS patients include young adults.

A recent study showed that thalamic volume loss in MS patients correlated with disability after adjusting for natural aging and whole brain lesion volume, suggesting that MS thalamic pathology has a neurodegenerative component independent from the white matter lesions (84). These findings suggest that thalamic atrophy is a central component in normal aging as well as in MS-associated neurodegeneration. Therefore, it can be anticipated that the aging process in MS patients will have a more deleterious effect than in aging individuals without MS. Accordingly, a similar decline in processing speed was documented in both MS patients and controls as age

increases, indicating that both processes, aging and MS, advance separately but may have an additive effect on the overall cognitive status (85).

> Evidence suggests that thalamic atrophy is a central component in normal aging as well as in MS-associated neurodegeneration.

Aging and Cognition in MS

Cognitive impairment, mostly affecting cognitive processing speed and episodic memory, is common among MS patients (86). However, we do not have a good understanding of how these cognitive deficits progress in the aging MS patient. It is also unclear if MS neuropathology makes the elderly patient more vulnerable to age-related cognitive disorders such as Alzheimer's disease (AD) and other dementias. As these topics have only recently emerged as areas of research focus, only a few cross-sectional studies have been published at this time. Two separate studies examining the interaction of age and MS on processing speed found that the magnitude of impairment was not magnified by age (87). More specifically, it appears that aging does not differentially impact the rate of cognitive decline among nondemented MS patients. Thus, evidence of rapid cognitive decline in an older MS patient may indicate the presence of a secondary neurodegenerative process such as AD. However, it may be challenging for clinicians to distinguish between cognitive impairment related to MS and emerging AD due to the lack of research in this area. An early study directly comparing the cognitive profiles of MS and AD found that the degree of cognitive impairment in MS was less severe and also affected fewer domains than in AD (88). More recently, a study compared the cognitive profiles of patients with MS to patients with amnestic mild cognitive impairment (aMCI), the prodromal stage of AD (89). The authors reported that memory impairment in the MS group was more reflective of executive dysfunction rather than a consolidation deficit demonstrated by the aMCI group. Another study conducted at our center, compared cognitive profiles of both cognitively impaired and unimpaired older MS patients with healthy age-matched controls, AD patients, and aMCI patients (under review). Overall, our findings showed that cognitive profiles of AD and MS patients were distinct, with some overlap between MS patients and aMCI patients. Therefore, it is critical that older MS patients showing rapid cognitive decline, or a profile questionable of AD/aMCI, be referred for comprehensive dementia workup. With respect to treatment options, findings on the effects of donepezil in MS have been inconsistent (90), although it is possible that older patients with comorbid AD may show some benefit. Further research is needed to both improve diagnostic specificity and evaluate interventions for this subgroup of MS patients. Future work should include longitudinal designs, neuroimaging techniques, as well as genetics testing—all commonly implemented procedures in studies on AD.

> *Referral for comprehensive dementia workup should be considered for older MS patients showing rapid cognitive decline.*

MS Diagnosed in the Elderly

In a recent work, Bermel et al. (91) described the clinical characteristics of patients diagnosed with MS after the age of 60 years (n = 111). At the time of diagnosis, 8% of patients had a CIS, 33% were in the relapsing–remitting stage, whereas 23% had a secondary progressive course, and 32% had a primary progressive course. Acute partial transverse myelitis was the most common initial clinical presentation (46%), followed by progressive myelopathy (38%). Finally, 46% of patients with RRMS or a CIS exhibited MRI gadolinium enhancement (brain and/or spine). These findings support the opinion that elderly patients, diagnosed after the age of 60 years, can still experience significant inflammatory processes. Another study analyzing time trends and disability milestones among enrollees in a large international database found that the more recent enrollees were significantly older than the earlier enrollees, raising the awareness to what appears as a new trend of relative increase in the age of onset in the MS population (92).

An older age of onset was also shown to be associated with a faster rate of functional decline compared to patients with early age of onset in several studies, and independent of other risk factors (gender and initial disease course type) (93,94). Similarly, a recent study comparing the outcomes in animal experimental autoimmune encephalomyelitis (EAE) at different ages (95) showed that older age groups developed onset of clinical signs simultaneously with the acute CNS lesions, while the younger mice groups showed some delay in the occurrence of clinical symptoms. This could be explained by a decreased nervous tissue reserve, with shorter time to reach a certain disease progression and/or decreased ability to repair in aging individuals (96). Myelin repair mechanisms might be impaired in older age groups, as shown in an animal model and attributed to decreased recruitment of oligodendrocyte precursors (97). An opposite effect of younger age may be responsible for the delay (up to 10 years) in reaching specific progression thresholds as well as conversion to SPMS in pediatric MS patients, compared to adults with MS (96,98).

> *Late age onset MS is associated with a faster rate of functional decline compared to early age onset MS.*

CONCLUSIONS AND FUTURE DIRECTIONS

There is mounting evidence linking the risk and progression of MS to various environmental risk factors and preexisting and coexisting comorbidities. Heterogeneity in disease severity, including cognition and ambulation, can also be partially attributed to associated vascular risk factors and other comorbidities.

Identifying comorbidities and their impact in MS patients will help tailor more individualized treatment plans. Practice guidelines were implemented in other specialties in the last decade, including the 2003 national hypertension (99) and hyperlipidemia guidelines, that take into account the existence of comorbid conditions (stroke, diabetes mellitus, ischemic heart disease, etc.). Similar therapeutic guidelines will probably be necessary to facilitate a comprehensive management strategy for MS in the future. Further research studies are needed to better understand the incidence and impact of comorbidities as well as the role of aging on MS.

KEYPOINTS FOR PATIENTS AND FAMILIES

- MS patients very often have other diseases besides MS, which can affect quality of life and survival and these should be addressed as well (among them cardiovascular diseases, pulmonary diseases, depression, hypothyroidism).
- Smoking has been reported to adversely affect the risk for MS disease progression.
- Autoimmune hypothyroidism is a relatively common disease often found among MS patients and should be checked for as well, as it can affect the well-being and increase fatigue.

REFERENCES

1. Gijsen R, Hoeymans N, Schellevis FG, et al. Causes and consequences of comorbidity: a review. *J Clin Epidemiol.* 2001;54(7):661–674.
2. Dean G. How many people in the world have multiple sclerosis? *Neuroepidemiology.* 1994;13(1-2):1–7.
3. Marrie RA, Cohen J, Stuve O, et al. A systematic review of the incidence and prevalence of comorbidity in multiple sclerosis: overview. *Mult Scler.* 2015;21(3):263–281.
4. Conway DS, Thompson NR, Cohen JA. Influence of hypertension, diabetes, hyperlipidemia, and obstructive lung disease on multiple sclerosis disease course. *Mult Scler.* 2017;23(2):277–285.
5. Marrie RA, Horwitz R, Cutter G, et al. Comorbidity delays diagnosis and increases disability at diagnosis in MS. *Neurology.* 2009;72(2):117–124.
6. Salter A, Tyry T, Wang G, et al. Examining the joint effect of disability, health behaviors, and comorbidity on mortality in MS. *Neurol Clin Pract.* 2016;6(5):397–408.
7. Marrie RA, Elliott L, Marriott J, et al. Comorbidity increases the risk of hospitalizations in multiple sclerosis. *Neurology.* 2015;84(4):350–358.
8. Thormann A, Sorensen PS, Koch-Henriksen N, et al. Comorbidity in multiple sclerosis is associated with diagnostic delays and increased mortality. *Neurology.* 2017;89(16):1668–1675.
9. Marrie RA, Rudick R, Horwitz R, et al. Vascular comorbidity is associated with more rapid disability progression in multiple sclerosis. *Neurology.* 2010;74(13):1041–1047.
10. Bronnum-Hansen H, Koch-Henriksen N, Stenager E. Trends in survival and cause of death in Danish patients with multiple sclerosis. *Brain.* 2004;127(pt 4):844–850.
11. Koch-Henriksen N, Bronnum-Hansen H, Stenager E. Underlying cause of death in Danish patients with multiple sclerosis: results from the Danish Multiple Sclerosis Registry. *J Neurol Neurosurg Psychiatry.* 1998;65(1):56–59.
12. Hirst C, Swingler R, Compston DA, et al. Survival and cause of death in multiple sclerosis: a prospective population-based study. *J Neurol Neurosurg Psychiatry.* 2008;79(9):1016–1021.
13. Christiansen CF, Christensen S, Farkas DK, et al. Risk of arterial cardiovascular diseases in patients with multiple sclerosis: a population-based cohort study. *Neuroepidemiology.* 2010;35(4):267–274.
14. Motl RW, Fernhall B, McAuley E, et al. Physical activity and self-reported cardiovascular comorbidities in persons with multiple sclerosis: evidence from a cross-sectional analysis. *Neuroepidemiology.* 2011;36(3):183–191.
15. Christiansen CF. Risk of vascular disease in patients with multiple sclerosis: a review. *Neurol Res.* 2012;34(8):746–753.
16. Weinstock-Guttman B, Zivadinov R, Mahfooz N, et al. Serum lipid profiles are associated with disability and MRI outcomes in multiple sclerosis. *J Neuroinflammation.* 2011;8:127.
17. Giubilei F, Antonini G, Di Legge S, et al. Blood cholesterol and MRI activity in first clinical episode suggestive of multiple sclerosis. *Acta Neurol Scand.* 2002;106(2):109–112.
18. Cybulsky MI, Gimbrone MA, Jr. Endothelial expression of a mononuclear leukocyte adhesion molecule during atherogenesis. *Science.* 1991;251(4995):788–791.
19. Sitia S, Tomasoni L, Atzeni F, et al. From endothelial dysfunction to atherosclerosis. *Autoimmun Rev.* 2010;9(12):830–834.
20. Stokes KY, Calahan L, Hamric CM, et al. CD40/CD40L contributes to hypercholesterolemia-induced microvascular inflammation. *Am J Physiol Heart Circ Physiol.* 2009;296(3):H689-H697.
21. Esteve E, Ricart W, Fernandez-Real JM. Dyslipidemia and inflammation: an evolutionary conserved mechanism. *Clin Nutr.* 2005;24(1):16–31.
22. Torres A, Askari AD, Malemud CJ. Cardiovascular disease complications in systemic lupus erythematosus. *Biomark Med.* 2009;3(3):239–252.
23. Boyer JF, Gourraud PA, Cantagrel A, et al. Traditional cardiovascular risk factors in rheumatoid arthritis: a meta-analysis. *Joint Bone Spine.* 2011;78(2):179–183.
24. von Eckardstein A, Sibler RA. Possible contributions of lipoproteins and cholesterol to the pathogenesis of diabetes mellitus type 2. *Curr Opin Lipidol.* 2011;22(1):26–32.
25. Li Y, Wang H, Hu X, et al. Serum lipoprotein levels in patients with neuromyelitis optica elevated but had little correlation with clinical presentations. *Clin Neurol Neurosurg.* 2010;112(6):478–481.
26. Di Pauli F, Reindl M, Ehling R, et al. Smoking is a risk factor for early conversion to clinically definite multiple sclerosis. *Mult Scler.* 2008;14(8):1026–1030.
27. Zivadinov R, Weinstock-Guttman B, Hashmi K, et al. Smoking is associated with increased lesion volumes and brain atrophy in multiple sclerosis. *Neurology.* 2009;73(7):504–510.
28. Koch M, van Harten A, Uyttenboogaart M, et al. Cigarette smoking and progression in multiple sclerosis. *Neurology.* 2007;69(15):1515–1520.
29. Healy BC, Ali EN, Guttmann CR, et al. Smoking and disease progression in multiple sclerosis. *Arch Neurol.* 2009;66(7):858–864.
30. Hernan MA, Jick SS, Logroscino G, et al. Cigarette smoking and the progression of multiple sclerosis. *Brain.* 2005;128 (pt 6):1461–1465.
31. Sundstrom P, Nystrom L. Smoking worsens the prognosis in multiple sclerosis. *Mult Scler.* 2008;14(8):1031–1035.
32. Horstman LL, Jy W, Bidot CJ, et al. Antiphospholipid antibodies: paradigm in transition. *J Neuroinflammation.* 2009;6:3.
33. Tourbah A, Clapin A, Gout O, et al. Systemic autoimmune features and multiple sclerosis: a 5-year follow-up study. *Arch Neurol.* 1998;55(4):517–521.
34. Rovaris M, Viti B, Ciboddo G, et al. Brain involvement in systemic immune mediated diseases: magnetic resonance and magnetisation transfer imaging study. *J Neurol Neurosurg Psychiatry.* 2000;68(2):170–177.
35. Stosic M, Ambrus J, Garg N, et al. MRI characteristics of patients with antiphospholipid syndrome and multiple sclerosis. *J Neurol.* 2010;257(1):63–71.
36. Zivadinov R, Ramanathan M, Ambrus J, et al. Anti-phospholipid antibodies are associated with response to interferon-beta1a treatment in MS: results from a 3-year longitudinal study. *Neurol Res.* 2012;34(8):761–769.
37. Marrie RA, Reider N, Cohen J, et al. A systematic review of the incidence and prevalence of cardiac, cerebrovascular, and peripheral vascular disease in multiple sclerosis. *Mult Scler.* 2015;21(3):318–331.
38. Ho PP, Kanter JL, Johnson AM, et al. Identification of naturally occurring fatty acids of the myelin sheath that resolve neuroinflammation. *Sci Transl Med.* 2012;4(137):137ra173.
39. Gupta G, Gelfand JM, Lewis JD. Increased risk for demyelinating diseases in patients with inflammatory bowel disease. *Gastroenterology.* 2005;129(3):819–826.
40. Broadley SA, Deans J, Sawcer SJ, et al. Autoimmune disease in first-degree relatives of patients with multiple sclerosis. A UK survey. *Brain.* 2000;123(pt 6):1102–1111.
41. Seyfert S, Klapps P, Meisel C, et al. Multiple sclerosis and other immunologic diseases. *Acta Neurol Scand.* 1990;81(1):37–42.
42. Jacobs LD, Wende KE, Brownscheidle CM, et al. A profile of multiple sclerosis: the New York State Multiple Sclerosis Consortium. *Mult Scler.* 1999;5(5):369–376.
43. Barcellos LF, Kamdar BB, Ramsay PP, et al. Clustering of autoimmune diseases in families with a high-risk for multiple sclerosis: a descriptive study. *Lancet Neurol.* 2006;5(11):924–931.
44. Niederwieser G, Buchinger W, Bonelli RM, et al. Prevalence of autoimmune thyroiditis and non-immune thyroid disease in multiple sclerosis. *J Neurol.* 2003;250(6):672–675.
45. Sloka JS, Phillips PW, Stefanelli M, et al. Co-occurrence of autoimmune thyroid disease in a multiple sclerosis cohort. *J Autoimmune Dis.* 2005;2:9.
46. Edwards LJ, Constantinescu CS. A prospective study of conditions associated with multiple sclerosis in a cohort of 658 consecutive outpatients attending a multiple sclerosis clinic. *Mult Scler.* 2004;10(5):575–581.

47. Midgard R, Gronning M, Riise T, et al. Multiple sclerosis and chronic inflammatory diseases. A case-control study. *Acta Neurol Scand*. 1996;93(5):322–328.

48. Marrie RA. Autoimmune disease and multiple sclerosis: methods, methods, methods. *Lancet Neurol*. 2007;6(7):575–576.

49. Durelli L, Ferrero B, Oggero A, et al. Autoimmune events during interferon beta-1b treatment for multiple sclerosis. *J Neurol Sci*. 1999;162(1):74–83.

50. Kreisler A, de Seze J, Stojkovic T, et al. Multiple sclerosis, interferon beta and clinical thyroid dysfunction. *Acta Neurol Scand*. 2003;107(2):154–157.

51. Okanoue T, Itoh Y, Yasui K. Autoimmune disorders in interferon therapy [in Japanese]. *Nihon Rinsho*. 1994;52(7):1924–1928.

52. Nousari HC, Kimyai-Asadi A, Tausk FA. Subacute cutaneous lupus erythematosus associated with interferon beta-1a. *Lancet*. 1998;352(9143):1825–1826.

53. Crispin JC, Diaz-Jouanen E. Systemic lupus erythematosus induced by therapy with interferon-beta in a patient with multiple sclerosis. *Lupus*. 2005;14(6):495–496.

54. Dionisiotis J, Zoukos Y, Thomaides T. Development of myasthenia gravis in two patients with multiple sclerosis following interferon beta treatment. *J Neurol Neurosurg Psychiatry*. 2004;75(7):1079.

55. Charach G, Grosskopf I, Weintraub M. Development of Crohn's disease in a patient with multiple sclerosis treated with copaxone. *Digestion*. 2008;77(3-4):198–200.

56. Zheng B, Switzer K, Marinova E, et al. Exacerbation of autoimmune arthritis by copolymer-I through promoting type 1 immune response and autoantibody production. *Autoimmunity*. 2008;41(5):363–371.

57. Frese A, Bethke F, Ludemann P, et al. Development of myasthenia gravis in a patient with multiple sclerosis during treatment with glatiramer acetate. *J Neurol*. 2000;247(9):713.

58. Heesen C, Gbadamosi J, Schoser BG, et al. Autoimmune hyperthyroidism in multiple sclerosis under treatment with glatiramer acetate—a case report. *Eur J Neurol*. 2001;8(2):199.

59. Costelloe L, Jones J, Coles A. Secondary autoimmune diseases following alemtuzumab therapy for multiple sclerosis. *Expert Rev Neurother*. 2012;12(3):335–341.

60. Cossburn M, Pace AA, Jones J, et al. Autoimmune disease after alemtuzumab treatment for multiple sclerosis in a multicenter cohort. *Neurology*. 2011;77(6):573–579.

61. Marrie RA, Horwitz RI. Emerging effects of comorbidities on multiple sclerosis. *Lancet Neurol*. 2010;9(8):820–828.

62. Centers for Disease Control and Prevention. Prevalence of disabilities and associated health conditions—United States, 1991–1992. *MMWR Morb Mortal Wkly Rep*. 1994;43(40):730–731, 737–739.

63. Warren S, Turpin KV, Warren KG. Health-related quality of life in MS: issues and interventions. *Can J Neurol Sci*. 2009;36(5):540–541.

64. Brass SD, Duquette P, Proulx-Therrien J, et al. Sleep disorders in patients with multiple sclerosis. *Sleep Med Rev*. 2010;14(2):121–129.

65. Ajayi OF, Chang-McDowell T, Culpepper WJ, et al. High prevalence of sleep disorders in veterans with multiple sclerosis. *Neurology*. 2008;70(suppl 1):A333.

66. Italian REMS Group, Manconi M, Ferini-Strambi L, et al. Multicenter case-control study on restless legs syndrome in multiple sclerosis: the REMS study. *Sleep*. 2008;31(7):944–952.

67. Gomez-Choco MJ, Iranzo A, Blanco Y, et al. Prevalence of restless legs syndrome and REM sleep behavior disorder in multiple sclerosis. *Mult Scler*. 2007;13(6):805–808.

68. Brass SD, Li CS, Auerbach S. The underdiagnosis of sleep disorders in patients with multiple sclerosis. *J Clin Sleep Med*. 2014;10(9):1025–1031.

69. Marrie R, Horwitz R, Cutter G, et al. High frequency of adverse health behaviors in multiple sclerosis. *Mult Scler*. 2009;15(1):105–113.

70. Francis G. Benefit-risk assessment of interferon-beta therapy for relapsing multiple sclerosis. *Expert Opin Drug Saf*. 2004;3(4):289–303.

71. Rudick RA, Stuart WH, Calabresi PA, et al. Natalizumab plus interferon beta-1a for relapsing multiple sclerosis. *N Engl J Med*. 2006;354(9):911–923.

72. Gulick EE. Emotional distress and activities of daily living functioning in persons with multiple sclerosis. *Nurs Res*. 2001;50(3):147–154.

73. US Food and Drug Administration. FDA Drug Safety Communication: Revised recommendations for cardiovascular monitoring and use of multiple sclerosis drug Gilenya (fingolimod), 2012. https://www.fda.gov/Drugs/DrugSafety/ucm303192.htm Accessed 6 June 2018.

74. Cornblath DR, Bienen EJ, Blight AR. The safety profile of dalfampridine extended release in multiple sclerosis clinical trials. *Clin Ther*. 2012;34(5):1056–1069.

75. Wallin MT, Culpepper WJ, Campbell J, et al. The prevalence of multiple sclerosis in the United States: a population-based healthcare database approach. Poster presented at: 2017 European Committee for Treatment and Research in Multiple Sclerosis Congress; October 2017; Paris, France.

76. Schumacher GA, Beebe G, Kibler RF, et al. Problems of experimental trials of therapy in multiple sclerosis: report by the panel on the evaluation of experimental trials of therapy in multiple sclerosis. *Ann N Y Acad Sci*. 1965;122:552–568.

77. Polliack ML, Barak Y, Achiron A. Late-onset multiple sclerosis. *J Am Geriatr Soc*. 2001;49(2):168–171.

78. Fleming ST, Blake RL, Jr. Patterns of comorbidity in elderly patients with multiple sclerosis. *J Clin Epidemiol*. 1994;47(10):1127–1132.

79. Zivadinov R. Can imaging techniques measure neuroprotection and remyelination in multiple sclerosis? *Neurology*. 2007;68(22)(suppl 3):S72–S82;discussion S91–S96.

80. Mesaros S, Rocca MA, Absinta M, et al. Evidence of thalamic gray matter loss in pediatric multiple sclerosis. *Neurology*. 2008;70(13)(pt 2):1107–1112.

81. Henry RG, Shieh M, Amirbekian B, et al. Connecting white matter injury and thalamic atrophy in clinically isolated syndromes. *J Neurol Sci*. 2009;282(1-2):61–66.

82. Ostby Y, Tamnes CK, Fjell AM, et al. Heterogeneity in subcortical brain development: a structural magnetic resonance imaging study of brain maturation from 8 to 30 years. *J Neurosci*. 2009;29(38):11772–11782.

83. Walhovd KB, Westlye LT, Amlien I, et al. Consistent neuroanatomical age-related volume differences across multiple samples. *Neurobiol Aging*. 2011;32(5):916–932.

84. Hasan KM, Walimuni IS, Abid H, et al. Multimodal quantitative magnetic resonance imaging of thalamic development and aging across the human lifespan: implications to neurodegeneration in multiple sclerosis. *J Neurosci*. 2011;31(46):16826–16832.

85. Bodling AM, Denney DR, Lynch SG. Cognitive aging in patients with multiple sclerosis: a cross-sectional analysis of speeded processing. *Arch Clin Neuropsychol*. 2009;24(8):761–767.

86. Benedict RH, Fischer JS, Archibald CJ, et al. Minimal neuropsychological assessment of MS patients: a consensus approach. *Clin Neuropsychol*. 2002;16(3):381–397.

87. Roy S, Frndak S, Drake AS, et al. Differential effects of aging on motor and cognitive functioning in multiple sclerosis. *Mult Scler*. 2017;23(10):1385–1393.

88. Filley CM, Heaton RK, Nelson LM, et al. A comparison of dementia in Alzheimer's disease and multiple sclerosis. *Arch Neurol*. 1989;46(2):157–161.

89. Muller S, Saur R, Greve B, et al. Recognition performance differentiates between elderly patients in the long term course of secondary progressive multiple sclerosis and amnestic mild cognitive impairment. *Mult Scler*. 2013;19(6):799–805.

90. Krupp LB, Christodoulou C, Melville P, et al. Multicenter randomized clinical trial of donepezil for memory impairment in multiple sclerosis. *Neurology*. 2011;76(17):1500–1507.

91. Bermel RA, Rae-Grant AD, Fox RJ. Diagnosing multiple sclerosis at a later age: more than just progressive myelopathy. *Mult Scler*. 2010;16(11):1335–1340.

92. Kister I, Chamot E, Cutter G, et al. Increasing age at disability milestones among MS patients in the MSBase Registry. *J Neurol Sci*. 2012;318(1-2):94–99.

93. Trojano M, Liguori M, Bosco Zimatore G, et al. Age-related disability in multiple sclerosis. *Ann Neurol.* 2002;51(4):475–480.

94. Guillemin F, Baumann C, Epstein J, et al. Older age at multiple sclerosis onset is an independent factor of poor prognosis: a population-based cohort study. *Neuroepidemiology.* 2017;48(3-4):179–187.

95. Smith ME, Eller NL, McFarland HF, et al. Age dependence of clinical and pathological manifestations of autoimmune demyelination. Implications for multiple sclerosis. *Am J Pathol.* 1999;155(4):1147–1161.

96. Pedre X, Mastronardi F, Bruck W, et al. Changed histone acetylation patterns in normal-appearing white matter and early multiple sclerosis lesions. *J Neurosci.* 2011;31(9):3435–3445.

97. Sim FJ, Zhao C, Penderis J, et al. The age-related decrease in CNS remyelination efficiency is attributable to an impairment of both oligodendrocyte progenitor recruitment and differentiation. *J Neurosci.* 2002;22(7):2451–2459.

98. Kuhlmann T, Miron V, Cui Q, et al. Differentiation block of oligodendroglial progenitor cells as a cause for remyelination failure in chronic multiple sclerosis. *Brain.* 2008;131(pt 7):1749–1758.

99. Lenfant C, Chobanian AV, Jones DW, et al. Seventh report of the Joint National Committee on the prevention, detection, evaluation, and treatment of high blood pressure (JNC 7): resetting the hypertension sails. *Hypertension.* 2003;41(6):1178–1179.

100. Bernstein CN, Wajda A, Blanchard JF. The clustering of other chronic inflammatory diseases in inflammatory bowel disease: a population-based study. *Gastroenterology.* 2005;129(3):827–836.

101. Kimura K, Hunter SF, Thollander MS, et al. Concurrence of inflammatory bowel disease and multiple sclerosis. *Mayo Clin Proc.* 2000;75(8):802–806.

36 Work, Insurance, and Disability Issues in Multiple Sclerosis

Matthew H. Sutliff and Deborah M. Miller

KEY POINTS FOR CLINICIANS

- Multiple sclerosis (MS) is often associated with loss of employment.
- Reasons for loss of employment include MS-related symptoms and functional limitations, as well as demographical and environmental factors.
- A multidisciplinary team is needed to help patients maintain or gain employment.
- Physical therapists, occupational therapists, social workers, speech–language pathologists, behavioral health psychologists, and vocational rehabilitation specialists are important members of this team as they specialize in gaining skills and helping to connect patients with appropriate resources, whether they seek to maintain employment or in the event that they become unable to work.
- Issues related to various types of insurance (health, disability, long-term care, and life insurance) must be discussed with MS patients, in order to minimize as much as possible the financial impact of the disease, and to help protect their access to appropriate care.
- Proper documentation of all impairments is imperative in order to support needed accommodations or to document the need for disability.

MS is a disease that is most commonly diagnosed when individuals are between 20 and 40, although it can also be diagnosed in childhood or in ages well over 40. MS affects physical, cognitive, emotional, and social well-being. One of the most common aspects of social functioning that can be affected is working (1). Many young- to middle-age adults define themselves in terms of the work they do. It provides self-definition, structure to daily life, social interaction, and a means of financial independence for now and in the future (2). Importantly, for persons with a chronic disease including MS, working is a primary source of health, disability, and long-term care (LTC) insurance. It is well established that persons with MS can be compromised in their ability to work (3), and the emotional, financial, and social cascade of loss of work can be devastating. To date, there has been no systematic assessment of the relationship between the use of disease-modifying therapies and job retention.

For all of these reasons, it is essential for MS care specialists to routinely review with their patients, from the time of diagnosis, how MS is affecting their work lives. It is not expected that healthcare providers will actively help patients to navigate the complex laws and institutions that are intended to help persons with disabilities maintain

employment and manage the consequences of loss of work. However, clinicians do need to understand the factors that influence their patients' ability to work, and to be knowledgeable about available resources that can help maintain employment and build a financial safety net, if and when the time comes when employment is no longer feasible.

Key resources within the care team for addressing these issues are the health social worker and rehabilitation specialists, including physical therapists, occupational therapists, and vocational counselors as well as behavioral health psychologists and neuropsychologists to help clients maintain employment. Social workers in healthcare settings provide a formal psychosocial evaluation of patients and, when indicated, their family members. They will provide essential support by engaging the patient and family through counseling, advocacy, practical support, and linkages with important community resources. These interventions remove barriers to care and help patients and family manage distress and successfully negotiate the complex systems that they will have to engage.

The rehabilitation team can provide a variety of critical services to help maintain employment, such as improving mobility, enhancing arm and hand function, learning strategies to cope with visual deficits, or for

TABLE 36.1 Factors Associated With Labor Force Participation

FACTOR	COMMENTS
Gender	In general, women have higher rates of unemployment and MS is more common in women
Socioeconomic status	Persons with higher education and less physical employment are more likely to remain employed
Age	Generally, older individuals are more likely to be unemployed compared to their younger counterparts, most likely due to the association of increased disability and time since diagnosis
Physiological symptoms	Several reports indicate that exacerbations and symptom severity, especially fatigue, are associated with work discontinuation.
Course and disease progression	More aggressive forms of MS and persistence of symptoms make work continuation difficult
Cognitive dysfunction	Perceived cognitive dysfunction is a major predictor of unemployment
Psychological and emotional factors	Research indicates that persons with MS do not commonly attribute these symptoms to loss of work.
Variability of symptoms and "invisible disability"	Many of the symptoms of MS are not obvious but disruptive to job performance (e.g., fatigue, paresthesias, and bladder dysfunction).
Workplace discrimination	Many individuals worry about the impact of diagnosis disclosure on how they are perceived and treated. While many persons with MS leave the workforce voluntarily, they often report that the departure is the result of both subtle and explicit discrimination by supervisors and coworkers.

MS, multiple sclerosis.
Source: Adapted from Rumrill PD, Nissen SW. Employment and career development considerations. In: Giesser BS, ed. *Primer on Multiple Sclerosis.* New York, NY: Oxford; 2011:401-418.

managing multiple tasks at work. In the event that a client is unfortunately unable to work, the rehabilitation team can help facilitate the process to obtain disability approval through clear and concise documentation of the client's functional deficits that prevent gainful employment.

Data regarding high unemployment rates for persons with MS is an indication of why this topic is so important. It has been reported that at least 90% of Americans with MS had some work experience at some point,[1] approximately 60% were employed at diagnosis (4), but that only 20% to 30% were employed 15 years beyond diagnosis (5–7). A recent study of the cost of MS in 16 European countries found that the proportion of respondents of working age who were not working due to MS ranged from 28% (Russia and France) to 65% (the Netherlands) (8); Rumrill and Nissen note that there are many demographic and environmental factors that affect employment (1). In the United States, the socioeconomic burden of MS has been estimated to be $2.2 million over a person's lifetime, which includes both direct (approximately 63%) and indirect (approximately 37%) costs. Indirect costs have been reported to be as high as 57% of the total cost of care. These costs may include alterations to accommodate disability, caregiving, and loss of earnings. In particular, productivity loss has been reported to be the single highest contributor to the societal burden associated with MS (3). This emphasizes the importance of building a multidisciplinary care team to help patients maintain employment (Table 36.1).

DISCLOSING THE DIAGNOSIS

As gaining or maintaining employment should be considered an important component of a comprehensive MS

treatment plan, there are several issues clinicians need to address with patients. These include issues of disclosing the diagnosis to employers, knowing what resources are available to help gain or maintain employment, and insurance-related questions they should be asking of their employer's human resources department.

Persons with MS may be ambivalent about disclosing their diagnosis to an existing or potential employer for fear of losing or not being accepted for a position, whether that individual is **already employed** or **seeking a new position**. Let us first consider guidance a clinician might give individuals who are applying for a position with a new company. There is no legal requirement to disclose a chronic condition or specifics about it, during the early phases of the interview process. However, as potential employee and employer are in the "postoffer" negotiation phases of hiring, potential employers have the right to ask about medical conditions and the potential employee must provide accurate information that is "job related and consistent with business necessity." Given the subtleties of the different phases of job negotiation, it is important for patients to have an opportunity to discuss with a member of their clinical team how they will disclose the symptoms and diagnosis of MS.

For employed individuals who are covered by the Americans with Disabilities Act (ADA) or the Family and Medical Leave Act and who are requesting a medical leave of absence, medical documentation is required. For those requesting reasonable job accommodations because they are experiencing MS symptoms affecting their ability to perform key aspects of their job, it is important for the employee to educate their Human Resources department or supervisor about their symptoms and the specific accommodations that can help them remain productive employees. In preparation for this discussion, it is useful to have

[1] Employment is very common (>90%) in people with MS, at least early in the disease. The work challenges that may develop with disease progression is later outlined in the chapter.

members of the rehabilitative team assess what accommodations to recommend and to provide documentation of those recommendations. Because there are so many variables that are unique to each work site, it is recommended that each patient develop an appropriate disclosure plan with a social worker, psychologist, or vocational counselor. A list of MS organizations is provided at the end of this chapter. The decision to disclose one's medical condition is a very personal matter. The National Multiple Sclerosis Society (NMSS) (9,10) offers a very thorough discussion of the pros and cons of disclosure, when in one's employment history to make the disclosure and who in the organization should be advised. The joint publication of the Washington Appleseed Center for Law in the Public Interest and the NMSS are excellent resources regarding a range of legal issues people with MS encounter (10).

GAINING AND MAINTAINING EMPLOYMENT IN THE UNITED STATES OF AMERICA

Vocational Rehabilitation Services

In the United States, there are multiple agencies and legal statutes intended to help individuals with disabilities gain or maintain employment, and to help prevent work place discrimination. The Rehabilitation Services Administration is a federally mandated agency authorized, in part, to carry out Title V of the Rehabilitation Act of 1973. Their mission is to provide leadership and resources to assist state and other agencies in providing vocational rehabilitation (VR) and other services to individuals with disabilities to maximize their employment, independence, and integration into the community and competitive labor markets (11). These federally funded services are administered by individual State Vocational Rehabilitation Agencies that are mandated to prioritize services to the most seriously disabled. In addition to these mandated VR agencies, there are a wealth of private and not-for-profit agencies that provide similar services to individuals with disability. Regardless of where they are located, vocational counselors' responsibilities typically include the following:

—Vocational evaluation to assess interests, abilities, and needed accommodations
—Career counseling
—Training and education
—Job seeking skills
—Assistance with job placement (12)

Federal Laws That Protect Persons With Disabilities in the Work Place

Important among the legal statues that protect the persons with MS in work place are ADA, which is enforced by the Equal Opportunity Employment Commission, and the Family Medical Leave Act, which is enforced by the Department of Labor. The ADA of 1990 and the ADA Amendments Act of 2008 give civil rights protections

to persons with disability in regards to employment, transportation, public accommodations, public services, and telecommunications. Title 1 of this act addresses employment issues and provides a definition of disability. Under this law, a "qualified individual with disabilities" "meets legitimate skill, experience, education, or other requirements of an employment position that she or he holds or seeks, and who can perform the essential functions of the position with or without reasonable accommodation. Requiring the ability to perform 'essential' functions assures that an individual with a disability will not be considered unqualified simply because of inability to perform marginal or incidental job functions" (13). The law relates to individuals who work for private employers who have 15 or more employees as well as Federal and State agencies, employment agencies, and unions. A key interpretation of this law is defining reasonable accommodations that include modifications to the job or work environment but does not modify the essential function of the job (14).

The Equal Employment Opportunity Commission (EEOC) is the federal agency that enforces laws prohibiting employment discrimination including Title 1 of ADA. A person who believes he or she has been discriminated against generally has 180 days to file a complaint. EEOC becomes involved when a person who believes he or she has been discriminated against files charges either in person, by telephone or by mail. Once the complaint is received, the EEOC will inform the employer of the complaint and then several different courses of action may occur. It is typical that the EEOC recommend mediation which it helps conduct. If mediation is declined or unsuccessful, the EEOC will investigate the claim in more detail and if it finds merit in the claim, is able to bring suit on behalf of the claimant. If they do not find grounds for discrimination, the claimant may file his own lawsuit with a private lawyer. Neath and colleagues (15) examined EEOC data regarding 1,028 persons with MS who filed charges with that agency during 1992 to 2003. The majority of the "charging parties" (those filing complaints) were predominantly women ($n = 687$, 67%) and white ($n = 769$, 76%). The most common allegations made by charging parties with MS included discharge, reasonable accommodation, terms and conditions of employment, and harassment, and two thirds of those reporting to the EEOC made more than one charge at a time. The authors conclude that these are the key issues for clinicians to address with our patients so as to position them to be proactive in addressing them.

Another important law is the Family and Medical Leave Act of 1993, a federal law that requires covered employers to provide eligible, covered employees with up to 12 weeks of absence from work that are job protected and unpaid, and the employee's group health benefits must remain active during the leave. This law is administered by the Employment Standards Administration's Wage and Hour Division of the U.S. Department of Labor.

The types of conditions that are covered under this law are less restrictive than those covered by the ADA and include the following:

1. Birth or placement for foster care or adoption if a child of the employee
2. Care of a spouse, child, or parent who has a serious health problem, which maybe temporary or permanent
3. Care of an employee's own health problems
4. Specific situation related to the call to active duty of an immediate family member.

This law has important implications for working families living with MS as it allows a person with MS to utilize the Family and Medical Leave Act (FMLA) during a worsening of the disease or an extended medical treatment and also covers family members who need to be away from work in order to care for their immediate family member who has MS. This leave may be taken in one block or intermittently over a 12-month period.

Employers covered by the FMLA provision include the following:

1. Those who participate in the public sector who engage in commerce or industry affecting commerce and have 50 or more employees each working day during, at minimum, the previous 20 calendar weeks.
2. All public agency and education employers regardless of the number of employees.

Employees covered by the FMLA must:

1. Be employed by a covered employer and work within 75 miles of a worksite that employs at least 50 people
2. Have worked at least 12 months, even if nonconsecutive, for the employer
3. Worked at least 1,250 hours for the employer before the FMLA begins

It is likely that a family member living with MS will request documentation from his treating physician of the serious medical condition they experience.

INSURANCE

Types

There are several types of insurance that are important for patients and their families to have and it is useful for the clinicians to be familiar with these insurances because their terms of coverage will significantly influence the ability to carry out treatment plans for individual patients. The primary types of insurance include Health, Disability, LTC, and Life. Clinicians should encourage their patients understand how to obtain, maintain, and afford these insurances and to be familiar with the exact terms of each type of policy. Health insurance covers some portion of the cost of medical and surgical care and may include coverage for prescription, vision, and dental costs as well as durable medical equipment. Disability insurance provides a source of income for individuals who become unable to perform gainful activity. The definition of disability as well as the duration and amount that is paid is highly variable. LTC insurance covers many of the costs of an extended illness, including help with activities of daily living that are not covered by Health insurance. Life insurance provides cash benefits to a named beneficiary (usually a spouse or other family member) in the event of the insured's death. This type of insurance assures a source of income to the beneficiary when the insured is no longer able to provide that support. It is available only if privately purchased.

Sources

Most individuals in the United States have access to these insurances as group policies through their or a family member's employer. As previously suggested, access to these benefits through work is an important reason to remain employed as long as one is able. If a person becomes unemployed or their employer does not offer these types of coverage, there are often options for continuing health, disability, LTC, or life insurance on a private pay basis but that can prove to be very expensive. For eligible individuals there are Federal and State programs that provide for health (Medicare and Medicaid), disability (Social Security Disability and Supplemental Security Income [SSI]) and LTC (Medicaid) insurance.

Obtaining and maintaining **health insurance** is a major concern for anyone diagnosed with a chronic illness, including MS, regardless of how minimal their disability. Access to health insurance for individuals with chronic illness was improved greatly with the passage and enactment of the Patient Protection and Affordable Care Act (ACA) of 2010. One of the most important provisions of this law is that people with preexisting illnesses or chronic conditions cannot be denied health insurance, have insurance coverage withdrawn or premiums unreasonably increased. The current legislative environment points to likely reductions in access to and limitations in coverage provided by the ACA of 2010 and this is a point of uncertainty for patients and healthcare providers alike. There are two existing laws that provide means, although expensive, to continue coverage if a person loses employer-based insurance. The Consolidated Omnibus Budget Reconciliation Act of 1985 (COBRA) offers qualified individuals who lose employment-based group insurance to pay the full cost of the group rate plus an administrative fee for a specified period of time. The Health Insurance and Portability Act (HIPPA), among its other provisions, provides protections for individuals participating in group health plans that limit exclusions for preexisting conditions, and provides for individual coverage if no group plan is available or COBRA has been exhausted. Although there are many U.S. governmental insurance plans for disabled civilians, federal employees, members of the armed forces, and veterans, we will limit our discussion to the two programs for disabled civilians, Medicare and Medicaid. Medicare is typically thought of as the federal government's insurance program for the elderly but it also is the insurance offered to younger age individuals 24 months after they have been determined eligible for Social Security Disability. It is important to understand that this insurance covers many aspects of healthcare but not all expenses or the cost of LTC. Medicaid is the federally funded and state-administered medical assistance program for individuals and families with very limited assets and is made available to individuals who receive SSI. In addition to providing comprehensive medical and hospital care, unlike Medicare, Medicaid also provides access to **LTC**. As this is a state-administered program, the extent of Medicaid coverage varies from state to state. A more exhaustive discussion of the health insurance and related laws can be found elsewhere (16).

Disability Insurance

This insurance is intended to replace wage income for individuals who are disabled. There are private policies that are available through employers or private purchase and these policies are highly variable in terms of cost and coverage and how long the individual must be unable to work before becoming eligible for the benefit. It is very important to encourage patients to become familiar with the existence and extend of any private disability policy because, if they become totally and permanently disabled under the terms of the Social Security Administration (SSA), this may be their only source of personal income until a SSA determination is made. The SSA administers two types of income assistance. Social Security Disability Insurance (SSDI), which is based on prior work history, and SSI, which is based on significant financial need. Medical determination of eligibility for both of these programs is based on federal criteria that a person is totally and permanently disabled from any type of gainful employment. The criteria for MS are outlined in Table 36.2.

In order to receive SSDI, a person must have earned this insurance by working and paying Federal Social Security Taxes (FICA) for a certain period of time. The work credit requirements are based on the amount earned per year. The criteria for earning credits change from year to year and are dependent on the age of the disabled worker, but generally an individual needs 40 credits, 20 of which were earned in the past 10 years (18). In addition to the work credit requirements, a person will not be eligible to be determined disabled until they have not been "gainfully employed" for 5 months. It typically takes several months to receive an SSDI determination once one becomes not gainfully employed. Given the potential delay between loss of gainful employment and completion of the determination process, the significance of having a private disability policy, if at all possible, becomes clear. There is no similar work credit contributions or wait period to be eligible for SSI but the financial criteria for household income are stringent.

SSA GUIDELINES PERTAINING TO THE DIAGNOSIS OF MS
The SSA defines disability as "the inability to engage in any substantial gainful activity (SGA) by reason of any medically determinable physical or mental impairment(s) which can be expected to result in death or which has lasted or can be expected to last for a continuous period of not less than 12 months" (19,17). In their assessment, the SSA considers both medical criteria and nonmedical criteria when assessing an individual's eligibility to receive disability benefits. The medical criteria includes two domains: (a) disorganization of motor function in two extremities and (b) marked limitation in physical functioning. An individual needs to meet at least one of the criteria to qualify for disability benefits.

TABLE 36.2 Medical Criteria for Disability for MS per U.S. SSA

1) Disorganization of motor function in two extremities: disorganization of motor function means interference with movement of two extremities. By "two extremities," the SSA defines this as both lower extremities, or both upper extremities, or one upper extremity and one lower extremity. Criteria for disorganization of motor function that results in an *extreme limitation* in the ability to:
   a) Stand up from a seated position
   b) Balance while standing or walking
   c) Use the upper extremities that very seriously limits the ability to independently initiate, sustain, and complete work-related activities

2) Marked limitation in physical functioning: Examples of this criterion include specific motor abilities, such as independently initiating, sustaining, and completing the following activities: standing up from a seated position, balancing while standing or walking, or using both your upper extremities for fine and gross movements. Physical functioning may also include functions of the body that support motor abilities, such as the abilities to see, breathe, and swallow.

   To satisfy the requirements of the functional criteria, the neurological disorder must result in a marked limitation in physical functioning and a marked limitation in one of the four areas of mental functioning:
   a) Understanding, remembering, or applying information (the ability to learn, recall, and use information to perform work activities)
   b) Interacting with others (the ability to relate to and work with supervisors, coworkers, and the public)
   c) Concentrating, persisting, or maintaining pace (the ability to focus attention on work activities and to stay on task at a sustained rate)
   d) Adapting or managing oneself (the ability to regulate emotions, control behavior, and maintain well-being in a work setting)

MS, multiple sclerosis; SSA, Social Security Administration.

Source: Social Security Administration: Disability Evaluation Under Social Security. Avaialble at: https://www.ssa.gov/disability/professionals/bluebook/11.00-Neurological-Adult.htm#11_09. Accessed November 6, 2017.

Although the SSA does not require the use of such a scale, "marked" would be the fourth point on a five-point scale consisting of no limitation, mild limitation, moderate limitation, marked limitation, and extreme limitation. For this criterion, a marked limitation means that, due to the signs and symptoms of MS, an individual is seriously limited in the ability to independently initiate, sustain, and complete work-related physical activities. An individual does need not be totally precluded from performing a function or activity to have a marked limitation, as long as the degree of limitation seriously limits the ability to independently initiate, sustain, and complete work-related physical activities.

The SSA may also find that there is a "marked" limitation in this area if, for example, symptoms such as pain or *fatigue*, as documented in the individual's medical record, and caused by the neurological disorder or its treatment, seriously limit the ability to independently initiate, sustain, and complete these work-related motor functions, or the other physical functions or physiological processes that support those motor functions.

Fatigue is one of the most common and limiting symptoms of MS. MS may result in physical fatigue (lack of muscle endurance) or mental fatigue (decreased energy, awareness, or attention). The SSA does not look at fatigue as a stand-alone symptom. Instead, as the SSA evaluates fatigue, it considers the intensity, persistence, and effects of fatigue on functioning. The SSA considers the effects of physical and mental fatigue when evaluating physical and mental functioning using the criteria described earlier.

A separate category for Social Security Disability that can unfortunately affect some individuals with MS is blindness. Blindness is defined as having central visual acuity of 20/200 or less in the better eye with best correction, or a limitation in the field of vision in the better eye so that the widest diameter of the visual field subtends an angle of 20 degrees or less. Under SSDI, this condition has to have lasted or be expected to last at least 12 months. Of note, there is no duration requirement for blindness under SSI.

ASSESSMENT OF FUNCTION THROUGH AN MS-SPECIFIC FUNCTIONAL CAPACITY EVALUATION

The ideal method to assess vocational function is through an MS-specific functional capacity evaluation (FCE) (20). The components of the MS-specific FCE provide a thorough assessment of the functional abilities of the person with MS. It also allows a clear comparison of the client's physical limitations to the disability criteria as outlined by the SSA.

The FCE is used primarily for either of two purposes:

1. As a client prepares to return to work or adapt their work using reasonable accommodations that enhance their ability to perform the essential functions of their job
2. To provide detailed documentation of impairments in the event that the client is no longer able to perform sustained, gainful work

The components of the FCE in our clinic are listed in Tables 36.3, 36.4, and 36.5.

In the event of suspected cognitive impairment, a thorough neuropsychological exam can be very helpful to determine the severity of impairment and its effect on vocational performance. In many cases the client will report trouble at work with mental functioning, but the Symbol Digit Modalities Test (SDMT) can be a helpful tool to screen for cognitive impairment and may act as a guide to refer the client for further assessment or for cognitive rehabilitation.

The MS-specific FCE uses these subjective and objective components to document a client's functional abilities while also assessing their degree of limitation as it pertains to the disability criteria established by the SSA. This can streamline the process to work with job accommodations, offer guidance to a client when they are considering disability, or to provide proper documentation in the event that they must apply for disability.

TABLE 36.3 Patient-Reported Components of FCE for MS

- Subjective level of fatigue prior to FCE, rated on 0–10 ordinal scale
- Source of current income (is client currently on short- or long-term disability? If so, who is the insurer and what are the terms and criteria for disability?)
- Fall history
- Living/home situation
- Bracing
- Adaptive equipment (home and work)
- Driving ability and current adaptations
- Education level, including all vocational skill training
- Employment history:
  - Employer
  - Occupation
  - Term of employment (including a determination of work credits earned in last 10 years, if applicable)
  - Is client currently covered under Workers Compensation?
  - Physical duties and responsibilities of the job
- Bowel and bladder function
- Depression
- Cognitive function (short- and long-term memory, concentration)
- Effects of environmental exposure to heat, cold
- Ability and confidence regarding exposure to heights (e.g., safety on elevated platforms, ladders)

FCE, functional capacity evaluation; MS, multiple sclerosis.

TABLE 36.4 Evaluator-Rated Components of the FCE for MS

- Strength, using manual muscle testing, including grip testing with a hand dynamometer
- Range of motion
- Spasticity, as measured by the Modified Ashworth Scale
- Balance, as measured by the Berg Balance Scale
- Gait, as measured via the Timed 25 Foot Walk, the Timed Up and Go Test, the Dynamic Gait Index, and the Six-Minute Walk Test. Visual gait analysis at baseline and after potentially fatiguing activities are noted within the exam.
- Gait on stairs, ramps, curbs
- Crawling test (if applicable to job description)
- Ladder test on 6-foot step ladder (if applicable to job description)
- Palpation and sensation testing
- Bed mobility status
- Transfer ability
- Coordination testing
  - Finger to nose testing
  - Rapid forearm alternating pronation and supination
  - Observations regarding the presence or absence of tremor or other movement disorders
  - Nine-Hole Peg Test
- Hand tests
  - Five-position JAMAR grip test
  - Typing test
- Cognitive Screen
  - Symbol Digit Modalities Test
- Repetitive motion testing
  - Overhead reaching
  - Bending
  - Squatting
- Visual acuity
- 3-minute Step Test
- Stand/Walk Test
- Occasional Material Handling Tests
  - Leg Lift
  - 12-inch Leg Lift
  - Shoulder Lift
  - Overhead Lift
  - 30-foot Carry

FCE, functional capacity evaluation; MS, multiple sclerosis.

TABLE 36.5 Patient Reported Outcome Measures Within the FCE

- Numeric Pain Rating Scale
- Interference scale of the Brief Pain Inventory, modified
- Pain Drawing
- Multiple Sclerosis Walking Scale-12
- Modified Fatigue Impact Scale
- Fatigue Severity Scale
- **Patient Health Questionnaire-9**

FCE, functional capacity evaluation.

LTC Insurance

This insurance is intended to cover the medical, social, and personal care services that can be essential for persons living with a chronic progressive disease like MS but are not included in traditional health insurance. The only way that most individuals can access LTC insurance is by purchasing a private policy through an employer or privately. The younger in life this type of policy is purchased, the less expensive it is. It has proven difficult for persons diagnosed with chronic diseases to purchase such a policy but it may be an important consideration for family members who may have similar needs in the future. For those who are financially indigent and meet criteria for Medicaid, this is a source of LTC insurance.

Life Insurance

There is no federal program that offers this type of coverage, it is available only through private purchase. If patients are exploring this option, it is important for them to work with an independent insurance broker who is aware of their diagnosis and can negotiate with many different insurance providers.

FINANCIAL PLANNING

MS is an expensive disease that has minimal impact on life expectancy but can cause significant disruption in one's work life. This can have profound implications for the entire family. While employment plays a central role in the well-being of an individual and family, loss of employment can have just as significant consequences, not the least of which is financial. As most newly diagnosed people with mild to moderate disability do not anticipate the economic impact MS can have, one additional recommendation MS healthcare providers should routinely raise with their patients is working with a financial adviser to prepare for their and their families' security for current expenses, potential loss of employment and to assist with LTC needs as they arise.

CONCLUSION

This chapter is intended to be an overview of the work and insurance issues MS patients face. Expertise in these areas is not typical of most healthcare professionals providing MS care. Therefore it is very important to encourage patients to include rehabilitation professionals, lawyers, and financial planners as members of their care team. Members of the healthcare team should be prepared to make these recommendations as these are highly technical issues. Without adequate guidance individuals living with MS may face significant social and financial consequences.

KEY POINTS FOR PATIENTS AND FAMILIES

- MS is often associated with loss of employment.

- There are combinations of factors that may lead to this loss of employment for people with MS. These factors include MS symptoms that impair the ability to perform job duties, environmental barriers in the work place, and the type of work the person usually performed.

- Persons with MS who want to maintain their employment or develop new job skills will benefit from a variety of specialists in addition to their neurologists. These specialists include physical therapists, occupational therapists, social workers, speech–language pathologists, behavioral health psychologists, and vocational rehabilitation specialists.

- It is important for persons with MS to ask their healthcare professionals about reasonable accommodations that may help them continue to perform their job.

- Persons with MS should talk to healthcare professionals regarding resources to help them better understand various types of insurance (health, disability, long-term care (LTC), and life insurance).

- In pursuing work place accommodations or applying for disability, it is the detailed documentation of their impairments in the medical record that will lead to a successful outcome for the person with MS

KEY MS ORGANIZATIONS RESOURCES FOR CLINICIANS AND FAMILIES REGARDING WORK, INSURANCE, AND DISABILITY ISSUES

Consortium of Multiple Sclerosis Centers (www.mscare.org/)

Multiple Sclerosis Association of America (mymsaa.org/)

National Multiple Sclerosis Society (www.nationalmssociety.org/)

Multiple Sclerosis Foundation (msfocus.org/)

KEY WEB RESOURCES

www.medicaid.gov/Medicaid-CHIP-Program-Information/By-Topics/Eligibility/ Eligibility.html

www.nationalmssociety.org/living-with-multiple-sclerosis/employment/knowing-your- rights/index.aspx

www.nationalmssociety.org/nationalmssociety/media/msnationalfiles/brochures/ guidebook-social-security-disability-for-people-with-ms.pdf

www.dol.gov/ebsa/healthreform/

www.dol.gov/dol/topic/health-plans/portability.htm

www.dol.gov/ebsa/cobra.html

www.dol.gov/whd/regs/compliance/whdfs28.htm

www.eeoc.gov/

ssa.gov/pgm/disability.htm

www.ssa.gov/pgm/medicare.htm

www.supremecourt.gov/opinions/11pdf/11-393c3a2.pdf

my.clevelandclinic.org/ccf/media/files/Neurological-Institute/mellen-center/13-neu- 542-disability-issues-fact-sheet.pdf

REFERENCES

1. Rumrill PD, Nissen SW. Employment and career development considerations. In: Giesser BS, ed. *Primer on Multiple Sclerosis*. New York, NY: Oxford; 2011:401–418.

2. Johnson KL, Yorkston KM, Klasner ER, et al. The cost and benefits of employment: a qualitative study of experiences of persons with multiple sclerosis. *Arch Phys Med Rehabil*. 2004;85:201–209.

3. Sutliff MH. Contribution of impaired mobility to patient burden in multiple sclerosis. *Curr Med Res Opin*. 2010;26:109–119.

4. LaRocca NG. *Employment and Multiple Sclerosis*. Report. New York, NY: National Multiple Sclerosis Society; 1995.

5. Fraser R, Clemmons D, Bennet F. *Multiple Sclerosis: Psychosocial and Vocational Interventions*. New York, NY: Demos Medical; 2002.

6. Johnson KL, Fraser RT. Mitigating the impact of multiple sclerosis on employment. *Phys Med Rehabil Clin N Am*. 2005;16:571-582, x–xi.

7. Roessler RT, Rumrill PD, Jr. Multiple sclerosis and employment barriers: a systemic perspective on diagnosis and intervention. *Work*. 2003;21:17–23.

8. Kobelt G, Thompson A, Berg J, et al. New insights into the burden and costs of multiple sclerosis in Europe. *Mult Scler*. 2017;23:1123–1136.

9. National Multiple Sclerosis Society. Disclosure decisions. Available at: http://www.nationalmssociety.org/Living-Well-With-MS/Work-and-Home/Employment/Disclosure-Decisions. Accessed November 11, 2017.

10. Washington Appleseed Center for Law in the Public Interest, National multiple Sclerosis Society GWC. Know Your Rights: A legal guide for people living with multiple sclerosis. In: Society NMS, ed. 2014. http://www.waappleseed.org/, accessed November 7, 2017.

11. Government U. Available at: https://rsa.ed.gov/, accessed June 8, 2018.

12. Khan F, Ng L, Turner-Stokes L. Effectiveness of vocational rehabilitation intervention on the return to work and employment of persons with multiple sclerosis. *Cochrane Database of Systematic Reviews* 2009, Issue 1. Art. No.: CD007256. DOI: 10.1002/14651858.CD007256.pub2.

13. Government U. Available at: https://www.ada.gov/hiv/ada_q&a_aids.htm.

14. Government U. Available at: https://www.ada.gov/regs2010/titleIII_2010/titleIII_2010_regulations.htm.

15. Neath J, Roessler RT, McMahon BT, et al. Patterns in perceived employment discrimination for adults with multiple sclerosis. *Work*. 2007;29:255–274.

16. Calder K. Managing the insurance maze. In: Kalb R, ed. *Multiple Sclerosis: The Questions You Have, the Answers You Need*. New York, NY: Demos Medical; 2012: 317–333.

17. Social Security Administration.Disability evaluation under social security. Avaialble at: https://www.ssa.gov/disability/professionals/bluebook/11.00-Neurological-Adult.htm#11_09. Accessed November 6, 2017.

18. Social Security Administration. Available at: https://www.ssa.gov/pubs/EN-05-10072.pdf. Accessed June 8, 2018.

19. Sutliff MH, Miller DM, Forwell S. Developing a functional capactiy evalution specific to multiple sclerosis. *Int J MS Care*. 2012;14:17–27.

20. Sutliff MH. Developing a functional capacity evaluation specific to multiple sclerosis. *Int J MS Care*. 2012;14:17–28.

37

Caregiving in Multiple Sclerosis

Amy Burleson Sullivan

KEY POINTS FOR CLINICIANS

- Caregiving for a loved one with a chronic condition can often be fulfilling, as many times individuals move closer together when challenges arise.
- Caregiving can also become overwhelming, physically and emotionally challenging, and isolating. At times it can be thought of as a burden.
- Caregivers must learn to take care of themselves physically and emotionally.
- The multidisciplinary care model used in the treatment of multiple sclerosis (MS) is important not only for the patient, but also for the caregiver. This care model allows for several practitioners to interact with the caregiver to assess and determine the optional interventions.
- Physical, emotional, and financial abuses secondary to the profound challenges inherent in caring for a relative with a disabling chronic illness are not uncommon. Assessing for abuse is an important component in the clinical management of MS.

MS is a chronic, unpredictable, and progressive neurological disease that most commonly starts in young adulthood (1). It is also the most common nontraumatic cause of disability in young adulthood (2). The course of the disease is unpredictableas are the duration of relapses. As the disease progresses, the often numerous and variable symptoms such as fatigue, impaired mobility and vision, bladder and bowel dysfunction, cognitive impairment, and depression, can create a need for family members or others to provide care. This responsibility often falls on family members, typically the partner/spouse or child. Because MS often affects young women, the caregiver, unlike caregivers of loved ones with Alzheimer's dementia, stroke, or other disabling conditions occurring later in life, is often a young parent, with children at home, and who is in the early part of their career development. The long course and duration of MS frequently requires family members to play multiple roles: that of caregiver *and* of assuming the financial and household responsibilities. In many patients, MS does not shorten life span, and so a caregiver's role can encompass a lifetime. Caregiving can be deeply satisfying as partners and family members can be drawn closer together. However, as the caregiving demands increase for the person with MS, often less time is available to be devoted to the caregiver's own needs, the children's needs, the care of the home, or a career. Thus, caregivers often feel a significant demand and burden to their own endurance and coping mechanisms. Caregivers commonly report a plethora of their own physical and psychological symptoms. The aim of this chapter is to review common caregiver challenges and provide suggestions for how caregivers can more effectively care for themselves while maintaining their responsibility to the MS patient.

CAREGIVERS

A *caregiver*, by definition, is an individual who helps with physical and psychological care for a person in need (3). As is the case for most caregivers, they are often family members (i.e., spouse, partner, child, and parent) and they are likely unpaid. Caregivers can be called upon to provide a wide variety of assistance with activities of daily living, including bathing, toileting, dressing, transferring, cooking, eating, dispensing medications, and managing the home. Demographically, 66% of family caregivers are women, and interestingly, 65% of care recipients are women. In addition, the typical caregiver spends no less than 20 hours per week in a caregiving role (4,5).

A caregiver by definition is an individual who helps with physical and psychological care for a person in need.

Caregiving for a loved one with a chronic condition can be profoundly fulfilling, as individuals often move closer together when challenges arise. However, caregiving can also be daunting, physically and emotionally challenging, and isolating. At times, caregiving may be referred to as *caregiver burden*, which Buhse defines as "a multidimensional response to physical, psychological, emotional, social, and financial stressors associated with the caregiving experience" (6). The challenges of caregiving are widespread and encompass much more than the care of the recipient, as will be noted here.

Caregiving can be daunting, physically and emotionally challenging, and isolating.

In a recent study published in the International Journal of MS Care (2015) about the far reaching impact of being a caregiver to a person with MS, individuals participating in the North American Research Consortium on Multiple Sclerosis (NARCOMS) registry were invited to answer an online questionnaire looking at demographic data, health status, caregiver burne, and the impact of caregiving on employment. The findings showed female caregivers reporting higher levels of burden and stress and more medication use for anxiety/stress and mood disorders. The male counterparts reported more physical concerns. Caregivers of those with primary progressive MS reported greater perceived caregiver burden, as measured by the Zarit Caregiver Burden Interview. Finally, over 40% of caregivers reported missing work over the past year (7).

Economically, many caregivers juggle both work and caregiving, as 58% are currently employed, and the majority of those are men. However, their median incomes are 15% lower than noncaregiving families. In addition, a caregiver is more than 2½ times as likely to live in poverty as noncaregivers; and the average family caregiver spends $5,531 per year on out of pocket expenses, which is 10% of their median family income (4,5). A 2013 study by Buchanan, Huang, and Zheng found that, of 530 MS caregivers interviewed, poorer cognitive ability in the care recipient predicted reduced caregiver employment. In addition, better caregiver physical health and quality of life was associated with lower odds of reduced employment (8).

Caregiving reaches far beyond economics, as it may also have an impact on a caregiver's health. The added stress inherent in caregiving may increase the stress hormone, which can lead to high blood pressure and glucose levels and also by weakening the immune system, making individuals more susceptible to infections (9). This effect has been seen up to 3 years after the caregiving role has ended, thus putting the individual at an increased risk for chronic illness themselves (9). Seventy-two percent of family caregivers report not taking care of their own health issues, and frequently forgo their own medical appointments (4,5). In addition, they report poor eating and self-care, and less routine exercise. Not surprisingly, the extreme stress of caregiving leads to premature aging, and may decrease the caregiver's life expectancy by as much as 10 years (4,5). Emotionally, caregivers may find themselves with significant depression and anxiety, due to not only the loss of their expectations for their family, but also due to social isolation, lack of support from coworkers, or participation in previous hobbies or activities (6).

Finally, it is important to look at the needs of each member of the family. A study in Sweden sought to understand how healthcare services can support the children of people with MS. The team completed focus group discussions with adolescents and parents with MS. The findings were that the adolescents had a need to be well informed about the disease, specifically around the time of diagnosis and then throughout the disease process. The authors caution that the information should be age appropriate and individualized based on the family member with MS (10).

As discussed earlier, family caregivers have several needs that warrant attention, but are often overlooked because of the care being focused on the MS patient (11). The rest of the chapter focuses on caregiver issues and gives specific and tangible guidelines for caring not only for the MS patient, but also for the caregiver.

STAGES OF CAREGIVING

The natural ebb and flow of life calls for taking care of infants and the elderly, but the care of an adult who suffers a chronic condition is usually unexpected (12). The course of MS is generally unpredictable, as caregivers are unable to predict a relapse, progression of the disease, and sometimes even a patient's functional ability or emotional response throughout a day. Caregivers may become concerned with both the person with MS and with how the disease has an impact on the caregiver's own life (13).

Caregiving, especially in a disease with an unpredictable course, is a dynamic and ever-changing phenomenon. As each family member presents in the medical team's office, each individual, from the patient to individual family members, will have their own unique reaction to new roles and identity due to the chronic disease. Although in the past, the family may have developed a certain identity and rhythm, the development of a disease challenges, and may even disrupt, the family identity. Often, the original family "caregiver" becomes the "caretaker," or the primary "bread winner" no longer holds that role. These new roles can present significant challenges to both individuals.

In many significant ways, a family benefits from progressing through the grieving process of the loss of role and identity and comes to some form of acceptance of the disease. Elisabeth Kubler-Ross is widely known for her grief/acceptance model, which she presented in her book *On Death and Dying* (14). In this model, a person or family who is presented with a major life loss or change engages in a series of emotional reactions. She describes these reactions as shock, denial, anger, bargaining, depression, and acceptance. Each person will engage in their own feelings and reactions and the cycle is not meant to be chronological, but rather a framework for grief and eventual acceptance.

Caregivers themselves also progress through caregiving stages. Lindegren, in 1993, in a study of spouses caring for partners with dementia (15), described "a caregiving career," where the specific stages include the *encounter phase*, wherein the couple confronts the diagnosis, then grieves the loss of their previous life, and acquires the skills necessary to properly care for the family member. In the next phase, the *enduring phase*, the caregiver is submersed in caregiving to a substantial degree, oftentimes to the detriment of their own self-care. In this phase, caregivers must learn to cope with social isolation and their own mental pain. Finally, in the *exit phase*, the "caregiving career" is somewhat relinquished because of either death or institutionalization of the patient.

> *Caregivers progress through caregiving stages: the* encounter phase, *the* enduring phase, *and the* exit phase.

As independent observers, the medical team is in a unique position to identify and discuss these cycles with both the patient and the caregiver. If a member of the medical team becomes aware of a patient or family member's difficulty or if there are unaddressed needs, coordination of care can begin to address these issues.

NEEDS OF THE CAREGIVER

Significant and healthy human relationships are successful only when they are reciprocal and mutual. The MS patient may need a great deal of assistance, but the needs of the caregiver must also be met in order for the relationship to remain healthy. Although several directions could be taken regarding the importance of self-care, this section addresses what one might consider the *trifecta of self-care* (Figure 37.1).

> *The MS patient may need a great deal of assistance, but the needs of the caregiver must also be met in order for the relationship to remain healthy.*

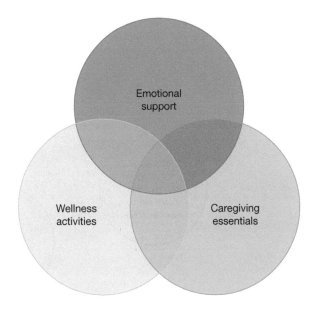

FIGURE 37.1 The trifecta of caregivers' self-care.

Emotional Support

Caring for someone with a chronic illness can lead to a decreased quality of life, a decline in psychological health, increased stress, and depression and anxiety (6,16–18). Research has clearly demonstrated the negative emotional consequences of caregiving, which can lead to dysfunctional coping skills, strained relationships, reduced life satisfaction, and emotional and physical sickness (19–21). In addition, the stress of caregiving can precipitate affective disorders such as anxiety and depression. It is not uncommon for caregivers to identify a need for treatment from a mental health provider, but few actually seek the needed help (18,19,22). Related to identifying the need for and seeking mental health treatments, one study using the NARCOMS registry found that older age of caregivers significantly decreased the perceived need for mental health treatment. In comparison, the caregivers feeling of emotional drain and burden was linked to the increased odds of the perceived need for mental health counselling (23) Recognizing the issue is important, but following through is vital. Failure to seek help has been identified as a factor in caregiver burnout and mental health disorders.

In the proposed medical team model or multidisciplinary model (Figure 37.2), support is built-in. Any member of the team can identify and validate the need for support that can be supplied by the appropriate team member. If practicing outside a Team Model, appropriate referrals can be made.

Mental health practitioners have specific interventions with the aim of reducing caregiver burden and improving mental and physical health. Sharing emotions with others relieves stress and may offer a different perspective on problems. These are helpful steps to improve the emotional and physical health of caregivers. The National Multiple Sclerosis Society (NMSS, United States) offers a variety of

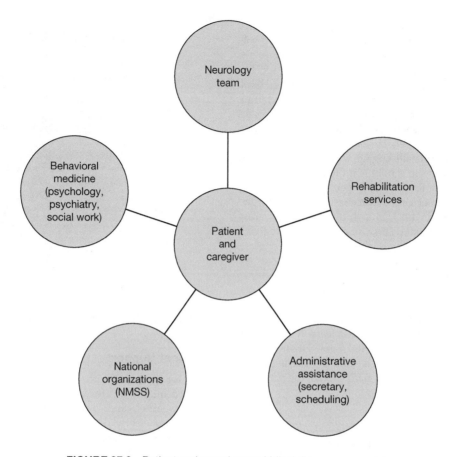

FIGURE 37.2 Patient and caregiver multidisciplinary care model.

programs aimed at helping ease the emotional burden such as support groups, psychoeducational programming, referrals to mental health providers, and web chats. The NMSS offers a program called "Relationship Matters" (RM), which is an 8-hour relationships enrichment program aimed at increasing relationship satisfaction in couples living with MS. The program integrates information on MS, the NMSS, and empirically based marriage education. The program is an in-person workshop that is delivered across the country by the local chapters of the NMSS. Outcomes were collected on this program with individuals who participated and were compared to a control group and the RM course showed significant improvements in relationship satisfaction over time compared to no intervention control group. Additionally, the program showed improvements in mental health–related quality of life, communication, conflict resolution, and the ability to handle MS-specific relationship issues. Overall, this program is of great benefit for individuals and partners of MS (24).

When referring to a mental health practitioner, it is important to pick a provider who has extensive experience in chronic disease management and understands the complexities of how MS affects the entire family. Early recognition by a clinician or by the caregiver themselves are linked with more successful outcomes (25).

Caregiving Essentials

Caregivers often come into the role of caregiving as a necessity and have no previous knowledge of skill. They may take the "learn as you go" approach, which can create more stress. In addition, oftentimes being the sole care provider comes with additional responsibilities, including, but not limited to, career, parenting, and household chores. As highlighted earlier, the relaying of information and referral to services such as the NMSS, the Multiple Sclerosis Association of America, or the Multiple Sclerosis Foundation, can be helpful in providing caregivers with useful skills. In addition, healthcare providers should be open to discussing and brainstorming ways to help ease these household task burdens (e.g., hired help, enlisting other family members or friends) (25,26).

Wellness Programs

The behavioral medicine literature is full of studies which show the power of physical activity and wellness in self-care. In general, research has demonstrated that engaging in exercise and physical activity significantly enhances both physiological and psychological health (27-30). The benefits of exercise and physical activity have been documented across a wide array of health areas, including chronic disease prevention and control, mental health, and health-related quality of life (27–30). Many caregivers neglect their own emotional, physical, and spiritual needs. Wellness encompasses healthy all-around living. Some studies suggest eating a balanced diet, getting at least 7 hours of restorative sleep, regular exercise (i.e., 30 minutes or aerobic exercise 4 or more days a week with a doctor's approval), caring for emotional health by way of a mental health provider, maintaining friendships and hobbies, and for those with a spiritual alignment, spending some time on that (25,26).

Within the multidisciplinary team of MS professionals, each and every member should take a moment to assess and address caregiver needs. When assessing a caregiver, "Ten Tips for Caregivers to Avoid Burnout" (Table 37.1) can be helpful.

ABUSE

The physical, financial, and emotional toll brought by caregiving can turn even the most loving family members into individuals who struggle with strong emotions and urge to harm. In people with MS or other disabling conditions, members of the multidisciplinary care team must become comfortable at assessing for abuse by spouse or caregiver, as individuals with disabilities may identify abuse as the most important health issue that they face (31). In fact, in 2005, the American Medical Association recommended that all patients be screened for domestic

violence and safety in their homes (32). Three types of abuse are described: (a) physical (including sexual and neglect), (b) psychological (including both verbal and nonverbal), and (c) financial. Oftentimes, overlap may occur within the types of abuse.

Physical abuse and emotional abuse are the most common types of abuse in a chronic care population. The care recipient is often frail and becomes an easy target for aggression. Physical abuse generally starts during caregiving. The caregiver can become rough during grooming or transfers. Scratches, bruises, and even the more obvious signs of abuse (e.g., black eyes or broken bones) can be noticed on the person. Neglect is often characterized in terms of physical abuse. This neglect can occur when a caregiver is burned out and decides to forgo on his or her duties to the family members without seeking help outside. A caregiver might leave the care recipient for long periods of time meeting his or her basic needs such as, toileting, eating, and transfers. The care recipient may miss appointments or become malnourished, or medications become mismanaged. These signs can be warning signs for the MS professional to seek immediate help. If the abuse happens once, it likely will happen again.

Emotional abuse is often more difficult to detect. It may happen in the home through degrading language, harsh comments, and humiliation. The abuser may control the victim through language and emotional reactions such as ignoring the person, and may cause the victim psychological damage. Emotional abuse may happen when a caregiver is overburdened, overextended,

TABLE 37.1 Ten Important Tips for Caregivers to Avoid Burnout

1) **Become Educated About MS**. The more one knows about the disease, the more empowered he or she will feel, and the more comfortable he or she will feel with role changes. Ask as many questions as you need when you are in appointments. No question is a stupid question, and all questions are important.

2) **Take Care of Yourself**. As airline stewardesses say, "You must put on your own oxygen mask, before putting on the mask of another," this philosophy stands for caregiving. If you are unhealthy emotionally, physically, or spiritually, you will be of no help to anyone else.

3) **Practice Healthy Living**. One is much more capable of being of help to others when you eat a healthy, balanced diet, you exercise regularly, you are involved with your own interests, and you get enough sleep.

4) **Stay Social**. Connecting with others in similar situations is powerful because you no longer feel isolated and you can learn from others. In addition, make sure you maintain other important relationships such as with children, family members, and close friends.

5) **Accept Help**. As difficult as it is to ask for help from others, realize that you need a break and that others may want to help. You do not have to do it all, nor is it healthy to do it all. The best way to avoid burnout is to accept help. People often want to help, just ask.

6) **Acknowledge Your Emotions**. If you are feeling hopeless, worthless, helpless, sad, anxious, or fearful, acknowledge these emotions. These are all normal reactions to your situation.

7) **Allow for Healthy Expression of Your Feelings With Each Other**. Just because you are now a caregiver does not take away that you had a relationship with this person in the past. You are still a spouse, partner, child, and so on, and with that comes the responsibility to speak respectfully open. Should difficulties arise, seek couples or family counseling. Your MS neurology team will have a list of qualified mental health professionals.

8) **Allow for Caregiving Holidays**. This simply means take some time away. You will be a better caregiver to your loved one if you take time away.

9) **Encourage Healthy Independence of Your Loved One**. Help your loved one be as independent as he or she can for as long as they can. This may involve assistive devices or new technologies, and so seek these out.

10) **Seek Help Through Your Local Organizations**. Each territory or state has their own MS society, which you can find in the United States by calling 1-800-344-4867. The National MS Society has an MS Navigator Program which will help guide you toward available resources for both you and your loved one with MS.

MS, multiple sclerosis.

and not taking care of their own emotional needs. Abuse of any kind generally occurs when there is a power differential.

Finally, financial abuse is less likely than the other forms of abuse and generally manifests through exploitation or theft. Examples of this include the abuser improperly, illegally, or without permission, using money or goods that are not their own.

> *If abuse of any kind is suspected, referrals should be made through local social services, adult protective services, social work, mental health providers, or nonprofit organizations such as the NMSS.*

O'Leary and colleagues (33) created "REACH" as an innovative program through their local chapter of the NMSS. REACH provides Respite, Education, Awareness, Change, and Hope. This educational and outreach program was designed to help medical providers assess for abuse and provide subsequent crisis care to those involved. If abuse of any kind is suspected, referrals should be made through local social services, adult protective services, social work, mental health providers, or the NMSS. Table 37.2 presents a list of resources that can be helpful to caregivers.

MULTIDISCIPLINARY MEDICAL TEAM

The most efficacious management of chronic disease benefits from access to high-quality comprehensive care teams of skilled professionals that include attention to symptom management and quality of life (Figure 37.2).

TABLE 37.2   Resources

Books

Carter R. *Helping Yourself Help Others: A Book for Caregivers*. Random House/Time Books; 1995
Provides basic information for caregivers

Kalb R. *Multiple Sclerosis: A Guide for Families*, 3rd ed. Demos Health; 2006
Provides information on a variety of caregiving issues such as emotions, cognitive issues, sexuality, intimacy, and life planning

Caregiving Support

National MS Society's MS Navigator Program
Tel: 800-344-4867.
www.nationalmssociety.org/living-with-multiple-sclerosis/relationships/carepartners/index.aspx
Provides information on educational programs and self-help groups.

Caregiver.com
www.caregiver.com

- Is the most visited caregiver site on the internet
- Publishes *Today's Caregiver Magazine*
- Provides many links to resources and agencies of interest

Today's Caregiver Magazine
Tel: 800-829-2734. www.caregiver.com/magazine
Is a bimonthly magazine resource for caregivers

The Well Spouse Association
63 West Main Street, Suite H, Freehold, NJ 07728
Tel: 800-838-0879. www.wellspouse.org

- Advocates and addresses the needs of individuals caring for the chronically ill
- Publishes *Mainstay*, a quarterly newsletter

Caregiver Action Network1130 Connecticut Ave., NW, Suite 300, Washington, DC 20036-3904
Tel: 202-454-3970 http://caregiveraction.org/ or e-mail info@caregiveraction.orgeducates, supports, and empowers more than 90 million Americans who are caregivers to the chronically ill

United Way
www.unitedway.org
Provides help for individuals and families to achieve their human potential through education, income stability, and healthy lives

Home Care Agencies/Hiring Help

National Association for Home Care and Hospice
228 Seventh Street, SE, Washington, DC 20003
Tel: 202-547-7424. www.nahc.org
Provides referrals to state associations

Hiring Help at Home
A fact sheet from the National MS Society
Tel: 1-800-344-4867

Adapted from the National MS Society: MS and Carepartners at
https://www.nationalmssociety.org/NationalMSSociety/media/MSNationalFiles/Brochures/Brochure-HiringHelpAtHome-BasicFacts-FINAL.pdf

This level of care is not always available and requires a shift from the traditional "medical" model to a more "functional" model of care, incorporating the concerns of patient, family member, and caregiver. This care may occur in the same medical setting or each provider may be housed in different facilities, yet work together collaboratively. Included in a successful multidisciplinary team for the management of MS are the physician, advanced practice clinicians, psychologist, psychiatrist, physical therapist, occupational therapist, social worker, nurses, speech therapist, national associations, and administrative support (Figure 37.1). This model allows for several practitioners, organizations, and even the administrative support to interact with, assess, and determine what types of interventions to recommend for the caregiver. When this type of a team can be assembled, an optimal level of care for both the patient and their family of caretakers can be provided. For those who are unable to practice within a team setting, developing referral listings and partnering with local organizations with the common interest in MS care are highly recommended.

SUMMARY

MS is a chronic, complex illness which can potentially have expansive and profound effects on the entire family. Although caregiving can be greatly rewarding, it also presents challenges. Caregivers can become overburdened with the care of the person with MS and care of the household, finances, and their own self. Caregivers must make it a point to care for themselves emotionally and physically. Although clinical visits are often focused on the MS patient, care providers must make it a point to assess and provide recommendations to the caregiver, particular if that caregiver is experiencing burnout or sometimes even abusing the MS patient. Table 37.2 presents a list of resources that can be helpful to health.

KEY POINTS FOR PATIENTS AND FAMILIES

- Caregiving for a loved one with a chronic condition can often be profoundly fulfilling, as many times individuals move closer together when challenges arise.
- Caregiving can become overwhelming, physically and emotionally challenging, and isolating. At times it can be thought of as a burden.
- Caregivers must learn to take care of themselves physically and emotionally.
- The multidisciplinary care model used in the treatment of MS is important not only for the patient, but also for the caregiver. This care model allows for several practitioners to interact with the caregiver to assess and determine the optional interventions.
- Physical, emotional, and financial abuses secondary to the profound challenges inherent in caring for a relative with a disabling chronic illness are not uncommon. Assessing for abuse is an important component in the clinical management of MS.

REFERENCES

1. Frohman EM. Multiple sclerosis. *Med Clin North Am*. 2003;87:867–897.
2. Pooyania MD, Lobchuk M, Chernomas W, et al. Examining the relationship between family caregiver's emotional states and ability to empathize with patients with multiple sclerosis. *Int J MS Care*. 2016;18(3):122–128.
3. Hileman J, Lackey N, Hassaneien R. Identifying the needs of home caregivers of patients with cancer. *Oncol Nurs Forum*. 1992;19:771–777.
4. Family Caregiver Alliance. Caregiving Statistics. Retrieved June 7, 2018. Available at: https://www.caregiver.org/caregiver-statistics-demographics
5. Pandya S. Caregiving in the United States. Retrieved November 7, 2017. Available at: http://assets.aarp.org/rgcenter/il/fs111_caregiving.pdf.
6. Buhse M. Assessment of caregiver burden in families of persons with multiple sclerosis. *J Neurosci Nurs*. 2008;40(1):25–31.
7. McKenzie T, Quig ME, Tyry T, et al. Care partners and multiple Sclerosis: Differential effect on men and women. *Int J MS Care*. 2015;17(6):253–260.
8. Buchannan R, Huang C, Zheng Z. Factors affecting employment among informal caregivers assisting people with multiple sclerosis. *Int J MS Care*. 2013;15(4):203–210.
9. American Psychological Association. The high cost of caregiving. Retrieved November 7, 2017. Available at: www.apa.org/research/action/caregiving.aspx.
10. Nilsagård Y, Boström K. Informing the children when a parent is diagnosed as having multiple sclerosis. *Int J MS Care*. 2015;17(1):42–48.
11. Dewis MEM, Niskala H. Nurturing a valuable resource: family caregivers in multiple sclerosis. *Axone*. 1992;13:87–94.
12. Bellou M, Vouzavali FJD, Koutroubas A, et al. The 'care' in caregiving: the multiple sclerosis experience for the healthy family members. *Existental Anal*. 2012;23(1):149–161.
13. McKeown L, Porter-Armstrong A, Baxter G. Caregivers of people with multiple sclerosis: experiences of support. *Mult Scler*. 2004;10:219–230.
14. Kübler-Ross, E. *On Death and Dying*. Macmillan Publishing Company; New York 1969.
15. Lindgren CL. The caregiver career. *Image J Nurs Sch*. 1993;25:214–219.
16. Patti F, Amato MP, Battaglia MA, et al. Caregiver quality of life in multiple sclerosis: a multicentre Italian study. *Mult Scler*. 2007;13:412–419.
17. Figved N, Myhr K, Larsen J, et al. Caregiver burden in multiple sclerosis: the impact of neuropsychiatric symptoms. *J Neurol Neurosurg Psychiatry*. 2007;78:1097–1102.

18. Sherman TE, Rapport IJ, Hanks RA, et al. Predictors of well-being among significant others of person with multiple sclerosis. *Mult Scler*. 2007;13:238–249.

19. O'Brien MT. Multiple sclerosis: stressors and coping strategies in spousal caregivers. *J Community Health Nurs*. 1993;10:123–135.

20. O'Brien RA, Wineman NM, Nealon NR. Correlates of the caregiving process in multiple sclerosis. *Sch Inq Nurs Pract*. 1995;9:323–338.

21. Gulick EE. Coping among spouses or significant others of persons with multiple sclerosis. *Nurs Res*. 1995;44:220–225.

22. Buchanan RJ, Radin D, Chakravorty B, et al. Informal care giving to more disable people with multiple sclerosis. *Disabil Rehabil*. 2009;31:1244–1256.

23. Buchanan R, Huang C. The need for mental health care among informal caregivers assisting people with multiple sclerosis. *Int J MS Care*. 2013;15(2):56–64.

24. Tompkins SA, Roeder JA, Thomas JJ, et al. Effectiveness of a relationship enrichment program for couples living with multiple sclerosis. *Int J MS Care*. 2013;15(1):27–34.

25. National MS Society. A guide for caregivers: managing major changes. Retrieved November 7, 2017. Available at: https://www.nationalmssociety.org/Resources-Support/Library-Education-Programs/Brochures/Managing-Major-Changes.

26. Holland NJ, Schneider DM, Rapp R, et al. Meeting the needs of people with primary progressive multiple sclerosis, their families, and the health-care community. *Int J MS Care*. 2011;13:5–74.

27. Sullivan AB, Covington E, Scheman J. Immediate benefits of a brief 10-minute exercise protocol in a chronic pain population: a pilot study. *Pain Med*. 2010;11(4):524–529.

28. Bouchard C, Shephard RJ, Stephens T. *Physical Activity, Fitness, and Health: International Proceedings and Consensus Statement*. Champaign, IL: Human Kinetics; 1994.

29. Brownell KD, O'Neil PM. Obesity. In: Barlow DH, ed. *Clinical Handbook of Psychological Disorders: A Step-by-Step Treatment Manual*. 2nd ed. New York, NY: Guilford; 1993:318–361.

30. Kirkcaldy BD, Shephard RJ, Siefen RG. The relationship between physical activity and self-image and problem behaviour among adolescents. *Soc Psychiatry Psychiatr Epidemiol*. 2002;37:544–550.

31. Berkeley Planning Associates. *Priorities for Future Research: Results of BPA's Delphi Survey of Disabled Women*. Oakland, CA: Berkley Planning Associates; 1996.

32. Chalk R, King PA, eds, Committee on the Assessment of Family Violence Interventions, National Research Council, Institute of Medicine. *Violence in Families: Assessing Prevention and Treatment Programs*. Washington DC: National Academies Press; 1998.

33. O'Leary M, Lammers S, Mageras A, et al. Relationship between domestic violence and multiple sclerosis. *Int J MS Care*. 2008;10:27–32.

38

Neuromyelitis Optica

Amanda L. Piquet and John R. Corboy

KEY POINTS FOR THE CLINICIAN

- Neuromyelitis optica (NMO) is a distinct clinical–pathological disease that is different from multiple sclerosis (MS).
- NMO occurs as acute attacks, and only rarely may evolve into a slow progressive phase of disability accumulation.
- NMO typically targets the optic nerves and spinal cord; however, it may also involve the hypothalamus, area postrema (intractable nausea and vomiting, or hiccoughs), or cerebral locations, hence the terminology neuromyelitis optica spectrum disorder (NMOSD) to include those individuals who do not have a classic presentation.
- NMOSD is defined by a pathogenic antibody, aquaporin-4 immunoglobulin G (AQP4-IgG).
- Treatment for acute attacks of NMOSD consists of high-dose methylprednisolone, +/− plasma exchange.
- Prophylactic treatment for NMOSD includes aggressive, early intervention given the high disability that is directly related to clinical relapses, with rituximab or azathioprine as first-line therapies for relapse prevention. Duration of prophylactic therapy remains unclear.

NMO, also known as Devic's disease, is an autoimmune demyelinating disease of the central nervous system (CNS). Once thought to be a form of MS, NMO has now been defined as a distinct clinical–pathological disorder, although the initial clinical presentation often mimics MS. Clinically, NMO preferentially targets the optic nerves and spinal cord; however, over time, the clinical spectrum has expanded and NMO is now known to affect the brain in a substantial minority of patients. The diagnosis and pathogenesis of NMO have been greatly advanced by the discovery of the NMO-immunoglobulin G (IgG), an antibody directed against, and with high affinity to, the water channel aquaporin-4 (AQP4) in the CNS. The NMO-IgG, also known as the AQP4-IgG, appears to be pathogenic. The term NMOSD was established to describe those individuals who are seropositive for the AQP4-IgG, but who do not have the classical presentation of isolated longitudinally extensive myelitis or optic neuritis. Given the clinical aggressiveness of NMO with the associated disability, rapid recognition and diagnosis is important to appropriately tailor both acute and long-term therapies, which are often different than therapies for MS and other related disorders.

NMO is a distinct disease, different than MS.

EPIDEMIOLOGY

Large studies defining the prevalence and incidence rate of NMO in populations are lacking; furthermore, incidence and prevalence varies between geographical regions and various ethnic populations. Data from systematic review of published peer-reviewed studies suggest a prevalence rate between 0.52 and 4.4 per 100,000 people per year and incidence rate of 0.053 to 0.40 per 100,000 people in various locations around the world (1–3). NMO prevalence is approximately 1% to 2% that of MS in the United States (4) and there is a higher representation of NMO among non-white populations (5). Given this observation, in a patient with a non-Caucasian background with severe optic neuritis or myelitis, NMO should be high on the differential diagnosis.

The median age of onset is 39 years old, which is later than MS (Table 38.1), although NMO has been described in both children and the elderly. The prevalence of NMO is three to nine times higher in women than men (1,8,9).

CLINICAL FEATURES

NMO most frequently presents as severe optic neuritis, transverse myelitis, or a combination of both. The diagnosis of NMO should be considered in patients with those presenting syndromes, especially if an MRI of the brain is normal or atypical for MS.

> NMO most often presents as severe optic neuritis, myelitis, or both.

NMO-associated optic neuritis is similar in clinical presentation to other causes of inflammatory optic neuritis. Vision loss typically occurs over hours to days and peaks within 1 to 2 weeks. Mild ocular pain, often associated with eye movement, is common. Dyschromatopsia (particularly red desaturation), central or paracentral scotoma, and photopsias may also occur. The vision loss in NMO is commonly more severe than in MS (10). Bilateral simultaneous or rapidly sequential optic neuritis may also be more indicative of NMO.

Transverse myelitis is often severe and complete and can present with a symmetric para, or tetra, paresis, spinal sensory level, and significant sphincter dysfunction early in the course. Myelitis is often heralded by severe spinal pain. In comparison, MS-related myelitis typically has a more mild, unilateral, and asymmetrical clinical presentation (Table 38.1). Approximately one third of NMO patients have associated Lhermitte's phenomenon, paroxysmal tonic spasms, or radicular pain associated with the myelitis (11).

Beyond the involvement of optic nerves and spinal cord, NMO may also present with brainstem symptoms such as intractable nausea and hiccupping (from area postrema involvement) (12), vertigo, trigeminal neuralgia, diplopia, and nystagmus. Cases have also been described with acute encephalopathy, cognitive changes, and hypothalamic dysfunction such as syndrome of inappropriate antidiuretic hormone secretion (SIADH) (13).

NMO may also be associated with organ-specific autoimmunity (e.g., myasthenia gravis, type 1 diabetes, pernicious anemia, and ulcerative colitis) and non-organ-specific autoimmune disease (e.g., systemic lupus erythematosus (SLE) and Sjögren's syndrome). Evidence suggests that

TABLE 38.1 NMO and MS Comparison

CLINICAL FACTORS	NMO	MS
Average age of onset	Late fourth to early fifth decade	Third to early fourth decade
Gender (Female: Male)	3:1 to 9:1	2:1
Population prevalence	Higher prevalence in nonwhite populations	Varies geographically, white populations more affected
Clinical features	Primarily severe optic neuritis and myelitis; greater than 90% with relapsing course, rarely monophasic course; slowly progressive symptoms are rare	Dissemination in time and space affecting multiple CNS sites, typically of milder severity; 85% relapsing–remitting, 15% progressive at onset; many relapsing patients later have a progressive course
Coexisting autoimmune disease MRI	Common (SLE, Sjögren's, myasthenia gravis)	Rare
Brain	Often normal, may have nonspecific T2 hyperintensities and hypothalamic, periventricular (third/fourth ventricle), or medullary lesions	Lesions are ovoid and periventricular, juxtacortical, callosal, and infratentorial locations
Spine	Lesions typically longitudinally extensive (three or more vertebral segments), centrally located with cord expansion	one to two vertebral segments, asymmetric, peripheral location
CSF profile	Pleocytosis in about 50%(up to 50–1,000 × 10⁶ WBC/L) (6) with increased neutrophils and eosinophils; increased protein; elevated IL-6 (7) and GFAP	Mild pleocytosis or normal
CSF oligoclonal bands	Uncommon (15–30%) (6)	Common (90%)
Serum AQP4-IgG	Present in majority	Absent

AQP4-IgG, aquaporin4-immunoglobulin G; CNS, central nervous system; CSF, cerebrospinal fluid; GFAP, glial fibrillary acidic protein; IL, interleukin; MS, multiple sclerosis; NMO, neuromyelitis optica; SLE, systemic lupus erythematosus; WBC, white blood cell.

systemic autoimmune diseases coexist with NMO rather than act as a direct cause. Autoantibodies to antinuclear antigen (ANA; 44%) and Sjögren's syndrome A autoantibody (SSA; 16%) are found more frequently in NMO patients than in seronegative individuals, while no patients with SLE or Sjögren's without manifestations consistent with NMO are AQP4-IgG seropositive (14). There is a high rate of coexisting neural-specific autoantibodies in NMOSD (35%), such as muscle acetylcholine receptor antibody (AChR), voltage-gated potassium channel complex antibodies (VGKC; LGI-1 and Caspr2), and collapsing response-mediator protein (CRMP-5) (10,15). NMO may present as a paraneoplastic syndrome, especially in the elderly. Neoplasms reported in NMO AQP4-IgG positive patients include breast, lung, thymic, uterine, ovarian teratoma, B-cell lymphoma, stomach carcinoid, and leiomyosarcoma (16–21).

Pediatric NMO

Children as young as 2 years old have been reported with NMO; however, pediatric NMO most commonly has onset between the ages of 10 to 14 years old (6). In pediatric cases, the brain tends to be more commonly involved than adults. Children may present with symptoms of encephalopathy, ataxia, seizure, and/or intractable nausea and vomiting. In seropositive NMO cases, 68% of children have brain abnormalities on MRI (22).

NMO and Pregnancy

Unlike MS, which tends to be quiescent during pregnancy with a decreased relapse rate, studies have shown an increase in relapse rate in NMO patients during pregnancy (23). Both NMO and MS have an increased risk of relapse rate within the immediate postpartum period. Additionally, patients with NMO have an increased rate of pregnancy complications with risks to both fetal and maternal health. Obstetric complications include spontaneous abortion, stillbirth, preterm delivery, low birth weight, and preeclampsia or pregnancy-induced hypertension (23).

IMAGING

MRI Spine

Spinal cord MRI is helpful in patients with signs and symptoms suggestive of a myelopathy. Lesions are typically longitudinally extensive (usually greater than three vertebral segments in length), centrally located, often occupy more than one-half of the cord area, and are associated with cord expansion and edema (Figure 38.1). T2 hyperintensities are best seen on short tau inversion recovery (STIR) or proton density sequences and may have associated T1 hypointensity. Gadolinium enhancement, often seen during the acute attack, is frequently homogenous and involves the central portion of the lesion (Figure 38.1). The pattern of T2 hyperintensity and gadolinium enhancement may help

differentiate NMO from other etiologies of longitudinally extensive myelitis, such as neurosarcoidosis, which is demonstrated in Figure 38.1. NMO will typically have central spinal cord involvement, often with relative sparing of the peripheral cord. In contrast, neurosarcoidosis often will have both central and peripheral involvement, classically sparing the small region between the central and peripheral cord. A small subset of patients may present with short MRI lesions, which should not exclude the diagnosis of NMO (25,26). On the contrary, rarely MS may actually mimic NMO with longitudinally extensive transverse myelitis (LETM) and this should be considered in the setting of AQP4 seronegativity (27). NMO patients with a history of a prior acute myelitis often can have extensive cord atrophy as chronic sequela (Figure 38.2).

> *Spinal cord lesions are typically greater than three vertebral segments in length.*

MRI Brain

Over time, it has been recognized that NMO is not limited to only the optic nerves and spinal cord, and there are reports of both symptomatic and asymptomatic brain lesions on neuroimaging. The lesions are often located within the areas of high AQP4 concentrations such as the hypothalamus, around the third and fourth ventricles, and in the brainstem, particularly the medulla near the area postrema, and are typically distinct from MS lesion appearance. Brain MRI early in the disease course is often normal, but up to 60% of NMO patients may develop brain MRI abnormalities over time, albeit many changes are often nonspecific (28). Optic nerve imaging may also help distinguish NMO from MS as MRI abnormalities often show extensive optic nerve involvement in NMO as well as enhancement of the optic chiasm; chiasmal involvement is not typical of MS (29).

DIAGNOSIS

The diagnosis of NMO is based on clinical features with paraclinical support from neuroimaging and serological testing. NMO should be considered in all patients with severe optic neuritis, longitudinally extensive transverse myelitis (> three vertebral segments long), recurrent episodes of isolated optic neuritis, or bilateral simultaneous or sequential optic neuritis. The current 2015 International Consensus Diagnostic Criteria offer guidance in the diagnosis of NMOSD (Table 38.2) (30). In 2006, as part of the revised Mayo Clinic criteria for NMO, the term NMOSD was introduced to describe individuals seropositive for AQP4-IgG, but with a form of CNS involvement beyond just longitudinally extensive transverse myelitis and/or bilateral simultaneous or recurrent optic neuritis (31). In 2015, the International Panel for NMO Diagnosis changed the nomenclature to unify the term NMO and

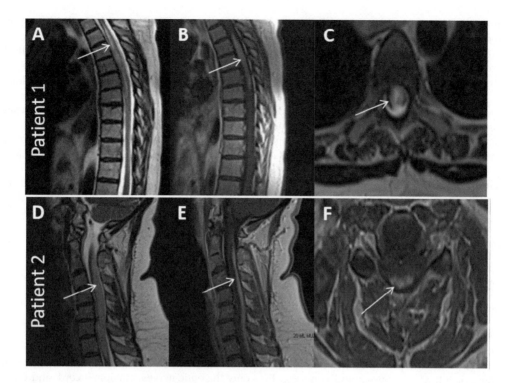

FIGURE 38.1 MRI for Patient 1 demonstrates a longitudinally extensive transverse myelitis in the setting of a positive AQP4-IgG. (A) T2-weighted sagittal image of the thoracic spine shows a longitudinally extensive T2 hyperintense lesion with the (B) T1-postcontrast sagittal image and (C) axial image demonstrating associated central cord enhancement. As seen in the axial image, it is common for spinal cord lesions to occupy more than half of the spinal cord in cross section. Patient 2 was diagnosed with neurosarcoidosis with biopsy-proven noncaseating granulomas of the lymph node, as well as a negative AQP4-IgG antibody. (D) T2-weighted sagittal image of cervical spine with longitudinally extensive myelitis and associated edema. (E and F) T1-postcontrast sagittal and axial images, respectfully, demonstrate posterior subpial enhancement. This pattern of dorsal subpial enhancement with central cord involvement (described as the "trident sign") in spinal neurosarcoidosis is distinctly different from NMO, which tends to have primarily central cord involvement, often with relative sparing of the peripheral and subpial regions.

Source: Images are original but source supports the terminology of the trident sign. Zalewski NL, Krecke KN, Weinshenker BG, et al. Central canal enhancement and the trident sign in spinal cord sarcoidosis. *Neurology.* 2016;87(7):743–744. (24)

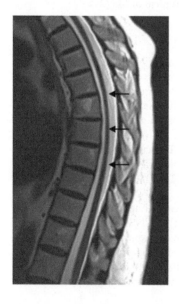

FIGURE 38.2 T2-weighted MRI of thoracic cord demonstrating thoracic cord atrophy extending greater than three vertebral segments in a patient with NMO.

NMO, neuromyelitis optica.

NMOSD and further stratify the disorder by serological testing (30). With a positive AQP4 antibody, one must have at least one of the six core clinical characteristics (Table 38.3). With a negative AQP4 antibody or unknown antibody status, a patient must meet more stringent clinical criteria (Table 38.2).

Other etiologies of optic neuritis and/or transverse myelitis must be considered and include MS, acute disseminated encephalomyelitis (ADEM), a systemic vasculitis such as SLE or Sjögren's syndrome (in the absence of an overlap syndrome with NMO supported by a negative AQP4 antibody), neurosarcoidosis, nutritional deficiency such as vitamin B_{12}, and infectious etiologies including neurosyphilis. Additionally, patients once thought to have seronegative NMOSD are now identified as having alternative autoantibodies such as myelin oligodendrocyte glycoprotein antibodies (MOG-IgG). Optic neuritis is the most common presentation with seropositive myelin oligodendrocyte glycoprotein (MOG)-IgG patients, followed by myelitis, and

TABLE 38.2   NMOSD Diagnostic Criteria

DIAGNOSTIC CRITERIA FOR NMOSD WITH POSITIVE AQP4-IGG
1) At least one core clinical characteristic (Table 38.3)
2) Positive test for AQP4-IgG using best available detection method
3) Exclusion of alternative diagnosis

DIAGNOSTIC CRITERIA FOR NMOSD WITHOUT AQP4-IgG (ANTIBODY NEGATIVE OR UNKNOWN STATUS DUE TO UNAVAILABLE TESTING)
1) At least two core clinical characteristics as one or more clinical attacks as well as:
a) At least one core clinical characteristic must be optic neuritis, acute myelitis with LETM, or area postrema syndrome
b) Dissemination in space (two or more different core clinical characteristics)
c) Additional MRI requirements as applicable:
1) Optic neuritis: requires brain MRI to show either normal findings OR T2-hyperintense lesion or T1-weighted gadolinium-enhanced lesion extending over half the optic nerve length or involving the optic chiasm
2) Acute myelitis: requires associated intramedullary MRI lesions extending over ≥ three continuous segments (LETM) OR ≥ contiguous segments of focal spinal cord atrophy in patients with a history of acute myelitis (Figure 38.1 and 38.2)
3) Area postrema syndrome: requires lesions in the dorsal medulla/area postrema
4) Acute brainstem syndrome: requires periependymal brainstem lesions
2) Exclusion of alternative diagnosis

AQP4-IgG, aquaporin-4 immunoglobulin G; LETM, longitudinally extensive transverse myelitis; NMOSD, neuromyelitis optica spectrum disorder.

Source: Wingerchuk DM, Banwell B, Bennett JL, et al., International consensus diagnostic criteria for neuromyelitis optica spectrum disorders. *Neurology.* 2015;85(2):177–189, p.179 and http://n.neurology.org/content/85/2/177.long

TABLE 38.3   Core Clinical Characteristics in NMOSD

- Optic neuritis
- Acute myelitis
- Area postrema syndrome (unexplained hiccups or nausea and vomiting)
- Acute brainstem syndrome
- Symptomatic narcolepsy or acute diencephalic clinical syndrome with associated radiographic lesions on MRI
- Symptomatic brain lesions typical of NMO such as hypothalamic, brainstem, and periventricular

NMO, neuromyelitis optica; NMOSD, neuromyelitis optica spectrum disorder.

Source: Wingerchuk DM, Banwell B, Bennett JL, et al., International consensus diagnostic criteria for neuromyelitis optica spectrum disorders. *Neurology.* 2015;85(2):177–189, p.179 and http://n.neurology.org/content/85/2/177.long

brainstem encephalitis (32). Unlike NMO, MOG-IgG seropositive disease is more likely to have a monophasic course (80%) and clinical or radiographic involvement of the brain, brainstem, or cerebellum (50%). Male-to-female ratio is 1:2 (32). Glial fibrillary acidic protein (GFAP)-IgG has also been recognized as a biomarker of autoimmune astrocytopathy with or without coexisting AQP4-IgG (33). Patients typically present with features of a subacute relapsing meningoencephalomyelitis. Unlike NMO, there is not a strong female predominance; in a study of 102 patients, only 54% were female (33).

LABORATORY STUDIES

The discovery of the autoantibody directed against AQP4 has aided in the distinction of NMO from other inflammatory demyelinating disorders. AQP4 is an osmosis-driven, water-selective transporter expressed on the astrocytic foot processes throughout the CNS and is involved in water homeostasis, astrocyte migration, neuronal signal transduction, and neuroinflammation. There are high concentrations of AQP4 in subpial, subependymal areas, and the hypothalamus, in addition to the optic nerve and spinal cord. The precise role of AQP4-IgG has not been fully elucidated; however, there is substantial evidence that this antibody has a pathogenic role in NMO (14,34). The original indirect immunofluorescence assay for AQP4-IgG, used with a composite substrate of mouse tissues, identified NMO patients with a sensitivity of 73% and specificity of 91% (35). Subsequently, the development of transfected cell-based assays (CBA) has increased the sensitivity of the test significantly, to almost 90% (6). The CBAs use either observer-based immunofluorescence or automated-flow cytometry for the detection of AQP4 antibodies. Currently, the AQP4-transfected CBA with fluorescence-activated cell sorting assay (FACS) is considered the best method for antibody detection. The CBA also has a lower rate of false positivity (specificity >99%)

(6) compared with the enzyme-linked immunosorbent assay (ELISA; sensitivity of 60%–65% and specificity of 99%) (36). AQP4-IgG testing should be performed on serum as the sensitivity is much better when compared to the cerebrospinal fluid (CSF) (6,14).

AQP4-IgG is a highly specific test for NMO.

CSF abnormalities are common in NMO. Elevation in white blood cells (WBC) is noted in approximately 50% and may be greater than 50×10^6 WBC/L, including a high proportion of neutrophils. Oligoclonal bands (OCBs) are present in only 15–30%, compared to approximately 90% in MS (6). Testing for AQP4-IgG in the CSF is not the preferred method of testing and while there is one study of 26 seronegative NMO patients with CSF AQP4 positivity (37), this was in the setting of older methodologies of testing and other recent studies have not supported this finding (6,10,38).

Seronegative NMO

There are patients who meet the clinical diagnostic criteria for NMOSD who do not have detectable AQP4-IgG (Table 38.2) and this can present as a diagnostic challenge. The reported prevalence of seronegative patients can vary due to multiple factors including the sensitivity of the assay used for diagnosis and concomitant use of immunotherapy. When using the best current method for antibody detection, the reported rate of seronegative patients is 12% (39). When a patient does not have a detectable AQP4-IgG, then additional workup including other antibody-mediated diseases such as MOG-IgG is essential.

CLINICAL COURSE AND PROGNOSIS

Approximately 90% of NMO patients have a relapsing course with further episodes of optic neuritis and/or myelitis, with the remainder being monophasic (40). In relapsing disease, attacks can be separated by months to years at unpredictable intervals. Predictors of a relapsing course includes older age of onset, longer interval between first and second clinical attacks, female gender, and less severe motor disability with the index event (41). Although counterintuitive, longer time between initial relapses is actually more predictive of a future relapsing course after the second attack (41); this observation suggests those with a short interval after initial relapse may simply represent a prolonged initial attack and subsequent lower risk of subsequent relapses over time. Fifty-five percent of relapsing NMO patients have their first relapse within 1 year and 90% within 5 years (42). Unlike MS, there does not appear to be a secondary or progressive form of NMO.

Most NMO patients have a relapsing course.

As in MS, the natural history of NMO is variable between individuals. Some have an aggressive, unrelenting, and ultimately fatal course from the outset, while others have a milder course that stabilizes over time. Overall, NMO attacks tend to be more severe with less recovery than MS. The disability of NMO is attack related rather than resulting from the accumulation of disability in a later, progressive phase of the disease as seen in MS (41). Higher attack frequency within the first 2 years, concomitant autoimmune disease, incomplete recovery from the index event, and sphincter signs at onset are associated with poorer outcomes (41). Without aggressive long-term therapy, 53% of patients presenting with optic neuritis had bilateral vision involvement and 63% were considered blind in one eye after 8 years (43). At 5 years, 65% of patients showed at least moderate disability and 42% required walking assistance (44). One study in the 1990s found a 5-year survival rate of 68% in relapsing disease with mortality secondary to respiratory failure from high cervical and medullary lesions (9). Patients who obtain an accurate diagnosis and are started on appropriate early immunotherapy have better outcomes; studies have shown reduced disability with less than 28% of NMO patients requiring a cane to walk and less than 8% wheelchair-bound after 5 years (39).

TREATMENT

Acute Relapse

The cornerstone of treatment of acute inflammatory demyelinating disease of the CNS is corticosteroids, and NMO is no different (Table 38.4 and Figure 38.3). Randomized controlled studies of corticosteroids in acute treatment of NMO exacerbations are lacking, and treatment is driven by clinical experience and studies of corticosteroids in MS and optic neuritis. Intravenous (IV) methylprednisolone dosage of 1,000 mg daily for 5 days, commonly followed by an oral prednisone taper of 2 to 8 weeks depending on the severity of the attack, is most commonly used based on a consensus among experts (45). If there is minimal or no response to corticosteroids, or if the attack is severe, then the use of plasma exchange (PLEX) has been shown to be beneficial (46,47) and is generally recommended. Predictors of favorable response to PLEX include minimal disability at baseline, preserved reflexes at time of diagnosis, and early initiation of treatment (46). Rescue therapy with early initiation of PLEX is recommended in steroid-unresponsive severe attacks, with three to seven exchanges (commonly five exchanges) performed daily to every other day based on tolerance. Clinical improvement may be noticed as early as one to two exchanges; nonetheless, treatment should continue for a full course.

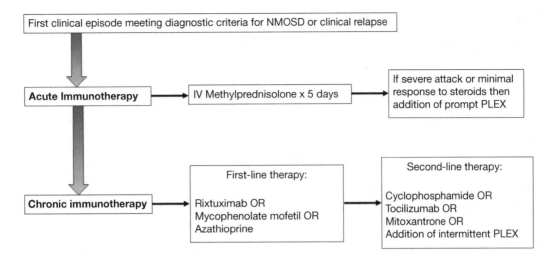

FIGURE 38.3 Treatment algorithm for NMOSD.

IV, intravenous; NMOSD, neuromyelitis optica spectrum disorder; PLEX, plasma exchange.

TABLE 38.4 Treatment Options for NMO

ACUTE RELAPSE		
MEDICATION	**TYPICAL DOSAGE**	**COMMON OR SERIOUS SIDE EFFECTS**
Methylprednisolone	1,000 mg IV daily for 5 days, usually followed by postinfusion oral prednisone taper for 2–8 wk depending on severity of attack	Insomnia, irritability, dysphoria, increased appetite, edema, heartburn, hyperglycemia, osteonecrosis
PLEX	three to seven exchanges over 1–2 weeks	Vagal reaction, hypotension, coagulopathy, hypocalcemia, deep vein thrombosis, infection

RELAPSE PREVENTION		
MEDICATION	**TYPICAL DOSAGE**	**COMMON OR SERIOUS SIDE EFFECTS**
First-line therapy		
Rituximab	1,000 mg IV two infusions, 2 wk apart OR 375 mg/m² weekly for 4 wk. Repeat infusion about every 6 mo, follow CD20 levels	Infusion reaction, infection, leukopenia, progressive multifocal leukoencephalopathy
Azathioprine±prednisolone	2–3 mg/kg/d in divided doses 1 mg/kg/d, begin tapering at 2–3 mo based on azathioprine effect	Nausea/vomiting, leukopenia, thrombocytopenia hepatotoxicity, infection
Mycophenolate mofetil	1–3 g oral/d in divided doses	Nausea/vomiting, diarrhea, peripheral edema, infections, elevated blood pressure, alopecia
Second-line therapy		
Mitoxantrone	12 mg/m² IV monthly for 6 mo, then 12 mg/m² every 3 mo for 9 mo	Nausea, amenorrhea, alopecia, leukopenia, hepatotoxicity, cardiotoxicity, acute leukemia, infection
Cyclophosphamide	500–1,000 mg/m² IV monthly for 6 mo pretreat with mesna	Nausea, vomiting, amenorrhea, leukopenia, infection, hemorrhagic cystitis, infertility
Methotrexate	50 mg IV weekly plus, prednisone 1 mg/kg/d	Nausea/vomiting, diarrhea, myelosuppression, renal dysfunction, liver dysfunction, infections
Tocilizumab infection, leukopenia, elevated LFTs, intermittent PLEX weekly to monthly	8 mg/kg IV once per month	Infusion reactions, thrombocytopenia, elevated cholesterol

CD20, cluster of differentiation 20; IV, intravenous; LFTs, liver functions tests; PLEX, plasma exchange.

Relapse Prevention

Owing to the relatively low prevalence of NMO, controlled studies of disease-modifying therapies in this disorder are very limited. The disability in NMO is directly related to relapses, often with incomplete recovery. Therefore, the preferred treatment approach in NMO and NMOSD is aggressive, early intervention.

Differentiating between NMO and MS becomes paramount when it comes to long-term immunotherapy for the prevention of relapse. It is not uncommon for NMO to be misdiagnosed as clinically isolated syndromes (CIS) or MS; thus, many NMO patients have been treated with conventional immunomodulatory therapies for MS. Several studies have reported poor efficacy or harmful effects of many MS therapies in NMO patients, by dramatically exacerbating NMO including IFN beta (42), natalizumab (48), fingolimod (49), and alemtuzumab (50). The exception to this observation is the emergence of anti-CD20 monoclonal antibodies (51,52), now being used in the treatment of MS. Recent evidence points to B-cell-mediated humoral immunity in the pathogenesis of NMO. Thus, rituximab therapy, which rapidly depletes B cells, has become a first-line treatment in NMO relapse prevention. Furthermore, with increased understanding of the pathogenic impact of the AQP4-IgG, there has been investigation of novel therapies targeting complement, interleukin-6 (IL-6) receptor, and CD19.

Clinical experience, further understanding of the pathophysiology of NMO, and increasing clinical study strongly argues for the use of long-term immunosuppression for relapse prevention. A number of therapies have been considered and include both oral and parenteral options (Table 38.4). There is no current biomarker for therapeutic response in NMOSD. While some observations may suggest that the antibody titer of the AQP4 antibody may correlate to effective immunotherapy (53), definitive studies are lacking (54). Additionally, the duration of preventative treatment in NMO has not been adequately studied, largely due to the lack of good natural history studies and the fact NMO has only recently been adequately defined as a distinct disease entity (55). Therefore, any decision to stop chronic immunotherapy must be taken with caution and careful clinical monitoring.

> *Prevention of attacks with immunosuppressants is important in relapsing NMO.*

Rituximab

Rituximab is a chimeric anti-CD20 monoclonal antibody that depletes precursor, and eventually mature, antibody-producing plasma cells. The CD20 antigen is an epitope that is expressed on the B-cell lineage cells with the exception of plasma cells. While the rational of using rituximab

for NMO is based on evidence of a pathogenic antibody, this drug does not target mature plasma cells; therefore, the rapid effect of rituximab suggests there is an antibody-independent pathway playing a role in the therapeutic response (55,56). In 2005, the first open-label study of rituximab in the treatment of NMOSD demonstrated promise (57), which was further supported by multiple additional prospective and retrospective studies. A retrospective study of 25 NMO patients treated with rituximab in doses of either 375 mg/m² once per week for 4 weeks or 1,000 mg for two treatments 2 weeks apart, led to a reduction of median annualized relapse rate (ARR) from 1.7 to 0 over 19 months, and stabilization or improvement in disability in 80% (58). A second study had similar results with reduction in median RR from 1.87 to 0 and stabilization or improvement in disability in all 23 patients (59). In a 2-year prospective open label study, 30 patients were treated with rituximab; there was a decline in the mean ARR from 2.4 to 0.3, 70% were relapse free on treatment over 2 years, and all but one patient had a decline in disability (60). Although there are no placebo-controlled studies, there appears to be a sustained benefit in the treatment of NMO with rituximab. Furthermore, in retrospective studies, comparing azathioprine, mycophenolate, and rituximab in NMO, rituximab was the most effective option followed by mycophenolate and then azathioprine (61).

Overall, rituximab seems to be well tolerated and safe (62) with the most common adverse effect being an infusion-related reaction, which can include fever, rash, headache, flu-like symptoms, and bronchospasm. The incidence is highest after the first infusion, occurring in approximately 25% of patients. Prevention of this reaction includes treatment with acetaminophen 1,000 mg by mouth (po), diphenhydramine 50 mg po, and methylprednisolone 100 mg IV prior to the infusion. Up to 30% of rituximab-treated patients can develop infections; however, only 2% are considered severe (63). There is a very low, not well-defined, risk of progressive multifocal leukoencephalopathy (PML) primarily seen in RA and B-cell lymphoma patients treated with rituximab, but there have only been very rare case reports of PML in rituximab-treated MS patients who have come off of natalizumab, a known risk factor for PML. There have been no reports of PML in NMO patients treated with rituximab. The estimated risk of PML in all patients treated with rituximab is approximately 1:25,000 (55). Ocrelizumab, a similar acting anti-CD20 monoclonal antibody that has U.S. Food and Drug Administration (FDA) approval for the treatment of MS, has potential to be used in NMO with a similar efficacy compared to rituximab, although its cost is currently much higher than rituximab.

Azathioprine

Azathioprine is the prodrug of 6-mercaptopurine (6-MP) and inhibits proliferation of lymphocytes. Treatment dose is 2 to 3 mg/kg/d, often combined with oral prednisone 1 mg/kg/d until peripheral WBC counts are suppressed

(~2 months after initiation), at which time the prednisone is slowly tapered. The effect of azathioprine in NMO has been demonstrated in a small open-label case series and two larger studies. One study of 29 Brazilian NMO patients had a 90% reduction in relapse rate and stabilization of EDSS scores over 28 months (63), whereas a second study of 99 patients showed a reduction of ARR by 76% with 37% of patients being relapse free over a median of 22 months (64). Doses less than 2 mg/kg/d have been associated with more frequent relapses. While patients are taking azathioprine, hematological monitoring for pancytopenia is recommended at least monthly initially and then every 2 to 3 months with longer duration of therapy. Occasionally, dose adjustments are necessary with hematological monitoring when lymphopenia is present ($<3,000/mm^3$) or thrombocytopenia ($<100,000/mm^3$). A small portion of the population have a mutation of thiopurine methyltransferase (TPMT), an enzyme that deactivates 6-MP, which leads to accumulation of 6-MP and increased risk for myelosuppression and infection. TPMT activity can be determined prior to initiating therapy and if suppressed or absent, alternative therapies may be considered. There may be an associated increased risk of cancer, particularly lymphoma, with longer duration and increasing cumulative dosing.

Mycophenolate Mofetil

Oral mycophenolate inhibits proliferation, and transendothelial migration, of B and T lymphocytes. In a retrospective study of 24 NMO patients, treatment with a median dose of 2,000 mg/d led to a reduction in relapse rates in 79% of patients and stabilization or improvement of EDSS in 91% over an average of 27 months (65). Of note, prednisone was coadministered in nine out of the 24 patients. Treatment effect may be delayed in mycophenolate, but is thought to be more rapid than azathioprine. Side effects include GI symptoms (diarrhea, nausea, and vomiting), myelosuppression, and increased risk for development of lymphomas or other malignancies.

Low-Dose Corticosteroids

In a retrospective study of nine NMO patients, long-term oral prednisolone 5 to 20 mg monotherapy was associated with a lower rate of relapses. A dose effect was suggested, as relapses occurred more often in doses less than 10 mg/d (66). The chronic use of corticosteroids is associated with various adverse effects (Table 38.4), and thus steroid sparing agents are preferred. Those patients maintained on long-term steroids should be given prophylaxis treatment for gastrointestinal ulcers, *Pneumocystis jiroveci* pneumonia, and osteoporosis.

Others

Other immunosuppressant therapies, including mitoxantrone, methotrexate, cyclophosphamide, and tacrolimus, have less supporting data for use in NMO. Mitoxantrone,

an anthracenedione derivative that delays cell-cycle progression, is approved for rapidly progressive relapsing–remitting and secondary progressive MS. An open-label study of five patients suggested benefit on relapse rate and disability in NMO (67). Use, however, is limited by adverse events including cardiomyopathy, treatment-related acute leukemia, and bone marrow suppression, and lifetime dose is limited to 140 mg/m². IV methotrexate 50 mg weekly plus oral prednisone 1 mg/kg/d, showed stabilization of disease in eight NMO patients (68). A retrospective study in 25 NMOSD patients showed an 86.2% reduction in relapse and statistically significant improvement on the EDSS (69). IV cyclophosphamide is an alkylating chemotherapeutic agent with only case reports of effectiveness in NMO patients who also had other autoimmune diseases such as lupus and Sjögren's. A variety of treatment dosages have been used in the literature; however, treatment with 1,000 mg/m² monthly for 6 months has been effective in other autoimmune processes such as chronic inflammatory demyelinating polyneuropathy (CIDP), lupus, and MS. Treatment with mesna should be given prior to starting cyclophosphamide to prevent acute hemorrhagic cystitis. Intermittent PLEX in combination with immunosuppressants was shown to reduce relapses in a case report of two NMO patients (70).

Novel Investigational Immunotherapies

Future therapy is aimed at disease pathogenesis, as our understanding of the pathogenic impact of the AQP4 antibody continues to expand. Several novel therapeutic targets are now in development for the treatment of NMO.

COMPLEMENT INHIBITORS

The classical complement pathway is thought to play a crucial role in the inflammatory pathway in NMO by binding to the AQP4 antibody (6). Eculizumab is a humanized monoclonal IgG that neutralizes the C5 complement protein and is already approved for paroxysmal nocturnal hemoglobinuria and atypical hemolytic uremic syndrome. An open-label trial investigated the efficacy of eculizumab in NMO and after a 12-month period, 12 patients were relapse free and two patients had possible attacks (71). A multicenter, randomized, double-blind, placebo-controlled trial is evaluating eculizumab further.

CD19-TARGETED THERAPY

As discussed earlier, studies of CD20-depleting drugs such as rituximab demonstrate a decrease in the relapse rate in NMO. The onset of depletion of CD20 cells is rapid after starting therapy. However, there is no direct effect on antibody-producing plasma cells; thus, some individuals may experience breakthrough relapses early during treatment and there are reports of poor responsiveness to rituximab in more severe cases. It is thought that plasmablasts producing AQP4-IgG that lack CD20 receptors are resistant to rituximab. While all CD20-positive B cells express CD19, not all CD19-positive cells express CD20 (72). Therefore, targeted depletion of CD19-positive cells may be more beneficial than the CD20 targeting drugs. MEDI-551 is an anti-CD19 monoclonal antibody being evaluated in NMO.

IL-6 RECEPTOR TARGETED THERAPIES

IL-6 is crucial to the survival of plasmablasts, the primary source of AQP4 antibody production. IL-6 is elevated in the CSF during an NMO attack (73) and plasmablasts are also increased (34). Tocilizumab is an IL-6 receptor blocking antibody that has shown benefit in the treatment of refractory NMO in case reports and retrospective observational studies (74–76). In addition, SA237 is an IL-6 receptor antibody that is under study in NMO.

ANTIGEN-SPECIFIC TREATMENT

Aquaporumab is a human monoclonal antibody against AQP4 that has been designed to bind to the endogenous AQP4 to prevent NMO-IgG from binding its target antigen in the body. Although these therapies are still in development (77), it may provide a highly specific, nonimmunosuppressive approach to the treatment of this challenging disorder.

Treatment Recommendations

Therapies often considered first line for the long-term treatment of NMO include rituximab, azathioprine, and mycophenolate mofetil as summarized in Figure 38.3. The choice of initial therapy must be individualized, weighing the risk and benefits of the medications with each patient. The author's experience with IV rituximab has generally been positive with disease stabilization, limited adverse events, and the benefit of infrequent administration. Rituximab is often used first line. Lack of good natural history data and biomarkers of relapse risk combine to make difficult decisions about discontinuing chronic therapies.

KEY POINTS FOR PATIENTS AND FAMILIES

- NMO is a different disease process than MS, although the initial clinical presentation may be similar.
- NMO most often affects the optic nerves (causing decrease or loss of vision) and the spinal cord (causing weakness, sensory changes, trouble walking, and bladder/bowel dysfunction).
- The diagnosis is made based on classic clinical symptoms of optic neuritis and myelitis, neuroimaging, serum testing for NMO antibody, and excluding other possible causes.
- Most individuals with NMO have a relapsing course with repeat exacerbations over time.
- Relapses in NMO tend to be more severe than in MS and often result in residual disability.
- Acute treatment for an NMO relapse includes IV steroids and possibly PLEX based on response to steroids and severity of disability.
- Disability appears to be directly related to relapses, so prevention of attacks with either oral or IV immunosuppressive therapies should be started quickly after the diagnosis is made.
- Websites with further information:
  - www.guthyjacksonfoundation.org
  - www.nationalmssociety.org
  - www.msaa.com
  - www.myelitis.org

REFERENCES

1. Marrie RA, Gryba C. The incidence and prevalence of neuromyelitis optica: a systematic review. *Int J MS Care.* 2013;15(3):113–118.
2. Bukhari W, Prain KM, Waters P, et al. Incidence and prevalence of NMOSD in Australia and New Zealand. *J Neurol Neurosurg Psychiatry.* 2017;88(8):632–638.
3. Daniëlle van Pelt E, Wong YYM, Ketelslegers IA, et al. Incidence of AQP4-IgG seropositive neuromyelitis optica spectrum disorders in the Netherlands: about one in a million. *Mult Scler J Exp Transl Clin.* 2016;2:2055217315625652.
4. Mealy MA, Wingerchuk DM, Greenberg BM, et al. Epidemiology of neuromyelitis optica in the United States: a multicenter analysis. *Arch Neurol.* 2012;69(9):1176–1180.
5. Flanagan EP, Cabre P, Weinshenker BG, et al. Epidemiology of aquaporin-4 autoimmunity and neuromyelitis optica spectrum. *Ann Neurol.* 2016;79(5):775–783.
6. Pittock SJ, Lucchinetti CF. Neuromyelitis optica and the evolving spectrum of autoimmune aquaporin-4 channelopathies: a decade later. *Ann N Y Acad Sci.* 2016;1366(1):20–39.
7. Uzawa A, Mori M, Masuda H, et al. Interleukin-6 analysis of 572 consecutive CSF samples from neurological disorders: a

special focus on neuromyelitis optica. *Clin Chim Acta*. 2017;469: 144–149.

8. Hinson SR, Lennon VA, Pittock SJ. Autoimmune AQP4 channelopathies and neuromyelitis optica spectrum disorders. *Handb Clin Neurol*. 2016;133:377–403.

9. Quek AM, McKeon A, Lennon VA, et al. Effects of age and sex on aquaporin-4 autoimmunity. *Arch Neurol*. 2012;69(8):1039–1043.

10. Ratchford JN, Quigg ME, Conger A, et al. Optical coherence tomography helps differentiate neuromyelitis optica and MS optic neuropathies. *Neurology*. 2009;73(4):302–308.

11. Wingerchuk DM, Hogancamp WF, O'Brien PC, et al. The clinical course of neuromyelitis optica (Devic's syndrome). *Neurology*. 1999;53(5):1107–1114.

12. Popescu BF, Lennon VA, Parisi JE, et al. Neuromyelitis optica unique area postrema lesions: nausea, vomiting, and pathogenic implications. *Neurology*. 2011;76(14):1229–1237.

13. Pu S, Long Y, Yang N, et al. Syndrome of inappropriate antidiuretic hormone secretion in patients with aquaporin-4 antibody. *J Neurol*. 2015;262(1):101–107.

14. Jarius S, Wildemann B. AQP4 antibodies in neuromyelitis optica: diagnostic and pathogenetic relevance. *Nat Rev Neurol*. 2010;6(7):383–392.

15. McKeon A, Lennon VA, Jacob A, et al. Coexistence of myasthenia gravis and serological markers of neurological autoimmunity in neuromyelitis optica. *Muscle Nerve*. 2009;39(1):87–90.

16. Armağan H, Tüzün E, Içöz S, et al. Long extensive transverse myelitis associated with aquaporin-4 antibody and breast cancer: favorable response to cancer treatment. *J Spinal Cord Med*. 2012;35(4):267–269.

17. De Santis G, Caniatti L, De Vito A, et al. A possible paraneoplastic neuromyelitis optica associated with lung cancer. *Neurol Sci*. 2009;30(5):397–400.

18. Frasquet M, Bataller L, Torres-Vega E, et al. Longitudinally extensive transverse myelitis with AQP4 antibodies revealing ovarian teratoma. *J Neuroimmunol*. 2013;263(1-2):145–147.

19. Pittock SJ, Lennon VA. Aquaporin-4 autoantibodies in a paraneoplastic context. *Arch Neurol*. 2008;65(5):629–632.

20. Ontaneda D, Fox RJ. Is neuromyelitis optica with advanced age of onset a paraneoplastic disorder? *Int J Neurosci*. 2014;124(7):509–511.

21. Al-Harbi T, Al-Sarawi A, Binfalah M, et al. Paraneoplastic neuromyelitis optica spectrum disorder associated with stomach carcinoid tumor. *Hematol Oncol Stem Cell Ther*. 2014;7(3):116–119.

22. McKeon A, Lennon VA, Lotze T, et al. CNS aquaporin-4 autoimmunity in children. *Neurology*. 2008;71(2):93–100.

23. Davoudi V, Keyhanian K, Bove RM, et al. Immunology of neuromyelitis optica during pregnancy. *Neurol Neuroimmunol Neuroinflamm*. 2016;3(6):e288.

24. Zalewski NL, Krecke KN, Weinshenker BG, et al. Central canal enhancement and the trident sign in spinal cord sarcoidosis. *Neurology*. 2016;87(7):743–744.

25. Flanagan EP, Weinshenker BG, Krecke KN, et al. Short myelitis lesions in aquaporin-4-IgG-positive neuromyelitis optica spectrum disorders. *JAMA Neurol*. 2015;72(1):81–87.

26. Zhang J, Liu F, Wang Y, et al. Aquaporin-4-IgG-positive neuromyelitis optica spectrum disorder with recurrent short partial transverse myelitis and favorable prognosis: two new cases. *Mult Scler*. 2017:1352458517705479.

27. Whittam D, Bhojak M, Das K, et al. Longitudinally extensive myelitis in MS mimicking neuromyelitis optica. *Neurol Neuroimmunol Neuroinflamm*. 2017;4(3):e333.

28. Pittock SJ, Lennon VA, Krecke K, et al. Brain abnormalities in neuromyelitis optica. *Arch Neurol*. 2006;63(3):390–396.

29. Storoni M, Davagnanam I, Radon M, et al. Distinguishing optic neuritis in neuromyelitis optica spectrum disease from multiple sclerosis: a novel magnetic resonance imaging scoring system. *J Neuroophthalmol*. 2013;33(2):123–127.

30. Wingerchuk DM, Banwell B, Bennett JL, et al. International consensus diagnostic criteria for neuromyelitis optica spectrum disorders. *Neurology*. 2015;85(2):177–189.

31. Wingerchuk DM, Lennon VA, Pittock SJ, et al. Revised diagnostic criteria for neuromyelitis optica. *Neurology*. 2006;66(10):1485–1489.

32. Jarius S, Ruprecht K, Kleiter I, et al. MOG-IgG in NMO and related disorders: a multicenter study of 50 patients. Part 2: epidemiology, clinical presentation, radiological and laboratory features, treatment responses, and long-term outcome. *J Neuroinflammation*. 2016;13(1):280.

33. Flanagan EP, Hinson SR, Lennon VA, et al. Glial fibrillary acidic protein immunoglobulin G as biomarker of autoimmune astrocytopathy: analysis of 102 patients. *Ann Neurol*. 2017;81(2):298–309.

34. Bennett JL, Lam C, Kalluri SR, et al. Intrathecal pathogenic anti-aquaporin-4 antibodies in early neuromyelitis optica. *Ann Neurol*. 2009;66(5):617–629.

35. Lennon VA, Wingerchuk DM, Kryzer TJ, et al. A serum autoantibody marker of neuromyelitis optica: distinction from multiple sclerosis. *Lancet*. 2004;364(9451):2106–2112.

36. Waters PJ, McKeon A, Leite MI, et al. Serologic diagnosis of NMO: a multicenter comparison of aquaporin-4-IgG assays. *Neurology*. 2012;78(9):665–671; discussion 669.

37. Klawiter EC, Alvarez E, Xu J, et al. NMO-IgG detected in CSF in seronegative neuromyelitis optica. *Neurology*. 2009;72(12):1101–1103.

38. Pittock SJ, Lennon VA, de Seze J, et al. Neuromyelitis optica and non organ-specific autoimmunity. *Arch Neurol*. 2008;65(1):78–83.

39. Jiao Y, Fryer JP, Lennon VA, et al. Updated estimate of AQP4-IgG serostatus and disability outcome in neuromyelitis optica. *Neurology*. 2013;81(14):1197–1204.

40. Sellner J, Boggild M, Clanet M, et al. EFNS guidelines on diagnosis and management of neuromyelitis optica. *Eur J Neurol*. 2010;17(8):1019–1032.

41. Wingerchuk DM, Weinshenker BG. Neuromyelitis optica: clinical predictors of a relapsing course and survival. *Neurology*. 2003;60(5):848–853.

42. Kim W, Kim SH, Kim HJ. New insights into neuromyelitis optica. *J Clin Neurol*. 2011;7(3):115–127.

43. Papais-Alvarenga RM, Carellos SC, Alvarenga MP, et al. Clinical course of optic neuritis in patients with relapsing neuromyelitis optica. *Arch Ophthalmol*. 2008;126(1):12–16.

44. Bergamaschi R, Ghezzi A. Devic's neuromyelitis optica: clinical features and prognostic factors. *Neurol Sci*. 2004;25 (suppl 4):S364–S367.

45. Kessler RA, Mealy MA, Levy M. Treatment of neuromyelitis optica spectrum disorder: acute, preventive, and symptomatic. *Curr Treat Options Neurol*. 2016;18(1):2.

46. Aungsumart S, Apiwattanakul M. Clinical outcomes and predictive factors related to good outcomes in plasma exchange in severe attack of NMOSD and long extensive transverse myelitis: case series and review of the literature. *Mult Scler Relat Disord*. 2017;13:93–97.

47. Bonnan M, Valentino R, Olindo S, et al. Plasma exchange in severe spinal attacks associated with neuromyelitis optica spectrum disorder. *Mult Scler*. 2009;15(4):487–492.

48. Kleiter I, Hellwig K, Berthele A, et al. Failure of natalizumab to prevent relapses in neuromyelitis optica. *Arch Neurol*. 2012;69(2):239–245.

49. Min JH, Kim BJ, Lee KH. Development of extensive brain lesions following fingolimod (FTY720) treatment in a patient with neuromyelitis optica spectrum disorder. *Mult Scler*. 2012;18(1):113–115.

50. Azzopardi L, Cox AL, McCarthy CL, et al. Alemtuzumab use in neuromyelitis optica spectrum disorders: a brief case series. *J Neurol*. 2016;263(1):25–29.

51. Hauser SL, Bar-Or A, Comi G, et al. Ocrelizumab versus interferon beta-1a in relapsing multiple sclerosis. *N Engl J Med*. 2017;376(3):221–234.

52. Montalban X, Hauser SL, Kappos L, et al. Ocrelizumab versus placebo in primary progressive multiple sclerosis. *N Engl J Med*. 2017;376(3):209–220.

53. Takahashi T, Fujihara K, Nakashima I, et al. Anti-aquaporin-4 antibody is involved in the pathogenesis of NMO: a study on antibody titre. *Brain*. 2007;130(pt 5):1235–1243.

54. Bienia B, Balabanov R. Immunotherapy of neuromyelitis optica. *Autoimmune Dis*. 2013;2013:741490.

55. Kimbrough DJ, Fujihara K, Jacob A, et al. Treatment of neuromyelitis optica: review and recommendations. *Mult Scler Relat Disord.* 2012;1(4):180–187.

56. Hinson SR, Pittock SJ, Lucchinetti CF, et al. Pathogenic potential of IgG binding to water channel extracellular domain in neuromyelitis optica. *Neurology.* 2007;69(24):2221–2231.

57. Cree BA, Lamb S, Morgan K, et al. An open label study of the effects of rituximab in neuromyelitis optica. *Neurology.* 2005;64(7):1270–1272.

58. Jacob A, Weinshenker BG, Violich I, et al. Treatment of neuromyelitis optica with rituximab: retrospective analysis of 25 patients. *Arch Neurol.* 2008;65(11):1443–1448.

59. Bedi GS, Brown AD, Delgado SR, et al. Impact of rituximab on relapse rate and disability in neuromyelitis optica. *Mult Scler.* 2011;17(10):1225–1230.

60. Kim SH, Kim W, Li XF, et al. Repeated treatment with rituximab based on the assessment of peripheral circulating memory B cells in patients with relapsing neuromyelitis optica over 2 years. *Arch Neurol.* 2011;68(11):1412–1420.

61. Mealy MA, Wingerchuk DM, Palace J, et al. Comparison of relapse and treatment failure rates among patients with neuromyelitis optica: multicenter study of treatment efficacy. *JAMA Neurol.* 2014;71(3):324–330.

62. van Vollenhoven RF, Emery P, Bingham CO, et al. Longterm safety of patients receiving rituximab in rheumatoid arthritis clinical trials. *J Rheumatol.* 2010;37(3):558–567.

63. Bichuetti DB, Lobato de Oliveira EM, Oliveira DM, et al. Neuromyelitis optica treatment: analysis of 36 patients. *Arch Neurol.* 2010;67(9):1131–1136.

64. Costanzi C, Matiello M, Lucchinetti CF, et al. Azathioprine: tolerability, efficacy, and predictors of benefit in neuromyelitis optica. *Neurology.* 2011;77(7):659–666.

65. Jacob A, Matiello M, Weinshenker BG, et al. Treatment of neuromyelitis optica with mycophenolate mofetil: retrospective analysis of 24 patients. *Arch Neurol.* 2009;66(9):1128–1133.

66. Watanabe S, Misu T, Miyazawa I, et al. Low-dose corticosteroids reduce relapses in neuromyelitis optica: a retrospective analysis. *Mult Scler.* 2007;13(8):968–974.

67. Weinstock-Guttman B, Ramanathan M, Lincoff N, et al. Study of mitoxantrone for the treatment of recurrent neuromyelitis optica (Devic disease). *Arch Neurol.* 2006;63(7):957–963.

68. Minagar A, Sheremata W. Treatment of Devic's disease with methotrexate and prednisone. *Int J MS Care.* 2000;2:39–43.

69. Chen B, Wu Q, Ke G, et al. Efficacy and safety of tacrolimus treatment for neuromyelitis optica spectrum disorder. *Sci Rep.* 2017;7(1):831.

70. Miyamoto K, Kusunoki S. Intermittent plasmapheresis prevents recurrence in neuromyelitis optica. *Ther Apher Dial.* 2009;13(6):505–508.

71. Pittock SJ, Lennon VA, McKeon A, et al. Eculizumab in AQP4-IgG-positive relapsing neuromyelitis optica spectrum disorders: an open-label pilot study. *Lancet Neurol.* 2013;12(6):554–562.

72. Tedder TF. CD19: a promising B cell target for rheumatoid arthritis. *Nat Rev Rheumatol.* 2009;5(10):572–577.

73. Içöz S, Tüzün E, Kürtüncü M, et al. Enhanced IL-6 production in aquaporin-4 antibody positive neuromyelitis optica patients. *Int J Neurosci.* 2010;120(1):71–75.

74. Ringelstein M, Ayzenberg I, Harmel J, et al. Long-term therapy with interleukin 6 receptor blockade in highly active neuromyelitis optica spectrum disorder. *JAMA Neurol.* 2015;72(7):756–763.

75. Kieseier BC, Stüve O, Dehmel T, et al. Disease amelioration with tocilizumab in a treatment-resistant patient with neuromyelitis optica: implication for cellular immune responses. *JAMA Neurol.* 2013;70(3):390–393.

76. Ayzenberg I, Kleiter I, Schröder A, et al. Interleukin 6 receptor blockade in patients with neuromyelitis optica nonresponsive to anti-CD20 therapy. *JAMA Neurol.* 2013;70(3):394–397.

77. Tradtrantip L, Zhang H, Saadoun S, et al. Anti-aquaporin-4 monoclonal antibody blocker therapy for neuromyelitis optica. *Ann Neurol.* 2012;71(3):314–322.

39 Acute Disseminated Encephalomyelitis

Eliza Gordon-Lipkin and Brenda Banwell

KEY POINTS FOR CLINICIANS

- Acute disseminated encephalomyelitis (ADEM) is an inflammatory demyelinating disorder of the central nervous system that manifests as a polysymptomatic clinical presentation and must include encephalopathy.
- Multiphasic ADEM is a new event of ADEM 3 or more months after the first ADEM event.
- ADEM may be preceded by a viral infection, although specific infections have only rarely been directly identified.
- There is no single test that confirms the diagnosis of ADEM. As such, establishing the diagnosis requires both clinical and radiological features and the exclusion of other diseases that resemble ADEM.
- Repeat imaging studies are necessary to evaluate for accrual of subclinical lesions, or to evaluate patients with subsequent clinical attacks.
- Therapy for ADEM is based on expert consensus as there are no randomized controlled clinical trials to date. A course of 3 to 5 days of high-dose intravenous methylprednisolone is considered standard and can often provide significant clinical benefit.
- Rarely, an ADEM attack occurs as the first attack of multiple sclerosis. ADEM-like attacks can also be the first or subsequent attack in children with neuromyelitis optica spectrum disorder (NMOSD), and an increasingly recognized number of children with ADEM followed by recurrent optic neuritis (ON) have serum antibodies directed against myelin oligodendroglial protein (MOG).

ADEM is an inflammatory demyelinating disorder of the central nervous system (CNS) that is often preceded by an infection (1–3). The hallmark clinical presentation is a multifocal onset with encephalopathy manifesting as behavioral change or alteration in consciousness (1–3). ADEM can occur at any age, but tends to affect children more than adults, and usually strikes children younger than 10 years (4). There does not appear to be a clear gender predominance (5,6), although a possible increase in risk among males has been reported (1,3).

> *The hallmark clinical presentation for ADEM is a multifocal onset with encephalopathy manifesting as behavioral change or alteration in consciousness.*

A challenge in diagnosing and studying ADEM has been the lack of formal diagnostic criteria. In 2007, an international panel of experts was organized by the National Multiple Sclerosis Society. This International Pediatric Multiple Sclerosis Study Group proposed consensus definitions for demyelinating diseases of childhood, which included ADEM. These definitions were updated in 2012 (1). ADEM is defined as a clinical CNS event with a presumed inflammatory demyelinating cause associated with typical MRI findings and encephalopathy that is not explained by fever alone (1). Other diagnoses, such as CNS infection, must be excluded. Appearance of new neurological findings, or MRI changes, within 90 days of ADEM onset is considered to be part of the same ADEM event (see Table 39.1 for full criteria). Of note, ADEM frequently follows a monophasic disease course; however, this can only be confirmed retrospectively after longitudinal observation.

TABLE 39.1   International Pediatric MS Study Group Consensus Definitions

MONOPHASIC ADEM	MULTIPHASIC ADEM
A first polyfocal clinical CNS event with presumed inflammatory cause[a]	New event of ADEM (with encephalopathy) 3 or more months after the first ADEM event, with new or reemergence of prior clinical and MRI findings
Encephalopathy, that cannot be explained by fever, is defined as	
1) Behavioral change	
2) Alteration in consciousness	
No history of a clinical episode with features of a prior demyelinating event	
No other etiologies can explain the event	
New or fluctuating symptoms, signs, or MRI findings occurring within 3 mo of the inciting ADEM event are considered part of the acute event	
No new symptoms or new MRI findings after 3 mo of initial event	
Brain MRI is abnormal during the acute (3-mo) phase and shows "typical" features:	
1) Diffuse, poorly demarcated, large (>1–2 cm) lesions involving predominantly the cerebral white matter	
2) T1 hypointense lesions in the white matter are rare	
3) Deep gray matter lesions (thalamus, basal ganglia) may be present	

ADEM, acute disseminated encephalomyelitis; CNS, central nervous system; MS, multiple sclerosis.

[a]Presumed inflammatory cause infers exclusion of alternative etiologies (including infectious, metabolic/genetic, oncologic or vascular) and inclusion of supportive inflammatory features on diagnostic workup (see Imaging and Laboratory Findings sections).

Source: Adapted from Krupp LB, Tardieu M, Amato MP, et al. International Pediatric Multiple Sclerosis Study Group criteria for pediatric multiple sclerosis and immune-mediated central nervous system demyelinating disorders: revisions to the 2007 definitions. *Mult Scler.* 2013;19(10):1261–1267.

The incidence of ADEM is estimated to be about 0.4 to 0.6 per 100,000 per year among people younger than 20 years of age (6,7). More recent studies have grouped ADEM with other demyelinating diseases of childhood and have reported incidence rates of 0.9 to 1.6 per 100,000 person years (8–10). The incidence of ADEM does have seasonal peaks in the winter and spring, providing some suggestion of an infectious trigger (4,5,10,11). Reports of a prodromal illness preceding the onset of ADEM have ranged from 46% to 100% (3,6,12).

Many infections have been associated with ADEM. Nonspecific upper respiratory infections were reported as the most commonly associated infection, reported by 29% of patients (12,13). Other infectious presentations reported in this cohort were "gastrointestinal disturbance" in 9% of cases and a "nonspecific febrile illness" in 6% of cases. Specific infections were found in relatively few cases but included varicella (4%), herpes simplex virus (2%), mumps (1%), and rubella (1%) (12,13).

Table 39.2 describes the various infections that have been linked to ADEM. It is important to realize that while an antecedent infection may increase the likelihood of ADEM, its presence is not required (14). An antecedent infection may also occur in patients with a first presentation of multiple sclerosis (MS) (15). As such, antecedent infection should not be used as criteria to exclude MS as a diagnostic possibility.

Several cases in the literature have reported the occurrence of ADEM following vaccinations, sparking controversies surrounding immunization safety. However, large follow-up studies have specified this risk to be exceedingly rare and a coincidental versus causal relationship has yet to be determined (16). Therefore, prioritizing the protection against infectious diseases through immunizations as a public health safety measure outweighs the extremely small risk (if any) of ADEM.

> *Antecedent infection should not be used as a criterion to exclude multiple sclerosis as a diagnostic possibility.*

EVALUATION

There is no single test that confirms the diagnosis of ADEM. Establishing the diagnosis requires a combination of clinical and radiological features and most importantly, the exclusion of other diseases that resemble ADEM. It is important to recognize that the differential diagnosis of ADEM is broad (see Table 39.3). As such, a thorough workup should include infectious, immunological, and metabolic tests. Longitudinal follow-up with repeat MRI studies to evaluate for accrual of new lesions. Importantly, the second demyelinating event can occur years later and may manifest as Multiphasic ADEM, MS, or Neuromyelitis Optic Spectrum Disorder (NMOSD). Multiphasic ADEM is rare and occurs in 1% to 10% of children with an initial ADEM event, typically 2 to 8 years after the first attack (1).

> *Establishing the diagnosis requires a combination of clinical and radiological features and the exclusion of other diseases that resemble ADEM.*

TABLE 39.2 Infections That Have Been Associated With ADEM

VIRUSES	REPORTED FREQUENCY	BACTERIAL	REPORTED FREQUENCY
Coronavirus	Case report	*Borrelia burdoreri*	Case report
Coxsackie B	Case report	Chlamydia	Case report
Dengue virus	Case report	*Legionella*	Case reports
Epstein–Barr virus	Case reports	*Mycoplasma pneumoniae*	Case reports
Hepatitis A	Case reports	*Rickettsia rickettsii*	Case report
Hepatitis C	Case reports	*Streptococcus*	Case series
Herpes simplex virus	Case series	Tuberculosis	Case report
HIV	Case reports		
Human herpesvirus 6	Case report		
Measles	100/100,000		
Mumps	Case reports		
Parainfluenza virus	Case reports		
Rubella virus	1/10,000–20,000		
Varicella-zoster virus	1/20,000–20,000		
OTHER			
Plasmodium vivax	Case reports		
Plasmodium falciparum	Case reports		

ADEM, acute disseminated encephalomyelitis.
Source: Adapted from Menge T, Hemmer B, Nessler S, et al. Acute disseminated encephalomyelitis: an update. *Arch Neurol*. 2005;62(11):1673–1680.

TABLE 39.3 Differential Diagnosis of ADEM

CNS INFECTIONS	IMMUNE-MEDIATED DISORDERS
Viral encephalitis (herpes, Epstein–Barr, enterovirus, human T-cell lymphotropic virus type 1)	Multiple sclerosis
Bacterial encephalitis (mycoplasma) or abscesses	Neuromyelitis optica spectrum disorder
Fungal infection/encephalitis (cryptococcus)	Anti-myelin-oligodendrocyte-glycoprotein disease
Parasitic encephalitis or CNS infection	Behçet's disease
Rickettsial infection/encephalitis	Systemic lupus erythematosus
Progressive multifocal leukoencephalopathy (JC virus)	Primary angiitis of the CNS
METABOLIC/GENETIC LEUKOENCEPHALOPATHIES	Neurosarcoidosis
Adrenoleukodystrophy	Bickerstaff brainstem encephalitis
Adrenomyeloneuropathy	Anti-N-methyl-D-aspartate receptor encephalitis
Metachromatic leukodystrophy	Schilder's myelinoclastic diffuse sclerosis
Mitochodrial encephalomyopathy, lactic acidosis and stroke-like episodes	CNS hemophagocytic lymphohistiocytosis
Leber hereditary optic neuropathy	Sydenham's chorea
Cerebral autosomal dominant arteriopathy with subcortical infarcts and leukoencephalopathy	Acute cerebellar ataxia
	OTHER
	Metastatic neoplasm
	Acute necrotizing encephalomyelitis (associated with RANBP2 mutations)

ADEM, acute disseminated encephalomyelitis; CNS, central nervous system; JC, John Cunningham.

Clinical Features

Distinguishing ADEM from other demyelinating etiologies, such as MS or NMOSD, at initial presentation may be challenging clinically, but there are a few clinical features that can be helpful. In particular, the presence of fever, seizure, impaired consciousness, or a multifocal onset are more suggestive of ADEM than MS (17–19). ON is common in both ADEM and other demyelinating diseases of childhood. However, ON is more often bilateral in ADEM or NMOSD, whereas ON in MS is usually unilateral. The clinical presentation of ADEM has been documented to range from an isolated fever of unknown origin (20), to acute onset psychosis (21), but each of these presentations are rare and many case reports were written prior to identification of specific antibodies, such as the anti-N-methyl-D-aspartate receptor (NMDA-R) antibody and the anti-myelin oligodendrocyte glycoprotein (MOG) antibody, which may have actually been the cause for these unusual clinical presentations. Table 39.4 shows a breakdown of the commonly reported symptoms at clinical presentation among patients with ADEM.

Though clinical features may be helpful, laboratory and imaging studies are often essential in distinguishing

TABLE 39.4 Common Symptoms at Clinical Presentation of ADEM

SYMPTOM	PERCENT REPORTED
Impaired consciousness/encephalopathy (NOTE: NOW A REQUIRED COMPONENT OF THE DIAGNOSIS)	33%–75%[a]
Fever	39%–67%
Headache/vomiting	23%–58%
Motor disturbance/weakness	23%–85%
Ataxia—cerebellar dysfunction	28%–65%
Cranial neuropathy	13%–89%
Seizure	10%–47%
Meningismus	6%–43%
Sensory disturbance	2%–28%
Optic neuritis	11%–23%
Aphasia/language disturbance	2%–20%

ADEM, acute disseminated encephalomyelitis.

[a]Of note, these cohorts were described prior to the proposed consensus definition requiring encephalopathy for a diagnosis of ADEM.

Source: Tenembaum S, Chitnis T, Ness J, et al. Acute disseminated encephalomyelitis. Neurology. 2007;68(16 suppl 2):S23–S36; Dale RC, de Sousa C, Chong WK, et al. Acute disseminated encephalomyelitis, multiphasic disseminated encephalomyelitis and multiple sclerosis in children. Brain. 2000;123 Pt 12:2407–2422; Leake JAD, Albani S, Kao AS, et al. Acute disseminated encephalomyelitis in childhood: epidemiologic, clinical and laboratory features. Pediatr Infect Dis J. 2004;23(8):756–764; Hynson JL, Kornberg AJ, Coleman LT, et al. Clinical and neuroradiologic features of acute disseminated encephalomyelitis in children. Neurology. 2001;56(10):1308–1312; Tenembaum S, Chamoles N, Fejerman N. Acute disseminated encephalomyelitis: a long-term follow-up study of 84 pediatric patients. Neurology. 2002;59(8):1224–1231; Atzori M, Battistella PA, Perini P, et al. Clinical and diagnostic aspects of multiple sclerosis and acute monophasic encephalomyelitis in pediatric patients: a single centre prospective study. Mult Scler. 2009;15(3):363–370; Schwarz S, Mohr A, Knauth M, et al. Acute disseminated encephalomyelitis: a follow-up study of 40 adult patients. Neurology. 2001;56(10):1313–1318; Davis LE, Booss J. Acute disseminated encephalomyelitis in children: a changing picture. Pediatr Infect Dis J. 2003;22(9):829–831. (22); Koelman DLH, Chahin S, Mar SS, et al. Acute disseminated encephalomyelitis in 228 patients: a retrospective, multicenter US study. Neurology. 2016;86(22):2085–2093. (23)

ADEM from other demyelinating diseases. Table 39.5 summarizes key features that distinguish ADEM from other demyelinating etiologies.

Imaging Findings

When evaluating for ADEM, it is important to realize that CT scans of the brain are not optimal as they are frequently normal (5,6). MRI of the brain with and without contrast (gadolinium) is the imaging modality of choice. If ON is suspected, dedicated imaging of the orbits should also be included. In one ADEM cohort ($n = 42$), CT scans of the brain were normal in 68%, whereas 100% of the patients had abnormalities on MRI of the brain or spinal cord (6). MRI abnormalities are usually noted on the T2-weighted or fluid-attenuated inversion recovery (FLAIR) sequences within the basal ganglia, thalami, brain stem, cerebellum, periventricular white matter, or gray–white junction (6). Contrast (gadolinium) enhancement on T1-weighted images is variable. Prior to the updated definition, gadolinium enhancement was reported in 14% to 30% of ADEM cases (1). However, more recent studies have reported these rates as low as 10% (24). The pattern of enhancement is also variable and can be complete or incomplete ring-shaped, nodular, gyral, or spotty (see Figures 39.1 and 39.2). In contrast, meningeal enhancement in the brain or spinal cord is unusual and should prompt consideration of infection or vasculitis (3).

CT scans of the brain are frequently normal. MRI of the brain and spinal cord with and without contrast is the imaging modality of choice for evaluating ADEM.

Laboratory Findings

Erythrocyte sedimentation rate (ESR) and white blood cell (WBC) count can be elevated in patients with ADEM although this is nonspecific. ESR and WBC counts are typically normal in MS (5,19). Cerebrospinal fluid (CSF) analysis can also be helpful. CSF oligoclonal bands are rare in ADEM, whereas they are present in 43% to 92% of pediatric MS patients (4,25,26).

Antibodies to MOG, a protein expressed on the outer surface of myelin sheath exclusively in the CNS, have been found in some patients with demyelinating disease of the brain, optic nerve, and spinal cord (27–30). These antibodies were first described in a cohort of children with ADEM and have since been identified in subsets of patients with other CNS demyelinating presentations. Currently, live cell-based assays are the standard for detecting anti-MOG antibodies, and serum samples are more sensitive than CSF. While anti-MOG antibodies are infrequently found in the adult MS population, anti-MOG antibodies are detected in 15% to 40% of pediatric demyelinating patients (30–31). Anti-MOG antibodies have been detected in up to 40% of

TABLE 39.5 Comparison of Key Features Distinguishing ADEM from RRMS, NMOSD

FEATURE	ADEM	MULTIPHASIC ADEM	RRMS	NMOSD
Clinical course	First event; typically monophasic	Recurrent events	Recurrent events	Recurrent events
Encephalopathy	Yes	Yes	Rare	Rare
MRI features	Diffuse, poorly demarcated, large lesions in the cerebral white matter or deep gray matter	Diffuse, poorly demarcated, large lesions in the cerebral white matter or deep gray matter	Disseminated in space: ≥ one lesion in at least two of the four locations (periventricular, juxtacortical, infratentorial, and spinal cord) Disseminated in time: new T2 lesions on serial scans or simultaneous clinically silent enhancing and nonenhancing lesions[a]	Optic nerve (frequently bilateral) and spinal cord (frequently longitudinally extensive) lesions; may have brain lesions that do not meet MS criteria
Oligoclonal bands	Rare	Rare	Frequent	Frequent
Antibody	±Anti-MOG	±Anti-MOG	--	Anti-aquaporin-4 or anti-MOG

ADEM, acute disseminated encephalomyelitis; MOG, myelin oligodendroglial protein; MS, multiple sclerosis; NMOSD, neuromyelitis optica spectrum disorder; RRMS, relapsing remitting MS.

Note: Patients who do not meet clinical criteria for any of the above diagnoses are frequently referred to as clinically isolated syndrome or acute demyelinating syndrome until a definitive diagnosis is established either with additional clinical events or new lesions on MRI.

[a]2010 Revised McDonald Criteria.

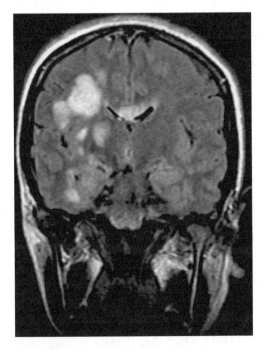

FIGURE 39.1 ADEM—coronal FLAIR sequences on brain MRI demonstrating T2 abnormal signal within the basal ganglia and periventricular white matter.

ADEM, acute disseminated encephalomyelitis; FLAIR, fluid-attenuated inversion recovery.

Image courtesy of Christopher Hess, MD, PhD, Associate Professor, University of California, San Francisco.

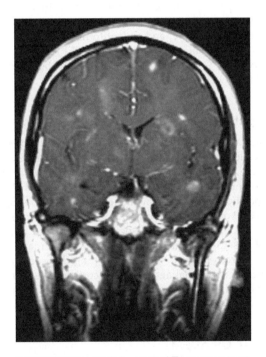

FIGURE 39.2 ADEM—coronal T1 postcontrast images on brain MRI demonstrating variable gadolinium contrast enhancement including one ring-shaped enhancing lesion.

ADEM, acute disseminated encephalomyelitis.

Image courtesy of Christopher Hess, MD, PhD, Associate Professor, University of California, San Francisco.

children with ADEM (30). When trended over time, anti-MOG antibody titers have been found to decrease and often become undetectable in children with monophasic ADEM but remain elevated in those children with recurrent demyelinating events (30,32). Thus far, research on patients with anti-MOG antibodies suggests three clinical trajectories—monophasic ADEM with transient titers that subsequently resolve, relapsing demyelination associated with both ADEM and ON, and NMOSD. It is important to note that at initial presentation, it is unknown which clinical trajectory any individual patient will take. While early data suggested that anti-MOG antibodies may be a marker of good outcome, subsequent studies have not confirmed that (28).

> *ADEM-like attacks can be the first or subsequent attack in children with NMOSD, and an increasing number of children with ADEM followed by recurrent ON have serum antibodies directed against MOG.*

Electrophysiologic Studies

Electroencephalography is of limited utility in ADEM. It may be abnormal, demonstrating diffuse slowing indicative of encephalopathy, and epileptiform spikes are rare in ADEM (33). Visual-evoked potentials (VEP) can be helpful to confirm ON, but does not distinguish between ON caused by ADEM, NMOSD, and MS (33).

Neuropathological Findings

Patients with ADEM rarely undergo biopsy and given the excellent survival rates, autopsy studies are exceedingly rare. Pathological findings include perivenular infiltrates of primarily macrophages as well as T and B cells in association with perivenular demyelination (34,35). By contrast, axons are relatively spared. Also notable is that lesions are of similar pathological age, implying uniform time of onset. A distinct finding in ADEM that may differentiate it from other CNS demyelinating disorders is the presence of microglial aggregates in cortical layer three. It is postulated that this may be the cause of encephalopathy in ADEM (34–36).

VARIANT OF ADEM

Acute Hemorrhagic Encephalomyelitis

Acute hemorrhagic leukoencephalitis (AHL), also known as acute hemorrhagic encephalomyelitis (AHEM), is considered to be a hyperacute variant of ADEM with rapidly progressive, usually fulminant, inflammatory, hemorrhagic demyelination in the CNS. While ADEM is most commonly seen in children, AHEM occurs more often in adults (37). Lesions on brain MRI tend to be large with surrounding edema and mass effect (38). AHL is often fatal, and death triggered by brain edema is common within 1 week of the onset of encephalopathy (37). Given the rapidly progressive nature of the disease, early and aggressive treatment using various combinations of corticosteroids, immunoglobulin, plasma exchange, and cyclophosphamide is recommended (37). As the level of evidence is limited to case reports, no formal recommendation can be given as to the acute treatment of AHEM. If intracranial pressure is increased, measures such as hyperventilation, mannitol, and even decompressive craniectomy have been reported as lifesaving (39–42). At times, corticosteroids are sufficient to arrest the disease (43), but prolonged immunosuppression with plasmapheresis, steroids, and cyclophosphamide are typically necessary and have been reported to result in a good outcome (44).

TREATMENT

The therapeutic approach in ADEM is based on expert consensus as there is a lack of evidence-based, prospective clinical trial data for ADEM management. If ADEM is suspected, standard of care includes empirical antibacterial and antiviral treatment while the workup for possible infectious encephalitis is ongoing. Antiepileptic medication should be used if there are seizures. Once a diagnosis of acute demyelinating disease has been established, the most common initial treatment approach for ADEM is high-dose intravenous methylprednisolone (IVMP) at a dosage of 20 to 30 mg/kg/d (maximum 1 g/d) for 3 to 5 days (2,45). If there is a good response but symptoms do not resolve fully, this is usually then followed by an oral corticosteroid taper over 10 days to 4 weeks (45). The side effects of high-dose corticosteroid treatment should also be managed, including hyperglycemia, hypokalemia, hypertension, facial flushing, and mood disorders. Finally, it is worth noting that high-dose IVMP is not without risk, as rare gastric perforation and death due to gastrointestinal bleeding related to IVMP treatment of ADEM have been reported (46).

> *The most common initial treatment approach for ADEM is high-dose IVMP at a dosage of 20 to 30 mg/kg/d (maximum 1 g/d) for 3 to 5 days.*

When treatment response to IVMP is inadequate, or in cases where corticosteroids are contraindicated, there are a few options to consider. Intravenous immunoglobulin G (IVIG) at a dosage of 2 g/kg divided over 2 to 5 days has been used successfully as monotherapy for the treatment of ADEM (47), even when corticosteroids failed (48,49). When the presentation of ADEM is more severe or life threatening, plasma exchange should be considered early in the disease course (45). One case series showed about 40% of patients with ADEM (n = 10) had moderate to marked improvement following plasma exchange (50). Within that study, early initiation of plasma exchange was associated with better outcome (50). As with high-dose corticosteroids, there are safety concerns with plasma exchange that need to be taken into consideration. Symptomatic hypotension, severe anemia, and heparin-induced thrombocytopenia have all been described as possible side effects of plasma exchange (50).

Rituximab may also be considered in refractory cases, particularly when anti-MOG antibodies are present. Finally, in severe cases of ADEM where there is significant edema, mass effect, and intracranial hypertension, decompressive craniectomy has been reported as a life-saving measure after maximal medical treatment (40).

PROGNOSIS

Risk for Recurrent Demyelinating Attacks

While approximately 70% to 97% of patients with ADEM have a monophasic disease course (24,51), it remains challenging to reliably identify those children for whom the incident ADEM attack is actually the first attack of MS, NMOSD, or whether they will be one of the children with MOG antibodies associated with relapsing ADEM. Several studies have prospectively examined MRI characteristics at initial presentation to predict the likelihood of later diagnosis of MS. These studies have cumulatively increased the sensitivity and specificity with which MRI features are predictive of MS versus ADEM and have guided the current clinical criteria for diagnosis put forth by the IPMSSG.

In 2004, the KIDMUS (Kids with MS) study group found that (a) lesions radiating perpendicularly to the long axis of the corpus callosum (also known as "Dawson's Fingers") and (b) the sole presence of well-defined lesions were predictive of further relapses leading to a diagnosis of MS. If both criteria were met, the specificity was 100%, but the sensitivity was only 21% (52). In 2009, Callen et al. proposed new criteria for distinguishing ADEM from MS including (a) two or more periventricular lesions, (b) presence of T1-weighted hypodensities within the white matter or "black holes," and (c) an absence of diffuse bilateral lesion distribution pattern. When any two out of these three Callen MS-ADEM criteria were present, it was predictive of subsequent confirmation of MS diagnosis with 95% specificity and 81% sensitivity (53).

Most recently, The International Pediatric Multiple Sclerosis Study Group revised their pediatric MS definitions to incorporate the 2010 McDonald criteria to optimize the sensitivity and specificity for diagnosis based on MRI features. The 2010 version of the McDonald criteria for MS diagnosis specifies that application of the criteria at the time of first attack to confirm MS diagnosis cannot be used when the first attack is consistent with ADEM and that dissemination in time must be evidenced by new clinically silent lesions and by a non-ADEM clinical attack (54). In a 2014 study of 82 children, the revised International Pediatric MS diagnostic criteria were found to be 80% sensitive and 100% specific (55).

Several epidemiological studies have also examined risk factors associated with later diagnosis of MS after an initial demyelinating event. Female sex, age 12 or older at presentation, high body mass index, younger age at menarche, low serum vitamin D, secondhand smoke exposure, remote Epstein-Barr virus infection, and HLA-DRB1*15:01 alleles have all been found more frequently in children with MS as compared to children with monophasic demyelination, including ADEM (56,57). In one study by van Pelt et al., 57 single nucleotide polymorphisms were analyzed to assess weight genetic risk scores in 188 children with demyelinating events. These scores significantly differed between children with a monophasic demyelinating event and children with MS (58).

Outcome and Disability

Prognosis after ADEM is generally considered favorable with over 90% of patients making a full and rapid recovery in neurologic exam (59). Death is rare, occurring in less than 2% of patients (24). However, some children with ADEM have cognitive or behavioral deficits long term. One study of 43 children with ADEM reported attention deficit hyperactivity disorder (ADHD) in 44% and motor impairment in 19% after mean follow-up of 5.5 years (60). A meta-analysis of 105 ADEM patients in seven publications reported by Burton et al. identified individual impairments in intellectual quotient, attention, executive function, processing speed, learning and memory, visuospatial skills, and internalizing symptoms (61). A single demyelinating event also may impact brain growth. A recent longitudinal study of 83 children with monophasic demyelination demonstrated reduced age-expected brain growth with particular volume differences in children with ADEM (62). The long-term effect of ADEM on the developing brain, the impact into adulthood, and the potential for neuroplasticity are currently unknown and are an important area for future research.

> ## KEY POINTS FOR PATIENTS AND FAMILIES
>
> - ADEM is a rare condition usually seen in children.
>
> - Symptoms include drowsiness or confusion, weakness of arms or legs, loss of balance or tremor, and loss of vision, often with multiple symptoms at once.
>
> - MRI shows changes in the white matter of the brain and sometimes in the spinal cord or optic nerves (the nerves that connect the eyes to the brain).
>
> - Treatment is usually intravenous (IV) high-dose steroids for a few days. Sometimes a blood-cleaning treatment called plasmapheresis is needed.
>
> - Many patients with ADEM recover, but some may be left with behavioral issues.
>
> - Most cases of ADEM occur only once, but sometimes it recurs.

REFERENCES

1. Krupp LB, Tardieu M, Amato MP, et al. International Pediatric Multiple Sclerosis Study Group criteria for pediatric multiple sclerosis and immune-mediated central nervous system demyelinating disorders: revisions to the 2007 definitions. *Mult Scler.* 2013;19(10):1261–1267.

2. Pohl D, Alper G, Van Haren K, et al. Acute disseminated encephalomyelitis: updates on an inflammatory CNS syndrome. *Neurology.* 2016;87(9 suppl 2):S38–S45.

3. Tenembaum S, Chitnis T, Ness J, et al. Acute disseminated encephalomyelitis. *Neurology.* 2007;68(16 suppl 2):S23–S36.

4. Banwell B, Ghezzi A, Bar-Or A, et al. Multiple sclerosis in children: clinical diagnosis, therapeutic strategies, and future directions. *Lancet Neurol.* 2007;6(10):887–902.

5. Dale RC, de Sousa C, Chong WK, et al. Acute disseminated encephalomyelitis, multiphasic disseminated encephalomyelitis and multiple sclerosis in children. *Brain.* 2000;123 Pt 12:2407–2422.

6. Leake JAD, Albani S, Kao AS, et al. Acute disseminated encephalomyelitis in childhood: epidemiologic, clinical and laboratory features. *Pediatr Infect Dis J.* 2004;23(8):756–764.

7. Torisu H, Kira R, Ishizaki Y, et al. Clinical study of childhood acute disseminated encephalomyelitis, multiple sclerosis, and acute transverse myelitis in Fukuoka Prefecture, Japan. *Brain Dev.* 2010;32(6):454–462.

8. Banwell B, Kennedy J, Sadovnick D, et al. Incidence of acquired demyelination of the CNS in Canadian children. *Neurology.* 2009;72(3):232–239.

9. Pohl D, Hennemuth I, von Kries R, et al. Paediatric multiple sclerosis and acute disseminated encephalomyelitis in Germany: results of a nationwide survey. *Eur J Pediatr.* 2007;166(5):405–412.

10. Langer-Gould A, Zhang JL, Chung J, et al. Incidence of acquired CNS demyelinating syndromes in a multiethnic cohort of children. *Neurology.* 2011;77(12):1143–1148.

11. Hynson JL, Kornberg AJ, Coleman LT, et al. Clinical and neuroradiologic features of acute disseminated encephalomyelitis in children. *Neurology.* 2001;56(8):1308–1312.

12. Tenembaum S, Chamoles N, Fejerman N. Acute disseminated encephalomyelitis: a long-term follow-up study of 84 pediatric patients. *Neurology.* 2002;59(8):1224–1231.

13. Menge T, Hemmer B, Nessler S, et al. Acute disseminated encephalomyelitis: an update. *Arch Neurol.* 2005;62(11):1673–1680.

14. Young NP, Weinshenker BG, Lucchinetti CF. Acute disseminated encephalomyelitis: current understanding and controversies. *Semin Neurol.* 2008;28(1):84–94.

15. Marrie RA, Wolfson C, Sturkenboom MC, et al. Multiple sclerosis and antecedent infections: a case-control study. *Neurology.* 2000;54(12):2307–2310.

16. Miravalle AA, Schreiner T. Neurologic complications of vaccinations. In: Biller J, Ferro JM, eds. *Handbook of Clinical Neurology.* Vol 121 (3rd series) Neurologic Aspects of Systemic Disease Part III. Amsterdam, The Netherlands: Elsevier B.V.; 2014.

17. Atzori M, Battistella PA, Perini P, et al. Clinical and diagnostic aspects of multiple sclerosis and acute monophasic encephalomyelitis in pediatric patients: a single centre prospective study. *Mult Scler.* 2009;15(3):363–370.

18. Schwarz S, Mohr A, Knauth M, et al. Acute disseminated encephalomyelitis: a follow-up study of 40 adult patients. *Neurology.* 2001;56(10):1313–1318.

19. Dale RC, Branson JA. Acute disseminated encephalomyelitis or multiple sclerosis: can the initial presentation help in establishing a correct diagnosis? *Arch Dis Child.* 2005;90(6):636–639.

20. Costanzo MD, Camarca ME, Colella MG, et al. Acute disseminated encephalomyelitis presenting as fever of unknown origin: case report. *BMC Pediatr.* 2011;11:103.

21. Nasr JT, Andriola MR, Coyle PK. ADEM: literature review and case report of acute psychosis presentation. *Pediatr Neurol.* 2000;22(1):8–18.

22. Davis LE, Booss J. Acute disseminated encephalomyelitis in children: a changing picture. *Pediatr Infect Dis J.* 2003;22(9):829–831.

23. Koelman DLH, Chahin S, Mar SS, et al. Acute disseminated encephalomyelitis in 228 patients: a retrospective, multicenter US study. *Neurology.* 2016;86(22):2085–2093.

24. Verhey LH, Shroff M, Banwell B. Pediatric multiple sclerosis: pathobiological, clinical, and magnetic resonance imaging features. *Neuroimaging Clin N Am.* 2013;23(2):227–243.

25. Pohl D, Rostasy K, Reiber H, et al. CSF characteristics in early-onset multiple sclerosis. *Neurology.* 2004;63(10):1966–1967.

26. Huppke B, Ellenberger D, Rosewich H, et al. Clinical presentation of pediatric multiple sclerosis before puberty. *Eur J Neurol.* 2013;21(3):441–446.

27. Reindl M, Rostasy K. MOG antibody-associated diseases. *Neurol Neuroimmunol Neuroinflamm.* 2015;2(1):e60.

28. Hennes E-M, Baumann M, Schanda K, et al. Prognostic relevance of MOG antibodies in children with an acquired demyelinating syndrome. *Neurology.* August 2017. doi:10.1212/WNL.0000000000004312.

29. Hacohen Y, Absoud M, Deiva K, et al. Myelin oligodendrocyte glycoprotein antibodies are associated with a non-MS course in children. *Neurol Neuroimmunol Neuroinflamm.* 2015;2(2):e81.

30. Ramanathan S, Dale RC, Brilot F. Anti-MOG antibody: the history, clinical phenotype, and pathogenicity of a serum biomarker for demyelination. *Autoimmun Rev.* 2016;15(4):307–324.

31. Fernandez-Carbonell C, Vargas-Lowy D, Musallam A, et al. Clinical and MRI phenotype of children with MOG antibodies. *Mult Scler.* 2016;22(2):174–184.

32. Baumann M, Sahin K, Lechner C, et al. Clinical and neuroradiological differences of paediatric acute disseminating encephalomyelitis with and without antibodies to the myelin oligodendrocyte glycoprotein. *J Neurol Neurosurg Psychiatry.* 2015;86(3):265–272.

33. Dale RC. Acute disseminated encephalomyelitis. *Semin Pediatr Infect Dis*. 2003;14(2):90–95.
34. Hardy TA, Reddel SW, Barnett MH, et al. Atypical inflammatory demyelinating syndromes of the CNS. *Lancet Neurol*. 2016;15(9):967–981.
35. Popescu BFG, Lucchinetti CF. Pathology of demyelinating diseases. *Annu Rev Pathol*. 2012;7:185–217.
36. Young NP, Weinshenker BG, Parisi JE, et al. Perivenous demyelination: association with clinically defined acute disseminated encephalomyelitis and comparison with pathologically confirmed multiple sclerosis. *Brain*. 2010;133(Pt 2):333–348.
37. Borlot F, da Paz JA, Casella EB, et al. Acute hemorrhagic encephalomyelitis in childhood: case report and literature review. *J Pediatr Neurosci*. 2011;6(1):48–51.
38. Kuperan S, Ostrow P, Landi MK, et al. Acute hemorrhagic leukoencephalitis vs ADEM: FLAIR MRI and neuropathology findings. *Neurology*. 2003;60(4):721–722.
39. Ahmed AI, Eynon CA, Kinton L, et al. Decompressive craniectomy for acute disseminated encephalomyelitis. *Neurocrit Care*. 2010;13(3):393–395.
40. Dombrowski KE, Mehta AI, Turner DA, et al. Life-saving hemicraniectomy for fulminant acute disseminated encephalomyelitis. *Br J Neurosurg*. 2011;25(2):249–252.
41. Refai D, Lee MC, Goldenberg FD, et al. Decompressive hemicraniectomy for acute disseminated encephalomyelitis: case report. *Neurosurgery*. 2005;56(4):E872.
42. Meilof JF, Hijdra A, Vermeulen M. Successful recovery after high-dose intravenous methylprednisolone in acute hemorrhagic leukoencephalitis. *J Neurol*. 2001;248(10):898–899.
43. Klein CJ, Wijdicks EF, Earnest F 4th. Full recovery after acute hemorrhagic leukoencephalitis (Hurst's disease). *J Neurol*. 2000;247(12):977–979.
44. Seales D, Greer M. Acute hemorrhagic leukoencephalitis. A successful recovery. *Arch Neurol*. 1991;48(10):1086–1088.
45. Pohl D, Tenembaum S. Treatment of acute disseminated encephalomyelitis. *Curr Treat Options Neurol*. 2012;14(3):264–275.
46. Thomas GST, Hussain IHMI. Acute disseminated encephalomyelitis: a report of six cases. *Med J Malaysia*. 2004;59(3):342–351.
47. Nishikawa M, Ichiyama T, Hayashi T, et al. Intravenous immunoglobulin therapy in acute disseminated encephalomyelitis. *Pediatr Neurol*. 1999;21(2):583–586.
48. Marchioni E, Marinou-Aktipi K, Uggetti C, et al. Effectiveness of intravenous immunoglobulin treatment in adult patients with steroid-resistant monophasic or recurrent acute disseminated encephalomyelitis. *J Neurol*. 2002;249(1):100–104.
49. Pradhan S, Gupta RP, Shashank S, et al. Intravenous immunoglobulin therapy in acute disseminated encephalomyelitis. *J Neurol Sci*. 1999;165(1):56–61.
50. Keegan M, Pineda AA, McClelland RL, et al. Plasma exchange for severe attacks of CNS demyelination: predictors of response. *Neurology*. 2002;58(1):143–146.
51. Verhey LH, Branson HM, Shroff MM, et al. MRI parameters for prediction of multiple sclerosis diagnosis in children with acute CNS demyelination: a prospective national cohort study. *Lancet Neurol*. 2011;10(12):1065–1073.
52. Mikaeloff Y, Adamsbaum C, Husson B, et al. MRI prognostic factors for relapse after acute CNS inflammatory demyelination in childhood. *Brain*. 2004;127(Pt 9):1942–1947.
53. Callen DJA, Shroff MM, Branson HM, et al. Role of MRI in the differentiation of ADEM from MS in children. *Neurology*. 2009;72(11):968–973.
54. Polman CH, Reingold SC, Banwell B, et al. Diagnostic criteria for multiple sclerosis: 2010 revisions to the McDonald criteria. *Ann Neurol*. 2011;69(2):292–302.
55. van Pelt ED, Neuteboom RF, Ketelslegers IA, et al. Application of the 2012 revised diagnostic definitions for paediatric multiple sclerosis and immune-mediated central nervous system demyelination disorders. *J Neurol Neurosurg Psychiatry*. 2014;85(7):790–794.
56. Banwell B, Bar-Or A, Arnold DL, et al. Clinical, environmental, and genetic determinants of multiple sclerosis in children with acute demyelination: a prospective national cohort study. *Lancet Neurol*. 2011;10(5):436–445.
57. Waubant E, Ponsonby A-L, Pugliatti M, et al. Environmental and genetic factors in pediatric inflammatory demyelinating diseases. *Neurology*. 2016;87(9 suppl 2):S20–S27.
58. van Pelt ED, Mescheriakova JY, Makhani N, et al. Risk genes associated with pediatric-onset MS but not with monophasic acquired CNS demyelination. *Neurology*. 2013;81(23):1996–2001.
59. O'Mahony J, Marrie RA, Laporte A, et al. Recovery from central nervous system acute demyelination in children. *Pediatrics*. 2015;136(1):e115–e123.
60. Shilo S, Michaeli O, Shahar E, et al. Long-term motor, cognitive and behavioral outcome of acute disseminated encephalomyelitis. *Eur J Paediatr Neurol*. 2016;20(3):361–367.
61. Burton KLO, Williams TA, Catchpoole SE, et al. Long-term neuropsychological outcomes of childhood onset acute disseminated encephalomyelitis (ADEM): a meta-analysis. *Neuropsychol Rev*. 2017;27(2):124–133.
62. Aubert-Broche B, Weier K, Longoni G, et al. Monophasic demyelination reduces brain growth in children. *Neurology*. 2017;88(18):1744–1750.

40

Transverse Myelitis

Isabella Strozzi and Michael Levy

KEY POINTS FOR CLINICIANS

- Incidence of acute transverse myelitis (TM) is reported at 1.34 to 4.6 new cases per million annually. It is estimated that there are about 1,400 new cases in the United States every year. Around 21% of all cases of TM are idiopathic. Other causes include multiple sclerosis (MS), neuromyelitis optica (NMO), and vascular lesions.

- The mechanism of TM, although still unknown, is presumed to be an immune-mediated attack of the spinal cord.

- Patients with TM usually present with paresis of the lower limbs that progresses from flaccid to spastic. Sensory deficits are typically loss of pain and temperature in the level of lesion and hyperesthesia in upper segments. Patients also commonly report preceding symptoms of infection and back pain.

- Diagnosis of TM begins with a comprehensive history and neurological exam, but it must be confirmed by MRI with gadolinium contrast, ideally within the first hours of presentation, and analysis of cerebrospinal fluid (CSF) cell count, oligoclonal bands (OCBs), and immunoglobulin G (IgG) index.

- Differential diagnoses include spinal cord trauma or compression, subacute combined degeneration (vitamin B12 deficiency), neurosyphilis, anterior spinal artery insufficiency, progressive MS, hereditary spastic paraplegia, and radiation myelitis.

- The first-line treatment for TM attacks is the administration of high-dose intravenous methylprednisolone. Plasma exchange is usually offered for patients with more severe presentations of TM or if the disease is unresponsive to steroid therapy.

- Classically, it is considered that about one-third of patients have a good outcome, another third has a fair outcome, and the other third have poor prognosis. Poor outcome is associated with back pain in adults, spinal shock, severe neurological deficits, longer duration of acute phase, and shorter interval between symptom onset and its peak.

- Recurrence of idiopathic TM varies in different international studies from 24% to 61%.

- Currently, mortality is around 5% to 10% and is more common in younger children or older adults, and with high cervical lesions, sepsis, respiratory failure, and pulmonary embolism.

INTRODUCTION

TM is a rare neuro-immune disease characterized by focal inflammation of the spinal cord, leading to acute or subacute onset of motor, and sensory and/or autonomic dysfunction (1). TM may occur independently or as a component of other diseases, such as MS, NMO, infections, and vasculitic disorders.

Descriptions of this disease have been present since 1882, initially mentioned as "acute myelitis" by British neurologist Henry Charlton Bastion in the section of Diseases of Spinal Cord of Quain's Dictionary of Medicine (2) and later on with a series of cases of "softening" of the spinal cord caused by either inflammation or vascular events, such as thrombosis (3). Other authors in the early 1900s published accounts of infectious, postinfectious, and postvaccine etiologies of acute myelitis (4,5). The actual term "acute transverse myelitis" was first used in 1948, in a case report of pneumonia evolving to weakness and loss of sensation of lower limbs with urinary retention (6). Other names used to refer to this disease were "acute myelomalacia" and "acute necrotic myelopathy" among others (7,8). Since 1953, the term "transverse myelopathy" has been ascribed to focal spinal cord lesions of multiple etiologies (9), whereas "transverse myelitis" is reserved for those attributed to inflammatory disease.

The most recent criteria for diagnosis of TM were proposed by the Transverse Myelitis Consortium Working Group, as described in Table 40.1. A diagnosis of idiopathic, monophasic acute TM requires the fulfilment of every inclusion criteria and none of the exclusion criteria. Conversely, for disease-associated TM, a patient must meet all of the inclusion and one of the exclusion criteria (1). The application of these proposed criteria has been validated by other groups; however, about a third of patients do not show confirmatory evidence of inflammation by CSF analysis or gadolinium enhancement on MRI (10). Some authors propose that when these signs are not present at symptom onset, patients should be reevaluated after 2 to 7 days to determine if these criteria are fulfilled (8).

TABLE 40.1   Diagnostic Criteria for Idiopathic Acute Transverse Myelitis

INCLUSION CRITERIA	EXCLUSION CRITERIA
• Development of sensory, motor, or autonomic dysfunction attributable to the spinal cord	• History of previous radiation to the spine within the last 10 y
• Bilateral signs and/or symptoms (though not necessarily symmetric)	• Clear arterial distribution clinical deficit consistent with thrombosis of the anterior spinal artery
• Clearly defined sensory level	• Abnormal flow voids on the surface of the spinal cord
• Exclusion of extra-axial compressive etiology by MRI or myelography (CT of spine is NOT adequate)	• Serologic or clinical evidence of connective tissue disease
• Inflammation within the spinal cord demonstrated by CSF or MRI findings[a]	• CNS manifestations of syphilis, Lyme disease, HIV, HTLV-1, *Mycoplasma* or other viral infections
• Progression to nadir between 4 hr and 21 d following the onset of symptoms	• Brain MRI abnormalities suggestive of MS
	• History of clinically apparent optic neuritis

CSF, cerebrospinal fluid; HTLV-1, human T-lymphotropic virus, type 1; MS, multiple sclerosis.

[a]Diagnosis is still considered possible if patient meets all the inclusion criteria except for inflammatory findings in CSF analysis or spinal cord MRI.

Source: Adapted from Table 1 in Transverse Myelitis Consortium Working Group. Proposed diagnostic criteria and nosology of acute transverse myelitis. *Neurology.* 2002;59:499-505 and http://n.neurology.org/content/59/4/499.long.

EPIDEMIOLOGY

Incidence of acute TM is reported at 1.34 to 4.6 new cases per million annually (11). This incidence increases to 24.6 per million per year within populations with acquired demyelinating diseases such as MS (12). It is estimated that there are about 1,400 new cases in the United States every year (13) and 300 new cases per year in the United Kingdom (14). In children, the incidence is lower, at 0.4 per million per year (11). Out of all cases of TM, about 21% are of idiopathic etiology (15).

Although there are no records of incidence of TM by state, the Transverse Myelitis Association conducted an informal survey among its members from 1997 to 2001. They included 454 U.S. residents in their sample, distributed through the states as shown in Figure 40.1, where each state is colored according to the number of patients per 1,000,000 inhabitants. They did not find any difference among the states through statistical testing (16). Currently, there is no evidence of hereditary or ethnic predisposition for acute TM (17).

Although the disease affects individuals of any age, there is a bimodal distribution with peaks at 15 to 19 years and between 30 and 39 years (1,11,18), and about 20% of patients are under 18 years old (19). There also appears to be a peak within the pediatric patient group before the age of 3 (19). Through the same survey mentioned earlier, the Transverse Myelitis Association gathered information on the age at onset of TM patients based on the United States. The data are presented in Figure 40.2.

There are some reports of a slight predominance of the female sex, from 1.9:1 to 2.6:1 female/male ratio although not as pronounced as other autoimmune diseases (11,20–22), whereas other sources affirm there is no sex predominance in this disease (1,19). In the published literature, there is no difference in incidence among ethnic groups (13).

PATHOPHYSIOLOGY

The mechanism of TM, although still unknown, is presumed to be an immune-mediated attack of the spinal cord. This is based on inflammatory signs in the CSF, such as lymphocytosis and elevated IgG index, and gadolinium enhancement by MRI which suggests breakdown of the blood–brain barrier of the spinal cord (23). One theory proposes that there is molecular mimicry and consequently stimulation of T cells and autoantibodies involved, similar to the pathogenesis of Guillain–Barré syndrome (23). Another theory involves the overactivation of lymphocytes by nonspecific superantigens (23).

Much of the speculation around the pathophysiology of TM comes from related diseases, such as MS and NMO, and animal models, particularly with experimental autoimmune encephalomyelitis (EAE). In EAE, mice are injected with a myelin antigen that causes the animal's immune system to react against its own central nervous system (CNS), reproducing some of the features of MS or TM.

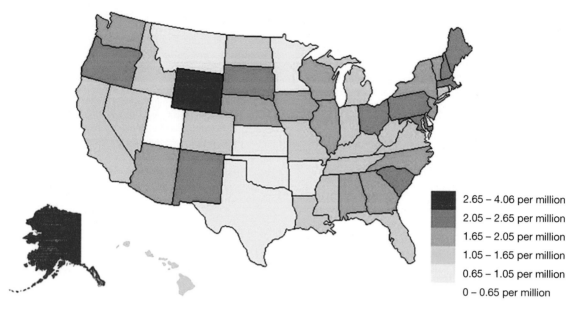

FIGURE 40.1 Patients with TM per state in the United States.
TM, transverse myelitis.

Source: Created based on data found in Siegel S, Wang D. The TMA study of transverse myelitis. *J For TR Myelitis Assoc*. 2001;4(2):24–29.

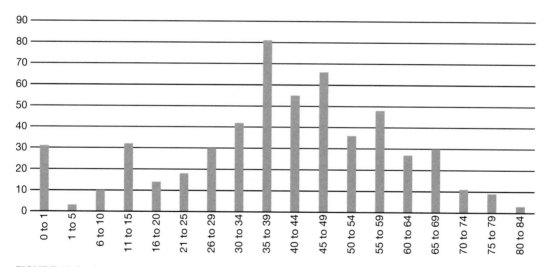

FIGURE 40.2 Age at onset of TM.
TM, transverse myelitis.

Source: Created based on data found in Siegel S, Wang D. The TMA study of transverse myelitis. *J TR Myelitis Assoc*. 2001;4(2):24–29.

Myelin antigens that are used include myelin basic protein (MBP), proteolipid protein (PLP), and myelin oligodendrocyte glycoprotein (MOG) (24). These antigens stimulate the proliferation and invasion of CD4+ T cells and macrophages, which consequently promote an immune response within the CNS. The role of B cells is still unclear, although there are higher circulating levels in EAE induced by anti-MOG antibodies (24).

Pathology of TM depends on the etiology, stratified by the type of lesion: demyelinating, necrotizing, or a mass lesion. Common causes for each category are listed in Table 40.2.

Demyelinating lesions are seen in animal models and autopsy from patients with TM through Luxol fast blue staining, combined with Cresyl violet acetate (see Figure 40.3), solochrome cyanin, black gold staining, or

TABLE 40.2 Types of Spinal Cord Pathology in TM

TYPE OF LESION	EXAMPLES
Demyelinating (most common)	• **Multiple sclerosis**
	• **Idiopathic transverse myelitis**
	• ADEM
	• HIV vacuolar myelopathy
	• Tropical spastic paraparesis (HTLV-1)
	• Progressive multifocal leukoencephalopathy (JC virus)
	• Neurosyphilis
Mass lesions	• **Systemic lupus erythematosus**
	• **Sjögren's syndrome**
	• **Enteroviral infection**
	• Sarcoidosis
	• Behçet's disease
	• Mixed connective tissue disorder
	• Lyme disease
	• Other viral infections (e.g., varicella-zoster virus, cytomegalovirus, Epstein–Barr virus, West Nile virus, Coxsackievirus)
Necrotizing	• **Neuromyelitis optica**
	• Herpes simplex virus acute necrotizing myelitis
	• Progressive necrotic myelopathy
	• Bacterial abscess
	• Neuroschistosomiasis

ADEM, acute disseminated encephalomyelitis; HTLV-1, human T-lymphotropic virus, type 1; JC, John Cunningham; TM, transverse myelitis.
Most common causes are in **bold**.
Source: Adapted from Table 6.4 found in Levy M, Kerr DA. Transverse myelitis. In Dale RC, Vincent A, eds. *Inflammatory and Autoimmune Disorders of the Nervous System in Children*. London, UK: Mac Keith Press; 2010:97–107. (25)

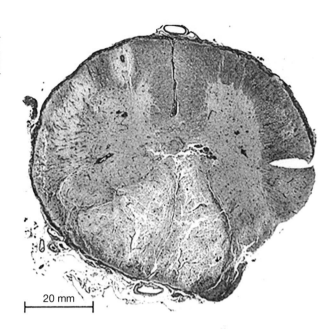

FIGURE 40.3 Luxol fast blue staining of demyelination in human spinal cord.

Source: Adapted from Figure 3 in Cox A, Coles A, Antoun N, et al. Recurrent myelitis and optic neuritis in a 29-year-old woman. *Lancet Neurol*. 2005;4(8):510–516. doi:10.1016/S1474-4422(05)70143-5.

immunofluorescence through anti-MBP antibodies (26–28). Loss of myelin is typically accompanied by lymphocytic infiltration, axonal degeneration, edema, and gliosis (29).

Studies have shown increased interleukin 6 (IL-6) levels within the CSF and correlation between markedly elevated IL-6 levels with worsening neurological disability. IL-6, synthesized mainly by astrocytes in response to inflammatory cytokines, may worsen spinal cord demyelination and axonal degeneration by activating the Janus kinase (JAK)/Signal Transducer and Activator of Transcription proteins (STAT) pathway and increasing inducible nitric oxide synthase (iNOS) activity. This results in high nitric oxide levels and free-radical production, causing cell membrane discontinuity and altered neurotransmitter production (30). It is also suggested that IL-17 might induce focal inflammation through the production of IL-6 (31).

ANATOMICAL AND CLINICAL FEATURES

Signs and symptoms of TM are diverse since they are determined by the location of the lesion within the spinal cord (see Table 40.3). In both adult and pediatric populations, the most common levels affected are from T7 to T12 (50–85), followed by the cervical region, and the lumbar spine is mostly preserved (8,18,19,21,32). Although this disease is called "transverse" myelitis, it does not necessarily affect the whole width of the spinal cord and may also involve more than one vertebral segment. In fact, some studies show that the median range of spinal involvement is 1.6 to 2 vertebral segments, ranging from zero to eight (33,34).

About 25% to 44% patients report preceding infectious symptoms, such as upper respiratory symptoms, fever, nausea and myalgia, and a significant amount prior to the neurological deficits (21,35,36). Most cases begin with ascending paresthesia and around half of patients report back ache at the level of the spinal cord that is affected (18,33). Sensory dysfunction may progress to loss of pain and temperature at the respective level. In contrast to MS, position and vibration senses are often preserved (37), especially with sparing of the posterior columns.

Motor impairment, which is present in up to 80% of patients (20) and is most common in lower limbs, is characterized by weakness that is initially flaccid. Over the subsequent weeks when the healing process begins, patients often develop spastic paresis and hyperreflexia. Weakness tends to follow a pyramidal distribution, affecting mostly the extensor muscles of the upper limbs and the flexors of the lower limbs (17). In up to 5% there may be respiratory weakness (37) due to either high cervical lesions affecting the phrenic nerve or thoracic lesions that cause intercostal muscle spasms. One study found that up to 89% of children with TM initially needed assisted ventilation (19).

TABLE 40.3 Transverse Myelitis Findings by Location Within the Spinal Cord

SPINAL CORD LEVEL	SIGNS AND SYMPTOMS
Cervical	• Weakness and hyperreflexia in **upper** and **lower** extremities • Numbness in **upper** and **lower** extremities • Sensory level in **neck or shoulder** • **Sympathetic** autonomic dysfunction • Bowel/bladder dysfunction • Muscle cramps • Difficulty walking
Thoracic (most common)	• Weakness and hyperreflexia in **lower** extremities • Numbness in **lower** extremities • Sensory level in **trunk or abdomen** • **Parasympathetic** autonomic dysfunction • Bowel/bladder dysfunction • Muscle cramps in legs • Difficulty walking
Lumbar	• Weakness and hyperreflexia in **lower** extremities • Numbness in **lower** extremities • Sensory loss in **lower** extremities • **Flaccid neurogenic bladder and constipation** • Difficulty walking

Source: Adapted from Table 6.2 found in Levy M, Kerr DA. Transverse myelitis. In Dale RC, Vincent A, eds. *Inflammatory and Autoimmune Disorders of the Nervous System in Children*. London UK: Mac Keith Press; 2010:97–107.

Acute sphincter dysfunction is found in 75% to 95% and nearly all TM patients have some form of bladder dysfunction, such as urgency, incontinence, or difficulty voiding (19,30,33). Other autonomic symptoms include varying severities of peaks in blood pressure, temperature dysregulation, sexual dysfunction, and sweating (11,12,17,37).

Typically, symptoms develop over hours or a few days, reach maximal severity an average of 3 to 7 days after onset, and then stabilize after 2 weeks (36). In hyperacute cases, the point of highest level of neurological deficit occurs within 4 hours (8,19,21,33,37). Many of these cases of TM involve a vasculopathy, such as arterial venous fistulas, strokes, or vasculitis. In these cases, two-third of patients present with disabling paresis or flaccid paralysis and arreflexia of the lower limbs and are unable to walk (18,21,37). This percentage is higher in children, reaching 90% of pediatric patients with TM (21).

DIAGNOSTIC INVESTIGATION

The evaluation of patients presenting with symptoms of TM begins with a comprehensive history, neurological exam, as well as imaging and blood/spinal fluid testing.

Once the history and exam localize to the spinal cord, there is a simple algorithm to narrow down the differential diagnoses.

First, one must exclude any form of physical compression of the spinal cord. The method of choice is MRI with gadolinium contrast, ideally performed within the first hours of presentation. MRI is a part of the formal diagnostic criteria of acute TM (1). MRI of the spinal cord could show a vertebral disk rupture or herniation, intraspinal tumors, vertebral fractures, spondylolisthesis, abscesses, or hematomas (12,25). If MRI is not available in due time, CT myelography is an alternative to ruling out compressive etiologies (1). In the absence of a compressive lesion, the MRI may show a lesion in the parenchyma of the spinal cord due to inflammatory, vascular, infectious, and metabolic etiologies.

For acute TM, the inflammatory lesion in the spinal cord will be evident as a gadolinium enhancing lesion in T1-weighted MRI and/or hyperintense signal in T2-weighted MRI, with or without local edema (38). However, in children with TM, up to 40% may not show classic MRI findings (25,1). TM lesions may be focal or long, but MS lesions are almost always less than two vertebral segments and usually peripheral and asymmetric (partial TM), whereas NMO creates longer cord lesions (>3 segments) and cord swelling (39,40). Consistent with these patterns on MRI, partial TM has a higher chance of transitioning to MS than complete TM (40). Brain MRI with "silent" T2 lesions in the brain at the time of the acute TM is also useful for the diagnosis of MS.

Diffusion tensor imaging (DTI) is an MRI technique sensitive to the motion of extracellular water molecules along the axons and can track the direction of nervous fibers. Through this method, a fractional anisotropy (FA) value, which extends from 0 to 1, can be obtained and it reflects tract orientation, axonal diameter, membrane thickness, and fiber myelination (41). It is proposed that FA values are more sensitive to spinal cord lesions than T2-weighted MRI and may be a prognostic marker (41). Although PET and single-photon emission computed tomography (SPECT) scans do not show TM lesions (except in a few cases of fulminant NMO attacks), they may be helpful to rule out malignancies, sarcoidosis, and other diseases (25). Spinal angiograms may be useful for excluding stroke or arteriovenous malformation in acute onset myelopathy (Figure 40.4) (42).

CSF analysis in TM may vary according to the etiology. Idiopathic TM classically elicits pleocytosis and at times increased IgG index (ratio of IgG in the CSF to serum IgG) with occasional OCBs. Immunoglobulins are more pronounced in the CSF in cases where MS is the underlying etiology. On the other hand, NMO usually does not present with elevations in IgG index or OCBs (<30% of cases) or it occurs transiently. NMO also shows marked pleocytosis (>50 cells/mm^3) with neutrophilic or eosinophilic predominance (39) compared to MS. CSF white blood cell counts higher than 10 cells/mm^3 might be useful for differentiating TM from spinal cord infarcts (40).

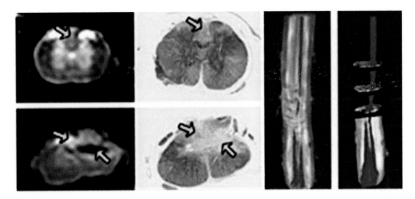

FIGURE 40.4 TM lesions in rat spinal cords.
TM, transverse myelitis.

Images obtained from rat with spinal cord injury induced by lipopolysaccharide (LPS) injection: T2-weighted MRI (left), Luxol fast blue staining (middle), and fractional anisotropy.

Source: Adapted from Figure 2B in DeBoy CA, Zhang J, Dike S, et al. High resolution diffusion tensor imaging of axonal damage in focal inflammatory and demyelinating lesions in rat spinal cord. *Brain*. 2007;130(8):2199–2210. With permission from Oxford University Press.

Transcranial magnetic stimulation (TMS), although not much used in adult TM patients, is often a relevant diagnostic method within the pediatric population. By stimulating the motor cortex through a magnetic field and measuring latency and amplitude in the muscles, TMS can identify flaws in descending motor tracts of the brain, spinal cord, and peripheral nerves, which may not be visualized by MRI or CT. Some authors propose that TMS can be considered as a prognostic tool with absence or gross abnormalities of latency and amplitude indicating a poor clinical outcome (43).

Other key differential diagnoses in TM include traumatic lesion of the spinal cord, compressive myelopathy, subacute combined degeneration (vitamin B12 deficiency), neurosyphilis, anterior spinal artery insufficiency, progressive MS, hereditary spastic paraplegia, radiation myelitis, and others (12,25).

TREATMENT AND MANAGEMENT

The first-line treatment for TM attacks is the administration of high-dose intravenous methylprednisolone for 3 to 7 days, which is reported to reduce symptoms and radiographic evidence of lesions (23,44,45). In children, some studies have reported continued improvement following corticosteroids up to 1 year after disease onset (46–48).

Plasma exchange (or plasmapheresis) is usually offered for patients with more severe presentations of TM or if the disease is unresponsive to steroid therapy. Plasma exchange is particularly beneficial, as monotherapy or complementary to corticosteroids, for patients with less than 20 days of evolution, males, and those without complete loss of function (23). Some sources suggest a combination of cyclophosphamide and plasma exchange for patients who develop total loss of motor and sensory function (49). In patients with TM caused by NMO or MS, mitoxantrone and rituximab may be helpful as well (40).

Nonpharmacological approaches, such as physical and occupational therapies, are essential for patients with neurological sequelae from TM. Therapy focused on specific symptoms should be emphasized for patients on an ongoing basis. Since many patients evolve to chronic neuropathic pain, gabapentin and tricyclic antidepressants can be considered to reduce neuropathic pain associated with recovery from TM. For spasticity, options such as baclofen, botulinum toxin, aquatic therapy, and physical exercises are available (23).

PROGNOSIS

Classically, it is considered that about one-third of patients have a good outcome, another third have a fair outcome, and the other third have poor prognosis (18). Studies have not found any correlation of poor outcome with sex, infectious symptoms, spinal fluid characteristics, or level of the lesion (18,32,33). Poor prognostic indicators include back pain in adult patients, spinal shock, severe neurological deficits, longer duration of acute phase, and shorter interval (particularly less than 8 days) between symptom onset and its peak (18,33,50). Recurrence of TM varies with different international studies from 24% to 61% (20) and is most commonly associated with serological presence of the anti-aquaporin-4 antibody in NMO.

In the 1940s, a time with less treatment options, the prognosis of acute transverse myelopathy was grim: every patient affected by it passed away from 10 to 90 days after symptom onset (7). Since then, mortality rates have been dropping due to proper care of autonomic dysfunction, use of antibiotics to treat infections and sepsis, and respiratory support when necessary (7). Currently, mortality is around 5% to 10% and is related to younger children or older adults, high cervical lesions, sepsis, respiratory failure, and pulmonary embolism (18,32).

KEY POINTS FOR PATIENTS AND FAMILIES

- TM is rare. It is estimated that there are about 1,400 new cases in the United States every year. Around 21% of all cases of TM are the idiopathic type, which is a single attack. Other causes include multiple sclerosis and rare causes of relapsing TM.

- The mechanism of TM is presumed to be an immune attack of the spinal cord.

- Patients with TM usually present with weakness of the legs, as well as sensory changes, tingling, and pain. Patients also commonly report preceding symptoms of infection and back pain.

- The diagnosis of TM begins with a thorough interview and neurological exam, and it must be confirmed by MRI, ideally within the first hours of presentation. Additional testing of the blood and spinal fluid analysis may be necessary as well.

- There are many other causes of spinal cord injury that mimic TM. These include spinal cord trauma or compression, subacute combined degeneration (vitamin B12 deficiency), neurosyphilis infection, spinal cord stroke, multiple sclerosis, hereditary spastic paraplegia, and radiation damage.

- Treatment for TM starts with the administration of high-dose intravenous methylprednisolone. Plasma exchange is usually offered for patients with more severe presentations of TM or if steroid therapy is not sufficient.

- Generally, about one-third of patients have a good outcome, another third have a fair outcome, and the other third have poor prognosis. Poor outcome may be predicted by back pain in adult patients, spinal shock, severity of neurological deficit, longer duration of acute phase, and shorter interval between symptom onset and its peak.

- The chance of a recurrence of idiopathic TM varies with different international studies, but can range from 24% to 61%.

- Currently, the chance of dying from a severe TM is around 5% to 10% and is related to younger children or older adults, lesions at the top of the spinal cord controlling the breathing muscles, and complications from hospitalization such as ventilation infections and blood clots.

REFERENCES

1. Transverse Myelitis Consortium Working Group. Proposed diagnostic criteria and nosology of acute transverse myelitis. *Neurology.* 2002;59:499–505.
2. Bastian HC. Diseases of the spinal cord. In: Murray HM, Harold J, Bosanquet WC, eds. *Quain's Dictionary of Medicine.* 3rd ed. London, UK: Longmans, Green and Co; 1882:1519–1565.
3. Bastian HC. Thrombotic softening of the spinal cord: a case of so-called "acute myelitis." *Lancet.* 1910;VII(4552):1894–1895. Available at: http://www.sciencedirect.com/science/article/pii/S0140673600527883. Accessed May 22, 2017.
4. Rivers TM. Viruses. 1929;*JAMA.* 92(14):1147–1151. Available at: http://jamanetwork.com/pdfaccess.ashx?url=/data/journals/jama/6674/. Accessed May 22, 2017.
5. Singer DH. The pathology of so-called acute myelitis. *Brain.* 1902;25(2):332–340. doi:10.1093/brain/25.2.332.
6. Suchett-Kaye AI. Acute transverse myelitis complicating pneumonia. *Lancet.* 1948;252(6524):417. doi:10.1016/S0140-6736(48)90987–8.
7. Altrocchi PH. Acute transverse myelopathy. *Arch Neurol.* 1963;9(2):111–119. doi:10.1001/archneur.1963.00460080021002.
8. Krishnan C, Kerr DA. Idiopathic transverse myelitis. *Arch Neurol.* 2005;62(6):1011–1013.
9. Paine RS, Byers RK. Transverse myelopathy in childhood. *AMA Am J Dis Child.* 1953;85(2):151–163.
10. de Sèze J, Lanctin C, Lebrun C, et al. Idiopathic acute transverse myelitis: application of the recent diagnostic. *Neurology.* 2005;65:1950–1953.
11. Bhat A, Naguwa S, Cheema G, et al. The epidemiology of transverse myelitis. *Autoimmun Rev.* 2010;9(5):A395-A399. doi:10.1016/j.autrev.2009.12.007.
12. Frohman EM, Wingerchuk DM. Transverse myelitis. *N Engl J Med.* 2010;363(6):564–572.
13. Berman M, Feldman S, Alter M, et al. Acute transverse myelitis: incidence and etiologic considerations. *Neurology.* 1981;31(8):966–971.
14. Hawke S, Alexander M. *Transverse Myelitis: A Guide for Patients and Carers.* London, UK: British Brain & Spine Foundation.
15. West TW, Hess C, Cree BAC. Acute transverse myelitis: demyelinating, inflammatory, and infectious myelopathies. *Semin Neurol.* 2012;32(2):97–113. doi:10.1055/s-0032–1322586.
16. Siegel S, Wang D. The TMA study of transverse myelitis. *J For TR Myelitis Assoc.* 2001;4(2):24–29.
17. West TW. Transverse myelitis—a review of the presentation, diagnosis, and initial management. *Discov Med.* 2013;16(88):167–177.
18. Christensen PB, Wermuth L, Hinge HH, et al. Clinical course and long-term prognosis of acute transverse myelopathy. *Acta Neurol Scand.* 1990;81:431–435.
19. Pidcock FS, Krishnan C, Crawford TO, et al. Acute transverse myelitis in childhood: center-based analysis of 47 cases. *Neurology.* 2007;68(1):1474–1480. doi:10.1212/01.wnl.0000260609.11357.6f.

20. Alvarenga MP, Thuler LCS, Neto SP, et al. The clinical course of idiopathic acute transverse myelitis in patients from Rio de Janeiro. *J Neurol.* 2010;257:992–998. doi:10.1007/s00415-009-5450-6.

21. Borchers AT, Gershwin ME. Transverse myelitis. *Autoimmun Rev.* 2012;11(3):231–248. doi:dd10.1016/j.autrev.2011.05.018.

22. Thomas T, Branson HM, Verhey LH, et al. The demographic, clinical, and magnetic resonance imaging (MRI) features of transverse myelitis in children. *J Child Neurol.* 2012;27(1):11–21. doi:10.1177/0883073811420495.

23. Krishnan C, Kaplin AI, Desphande DM, et al. Transverse myelitis: pathogenesis, diagnosis and treatment. *Front Biosci.* 2004;9:1483–1499.

24. Kishore A, Kanaujia A, Nag S, et al. Different mechanisms of inflammation induced in virus and autoimmune-mediated models of multiple sclerosis in C57BL6 mice. *Biomed Res Int.* 2013;2013:589048. doi:10.1155/2013/589048.

25. Levy M, Kerr DA. Transverse myelitis. In Dale RC, Vincent A, eds. *Inflammatory and Autoimmune Disorders of the Nervous System in Children.* London UK: Mac Keith Press; 2010:97–107.

26. Cox A, Coles A, Antoun N, et al. Recurrent myelitis and optic neuritis in a 29-year-old woman. *Lancet Neurol.* 2005;4(8):510–516. doi:10.1016/S1474-4422(05)70143-5.

27. Love S. Demyelinating diseases. *J Clin Pathol.* 2006;59(11):1151–1159. doi:10.1136/jcp.2005.031195.

28. McMillan MT, Pan X-Q, Smith AL, et al. Coronavirus-induced demyelination of neural pathways triggers neurogenic bladder overactivity in a mouse model of multiple sclerosis. *Am J Physiol Renal Physiol.* 2014;307(5):F612-F622. doi:10.1152/ajprenal.00151.2014.

29. DeBoy CA, Zhang J, Dike S, et al. High resolution diffusion tensor imaging of axonal damage in focal inflammatory and demyelinating lesions in rat spinal cord. *Brain.* 2007;130(8):2199–2210. doi:10.1093/brain/awm122.

30. Kaplin AI, Deshpande DM, Scott E, et al. IL-6 induces regionally selective spinal cord injury in patients with the neuroinflammatory disorder transverse myelitis. *J Clin Invest.* 2005;115(10):2731–2741. doi:10.1172/JCI25141.

31. Graber JJ, Allie SR, Mullen KM, et al. Interleukin-17 in transverse myelitis and multiple sclerosis. *J Neuroimmunol.* 2008;196:124–132. doi:10.1016/j.jneuroim.2008.02.008.

32. Miyazawa R, Ikeuchi Y, Tomomasa T, et al. Determinants of prognosis of acute transverse myelitis in children. *Pediatr Int.* 2003;45:512–516.

33. Bruna J, Martínez-Yélamos S, Martínez-Yélamos A, et al. Idiopathic acute transverse myelitis: a clinical study and prognostic markers in 45 cases. *Mult Scler.* 2006;12:169–173. doi:10.1191/135248506ms1260oa.

34. Chan KH, Tsang KL, Fong GCY, et al. Idiopathic inflammatory demyelinating disorders after acute transverse myelitis. *Eur J Neurol.* 2006;13(8):862–868. doi:10.1111/j.1468.

35. Kaplin AI, Krishnan C, Deshpande DM, et al. Diagnosis and management of acute myelopathies. *Neurologist.* 2005;11(1):2–18. doi:10.1097/01.nrl.0000149975.39201.0b.

36. Ropper AH, Poskanzer DC. The prognosis of acute and subacute transverse myelopathy based on early signs and symptoms. *Ann Neurol.* 1978;4:51–59.

37. Sá MJ. Acute transverse myelitis: a practical reappraisal. *Autoimmun Rev.* 2009;9(2):128–131. doi:10.1016/j.autrev.2009.04.005.

38. Desanto J, Ross JS. Spine infection/inflammation. *Radiol Clin North Am.* 2011;49(1):105–127. doi:10.1016/j.rcl.2010.07.018.

39. Jacob A, Weinshenker BG. An approach to the diagnosis of acute transverse myelitis. *Semin Neurol.* 2008;28:105–120. doi:10.1055/s-2007-1019132.

40. Scott TF, Frohman EM, De Seze J, et al. Evidence-based guideline: clinical evaluation and treatment of transverse myelitis. *Neurology.* 2011;77(12):2128–2134. doi:10.1212/WNL.0b013e31823dc535.

41. Lee JW, Park KS, Kim JH, et al. Diffusion tensor imaging in idiopathic acute transverse myelitis. *AJR Am J Roentgenol.* 2008;191(2):52–57. doi:10.2214/AJR.07.2800.

42. Mealy MA, Jimenez JA, Gailloud P, et al. Differentiating vascular myelopathy from transverse myelitis. In: *American Academy of Neurology Meeting.* San Diego, CA; 2013. Available here: https://archive.myelitis.org/wp/wp-content/uploads/2013/04/AAN-2013-myelopathy-poster.pdf. Accessed May 22, 2017.

43. Voitenkov VB, Klimkin AV, Skripchenko NV, et al. Diagnostic transcranial magnetic stimulation as a prognostic tool in children with acute transverse myelitis. *Spinal Cord.* 2016;54(3):226–228. doi:10.1038/sc.2015.129.

44. Kalita J, Misra UK. Is methyl prednisolone useful in acute transverse myelitis? *Spinal Cord.* 2001;39:471–476.

45. Kennedy PGE, Weir AI. Rapid recovery of acute transverse myelitis treated with steroids. *Postgrad Med J.* 1988;64:384–385.

46. Defresne P, Meyer L, Tardieu M, et al. Efficacy of high dose steroid therapy in children with severe acute transverse myelitis. *J Neurol Neurosurg Psychiatry.* 2001;71(1):272–274.

47. Lahat E, Pillar G, Ravid S, et al. Rapid recovery from transverse myelopathy in children treated with methylprednisolone. *Pediatr Neurol.* 1998;19(4):279–282.

48. Sébire G, Hollenberg H, Meyer L, et al. High dose methylprednisolone in severe acute transverse myelopathy. *Arch Dis Child.* 1997;76:167–168.

49. Greenberg BM, Thomas KP, Krishnan C, et al. Idiopathic transverse myelitis: corticosteroids, plasma exchange, or cyclophosphamide. *Neurology.* 2007;68(5):1614–1617. doi:10.1212/01.wnl.0000260970.63493.c8.

50. Defresne P, Hollenberg H, Husson B, et al. Acute transverse myelitis in children: clinical course and prognostic factors. *J Child Neurol.* 2003;18(6):401–406.

41

Autoimmune Encephalitis

Michel Toledano

KEY POINTS FOR CLINICIANS

- Autoimmune encephalitis (AE) describes a group of disorders associated with neural-specific autoantibodies.
- Antibodies can target either intracellular antigens or extracellular plasma membrane proteins such as ion channels or neurotransmitter receptors.
- Antibodies targeting intracellular antigens are usually associated with malignancy and are poorly responsive to immunotherapy.
- AE associated with antibodies targeting extracellular plasma membrane proteins are immunotherapy responsive.
- AE can present with distinct clinical syndromes but presentation is heterogeneous and selective antibody testing should be avoided.
- Anti-N-methyl-D-aspartate receptor (NMDAR) encephalitis can occur as a postinfectious syndrome following herpes simplex virus encephalitis.
- Antibodies should be tested in both serum and cerebrospinal fluid (CSF).
- Prompt initiation of immunotherapy improves outcome.

Clinically, encephalitis is characterized by the subacute onset of altered mental status, focal neurologic deficits, fever, and generalized or focal seizures. Historically, encephalitis was synonymous with infection but over the last decades it has become clear that central nervous system (CNS) autoimmunity is a common cause of encephalitis [1,2]. AE describes a heterogeneous group of neurologic disorders associated with neural-specific autoantibodies [3]. Establishing the diagnosis can be challenging given the wide range of clinical presentations, as well as the overlap with other causes of encephalitis such as infection.

Understanding the pathophysiology of AE is helpful in guiding diagnostic testing and management (Figure 41.1). AE can be subdivided into two major groups based on the location of the antigenic target of the associated neural autoantibody. The first group includes the classic paraneoplastic disorders, which are associated with antibodies targeting intracellular antigens (nuclear and cytoplasmic enzymes, ribonucleic acid (RNA)-binding proteins, and transcription factors) [4,6]. These antibodies have a strong association with neoplasms but are not considered pathogenic. Rather, it is thought that CD8+ T cell mediated inflammation is the likely responsible mechanism of

tissue injury [7]. Prognosis in these disorders tends to be poor and patients respond poorly to immunotherapy [8]. Not all autoantibodies targeting intracellular antigens are paraneoplastic. Antibodies to glutamic acid decarboxylase 65 (GAD65), an intracellular synaptic protein, are not usually associated with malignancy. Patients harboring these antibodies tend to have more variable response to immunotherapy.

The second group is associated with antibodies targeting extracellular plasma membrane proteins (neurotransmitter receptors, ion channels, water channels, and channel-complex proteins). Tumor associations in this group are variable but unlike antibodies targeting intracellular proteins, these antibodies can access their target antigen in vivo and alter their function and number to cause disease [9]. Consequently, neurologic syndromes associated with these antibodies tend to be immunotherapy responsive and have a much better prognosis.

WHEN TO SUSPECT AE

Patients with AE tend to present with subacute onset of alterations in level of consciousness, cognitive difficulties,

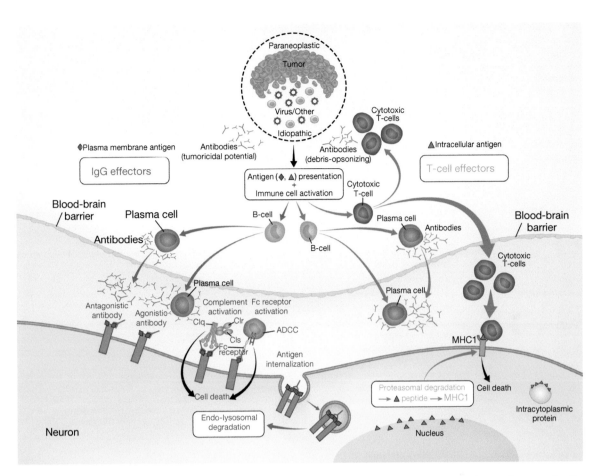

FIGURE 41.1 Immunopathogenic mechanisms of paraneoplastic and nonparaneoplastic (idiopathic) neural autoantibodies.

In cases of paraneoplastic autoimmunity, tumor-targeted immune responses are initiated by onconeural proteins expressed in the plasma membrane (red diamond) or in the cytoplasm, nucleus or nucleolus (green triangle) of certain tumors. These antigens are also expressed in neural cells and thus are coincidental targets. Although there is some evidence to support an analogous infectious-induced mimicry in nonparaneoplastic autoimmunity (e.g., anti-NMDAR encephalitis after encephalitis with certain herpes viruses) (5), the source of the antigen remains elusive in the majority of these cases. Antibodies targeting plasma membrane antigens are effectors of injury (red): antibodies (red) directed at neural cell plasma membrane antigens (e.g., leucine-rich glioma inactivated-1, NMDAR, or alpha-amino-3-hydroxy-5-methyl-4-isoxazoleproponic acid receptor are effectors of cellular dysfunction or injury through multiple effector mechanisms. These mechanisms include receptor agonist or antagonist effects, activation of the complement cascades, activation of Fc receptors (leading to antibody-dependent cell mediated cytotoxicity), and antigen internalization (antigenic modulation), thereby altering antigen density on the cell surface. Antibodies targeting nuclear or cytoplasmic antigens are serum markers of a T cell effector mediated injury (green): intracellular antigens (green triangles) are not accessible to immune attack in situ, but peptides derived from intracellular proteins are displayed on upregulated MHC class-I molecules in a pro-inflammatory cytokine milieu after proteasomal degradation, and are then accessible to peptide-specific cytotoxic T cells. Antibodies (green e.g., antineuronal nuclear antibody type-1, or collapsin response mediator protein-5) targeting these intracellular antigens (green) are detected in both serum and in CSF but are not pathogenic. In clinical practice, these antibodies serve as diagnostic markers of a T cell predominant effector process.

CSF, cerebrospinal fluid; NMDAR, N-methyl-D-aspartate receptor.

Source: Modified with permission from Figure 1 in Toledano M, Pittock SJ. Autoimmune epilepsy. *Semin Neurol*. 2015;35(3):246.

movement abnormalities, sleep disturbances, and seizures. Psychiatric disturbances including psychosis, hallucination, and agitation are common in some types of AE, particularly NMDAR encephalitis. Distinct clinical syndromes have been described and these can help narrow the differential of AE but the clinical spectrum is wide and many patients with AE do not fit neatly into any of the described syndromes (9,10) (Table 41.1).

Clinicians should suspect AE in patients presenting with

- Subacute onset of unexplained neuropsychiatric symptoms or the presence of a well-defined clinical syndrome such as limbic encephalitis, progressive encephalomyelitis with rigidity and myoclonus (PERM), or faciobrachial dystonic seizures
- Recent-onset cryptogenic epilepsy or new-onset refractory status epilepticus (including nonconvulsive status)

TABLE 41.1   Clinical Syndromes Associated With Neural Antibodies

SYNDROME	CLINICAL CHARACTERISTICS	ANTIBODIES	OTHER CAUSES
Limbic encephaliti	Memory deficits, hallucinations, delusions, Sleep disturbances, seizures	LGI1, NMDAR, AMPAR, GABA$_B$R, ANNA1, Amphiphysin, MA2, ANNA3, GAD65,	HSVE, HHV-6, gliomatosis cerebri
Psychosis, movement disorders, seizures	Delusions, aural hallucinations, paranoid ideation, oro-lingua or limb diskynesias, chorea, convulsive, nonconvulsive status epilepticus	NMDAR, AMPAR, GABA$_A$R (seizures predominate)	
Brainstem encephalitis	Alterations in awareness, cranial nerve abnormalities, ataxia	Ma2, Ma1, ANNA2, ANNA3, PCA2, CRMP5	Bickerstaff encephalitis, sarcoidosis, Lyme disease, listeriosis, TB, Whipple disease
Diencephalitis	Alterations in awareness, hypothalamic dysfunction	Ma2	Sarcoidosis, NMOSD, neoplastic
Basal ganglionitis	Chorea, dystonia, chorea	NMDAR, DR2, CRMP5	Sydenham chorea
Faciobrachial dystonic seizures	Paroxysmal posturing of the hemi-face and ipsilateral arm	LGI1	
Issacs/Morvans	Neuromyotonia/Neuromyotonia, sleep disturbances, muscle spasms, encephalopathy, dysautonomia	CASPR2	Inherited neuromyotonia
SPS	Truncal stiffness, hyperekplexia, painful spasms, paroxysmal autonomic dysfunction	GAD65, Aphiphysin, GlyαR	Idiopathic
PERM	Brainstem dysfunction, stiffness, hyperekplexia, myoclonus, encephalopathy, auronomic dysfunction, seizures	GlyαR, ANNA2, DPPX (with prominent gastrointestinal hyper-excitability)	
Cerebellar degeneration		PCA1, PCA2, GAD65, ANNA2, DNER, mGluR1, ZIC4	Prion disease, JC virus granule cell neuronopathy, alcoholic cerebellar degeneration, SCA, MSA-c, vitamin E deficiency
Opsoclonus-Myoclonus	Rapid, random eye movements in both vertical and horizontal directions (opsoclonus), myoclonus, dysarthria, ataxia, dysautonomia, and sleep disturbances.	NMDAR, ANNA2, GAD65	Seronegative paraneoplastic: neuroblastoma in children, lung and breast cancer adultsHIV, Whipple disease, idiopathic (presumed post-infectious)

AMPAR, alpha-amino-3-hydroxy-5-methyl-4-isoxazolepropionic acid receptor; ANNA1, antineuronal nuclear antibody type 1; ANNA2, antineuronal nuclear antibody type 2; ANNA3, antineuronal nuclear antibody type 3; Caspr2, contactin-associated protein-like 2; CRMP-5, collapsin response mediator protein 5; DNER, delta/notch-like epidermal growth factor-related protein receptor; DPPX, dipeptidyl-peptidase-like protein; DR2, dopamine 2 receptor; GABA$_A$R, gamma-aminobutyric acid-A receptor; GABA$_B$R, gamma-aminobutyric acid-B receptor; GAD65, glutamic acid decarboxylase 65; GlyαR, glycine-alpha receptor; HHV6, human herpes virus 6; HSVE; herpes-simplex virus encephalitis; LGI1, leucine rich glioma inactivated protein 1; MSA-c, multiple system atrophy-cerebellar type; mGluR1, metabotropic glutamate receptor 1; NMDAR, N-methyl-D-aspartate receptor; NMOSD, neuromyelitis optica spectrum disorder; SCA, spinal cerebellar ataxia; PCA1, Purkinje cell cytoplasmic antibody 1; PCA2, Purkinje cell cytoplasmic antibody-2; PERM, progressive encephalopathy with rigidity and myoclonus; SPS, stiff-person syndrome; TB, tuberculosis; ZIC4, zinc finger protein 4.

Supportive clinical features include

- Antiepileptic drug resistance
- Viral prodrome (but not persistent or periodic fevers which are suggestive of infectious encephalitis)
- Fluctuating course
- History of systemic autoimmunity
- History of smoking

- History of past or recent malignancy, particularly with a tumor known to be associated with AE

These patients should undergo evaluation for neural-specific antibodies. In addition to neural-antibody testing, patients should undergo a thorough evaluation for clinical and paraclinical markers supportive of a diagnosis of AE. Infectious, metabolic, neoplastic, and neurodegenerative causes of encephalopathy should be ruled out.

Supportive paraclinical biomarkers include

- Evidence of CNS inflammation on:
  - CSF (elevated protein [<100 mg/dL], pleocytosis [<100 cells/uL], oligoclonal bands, elevated synthesis rate or IgG index)
  - MRI brain scan demonstrating mesiotempotal, mesencephalic, or parenchymal fluid-attenuated inversion-recovery (FLAIR) T2-weighted hyperintensity. T1-gadolinium (GAD) enhancement can occur but is less common in AE
  - Fluorodeoxyglucose (FDG)-PET hypermetabolism or hypometabolism
  - Systemic markers of autoimmunity such as antinuclear antibody (ANA) or thyroid peroxidase (TPO) antibody positivity

MRI imaging is variable and partially dependent on the underlying antibody. Many patients with AE can have normal imaging. Normal CSF parameters, although uncommon, also do not rule out AE.

AUTOANTIBODIES SPECIFIC FOR PLASMA MEMBRANE ANTIGENS ASSOCIATED WITH AE

AE associated with antibodies targeting extracellular plasma membrane antigens (Table 41.2) tend to be immunotherapy responsive, as the antibodies themselves are likely pathogenic. Epidemiologic and clinical characteristics, as well as oncologic associations, vary among different antibodies and are discussed in the following section.

Voltage-Gated Potassium Channel Complex Antibodies

Both leucine-rich glioma inactivated-1 (LGI1) and contactin-associated protein-2 (CASPR2) are components of the macromolecular complex formed by voltage-gated channels (VGKCs) on the cell surface. Antibodies to LGI1 and CASPR2 comprise a majority of antibodies previously thought to target VGKCs themselves (11,12). Patients with these antibodies are predominately men, with a median age of 60 years. The incidence of cancer detection is less than 10% in cases of LGI1 encephalitis (13), but CASPR2 antibodies can be associated with thymoma in up to 40% of cases. Malignancy is more common in patients with dual LGI1/CASPR2 positivity (13).

Anti-LGI1 encephalitis is the second most common form of AE after anti-NMDA receptor encephalitis (14). Memory disturbances, seizures, hallucinations, myoclonus, and hyponatremia are common. Seizures tend to be focal and largely mesiotemporal in origin (15). A new type of seizure called faciobrachial dystonic seizures characterized by posturing of the hemi-face and ipsilateral arm can occur during or prior to the cognitive disturbances (16). Seizures respond well to immunotherapy but patients can be left with cognitive deficits in spite of adequate immunotherapy (13,17). CASPR-2 antibodies are associated with encephalitis, Morvan syndrome (sleep disturbances, dysautonomia, and peripheral nerve hyperexcitability), and acquired neuromyotonia (Isaacs syndrome) (9).

Up to 50% of patients with LGI1 and CASPR2 encephalitis have MRI evidence of inflammation manifested

TABLE 41.2 Antibodies Targeting Plasma Membrane Proteins Associated With AE

ANTIBODY	ONCOLOGICAL ASSOCIATION	FREQUENCY OF TUMOR	RESPONSE TO IMMUNOTHERAPY	NEUROLOGIC MANIFESTATIONS
NMDAR	Ovarian Teratomas, Testicular germinoma, neuroblastoma	Varies with age, gender, and ethnicity	Good	Psychiatric disturbances, orolingual/limb dyskinesias, catatonia, chorea, central hypoventilation and autonomic instability, opsoclonus-myoclonus
LGI1	Small-cell lung cancer, thymoma	<10%	Good	Limbic encephalitis, faciobrachial dystonic seizures, myoclonus (>60% hyponatremia)
Caspr2	Thymoma	~40%	Good	Encephalitis, Isaacs syndrome, Morvan syndrome
AMPAR	Thymic tumors, lung carcinoma, breast adenocarcinoma	70%	Good	Limbic encephalitis, psychosis
GABA$_A$R	Thymoma, small-cell lung cancer, rectal cancer	~40%	Good	Status epilepticus, epilepsia partialis continua, psychosis, behavioral disturbances, orolingual dyskinesias, chorea
mGluR5	Hodgkin lymphoma; can occur without tumor	>90%	Good	Limbic encephalitis, myoclonus

(continued)

TABLE 41.2 Antibodies Targeting Plasma Membrane Proteins Associated With AE *(continued)*

ANTIBODY	ONCOLOGICAL ASSOCIATION	FREQUENCY OF TUMOR	RESPONSE TO IMMUNOTHERAPY	NEUROLOGIC MANIFESTATIONS
DPPX	None described to date		Moderate	PERM, sleep disturbances, gastrointestinal hyperexcitability, ataxia
GlyαR	Thymoma, breast adenocarcinoma, B-cell lymphoma	Infrequent	Moderate	SPS, PERM, brainstem encephalitis, dysautonomia, seizure, cerebellar degeneration
VGCC (N, P/Q)	Small-cell carcinoma in LEMS	~50%	Variable	N and P/Q:LEMS P/Q: cerebellar degeneration seizures N: encephalitis, seizures
gAChR	Thymoma, adenocarcinoma, small-cell carcinoma	~10%	Variable	Autonomic dysfunction, peripheral neuropathy, encephalopathy, seizures
IgLON5	None described to date		Poor; recent data suggest higher rate of response	Obstructive sleep apnea, nocturnal stridor, abnormal motor behaviors of sleep, ocular motility abnormalities, chorea

AE, autoimmune encephalitis; AMPAR, alpha-amino-3-hydroxy-5-methyl-4-isoxazolepropionic acid receptor; Caspr2, contactin-associated protein-like 2; DPPX, dipeptidyl-peptidase-like protein-6; LEMS, Lamert-Eaton myasthenic syndrome; LGI1, leucine rich glioma inactivated protein 1; GABA$_A$R, gamma-aminobutyric acid-A receptor; GABA$_B$R, gamma-aminobutyric acid-B receptor; gAChR, ganglionic acetylcholine receptor; GlyαR, glycine-alpha receptor; mGluR5, metabotropic glutamate receptor 5; NMDAR, N-methyl-D-aspartate receptor; PERM, progressive encephalomyelitis with rigidity and myoclonus; SPS, stiff-person syndrome; VGCC, voltage-gated calcium channel.

Source: Modified with permission from Table 2 in Toledano M, Pittock SJ. Autoimmune epilepsy. *Semin Neurol.* 2015;35(3):248.

as enlargement and T2 FLAIR hyperintensity of the mesial temporal lobe structures in the acute phase (18). Enhancement and restricted diffusion can occur but are less common. Basal ganglia nonenhancing T1 hyperintensity is sometimes associated with faciobrachial dystonic seizures in anti-LGI1 encephalitis (Figure 41.2) (19). Serial MRI frequently demonstrate mesial temporal sclerosis, even in patients who have been treated successfully (Figure 41.2) (18). Mesiotemporal sclerosis may account in part for the persistence of cognitive deficits in successfully treated patients, as well as the need for long-term therapy with antiepileptic drugs in these patients (13,17).

Ionotropic Glutamate Receptor Antibodies

Anti-NMDAR encephalitis was first described in young women with ovarian teratomas (20), but it can affect males, infants, and older patients as well (21). About one-third of women over 18 with this disorder have an ovarian teratoma but the likelihood of finding a tumor varies according to sex, age, and ethnicity. Ovarian teratomas are more frequent in African Americans and Asians and approximately 5% of men have testicular germ-cell tumors (21). Anti-NMDAR encephalitis can also occur as a postinfectious complication in patients with successfully treated herpes simplex virus (HSV) encephalitis (5). This phenomenon has also been described with encephalitis caused by other herpes viruses (22,23). Possible mechanisms include molecular mimicry or an immune response to neuronal damage.

Anti-NMDAR encephalitis classically presents with a viral prodrome followed by onset of psychiatric disturbances, orolingual/limb dyskinesias, and other abnormal movements. If untreated, dysautonomia, central hypoventilation, and coma can ensue (21). Children are more likely to present with abnormal movement disorders early in the course of the disease, and psychosis is less common compared with adults (21).

Seizures, including subclinical seizures, can occur early in the disorder. In a recent case series of 23 patients with anti-NMDAR encephalitis who underwent continuous EEG, 60% had electrographic seizures without clinical correlate. Up to 30% of patients in this series had a unique electrographic pattern that the investigators termed "extreme delta brush" because of similarities to waveforms seen in premature infants (24). Although the specificity of this finding is not yet established, its presence should raise suspicion for this disorder. Less than a third of patients have abnormalities on MRI brain, usually T2 FLAIR hyperintensity in cortical or subcortical regions, or in the cerebellum or brainstem (21).

Patients with antibodies to the alpha-amino-3-hydroxy-5-methyl-4-isoxazoleproponic acid receptor (AMPAR) have been associated with limbic encephalitis (25). Females appear to be more susceptible than men, with a median age of 60. In the initial case series only four of 10 had seizures and eight had MRI findings of mesiotemporal inflammation. Seventy percent had an associated malignancy (small-cell and non–small-cell lung cancer, thymoma, and breast cancer) (25). Relapses were common, occurring in about half of the patients.

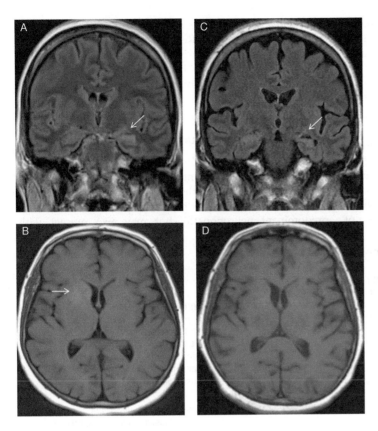

FIGURE 41.2 A 58-year-old woman with leucine-rich glioma inactivated-1 encephalitis presenting with faciobrachial dystonic seizures and encephalopathy. Imaging at presentation demonstrates increased T2 FLAIR signal (A) in the bilateral (left > right) hippocampi (arrowheads), as well as T1 hyperintensity (B) in the right basal ganglia (arrowhead). Follow-up coronal FLAIR (C) 6 months after treatment shows reduction in signal abnormality but development of left mesial temporal sclerosis (arrowheads). Following treatment, T1 hyperinstensity in the basal ganglia has resolved (D).

FLAIR, fluid-attenuated inversion-recovery.

Gamma-amino butyric acid B receptor (GABA$_B$R) antibodies have been recently recognized as a cause of epilepsy associated with limbic encephalitis. In the initial case series, men and women were equally affected and all patients had seizures (26). MRI imaging in most revealed evidence of mesiotemporal inflammation (26). Approximately 60% of them had an associated malignancy, most often small-cell lung cancer.

High titers of GABA$_A$R antibodies have been identified in patients presenting with seizures (frequently accompanied by status epilepticus), cognitive impairment, and movement abnormalities (more common in children) (23). MRI showed unilateral or bilateral multifocal T2 hyperintensities involving both gray and white matter (23). About 40% of patients had an associated neoplasm, mostly thymoma.

Autoantibodies to the metabotropic glutamate receptor 5 (mGluR5) were identified in the CSF of one woman and two men with Hodgkin lymphoma and limbic encephalitis (Ophelia syndrome) (27,28). Recently, a nonparaneoplastic case has been reported (29). Patients with anti-mGluR5 encephalitis display a relatively mild form of encephalitis without the dramatic psychosis, agitation, seizures, and autonomic instability seen with anti-NMDAR encephalitis.

Other Antibodies

Anti-glycine receptor (GlyR) antibodies should be considered in patients presenting with PERM (30), and stiff-person syndrome (SPS) (31). CNS hyper-excitability with

increased muscle tone, a pathologically exaggerated startle response, and spasms is the defining characteristic of these syndromes. Limbic encephalitis, seizures, cerebellar ataxia, and optic neuritis have also been described in association with this antibody. Most patients do not have associated malignancy.

Anti-dipeptidyl-peptidase-like protein-6 (DPPX6) antibodies are associated with a broad clinical spectrum including encephalopathy, central hyperexcitability, myelopathy, dysautonomia, and seizures (32,33). Gastrointestinal symptoms characterized by severe diarrhea and/or constipation are common.

Both neuronal ganglionic nicotinic acetylcholine receptor (gAChR) and voltage-gated calcium channel N-type and P/Q-type (VGCC N/VGCC P/Q) antibodies have been described in patients with suspected AE in a non-paraneoplastic context (15). The pathogenic role of these antibodies in AE is uncertain, and may be secondary to coexisting autoantibodies such as anti-GABA$_B$R, which are known to co-occur with VGCC antibodies (26).

Antibodies targeting IgLON5, an immunoglobulin-like cell adhesion molecule, have been associated with a progressive CNS disorder of insidious onset characterized by bulbar symptoms, sleep disturbances, central hyperexcitability, and movement abnormalities (34). Neuropathologic features include a lack of inflammatory infiltrates and neuronal accumulation of hyperphosphorylated tau protein (both 3-repeat and 4-repeat), leading some to question whether antibodies to IgLON5 are a marker of autoimmunity or epiphenomena of a primarily neurodegenerative process. In a recent case series, seven out of nine treated patients responded to immunotherapy supporting an autoimmune basis for this disorder (34).

ANTIBODIES TO INTRACELLULAR ANTIGENS ASSOCIATED WITH AE

Antigenic targets of autoantibodies targeting intracellular proteins include nuclear and cytoplasmic enzymes, RNA-binding proteins, transcription factors, as well as synaptic proteins (Table 41.3). With the exception of antibodies targeting GAD65 these antibodies have a strong association with malignancy. The antibodies themselves are not

pathogenic and symptoms result from cytotoxic T-cell mediated damage (7). Response to immunotherapy is poor, although response is more variable in AE associated with antibodies to intracellular synaptic antibodies, the reasons for which are discussed in the following section.

Autoantibodies to Neuronal Nuclear and Cytoplasmic Antigens

Antineuronal nuclear antibody type-1 (ANNA1, also known as anti-Hu) was the first type of onconeural antibody described (35). Most patients present with a sensory-predominant neuronopathy but may also present with

TABLE 41.3   Neuronal Nuclear and Cytoplasmic Antibodies Accompanying AE

ANTIBODY	ONCOLOGICAL ASSOCIATION	FREQUENCY OF TUMOR (%)	RESPONSE TO IMMUNOTHERAPY	NEUROLOGIC MANIFESTATIONS
ANNA1 (anti-Hu)	Small-cell carcinoma, rarely thymoma, prostate cancer Children: neuroblastoma	>80	Poor	Limbic, cortical encephalitis. Neuropathies (sensory, mixed sensorimotor, autonomic), status epilepticus, cerebellar degeneration, opsoclonus-myoclonus
ANNA2 (anti-Ri)	Small-cell carcinoma, breast adenocarcinoma, bladder cancer	>60	Poor	Brainstem encephalitis (opsoclonus-myoclonus, laryngospasm, trismus, cranial neuropathy), cerebellar degeneration
ANNA3	Small-cell carcinoma	>60	Poor	Limbic and brainstem encephalitis, sensory and sensorimotor neuropathies, myelopathy
AGNA (SOX-1)	Small-cell carcinoma	>90	Poor	LEMS most common but also limbic encephalitis
Amphiphysin	Small-cell carcinoma, breast adenocarcinoma	>85	Poor	Limbic encephalitis, SPS, cerebellar degeneration, opsoclonus-myoclonus, myelopathy
CRMP5	Small-cell carcinoma, thymoma	>75	Poor	Encephalitis, optic neuritis and retinitis, myelopathy, neuropathy, LEMS, basal ganglionitis
GAD65	Thymoma; neuroendocrine tumors, breast, or colon adenocarcinoma	<10	Moderate	Limbic encephalitis, brainstem encephalitis, seizures, opsoclonus myoclonus SPS, cerebellar degeneration
Ma2 (anti-Ta); Ma1	Ma2 testicular or extragonadal germ cell; Ma1 and Ma2 breast, lung (small-cell and non–small cell), colon, parotid	>90	Moderate	Ma2 Limbic encephalitis, diencephalitis, brainstem encephalitis; Ma1 and Ma2 brainstem encephalitis, cerebellar degeneration
PCA2	Small-cell carcinoma	>90	Poor	Brainstem or limbic encephalitis, cerebellar degeneration

AE, autoimmune encephalitis; ANNA1, antineuronal nuclear antibody type 1; ANNA2, antineuronal nuclear antibody type 2; ANNA3, antineuronal nuclear antibody type , AGNA, antiglial nuclear antibody; CRMP5, collapsin response mediator protein 5; GAD65, glutamic acid decarboxylase 65; LEMS, Lambert–Eaton myaesthenic syndrome; PCA2, Purkinje cell cytoplasmic antibody 2; SPS, stiff-person syndrome.

Source: Modified with permission from Table 1 in Toledano M, Pittock SJ. Autoimmune epilepsy. *Semin Neurol.* 2015;35(3):247.

limbic encephalitis, encephalomyelitis, and gastrointenstinal dysmotility. Seizures may occur in the absence of other syndromic manifestations of limbic encephalitis (36). The vast majority of cases is associated with small-cell carcinoma but can also occur with thymoma and neuroblastoma (in children).

Antineuronal nuclear antibody type-2 (ANNA2, also known as anti-Ri) has been associated with a broad spectrum of presentations, including cerebellar degeneration, brainstem encephalitis, and encephalomyelitis (37). Most patients have associated small-cell lung carcinoma or breast adenocarcinoma. Antineuronal nuclear antibody type-3 (ANNA3) can rarely present with encephalitis and is strongly associated with small-cell lung cancer (38).

Anti-glial neuronal antibody (AGNA, also known as SOX-1) is associated with Lambert–Eaton myasthenic syndrome but can present with limbic encephalitis (39). Purkinje cell cytoplasmic antibody type-2 (PCA2) usually presents with cerebellar degeneration but can also present with brainstem or limbic encephalitis (40). Both of these antibodies are strongly associated with small-cell lung cancer.

Anti-collapsin response mediator protein-5 (CRMP5) antibodies are associated with a wide spectrum of neurologic presentations, including cerebellar degeneration, chorea (basal ganglionitis), optic neuropathy, retinopathy, myelopathy, radiculoneuropathy, encephalitis, and seizures (7). The most common associated neoplasms are small-cell lung carcinoma and thymoma (41).

Dual Ma-1/M-2 positivity (anti-Ma) is more common in females and associated with ovarian, breast, and colon cancer (42). Anti-Ma-2 (anti-Ta) is associated with testicular germ-line cancers in males (43). Patients with these antibodies usually present with brainstem encephalitis, diencephalic encephalitis, and/or limbic encephalitis (Figure 41.3). Presence of the antibody strongly suggests underlying malignancy and neoplastic workup (including biopsy) should be pursued even in cases when imaging is equivocal.

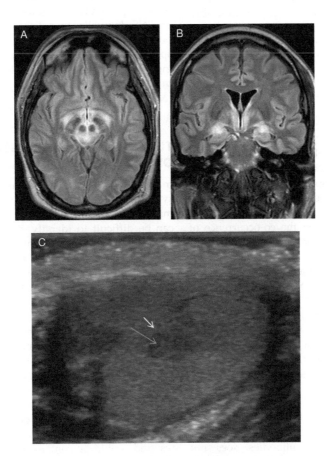

FIGURE 41.3 A 46-year-old man with anti-Ma2 antibodies presenting with encephalopathy and multiple cranial neuropathies. Brain imaging shows increased T2 fluid-attenuated inversion-recovery signal involving the diencephalon, mesencephalon, and limbic system (A and B). Ultasonography of his scrotum (C), demonstrated several hypoechoic regions in his left testicle (arrowhead) interpreted as representing prior ischemia or orchitis. Histopathology from left orchiectomy was consistent with seminoma, classic type (not shown).

Autoantibodies to Intracellular Synaptic Proteins

GAD65 is a synaptic vesicle-associated enzyme necessary to synthetize GABA. Antibodies to GAD65 are associated with diabetes mellitus type 1 but can also be detected in patients with autoimmune neurologic disease, although usually at an order of magnitude higher than in those with type 1 diabetes. Neurologically, GAD65 antibodies are associated with SPS, cerebellar ataxia, encephalomyelitis, extrapyramidal disorders, and seizures (4,44).

When occurring on its own, anti-GAD65 autoimmunity is rarely paraneoplastic; however, it frequently presents in association with other onconeural antibodies such as anti-GABA$_A$R and anti GABA$_B$R (45). Coexisting anti-GlyR antibodies in patients presenting with SPS has also been described (31).

Because GAD65 is an intracellular antigen, GAD65 autoantibodies are unlikely to be pathogenic. Nonetheless, 30% to 50% of these patients respond favorably to immunosuppression (15,46) even when it is the only autoantibody found. A possible explanation for this could be the coexistence of pathogenic autoantibodies targeting as of yet unrecognized plasma membrane antigens as described earlier.

Anti-amphyphisin antibodies are associated with limbic encephalitis and SPS. The most common associated malignancies are breast and small-cell lung carcinoma (47).

ANTIBODY TESTING IN AE

Most laboratories offer either targeted testing for single antigens (e.g., NMDAR) or a panel of autoantibodies packaged according to the clinical presentation (3). Unless a high degree of suspicion exists for a specific antibody, targeted antibody testing should be avoided, as there can be significant overlap between the signs and symptoms associated with each autoantibody. Also, given the co-occurrence of paraneoplastic and nonparaneoplastic autoantibodies, additional markers of occult malignancy may be missed with selective testing (3,41,48). It is important to note that panels vary between laboratories and that panels may be incomplete. Antibodies to Ma-1 and Ma-2, for example, are not included in many of the commercially available paraneoplastic panels. Clinicians need to be aware which antibodies are included in the panel they request and obtain additional antibodies if suspected on clinical grounds.

Although testing for antibodies in CSF is more sensitive in some cases, such as in anti-NMDAR encephalitis (49), sensitivity is not known for all autoantibodies and both serum and CSF should be sent for analysis in order to maximize detection.

The presence of neural autoantibodies does not always suffice to establish the diagnosis of AE. Several studies have confirmed the presence of anti-VGKC antibodies (usually low titers and without LGI1 or CASPR2 positivity) in patients without definitive associated symptoms (50). GAD65 antibodies can be found in around 10% of adults with long-standing epilepsy (4). The pathogenic role of the antibodies in these cases remains unclear. Conversely, failure to detect an autoantibody in patients presenting with a clinical picture highly suggestive of AE does not rule out the diagnosis. Response to an immunotherapy trial in these cases can support the diagnosis of AE (15). Such positive responses need to be interpreted with caution, however, as patients may report subjective improvement while on immunosuppression, particularly those trialed on corticosteroids.

OVERLAP WITH DEMYELINATING DISEASE

An overlap between patients with CNS demyelinating disease and anti-NMDAR encephalitis has been reported (51). In half of these patients, the disorders were concurrent whereas in the other half the demyelinating disease occurred either before or after the encephalitis. Most were positive for aquaporin-4 (AQP-4) or myelin oligodendrocyte glycoprotein (MOG) antibodies. This phenomenon likely represents co-occurrence of two disorders rather than atypical presentations of anti-NMDAR encephalitis or CNS demyelinating disease. By contrast, CRMP5 antibodies have been associated with paraneoplastic opticospinal disease that can mimic demyelinating syndromes, including progressive multiple sclerosis, acute transverse myelitis, and neuromyelitis optica spectrum disorder (NMOSD) (52).

TUMOR SCREENING BASED ON THE RESULTS OF ANTIBODY TESTING

In up to 70% of cases of paraneoplastic AE, neurologic symptoms present prior to the discovery of an underlying malignancy (53). Neoplasms associated with autoimmunity can be difficult to identify on conventional imaging, possibly due to immune-mediated inhibition of tumor growth (54). Subtle imaging abnormalities should be investigated further and there should be a low threshold for pursuing biopsies. Workup should be guided by the patient's risk factors and the antibody found. Paraneoplastic antibodies are more strongly predictive of tumor type than they are of specific neurologic syndromes (48). The discovery of a neoplasm atypical for the paraneoplastic antibody should alert clinicians to the possibility of a second more typical occult malignancy (48). If no malignancy is found, it is prudent to do periodic surveillance once or twice yearly for the next few years.

CT of the chest, abdomen, and pelvis can be used as a screening tool, but FDG-PET-CT is a more sensitive test and should be contained if the former is negative (55). FDG-PET-CT is not the test of choice in a young female with NMDAR encephalitis or in other patients suspected of having a germ-cell tumor such as those with anti-Ma/Ta antibodies. Ultrasonography or MRI is the preferred modality in these cases.

TREATMENT

Prompt initiation of immunotherapy improves outcome (15). Although randomized control data are lacking, therapeutic approaches have been extrapolated from treatments that have been successfully applied previously in a variety of systemic or neurologic autoimmune conditions. At our institution, we use a protocol divided into acute and chronic therapeutic phases (Figure 41.4).

Acute Therapy

Treatment for suspected AE is often initiated empirically before antibody status is known. Acute first-line therapies include high-dose intravenous methylprednisolone (IVMP), intravenous immunoglobulin (IVIG), and plasma exchange (PLEX) (Table 41.4). At our institution, we tend to reserve IVIG for children (due to its perceived favorable side effect profile in the pediatric population compared with corticosteroids), or for patients who are unable to tolerate corticosteroids. PLEX can be used in patients who have failed IVMP or when IVMP or IVIG are poorly tolerated. If CNS infection remains a concern before the diagnosis of AE has been fully established, IVIG and PLEX are unlikely to significantly worsen infectious encephalitis and can be given concurrently with antimicrobials. For patients who fail to respond to first-line therapies, second-line therapies include Rituximab or cyclophosphamide (Table 41.4).

The intensity and duration of the acute phase of treatment varies depending on presentation and severity

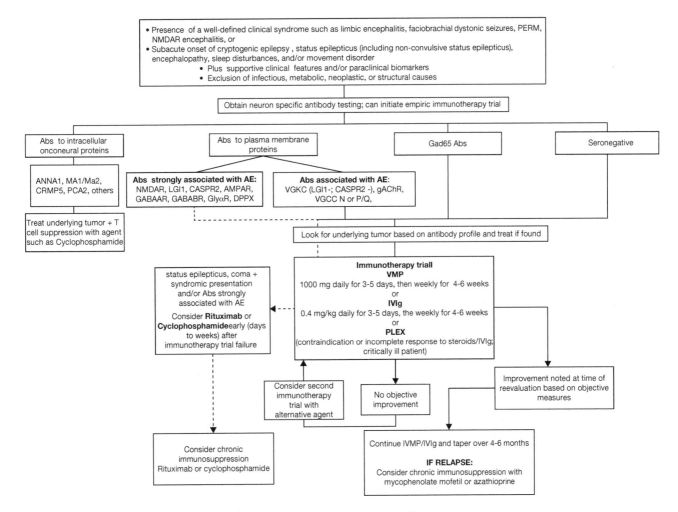

FIGURE 41.4 Diagnostic and therapeutic approach to autoimmune encephalitis.

AGNA, antiglial nuclear antibody; AMPAR, alpha-amino-3-hydroxy-5-methyl-4-isoxazolepropionic acid receptor; ANNA1, antineuronal nuclear antibody type 1; Caspr2, contactin-associated protein-like 2; CRMP5, collapsin response mediator protein 5; DPPX6, dipeptidyl-peptidase-like protein-6; GABA$_A$R, gamma-aminobutyric acid-A receptor; GABA$_B$R, gamma-aminobutyric acid-B receptor; gAChR, ganglionic acetylcholine receptor; GAD65, glutamic acid decarboxylase 65; GlyαR, glycine-alpha receptor; IVMP, intravenous methylprednisolone; IVIG, intravenous immunoglobulin; LGI1, leucine-rich glioma inactivated protein 1; NMDAR, N-methyl-D-aspartate receptor; PCA2, Purkinje cell cytoplasmic antibody 2; VGCC, voltage-gated calcium channel.

Source: Modified from Figure 3 in Toledano M, Pittock SJ. Autoimmune epilepsy. *Semin Neurol*. 2015;35(3):253.

TABLE 41.4 Therapeutic Options in Patients With Autoimmune Epilepsy

DRUG	DOSE	ROUTE	FREQUENCY	SOME COMMON AND SEVERE SIDE EFFECTS ENCOUNTERED	THERAPEUTIC PHASE
Methylprednisolone	1,000 mg	IV	Daily for 3–5 d, Then weekly for 4–8 wk, then gradually extend interval between infusions	Insomnia, increased appetite, psychiatric disturbance, Cushing syndrome, diabetes, cataracts, osteoporosis, hip avascular necrosis, skin thinning Addisonian crisis on rapid withdrawal of physiologic doses of corticosteroid	Acute and chronic, then taper
Immunoglobulin	0.4 g/kg	IV	Daily for 3 d, then alternate weeks for 6–8 wk, then gradually extend interval between infusions	Aseptic meningitis, deep venous thrombosis, headache, anaphylaxis, renal failure	Acute and chronic, then taper
Azathioprine	1–2 mg/kg/d	PO	Two daily divided doses aiming for a rise in mean corpuscular volume ≥5 femtoliters	Myelotoxicity, liver toxicity, hypersensitivity reaction, rash	Chronic
Mycophenolate mofetil	500–2,000 mg/d	PO	Two daily divided doses	Myelotoxicity, CNS lymphoma, diarrhea, hypertension, renal failure	Chronic
Rituximab	1,000 mg once, then again 2 wk later, or 375 mg/m^2 weekly for 4 wk	IV	Every 6 mo	Infusion reactions, edema, hypertension, fever, fatigue, chills, headache, insomnia, rash, pruritus, nausea, diarrhea, weight gain, cytopenias, neutropenic fever, liver toxicity, hepatitis B reactivation	Acute (second line) and chronic

(continued)

TABLE 41.4   Therapeutic Options in Patients With Autoimmune Epilepsy (*continued*)

DRUG	DOSE	ROUTE	FREQUENCY	SOME COMMON AND SEVERE SIDE EFFECTS ENCOUNTERED	THERAPEUTIC PHASE
Cyclophosphamide	(IV)500–1,000 mg/m²/mo(PO) 1–2 mg/kg/d	IV or PO	Monthly (IV) Daily (PO)	Chronic infertility, alopecia mucositis, hemorrhagic cystitis, myelotoxicity.	Acute (second line) and chronic

CNS, central nervous system; IV, intravenous; PO, by mouth.

Source: Modified with permission from Table 5 in Linnoila J, Pittock SJ. Autoantibody-associated central nervous system neurologic disorders. *Semin Neurol*. 2016;36(4):392.

of illness. A comatose patient with NMDAR antibody positivity or a patient with treatment refractory LGI1 limbic encephalitis may require more rapid escalation of treatment to second-line therapies such as Rituximab. In the outpatient setting, patients are typically treated with 5 days of IVMP 1,000 mg/d or IVIG 0.4 g/kg/d followed by weekly IVMP 1,000 mg or once weekly IVIG 0.4 g/kg for a total of 6 weeks. It is important to obtain objective measures of disability and treatment response (e.g., MRI, EEG, CSF, cognitive testing) (Table 41.5). Clinical response is a better indicator of treatment response than antibody titers.

Patients with antibodies to intracellular onconeural antigens can have treatment refractory AE. Underlying malignancy should be treated. A trial of immunotherapy as described earlier can be considered, although these patients may respond preferentially to agents targeting T-cell cytotoxic mechanisms such as cyclophosphamide. In practice, however, less than 10% of these cases experience substantial recovery (4).

Long-Term Therapy

Once objective and maximal improvement is achieved, long-term management should be addressed. The duration of long-term immunotherapy is based on the clinical syndrome and antibody profile. AE may be monophasic in nature, such as in the case of most NMDAR encephalitis

where the risk of relapse is approximately 12% over 2 years. Risk is highest in untreated patients and lowest in patients treated with second-line therapies during the acute phase (21). Relapses are more common in LGI1 encephalitis approximating 30% but care must be taken to distinguish true relapses from residual cognitive deficits (13,56). The risk of relapses in other forms of AE is less clearly established. Medium- to long-term treatment with corticosteroids or IVIG is usually required even in cases of monophasic illness. In our practice, we gradually extend the interval between infusions of either IVMP or IVIG over a period of 3 to 6 months from weekly, to fortnightly, and then monthly infusions. If using an oral corticosteroid instead, a slow taper over a period of months is advisable. Patients who relapse may require long-term treatment with an oral steroid sparing agent such as azathioprine or mycophenolate (Table 41.4). It is important to overlap corticosteroid or IVIG treatment with the steroid sparing agent as these drugs take time to take effect (~12 weeks for azathioprine and 8 weeks for mycophenolate mofetil). A minority of patients remain dependent on corticosteroid or IVIG despite initiation of long-term immunosuppression. Rituximab and cyclophosphamide can be considered as long-term therapies in patients who received these agents during the acute phase or in treatment-refractory cases. There are little data to guide duration of long-term immunosuppression in AE. In our practice we generally start a trial of immunosuppression after 2 years.

TABLE 41.5   Objective Tests to Monitor Treatment Response

SYMPTOMS /FINDINGS	OBJECTIVE TESTS TO FOLLOW
Seizures	EEG (sleep deprived, EMU, prolonged ambulatory), seizure diary.
CNS inflammation	Brain MRI, Brain FDG-PET, CSF
Autonomic dysfunction	Autonomic reflex testing, Thermoregulatory sweat test[a], GI transit study, gastric emptying study
Cognitive decline	ACE-III, MMSE, MoCA, other neuropsychometric studies
Movement disorder	Movement laboratory studies[a], video

[a]Specialized studies not available everywhere.

ACE-III, Addenbrooke's Cognitive Examination III; CSF, cerebrospinal fluid; EEG, electroencephalogram; EMU, epilepsy monitoring unit; FDG-PET, fluorodeoxyglucose-PET; GI, gastrointestinal; MMSE, Mini Mental Status Examination; MoCA, Montreal test of Cognitive Assessment.

Source: Modified with permission from Table 4 in Linnoila J, Pittock SJ. Autoantibody-associated central nervous system neurologic disorders. *Semin Neurol*. 2016;36(4):390.

KEY POINTS FOR PATIENTS AND FAMILIES

- Autoimmune encephalitis usually presents with subacute onset of confusion, hallucinations, seizures, sleep disturbances, and movement abnormalities.
- Brain imaging and CSF usually show signs of inflammation but can be negative.
- Detection of a neural autoantibody can be diagnostic.
- Neural autoantibodies should be tested for both in serum and in CSF.
- Some antibodies can be associated with an underlying malignancy. Imaging studies sometimes followed by biopsy may be needed to rule this possibility out.
- Prompt initiation of immunotherapy improves outcomes.

REFERENCES

1. Venkatesan A. Epidemiology and outcomes of acute encephalitis. *Curr Opin Neurol.* 2015;28(3):277–282.
2. Gable MS, Sheriff H, Dalmau J, et al. The frequency of autoimmune N-methyl-D-aspartate receptor encephalitis surpasses that of individual viral etiologies in young individuals enrolled in the California Encephalitis Project. *Clin Infect Dis.* 2012;54(7):899–904.
3. Tobin WO, Pittock SJ. Autoimmune neurology of the central nervous system. *Continuum (Minneap Minn).* 2017;23(3, Neurology of Systemic Disease):627–653.
4. Toledano M, Pittock SJ. Autoimmune epilepsy. *Semin Neurol.* 2015;35(3):245–258.
5. Galli J, Clardy SL, Piquet AL. NMDAR encephalitis following herpes simplex virus encephalitis. *Curr Infect Dis Rep.* 2017;19(1):1.
6. Wilkinson PC, Zeromski J. Immunofluorescent detection of antibodies against neurones in sensory carcinomatous neuropathy. *Brain.* 1965;88(3):529–583.
7. Dalmau J, Gultekin HS, Posner JB. Paraneoplastic neurologic syndromes: pathogenesis and physiopathology. *Brain Pathol.* 1999;9(2):275–284.
8. Gultekin SH, Rosenfeld MR, Voltz R, et al. Paraneoplastic limbic encephalitis: neurological symptoms, immunological findings and tumour association in 50 patients. *Brain.* 2000;123(pt 7):1481–1494.
9. Linnoila J, Pittock SJ. Autoantibody-associated central nervous system neurologic disorders. *Semin Neurol.* 2016;36(4):382–396.
10. Graus F, Titulaer MJ, Balu R, et al. A clinical approach to diagnosis of autoimmune encephalitis. *Lancet Neurol.* 15(4):391–404.
11. Irani SR, Alexander S, Waters P, et al. Antibodies to Kv1 potassium channel-complex proteins leucine-rich, glioma inactivated 1 protein and contactin-associated protein-2 in limbic encephalitis, Morvan's syndrome and acquired neuromyotonia. *Brain.* 2010;133(9):2734–2748.
12. Lai M, Huijbers MG, Lancaster E, et al. Investigation of LGI1 as the antigen in limbic encephalitis previously attributed to potassium channels: a case series. *Lancet Neurol.* 2010;9(8):776–785.
13. Gadoth A, Pittock SJ, Dubey D, et al. Expanded phenotypes and outcomes among 256 LGI1/CASPR2-IgG-positive patients. *Ann Neurol.* 2017;82(1):79–92.
14. Linnoila JJ, Rosenfeld MR, Dalmau J. Neuronal surface antibody-mediated autoimmune encephalitis. *Semin Neurol.* 2014;34(4):458–466.
15. Toledano M, Britton JW, McKeon A, et al. Utility of an immunotherapy trial in evaluating patients with presumed autoimmune epilepsy. *Neurology.* 2014;82(18):1578–1586.
16. Irani SR, Stagg CJ, Schott JM, et al. Faciobrachial dystonic seizures: the influence of immunotherapy on seizure control and prevention of cognitive impairment in a broadening phenotype. *Brain.* 2013;136(pt 10):3151–3162.
17. Finke C, Prüss H, Heine J, et al. Evaluation of cognitive deficits and structural hippocampal damage in encephalitis with leucine-rich, glioma-inactivated 1 antibodies. *JAMA Neurol.* 2017;74(1):50–59.
18. Kotsenas AL, Watson RE, Pittock SJ, et al. MRI findings in autoimmune voltage-gated potassium channel complex encephalitis with seizures: one potential etiology for mesial temporal sclerosis. *AJNR Am J Neuroradiol.* 2014;35(1):84–89.
19. Flanagan EP, Kotsenas AL, Britton JW, et al. Basal ganglia T1 hyperintensity in LGI1-autoantibody faciobrachial dystonic seizures. *Neurol Neuroimmunol Neuroinflamm.* 2015;2(6):e161.
20. Vitaliani R, Mason W, Ances B, et al. Paraneoplastic encephalitis, psychiatric symptoms, and hypoventilation in ovarian teratoma. *Ann Neurol.* 2005;58(4):594–604.
21. Titulaer MJ, McCracken L, Gabilondo I, et al. Treatment and prognostic factors for long-term outcome in patients with anti-NMDA receptor encephalitis: an observational cohort study. *Lancet Neurol.* 2013;12(2):157–165.
22. Schabitz WR, Rogalewski A, Hagemeister C, et al. VZV brainstem encephalitis triggers NMDA receptor immunoreaction. *Neurology.* 2014;83(24):2309–2311.
23. Spatola M, Petit-Pedrol M, Simabukuro MM, et al. Investigations in GABAA receptor antibody-associated encephalitis. *Neurology.* 2017;88(11):1012–1020.
24. Schmitt SE, Pargeon K, Frechette ES, et al. Extreme delta brush: a unique EEG pattern in adults with anti-NMDA receptor encephalitis. *Neurology.* 2012;79(11):1094–1100.
25. Lai M, Hughes EG, Peng X, et al. AMPA receptor antibodies in limbic encephalitis alter synaptic receptor location. *Ann Neurol.* 2009;65(4):424–434.
26. Lancaster E, Lai M, Peng X, et al. Antibodies to the GABA(B) receptor in limbic encephalitis with seizures: case series and characterisation of the antigen. *Lancet Neurol.* 2010;9(1):67–76.
27. Lancaster E, Martinez-Hernandez E, Titulaer MJ, et al. Antibodies to metabotropic glutamate receptor 5 in the Ophelia syndrome. *Neurology.* 2011;77(18):1698–1701.
28. Mat A, Adler H, Merwick A, et al. Ophelia syndrome with metabotropic glutamate receptor 5 antibodies in CSF. *Neurology.* 2013;80(14):1349–1350.
29. Pruss H, Rothkirch M, Kopp U, et al. Limbic encephalitis with mGluR5 antibodies and immunotherapy-responsive prosopagnosia. *Neurology.* 2014;83(15):1384–1386.
30. Hutchinson M, Waters P, McHugh J, et al. Progressive encephalomyelitis, rigidity, and myoclonus: a novel glycine receptor antibody. *Neurology.* 2008;71(16):1291–1292.
31. McKeon A, Martinez-Hernandez E, Lancaster E, et al. Glycine receptor autoimmune spectrum with stiff-man syndrome phenotype. *JAMA Neurol.* 2013;70(1):44–50.
32. Boronat A, Gelfand JM, Gresa-Arribas N, et al. Encephalitis and antibodies to dipeptidyl-peptidase-like protein-6, a subunit of Kv4.2 potassium channels. *Ann Neurol.* 2013;73(1):120–128.
33. Tobin WO, Lennon VA, Komorowski L, et al. DPPX potassium channel antibody: frequency, clinical accompaniments, and outcomes in 20 patients. *Neurology.* 2014;83(20):1797–1803.

34. Honorat JA, Komorowski L, Josephs KA, et al. IgLON5 antibody: neurological accompaniments and outcomes in 20 patients. *Neurol Neuroimmunol Neuroinflamm.* 2017;4(5):e385.

35. Lucchinetti CF, Kimmel DW, Lennon VA. Paraneoplastic and oncologic profiles of patients seropositive for type 1 antineuronal nuclear autoantibodies. *Neurology.* 1998;50(3):652–657.

36. Rudzinski LA, Pittock SJ, McKeon A, et al. Extratemporal EEG and MRI findings in ANNA-1 (anti-Hu) encephalitis. *Epilepsy Res.* 2011;95(3):255–262.

37. Brieva-Ruiz L, Diaz-Hurtado M, Matias-Guiu X, et al. Anti-Ri-associated paraneoplastic cerebellar degeneration and breast cancer: an autopsy case study. *Clin Neurol Neurosurg.* 2008;110(10):1044–1046.

38. Chan KH, Vernino S, Lennon VA. ANNA-3 anti-neuronal nuclear antibody: marker of lung cancer-related autoimmunity. *Ann Neurol.* 2001;50(3):301–311.

39. Stich O, Klages E, Bischler P, et al. SOX1 antibodies in sera from patients with paraneoplastic neurological syndromes. *Acta Neurol Scand.* 2012;125(5):326–331.

40. Vernino S, Lennon VA. New Purkinje cell antibody (PCA-2): marker of lung cancer-related neurological autoimmunity. *Ann Neurol.* 2000;47(3):297–305.

41. Horta ES, Lennon VA, Lachance DH, et al. Neural autoantibody clusters aid diagnosis of cancer. *Clin Cancer Res.* 2014;20(14):3862–3869.

42. Dalmau J, Gultekin SH, Voltz R, et al. Ma1, a novel neuron- and testis-specific protein, is recognized by the serum of patients with paraneoplastic neurological disorders. *Brain.* 1999;122(pt 1):27–39.

43. Ortega Suero G, Sola-Valls N, Escudero D, et al. Anti-Ma and anti-Ma2-associated paraneoplastic neurological syndromes. *Neurologia.* 2016;33(1):18–27.

44. Solimena M, Folli F, Denis-Donini S, et al. Autoantibodies to glutamic acid decarboxylase in a patient with stiff-man syndrome, epilepsy, and type I diabetes mellitus. *N Engl J Med.* 1988;318(16):1012–1020.

45. Boronat A, Sabater L, Saiz A, et al. GABA(B) receptor antibodies in limbic encephalitis and anti-GAD-associated neurologic disorders. *Neurology.* 2011;76(9):795–800.

46. Dalakas MC, Fujii M, Li M, et al. High-dose intravenous immune globulin for stiff-person syndrome. *N Engl J Med.* 2001;345(26):1870–1876.

47. Pittock SJ, Lucchinetti CF, Parisi JE, et al. Amphiphysin autoimmunity: paraneoplastic accompaniments. *Ann Neurol.* 2005;58(1):96–107.

48. Pittock SJ, Kryzer TJ, Lennon VA. Paraneoplastic antibodies coexist and predict cancer, not neurological syndrome. *Ann Neurol.* 2004;56(5):715–719.

49. Gresa-Arribas N, Titulaer MJ, Torrents A, et al. Antibody titres at diagnosis and during follow-up of anti-NMDA receptor encephalitis: a retrospective study. *Lancet Neurol.* 2014;13(2):167–177.

50. Paterson RW, Zandi MS, Armstrong R, et al. Clinical relevance of positive voltage-gated potassium channel (VGKC)-complex antibodies: experience from a tertiary referral centre. *J Neurol Neurosurg Psychiatry.* 2014;85(6):625–630.

51. Titulaer MJ, Höftberger R, Iizuka T, et al. Overlapping demyelinating syndromes and anti-N-methyl-D-aspartate receptor encephalitis. *Ann Neurol.* 2014;75(3):411–428.

52. Keegan BM, Pittock SJ, Lennon VA. Autoimmune myelopathy associated with collapsin response-mediator protein-5 immunoglobulin G. *Ann Neurol.* 2008;63(4):531–534.

53. Darnell RB, Posner JB. Paraneoplastic syndromes involving the nervous system. *N Engl J Med.* 2003;349(16):1543–1554.

54. Pignolet BS, Gebauer CM, Liblau RS. Immunopathogenesis of paraneoplastic neurological syndromes associated with anti-Hu antibodies: a beneficial antitumor immune response going awry. *Oncoimmunology.* 2013;2(12):e27384.

55. McKeon A, Apiwattanakul M, Lachance DH, et al. Positron emission tomography-computed tomography in paraneoplastic neurologic disorders: systematic analysis and review. *Arch Neurol.* 2010;67(3):322–329.

56. Arino H, Armangué T, Petit-Pedrol M, et al. Anti-LGI1-associated cognitive impairment: presentation and long-term outcome. *Neurology.* 2016;87(8):759–765.

42

Neurosarcoidosis

Brandon P. Moss and Jinny Tavee

KEY POINTS FOR THE CLINICIAN

- Neurologic complications are seen in 5% to 10% of patients with systemic sarcoidosis, but are the presenting symptom in half of these cases.
- Sarcoidosis can affect any part of the nervous system.
- Diagnosis relies on confirming nervous system involvement, excluding alternate diagnoses, and biopsy confirmation when possible.
- Hydrocephalus, intraparenchymal mass lesions, seizures at onset, multiple cranial neuropathies, spinal cord lesions, and chronic meningitis are associated with a worse prognosis.
- Tumor necrosis factor-alpha (TNF-alpha) antagonists have emerged as a promising treatment for refractory neurosarcoidosis.

INTRODUCTION

Sarcoidosis is a systemic inflammatory disorder characterized by nonnecrotizing granulomas on pathology. It causes neurologic complications in 5% to 10% of cases (1–4). Any part of the nervous system may be affected, leading to overlap in presentation with many other diseases. However, a systematic approach to establishing objective evidence of neurologic disease along with a careful evaluation for systemic involvement can expedite diagnosis and lead to appropriate treatment.

EPIDEMIOLOGY

Sarcoidosis has an estimated prevalence of 1 to 40 per 100,000 worldwide (1,5,6). Although the disease can affect all ethnic groups, it is more common in African Americans and people of Scandinavian descent (1,5,6). Peak incidence is in the third to fifth decades of life, although African Americans tend to present late in the fourth decade (1). Women also appear to have a later age of onset and more commonly have neurologic complications and systemic disease compared to men (1,5).

Sarcoidosis most commonly affects the lungs, skin, and lymph nodes. Neurologic complications are seen in 5% to 10% of patients with systemic sarcoidosis and are the presenting symptom in half of these cases (1–4). Extraneural manifestations eventually develop in over 80% of neurosarcoidosis cases (2).

> *Neurologic complications are seen in approximately 5% to 10% of patients with systemic sarcoidosis and are the presenting symptom in half of these cases.*

CLINICAL MANIFESTATIONS

Sarcoidosis can affect any part of the nervous system. The most commonly affected sites are the cranial nerves and meninges. Involvement of the brain parenchyma, spinal cord, and hypothalamic-pituitary axis may also be seen with the clinical presentation reflecting the location of the lesion. Large-fiber peripheral neuropathy and myopathy are rare, although muscle involvement may be underestimated due to subclinical disease.

> *Sarcoidosis can affect any part of the nervous system, but most commonly involves the cranial nerves and meninges.*

Cranial Neuropathy

Sarcoidosis can affect cranial nerves at the level of the nucleus or along the nerve tract. In addition, inflammation of the leptomeninges can cause both isolated and multiple cranial nerve involvement.

FACIAL NERVE PALSY

Facial nerve palsy is the most common neurologic manifestation, reported in 20% to 50% of neurosarcoidosis cases (2,4) with bilateral involvement seen in 30% to 40% of cases (4,7). Symptoms are typically self-limited and resolve within a few weeks with little to no residual deficits.

OPTIC NEUROPATHY

Optic neuropathy is reported nearly as frequently as facial nerve palsy, with some estimates over 20% (2). Outcomes are mixed, with some series reporting improvement with treatment (4,8), while others reporting marked long-term visual impairment (6,9).

VESTIBULOCOCHLEAR AND TRIGEMINAL NERVE INVOLVEMENT

Other cranial nerves are less frequently affected. Vestibulocochlear nerve involvement can cause severe and often acute hearing loss. Patients typically recover at least partially with corticosteroid treatment, although chronic hearing loss is common with bilateral involvement. Trigeminal nerve involvement most commonly presents with severe lancinating pain characteristic of trigeminal neuralgia.

OTHER CRANIAL NERVE INVOLVEMENT

Other cranial nerves can be involved as well, causing a variety of manifestations including vocal cord paralysis, dysphagia, diplopia, and olfactory disturbances.

Meningitis

Leptomeningeal inflammation is common in neurosarcoidosis (10). Most patients present with a subacute to chronic course predominantly involving the basal regions of the brain (11). Headache is a frequent manifestation. Hydrocephalus may also develop due to obstruction of the ventricles or impaired absorption of cerebrospinal fluid (CSF) by the arachnoid villi. This can lead to cognitive changes and, in severe cases, stupor or encephalopathy.

Intraparenchymal Brain Lesions

Intraparenchymal brain lesions have been reported in 20% to 45% of cases (7,9,12,13). Lesions are typically hyperintense on T2-weighted sequences with enhancement after administration of gadolinium contrast (12,14). Their frequent occurrence near areas of meningeal involvement suggests the possibility of local spread (12,14). Clinical presentation is variable depending on the location of the lesion, but can include headaches, focal neurological deficits, hydrocephalus, and seizures. Multiple nonenhancing white matter lesions are also common and may be indistinguishable from multiple sclerosis (MS) in some cases (15,16).

Myelopathy

Isolated spinal cord involvement is rare (17,18). The cervical and upper thoracic cords are the most commonly involved, although the entire cord may be affected (17,19–21). Compared to other neurologic manifestations, the prognosis for functional recovery with spinal cord involvement is often poor. Despite aggressive treatment, most patients are left with residual deficits (17,19).

Hypothalamic–Pituitary Dysfunction

Hypothalamic–pituitary dysfunction can occur as a result of direct structural invasion or basal meningeal inflammation (Figure 42.1). In the largest case series, the most common features were gonadotropin deficiency, thyroid stimulating hormone deficiency, and hyperprolactinemia (22). Most patients had long-standing endocrine dysfunction.

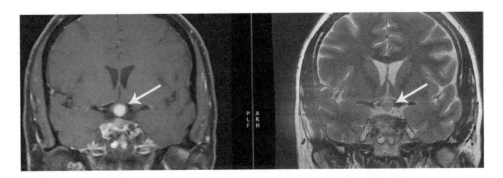

FIGURE 42.1 Hypothalamic-pituitary lesion. Left: Postcontrast T1-weighted coronal section showing enhancement of the pituitary gland. Right: Normal appearing T2-weighted coronal section of the same view.

Stroke

Ischemic stroke related to neurosarcoidosis is rare and may be caused by granulomatous infiltration of the endothelial wall resulting in stenosis or occlusion (23). Central nervous system (CNS) vasculitis, embolic infarcts related to cardiac sarcoidosis, and intracerebral hemorrhage have also been reported (23).

Peripheral Neuropathy

Estimates of the prevalence of peripheral nerve involvement in people with sarcoidosis vary widely. Because there are many other causes of peripheral neuropathy, it can be hard to determine which cases are sarcoidosis related. In addition, case series do not always distinguish between small fiber and large fiber neuropathy, which require different approaches to diagnosis and management.

LARGE FIBER NEUROPATHY

Large fiber nerve involvement typically presents as an axonal, non–length-dependent polyneuropathy caused by granulomatous compression or infiltration of the nerve fibers and vasculitis (24). The asymmetric distribution of findings as opposed to a distal stocking-glove pattern can help distinguish sarcoidosis-related neuropathy from more common causes, such as diabetes or vitamin deficiencies. Rarely, sarcoidosis can cause a demyelinating polyneuropathy similar to an acute or chronic inflammatory demyelinating polyradiculoneuropathy (25). With immunomodulatory treatment, the prognosis is favorable for a substantial number of patients with sarcoidosis-related peripheral neuropathy, especially when the presentation is less severe and the onset of symptoms is more recent (24).

SMALL FIBER NEUROPATHY

Estimates vary, but small fiber neuropathy symptoms have been reported in up to 40% of patients with sarcoidosis (26). Sarcoidosis-associated small fiber neuropathy typically presents with pain and paresthesias either in a distal stocking-glove pattern or patchy non–length-dependent pattern involving the face, trunk, and proximal limbs. Autonomic manifestations include orthostatic intolerance, gastrointestinal dysmotility, and sweating abnormalities. The pathogenesis is thought to be cytokine mediated rather than granulomatous in nature (27). Assessment of intraepidermal nerve fiber density (by skin biopsy or corneal confocal microscopy) and assessment of autonomic function (by quantitative sudomotor axonal reflex testing or quantitative sensory testing) can aid in the diagnosis (28,29). Other causes of small fiber neuropathy must be excluded such as diabetes and vitamin deficiencies. In a large case series, 76% of patients treated with intravenous immunoglobulin and 67% treated with TNF-alpha antagonists had symptomatic improvement (30). In addition, in a phase II, double-blind, randomized, placebo-controlled trial, cibinetide showed a significant improvement in pain control over the control arm as well as a significant increase in corneal nerve fiber area and regenerating nerve fibers at a dose of 4 mg/d (31).

Myopathy

Sarcoidosis myopathy typically presents with generalized weakness, myalgias, and fatigue. In some cases, intramuscular nodules can be palpated under the skin. There is likely a significant amount of subclinical disease as granulomatous muscle involvement has been found in up to 50% of sarcoidosis cases at autopsy (32).

DIAGNOSIS

Because there are many different manifestations of neurosarcoidosis, the differential diagnosis is broad (Table 42.1).

The modified Zajicek criteria are the most commonly used diagnostic criteria for neurosarcoidosis, defining three levels of diagnostic probability: definite, requiring biopsy

TABLE 42.1 Differential Diagnosis of Neurosarcoidosis

INFECTIOUS	AUTOIMMUNE	NEOPLASTIC	DEMYELINATING
—Cryptococcosis	—IgG4-related meningeal disease	—Lymphoma	—Multiple sclerosis
—Coccidioidomycosis	—CNS vasculitis	—Leptomeningeal carcinomatosis	—Neuromyelitis optica
—Histoplasmosis	—Wegener granulomatosis	—Leptomeningeal or dural metastases	—Acute disseminated encephalomyelitis
—Blastomycosis	—Sjogren's syndrome	—Meningioma	—Idiopathic transverse myelitis
—Toxoplasmosis	—Behcet's disease	—Glioma	—Idiopathic optic neuritis
—Tuberculosis	—Systemic lupus erythematosus	—Meningeal plasmacytoma	—Progressive multifocal leukoencephalopathy
—Syphilis	—Vogt-Koyanagi-Harada syndrome	—Spinal cord metastases	
—Borreliosis (Lyme disease)	—Lymphocytic hypophysitis	—Ependymoma	
—Brucellosis	—Rosai-Dorfman disease	—Astrocytoma	
—Listeriosis	—CLIPPERS	—Primitive neuroectodermal tumors	
—Whipple disease	—Paraneoplastic syndrome		
—HIV	—Idiopathic hypertrophic cranial pachymeningitis		
—HSV			
—VZV			

CLIPPERS, chronic lymphocytic inflammation with pontine perivascular enhancement responsive to steroids; CNS: central nervous system; HSV, herpes simplex virus; IgG, immunoglobulin G; VZV, varicella zoster virus.

confirmation from nervous system tissue; probable, requiring evidence of CNS inflammation and systemic sarcoidosis (histologic confirmation or at least two of the following indirect indicators: fluorodeoxyglucose-PET [FDG-PET], chest imaging, gallium scan, serum angiotensin converting enzyme [ACE]); and possible, for a clinical presentation suggestive of neurosarcoidosis that does not meet the first two criteria (33).

Biopsy

The gold standard for diagnosis of neurosarcoidosis is the presence of nonnecrotizing granulomas in nervous system tissue. However, given the potential morbidity associated with biopsy of eloquent nervous system structures in cases when tissue is not readily or safely available, the goal should be to confirm the presence of neurologic

involvement and evaluate for an extraneural source of biopsy or other supporting evidence of systemic sarcoidosis. See Table 42.2 for a general approach to diagnosis.

MRI

MRI with and without gadolinium contrast is the initial test of choice to establish CNS inflammation. The most common intracranial findings are parenchymal lesions, dural nodules or thickening, leptomeningeal enhancement, and cranial nerve enhancement (2).

LEPTOMENINGEAL ENHANCEMENT

The most common radiographic abnormality is leptomeningeal enhancement, which tends to affect the basal surfaces of the brain (34). Lesions often vary in appearance and may be smooth or nodular, diffuse or focal, or a

---

TABLE 42.2   Diagnostic Approach to Neurosarcoidosis

Step 1: Confirm neurologic involvement
- **CNS**
  - MRI brain with and without gadolinium
    - Cervical, thoracic, and lumbosacral spinal cord depending on index of suspicion for spinal cord involvement
  - CSF analysis
    - Cell count and differential
    - Protein
    - Glucose
    - IgG indices
    - Oligoclonal bands
- **PNS**
  - EMG
  - MRI muscle if indicated
  - Skin biopsy or corneal confocal microscopy for evaluation of intraepidermal nerve fiber density and small fiber neuropathy
  - Autonomic testing

Step 2: Evaluate for systemic disease and exclude alternative diagnoses
- CT chest, abdomen, and pelvis
- FDG-PET body
- Pulmonary function tests
- Comprehensive metabolic panel
- Soluble interleukin-2 receptor level
- Serum ACE level
- Screen for mimics
  - Serological studies
  - CSF studies
    - Fungal PCR
    - Fungal cultures
    - Cytology
    - Flow cytometry

Step 3: Tissue biopsy
- Bronchoscopy or endobronchial ultrasound with fine needle aspiration and lung biopsy
- Lymph node biopsy
- Nerve or muscle biopsy
- Brain meningeal or parenchymal biopsy for amenable target

ACE, angiotensin converting enzyme; CNS, central nervous system; CSF, cerebrospinal fluid; EMG, electromyography; FDG-PET, fluorodeoxyglucose-PET; IgG, immunoglobulin G; PCR, polymerase chain reaction; PNS, peripheral nervous system.

combination of features (34). See Figure 42.2 for an example of sarcoidosis-related leptomeningeal enhancement as seen on MRI.

DURAL THICKENING

Dural involvement is also common and can present as a focal mass similar to a meningioma or diffuse thickening as can be seen with lymphoma and idiopathic hypertrophic cranial pachymeningitis. Lesions typically enhance homogeneously on contrast-enhanced T1-weighted images and are dark on T2-weighted images, which can serve as a diagnostic clue (34).

INTRACRANIAL PARENCHYMAL LESIONS

Intraparenchymal brain involvement may present as a focal mass lesion, nonenhancing white matter changes, dense infiltration, or areas of patchy enhancement (34). Enhancing mass lesions are often associated with nearby leptomeningeal enhancement (Figure 42.3) and are thought to represent spread of leptomeningeal disease along the perivascular spaces.

INTRAMEDULLARY SPINAL CORD LESIONS

Intramedullary spinal cord lesions are often longitudinally extensive, affecting three or more spinal cord segments, and are associated with meningeal enhancement in about half of cases (Figure 42.4) (21).

MUSCLE INVOLVEMENT

MRI has utility in identifying granulomatous muscle involvement in patients with symptoms of myopathy and, in some cases, in identifying targets for biopsy that can help confirm the diagnosis.

CSF Studies

CSF analysis should be performed on every patient with suspected neurosarcoidosis to confirm CNS inflammation and exclude infection and malignancy. Seventy percent to 95% of neurosarcoidosis cases have abnormalities of one or more routine CSF parameters (35,36).

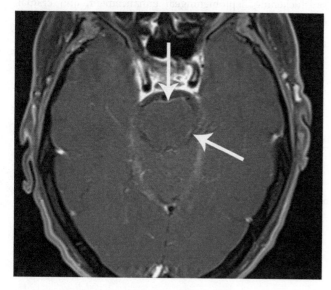

FIGURE 42.2 Basal meningeal enhancement. Postcontrast T1-weighted image showing mild pial enhancement along the margins of the brainstem.

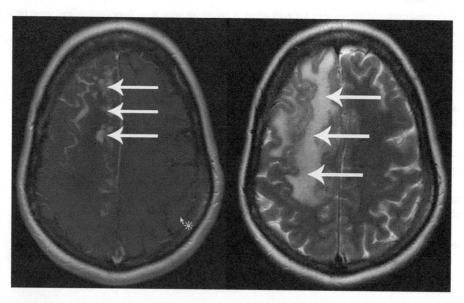

FIGURE 42.3 Intracranial mass lesion extending from the meninges. Left: Postcontrast T1-weighted axial section showing multiple enhancing masses extending from the meninges into the parenchyma of the brain. Right: T2-weighted axial section showing corresponding T2 signal change throughout a large region of the right cerebral hemisphere.

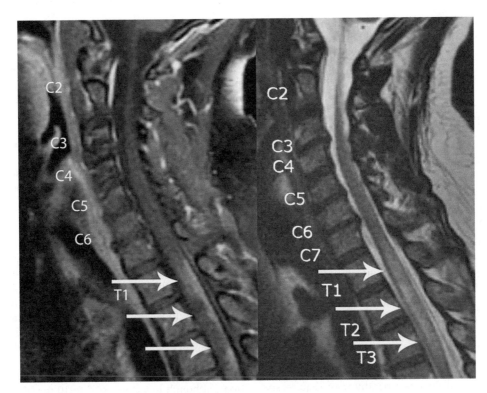

FIGURE 42.4 Longitudinally extensive meningeal-based spinal cord lesion. Left: Postcontrast T1-weighted sagittal section showing an enhancing intramedullary spinal cord lesion extending from C7 to T1 down. Right: T2-weighted sagittal section of the same view showing corresponding T2 signal change.

CELL COUNT AND PROTEIN

Elevated CSF protein and cell count are the most commonly reported CSF abnormalities (36). Although these findings are not specific for neurosarcoidosis, they establish the presence of CNS inflammation. In addition, protein levels ≥200 mg/dL and a white blood cell count ≥50 cells/mL have been found to correlate with clinically active disease (36).

GLUCOSE

Hypoglycorrhachia, or low CSF glucose, is seen in 10% to 30% of cases and is caused by disruption of the CSF glucose transport system (36–38). Its primary value is in distinguishing neurosarcoidosis from MS, which can overlap considerably in other CSF markers (39). Bacterial meningitis, tuberculosis, fungal infections, and carcinomatous meningitis can also present with hypoglycorrhachia and can be differentiated based on other CSF tests.

IMMUNOGLOBULIN G INDEX AND OLIGOCLONAL BANDS

Elevated immunoglobulin G (IgG) index and the presence of oligoclonal bands have been reported in 20% to 40% of neurosarcoidosis cases (2,7,9,36). These markers are also commonly elevated in MS (39).

SOLUBLE INTERLEUKIN-2 RECEPTOR

In one recent study, elevated CSF-soluble interleukin (IL)-2 receptor levels over 150 pg/mL were detected in untreated neurosarcoidosis patients with a 61% sensitivity and 93% specificity in comparison with healthy controls and other inflammatory diseases such as MS and CNS vasculitis (40). There was no significant difference when compared with infection (40).

ANGIOTENSIN CONVERTING ENZYME

CSF ACE is not helpful in the diagnosis of neurosarcoidosis given its poor sensitivity (36,41).

> *CSF ACE is not helpful in the diagnosis of neurosarcoidosis given its poor sensitivity.*

Systemic Evaluation

The initial evaluation for systemic disease should begin with a pulmonary evaluation and serological studies, including a comprehensive metabolic panel to evaluate for renal and liver involvement. Although the serum ACE level is still part of the diagnostic criteria, it may be affected by genetic polymorphisms and (42) is only elevated in 30% to 40% of individuals with neurosarcoidosis (43). In addition, it is a nonspecific finding that may be elevated in patients without sarcoidosis and does not correlate well with disease activity (44).

CT AND FDG-PET

A CT scan of the chest, abdomen, and pelvis should be done to evaluate lymphadenopathy and other lesions that are supportive of the diagnosis or amenable to biopsy. If no evidence of extraneural disease is found, a whole body FDG-PET scan may be considered to increase the sensitivity of subclinical systemic involvement. The sensitivity of whole body FDG-PET in detecting active sarcoidosis is 80% to 100%, but its main limitations are limited availability and cost (45). Although gallium scanning can be done as well, FDG-PET is more sensitive and is the preferred imaging modality (45).

ELECTROMYOGRAPHY NERVE CONDUCTION TESTING

Electromyography (EMG) nerve conduction testing is the primary diagnostic test for people with symptoms of neuromuscular involvement. In cases with peripheral nerve involvement it provides information about localization, demyelinating versus axonal pathophysiology, severity, and chronicity. It can also identify targets for nerve biopsy that can help confirm the diagnosis.

ADDITIONAL TESTING

The diagnosis of small fiber neuropathy may require specialized testing, such as skin biopsy or corneal confocal microscopy, to evaluate intraepidermal nerve fiber density, and quantitative sudomotor axonal reflex testing to assess autonomic function (28,29,31).

PROGNOSIS

Precise characterization of the disease course in neurosarcoidosis is difficult due to varying diagnostic criteria, changes in treatment strategy over time, referral bias for available case series, and lack of validated outcomes measures. In the overall neurosarcoidosis population, one 52-patient cross-sectional study found that 12% had minor disability, defined as neurological deficits causing minor interference in everyday life, and 17% had major disability, defined as neurological deficits causing failure to return to a job or school, the need for special equipment such as crutches or a wheelchair, or assistance with everyday activities (7).

Features associated with a poorer prognosis include hydrocephalus, intraparenchymal mass lesions, seizures at onset, multiple cranial nerve involvement, spinal cord lesions, and chronic meningitis (17,35,46).

TREATMENT

Symptomatic CNS disease is associated with significant morbidity and often requires immunosuppressive treatment (2,7,35,47). Given a lack of randomized controlled trials, treatment guidelines are largely based on anecdotal evidence and small case series. Gadolinium-enhancing brain

or spinal cord lesions, bilateral optic neuropathy, and multiple cranial neuropathies are more likely to be refractory to first-line therapies and may require more effective therapies such as TNF-alpha antagonists (42,48). Some authors have proposed stratifying CNS manifestations into mild (facial nerve palsy), moderate (optic neuritis, vestibular neuritis, myopathy, neuropathy, and dural meningeal involvement), and severe disease (brain and spinal cord lesions, leptomeningeal involvement, and hydrocephalus) as a guide to the intensity of therapy (49).

See Table 42.3 for a summary of the dose, side effects, and monitoring requirements for the commonly used maintenance therapies.

Corticosteroids

Corticosteroids are the first-line therapy for neurosarcoidosis. Although no studies have evaluated the optimal dose and length of treatment, 20 to 40 mg/d of oral prednisone is a reasonable starting dose for mild to moderate disease. In severe cases, 500 to 1,000 mg/d pulse dose intravenous (IV) methylprednisolone for 3 to 5 days followed by an oral prednisone maintenance dose of 60 mg/d is a typical approach. The dose may be slowly tapered over 6 to 12 months with close monitoring for disease exacerbations, although low doses of 5 to 10 mg/d may be required for a longer period of time. Side effects are the major limiting factor to the dose and duration of steroid therapy and are detailed in Table 42.3.

Steroid-Sparing Agents

Steroid-sparing agents are typically used as adjunct therapy to corticosteroids for patients with severe or refractory disease and to limit the dose and duration of steroid use. For patients with severe disease who are not candidates for TNF-alpha antagonists, azathioprine may be an effective alternative that can serve as monotherapy in some cases (50). Thiopurine methyltransferase genotype testing should be obtained before initiation of treatment to identify patients at risk for toxicity causing life-threatening myelosuppression. Methotrexate and hydroxychloroquine may be used as adjunct treatment to corticosteroids or other immunomodulatory therapies for treating neurosarcoidosis, but are typically insufficient as monotherapy (3,51). In contrast, mycophenylate mofetil has been effective as monotherapy in some cases of neurosarcoidosis (52) and can be used in conjunction with infliximab for severe disease (53).

TNF-alpha Antagonists

TNF-alpha antagonists, specifically infliximab and adalimumab, have emerged as a promising treatment for refractory neurosarcoidosis (54–57). These medications can be used as monotherapy, but some patients may not be candidates due to cost.

TABLE 42.3 Maintenance Therapies for Neurosarcoidosis

DRUG	DOSE	SIDE EFFECTS	PRINCIPAL MONITORING
Prednisone	5–60 mg/d	Weight gain, diabetes, hypertension, dyslipidemia, increased risk of infections, cataract formation, increased intraocular pressure, osteoporosis	Blood pressure, weight, glucose if indicated, bone density scans
Azathioprine	50–200 mg/d	GI side effects, rash, fever, malaise, lymphoma, bone marrow suppression, liver dysfunction, increased risk of infection, PML	CBC and LFTs every 1–3 mo Check thiopurine methyltransferase genetic testing prior to initiation
Mycophenolate mofetil	500–1,500 mg twice a day	Hypertension, hyperglycemia, hypercholesterolemia, GI side effects, lymphoma, skin cancer, bone marrow suppression, liver dysfunction, increased risk of opportunistic infections, PML	CBC and LFTs every 1–3 mo, regular skin checks
Methotrexate	5–25 mg/wk orally or SQ (prescribed with folate)	GI symptoms, acute renal failure, bone marrow suppression, severe skin reactions, hepatotoxicity including fibrosis and cirrhosis, lymphoma, increased risk of infections including PJP	CBC and LFTs every 1–3 mo
Hydroxychloroquine	200–400 mg/d	Cardiomyopathy, skin reactions, bone marrow suppression, severe hypoglycemia, retinal toxicity, proximal myopathy	Eye examination every 6–12 mo
Infliximab	3–5 mg/kg initially every 2 wk for two doses, then every 4–8 wk	GI symptoms, hepatic reactions, predisposition to a lupus-like syndrome, increased risk of opportunistic infections and reactivation of hepatitis B and tuberculosis, bone marrow suppression, hypersensitivity reactions, lymphoma, predisposition to demyelinating disease	Active and latent TB screening prior to initiating and during therapy, HBV screening prior to initiating therapy
Adalimumab	40–80 mg SQ every 1–2 wk	Skin reactions, predisposition to a lupus-like syndrome, increased risk of opportunistic infections and reactivation of hepatitis B and tuberculosis, heart failure, bone marrow suppression, hypersensitivity reactions, lymphoma, predisposition to demyelinating disease	Active and latent TB screening prior to initiating and during therapy, HBV screening prior to initiating therapy
Rituximab	Two 1,000-mg infusions 2 wk apart every 6 mo	Infusion-related reactions, sinusitis, UTIs, hepatitis B reactivation, PML, hypogamma-globulinemia	CBC and LFTs every 6 mo

CBC, complete blood count; GI, gastrointestinal; LFTs, liver function tests; PJP, *Pneumocystis jiroveci* pneumonia; HBV, hepatitis B virus; PML, progressive multifocal leukoencephalopathy; SQ, subcutaneous administration; TB, tuberculosis; UTI, urinary tract infection.

Cyclophosphamide

Cyclophosphamide is an effective therapy for the treatment of refractory neurosarcoidosis (3,48,50,58), but its use is mainly limited to treating disease exacerbations due to its risk of serious side effects with long-term use. Cancer risk, in particular, appears to be linked to the total cumulative dose (59,60). Other serious side effects include bone marrow suppression, hemorrhagic cystitis, cardiotoxicity, pulmonary toxicities, hepatotoxicity, sterility, and fetal anomalies.

Rituximab

Rituximab is an anti-CD20 monoclonal antibody used in the treatment of MS, neuromyelitis optica (NMO), and other autoimmune diseases. A few isolated case reports have described improvement with rituximab in patients with treatment-refractory neurosarcoidosis (9,61), but further studies are necessary to help characterize its utility.

Whole-Brain Radiation Therapy

Whole-brain radiation is another potential option for refractory neurosarcoidosis cases, but most reports were published before the advent of TNF-alpha antagonists (62). Given the long-term complications of radiation therapy, however, other therapeutic options should be tried prior to consideration of whole-brain radiation.

KEY POINTS FOR PATIENTS AND FAMILIES

- Neurologic involvement is rare in sarcoidosis but can be the presenting symptom.

- Facial weakness is the most common presentation of neurosarcoidosis and usually resolves on its own.

- Patients with sarcoidosis who develop neurologic symptoms, such as weakness, numbness, difficulty walking, and confusion, should be evaluated urgently with a brain and spinal cord MRI.

- A spinal tap, or lumbar puncture, is an important test in evaluating patients with neurosarcoidosis to look for inflammation and other diseases that may mimic sarcoidosis.

- Treatment with corticosteroids and other medications that suppress the immune system can result in improvement of neurologic disease.

REFERENCES

1. Baughman RP, Teirstein AS, Judson MA, et al. Clinical characteristics of patients in a case control study of sarcoidosis. *Am J Respir Crit Care Med*. 2001;164(10)(pt 1):1885–1889. doi:10.1164/ajrccm.164.10.2104046.

2. Fritz D, van de Beek D, Brouwer MC. Clinical features, treatment and outcome in neurosarcoidosis: systematic review and meta-analysis. *BMC Neurol*. 2016;16(1):220. doi:10.1186/s12883-016-0741-x.

3. Lower EE, Broderick J. P, Brott TG, et al. Diagnosis and management of neurological sarcoidosis. *Arch Intern Med*. 1997;157(16):1864–1868.

4. Stern BJ, Krumholz A, Johns C, et al. Sarcoidosis and its neurological manifestations. *Arch Neurol*. 1985;42(9):909–917.

5. Iannuzzi MC, Rybicki BA, Teirstein AS. Sarcoidosis. *N Engl J Med*. 2007;357(21):2153-2165. doi:10.1056/NEJMra071714.

6. Stern BJ, Aksamit A, Clifford D, et al. Neurologic presentations of sarcoidosis. *Neurol Clin*. 2010;28(1):185–198. doi:10.1016/j.ncl.2009.09.012.

7. Leonhard SE, Fritz D, Eftimov F, et al. Neurosarcoidosis in a tertiary referral center: a cross-sectional cohort study. *Medicine (Baltimore)*. 2016;95(14):e3277. doi:10.1097/MD.0000000000003277.

8. Ricker W, Clark M. Sarcoidosis; a clinicopathologic review of 300 cases, including 22 autopsies. *Am J Clin Pathol*. 1949;19(8):725–749.

9. Pawate S, Moses H, Sriram S. Presentations and outcomes of neurosarcoidosis: a study of 54 cases. *QJM*. 2009;102(7):449–460. doi:10.1093/qjmed/hcp042.

10. Chapelon C, Ziza JM, Piette JC, et al. Neurosarcoidosis: signs, course and treatment in 35 confirmed cases. *Medicine (Baltimore)*. 1990;69(5):261–276.

11. Christoforidis GA, Spickler EM, Recio MV, et al. MR of CNS sarcoidosis: correlation of imaging features to clinical symptoms and response to treatment. *AJNR Am J Neuroradiol*. 1999;20(4):655–669.

12. Nowak DA, Widenka DC. Neurosarcoidosis: a review of its intracranial manifestation. *J Neurol*. 2001;248(5):363–372.

13. Shah R, Roberson GH, Cure JK. Correlation of MR imaging findings and clinical manifestations in neurosarcoidosis. *AJNR Am J Neuroradiol*. 2009;30(5):953–961. doi:10.3174/ajnr.A1470.

14. Ginat DT, Dhillon G, Almast J. Magnetic resonance imaging of neurosarcoidosis. *J Clin Imaging Sci*. 2011;1:15. doi:10.4103/2156-7514.76693.

15. Miller DH, Kendall BE, Barter S, et al. Magnetic resonance imaging in central nervous system sarcoidosis. *Neurology*. 1988;38(3):378–383.

16. Smith AS, Meisler DM, Weinstein MA, et al. High-signal periventricular lesions in patients with sarcoidosis: neurosarcoidosis or multiple sclerosis? *AJR Am J Roentgenol*. 1989;153(1):147–152. doi:10.2214/ajr.153.1.147.

17. Cohen-Aubart F, Galanaud D, Grabli D, et al. Spinal cord sarcoidosis: clinical and laboratory profile and outcome of 31 patients in a case-control study. *Medicine (Baltimore)*. 2010;89(2):133–140. doi:10.1097/MD.0b013e3181d5c6b4.

18. Nozaki K, Scott TF, Sohn M, et al. Isolated neurosarcoidosis: case series in 2 sarcoidosis centers. *Neurologist*. 2012;18(6):373–377. doi:10.1097/NRL.0b013e3182704d04.

19. Durel CA, Marignier R, Maucort-Boulch D, et al. Clinical features and prognostic factors of spinal cord sarcoidosis: a multicenter observational study of 20 BIOPSY-PROVEN patients. *J Neurol*. 2016;263(5):981–990. doi:10.1007/s00415-016-8092-5.

20. Flanagan EP, Kaufmann TJ, Krecke KN, et al. Discriminating long myelitis of neuromyelitis optica from sarcoidosis. *Ann Neurol*. 2016;79(3):437–447. doi:10.1002/ana.24582.

21. Sohn M, Culver DA, Judson MA, et al. Spinal cord neurosarcoidosis. *Am J Med Sci*. 2014;347(3):195–198. doi:10.1097/MAJ.0b013e3182808781.

22. Langrand C, Bihan H, Raverot G, et al. Hypothalamo-pituitary sarcoidosis: a multicenter study of 24 patients. *QJM*. 2012;105(10):981–995. doi:10.1093/qjmed/hcs121.

23. Herring AB, Urich H. Sarcoidosis of the central nervous system. *J Neurol Sci*. 1969;9(3):405–422.

24. Burns TM, Dyck PJ, Aksamit AJ, et al. The natural history and long-term outcome of 57 limb sarcoidosis neuropathy cases. *J Neurol Sci*. 2006;244(1–2):77–87. doi:10.1016/j.jns.2006.01.014.

25. Said G, Lacroix C, Plante-Bordeneuve V, et al. Nerve granulomas and vasculitis in sarcoid peripheral neuropathy: a clinicopathological study of 11 patients. *Brain*. 2002;125(pt 2):264–275.

26. Hoitsma E, Marziniak M, Faber CG, et al. Small fibre neuropathy in sarcoidosis. *Lancet*. 2002;359(9323):2085–2086.

27. Judson MA, Costabel U, Drent M, et al. The WASOG sarcoidosis organ assessment instrument: an update of a previous clinical tool. *Sarcoidosis Vasc Diffuse Lung Dis*. 2014;31(1):19–27.

28. Chen X, Graham J, Dabbah MA, et al. Small nerve fiber quantification in the diagnosis of diabetic sensorimotor polyneuropathy: comparing corneal confocal microscopy with intraepidermal nerve fiber density. *Diabetes Care*. 2015;38(6):1138–1144. doi:10.2337/dc14–2422.

29. Tavee J, Culver D. Sarcoidosis and small-fiber neuropathy. *Curr Pain Headache Rep*. 2011;15(3):201–206. doi:10.1007/s11916-011-0180–8.

30. Tavee JO, Karwa K, Ahmed Z, et al. Sarcoidosis-associated small fiber neuropathy in a large cohort: clinical aspects and response to IVIG and anti-TNF alpha treatment. *Respir Med*. 2017;126:135–138. doi:10.1016/j.rmed.2017.03.011.

31. Culver DA, Dahan A, Bajorunas D, et al. Cibinetide improves corneal nerve fiber abundance in patients with sarcoidosis-associated small nerve fiber loss and neuropathic pain. *Invest Ophthalmol Vis Sci*. 2017;58(6):BIO52-BIO60. doi:10.1167/iovs.16–21291.

32. Iwai K, Tachibana T, Takemura T, et al. Pathological studies on sarcoidosis autopsy. I. Epidemiological features of 320 cases in Japan. *Acta Pathol Jpn.* 1993;43(7-8): 372–376.

33. Zajicek JP, Scolding NJ, Foster O, et al. Central nervous system sarcoidosis—diagnosis and management. *QJM.* 1999;92(2):103–117.

34. Smith JK, Matheus MG, Castillo M. Imaging manifestations of neurosarcoidosis. *AJR Am J Roentgenol.* 2004;182(2):289–295. doi:10.2214/ajr.182.2.1820289.

35. Oksanen V. Neurosarcoidosis: clinical presentations and course in 50 patients. *Acta Neurol Scand.* 1986;73(3):283–290.

36. Wengert O, Rothenfusser-Korber E, Vollrath B, et al. Neurosarcoidosis: correlation of cerebrospinal fluid findings with diffuse leptomeningeal gadolinium enhancement on MRI and clinical disease activity. *J Neurol Sci.* 2013;335(1–2):124–130. doi:10.1016/j.jns.2013.09.008.

37. Borucki SJ, Nguyen BV, Ladoulis CT, et al. Cerebrospinal fluid immunoglobulin abnormalities in neurosarcoidosis. *Arch Neurol.* 1989;46(3):270–273.

38. Reske D, Petereit HF, Heiss WD. Difficulties in the differentiation of chronic inflammatory diseases of the central nervous system—value of cerebrospinal fluid analysis and immunological abnormalities in the diagnosis. *Acta Neurol Scand.* 2005;112(4):207–213. doi:10.1111/j.1600-0404.2005.00414.x.

39. Komori M, Blake A, Greenwood M, et al. Cerebrospinal fluid markers reveal intrathecal inflammation in progressive multiple sclerosis. *Ann Neurol.* 2015;78(1):3–20. doi:10.1002/ana.24408.

40. Petereit HF, Reske D, Tumani H, et al. Soluble CSF interleukin 2 receptor as indicator of neurosarcoidosis. *J Neurol.* 2010;257(11):1855–1863. doi:10.1007/s00415-010-5623-3.

41. Khoury J, Wellik KE, Demaerschalk BM, et al. Cerebrospinal fluid angiotensin-converting enzyme for diagnosis of central nervous system sarcoidosis. *Neurologist.* 2009;15(2):108-111. doi:10.1097/NRL.0b013e31819bcf84.

42. Tomita H, Ina Y, Sugiura Y, et al. Polymorphism in the angiotensin-converting enzyme (ACE) gene and sarcoidosis. *Am J Respir Crit Care Med.* 1997;156(1):255–259. doi:10.1164/ajrccm.156.1.9612011.

43. Kellinghaus C, Schilling M, Ludemann P. Neurosarcoidosis: clinical experience and diagnostic pitfalls. *Eur Neurol.* 2004;51(2) 84-88. doi:10.1159/000076534.

44. Miyoshi S, Hamada H, Kadowaki T, et al. Comparative evaluation of serum markers in pulmonary sarcoidosis. *Chest.* 2010;137(6):1391-1397. doi:10.1378/chest.09–1975.

45. Mana J, Gamez C. Molecular imaging in sarcoidosis. *Curr Opin Pulm Med.* 2011;17(5):325-331. doi:10.1097/MCP.0b013e3283480d36.

46. Luke RA, Stern BJ, Krumholz A, et al. Neurosarcoidosis: the long-term clinical course. *Neurology.* 1987;37(3):461–463.

47. Judson MA, Boan AD, Lackland DT. The clinical course of sarcoidosis: presentation, diagnosis, and treatment in a large white and black cohort in the United States. *Sarcoidosis Vasc Diffuse Lung Dis.* 2012;29(2):119–127.

48. Scott TF, Yandora K, Valeri A, et al. Aggressive therapy for neurosarcoidosis: long-term follow-up of 48 treated patients. *Arch Neurol.* 2007;64(5):691–696. doi:10.1001/archneur.64.5.691.

49. Tavee JO, Stern BJ. Neurosarcoidosis. *Clin Chest Med.* 2015;36(4): 643–656. doi:10.1016/j.ccm.2015.08.007.

50. Agbogu BN, Stern BJ, Sewell C, et al. Therapeutic considerations in patients with refractory neurosarcoidosis. *Arch Neurol.* 1995;52(9):875–879.

51. Sharma OP. Effectiveness of chloroquine and hydroxychloroquine in treating selected patients with sarcoidosis with neurological involvement. *Arch Neurol.* 1998;55(9):1248–1254.

52. Androdias G, Maillet D, Marignier R, et al. Mycophenolate mofetil may be effective in CNS sarcoidosis but not in sarcoid myopathy. *Neurology.* 2011;76(13):1168–1172. doi:10.1212/WNL.0b013e318212aafb.

53. Moravan M, Segal BM. Treatment of CNS sarcoidosis with infliximab and mycophenolate mofetil. *Neurology.* 2009;72(4):337-340. doi:10.1212/01.wnl.0000341278.26993.22.

54. Marnane M, Lynch T, Scott J, et al. Steroid-unresponsive neurosarcoidosis successfully treated with adalimumab. *J Neurol.* 2009;256(1):139-140. doi:10.1007/s00415-009-0077–1.

55. Pereira J, Anderson NE, McAuley D, et al. Medically refractory neurosarcoidosis treated with infliximab. *Intern Med J.* 2011;41(4):354–357. doi:10.1111/j.1445-5994.2011.02457.x.

56. Santos E, Shaunak S, Renowden S, et al. Treatment of refractory neurosarcoidosis with Infliximab. *J Neurol Neurosurg Psychiatry.* 2010;81(3):241-246. doi:10.1136/jnnp.2008.149989.

57. Sodhi M, Pearson K, White ES, et al. Infliximab therapy rescues cyclophosphamide failure in severe central nervous system sarcoidosis. *Respir Med.* 2009;103(2):268-273. doi:10.1016/j.rmed.2008.08.016.

58. Doty JD, Mazur JE, Judson MA. Treatment of corticosteroid-resistant neurosarcoidosis with a short-course cyclophosphamide regimen. *Chest.* 2003;124(5):2023–2026.

59. Baker GL, Kahl LE, Zee BC, et al. Malignancy following treatment of rheumatoid arthritis with cyclophosphamide. Long-term case-control follow-up study. *Am J Med.* 1987;83(1):1–9.

60. Travis LB, Curtis RE, Glimelius B, et al. Bladder and kidney cancer following cyclophosphamide therapy for non-Hodgkin's lymphoma. *J Natl Cancer Inst.* 1995;87(7):524–530.

61. Bomprezzi R, Pati S, Chansakul C, et al. A case of neurosarcoidosis successfully treated with rituximab. *Neurology.* 2010;75(6):568–570. doi:10.1212/WNL.0b013e3181ec7ff9.

62. Motta M, Alongi F, Bolognesi A, et al. Remission of refractory neurosarcoidosis treated with brain radiotherapy: a case report and a literature review. *Neurologist.* 2008;14(2):120–124. doi:10.1097/NRL.0b013e31815b97ec.

Index

AARMS. *See* Association for the Advancement of Research into Multiple Sclerosis
abuse
  emotional, 347
  financial, 348
  physical, 347
acquired demyelinating syndromes, 297–298
ACTH. *See* adrenocorticotropic hormone
action research arm test (ARAT), 237–238
activities of daily livings (ADLs), 232
acupuncture, 290
acute disseminated encephalomyelitis (ADEM), 302–303
  clinical features, 365–366
  definition, 297, 363
  demyelinating attacks, risk for, 369
  differential diagnosis of, 365
  electrophysiologic studies, 368
  hallmark clinical presentation for, 363, 366
  imaging findings, 366
  incidence, 364
  infections, 365
  key features, 367
  laboratory findings, 366–368
  neuropathological findings, 368
  outcome and disability, 369
  treatment, 368–369
  variants, 368–369
acute hemorrhagic leukoencephalitis (AHL), 368
acute optic neuritis (AON), 56
acute relapse treatment, 356–357
acute sphincter dysfunction, 376
acute therapy, 389–391
ADA. *See* Americans with Disabilities Act
ADEM. *See* acute disseminated encephalomyelitis
adhesion molecules, 17
adjustment disorder, 186
ADLs. *See* activities of daily livings
adrenocorticotropic hormone (ACTH), 7, 110, 112, 127
advanced practice clinician (APC), 167, 168
AE. *See* autoimmune encephalitis
afferent demyelination, 213–214
afferent pathology, 208–212
AFOs. *See* ankle foot orthoses
aging, 328–330
AGNA. *See* anti-glial neuronal antibody
AHL. *See* acute hemorrhagic leukoencephalitis
aHSCT. *See* autologous hematopoietic stem cell transplant
Ai Chi therapy, 236
alemtuzumab, 102
alternative medicine, 9

ambulation
  assessment tools, 271–273
  assistive devices, 274–275
  common gait abnormalities, 273
  exercise, 273
  interventions, 273–276
  limitations, 274
  medications, 275
  orthoses, 274–275
  rehabilitation, 273
  surgical treatments, 275–276
American Academy of Neurology, 185
Americans with Disabilities Act (ADA), 335, 336
amiloride, 141
ANA. *See* antinuclear antibody
ankle foot orthoses (AFOs), 274
ANNA1. *See* antineuronal nuclear antibody type-1
ANNA2. *See* antineuronal nuclear antibody type-2
annualized relapse rate (ARR), 118, 130
antibodies
  anti-dipeptidyl-peptidase-like protein-6, 385
  anti-glycine receptor, 385
  extracellular plasma membrane antigens, 383–384
  gamma-amino butyric acid B receptor, 385
  intracellular antigens, 386–388
  ionotropic glutamate receptor, 384–385
  testing in, 388
  tumor screening, 388–389
  voltage-gated potassium channel complex, 383–384
antibodies targeting extracellular plasma membrane antigens, 383
anti-collapsin response mediator protein-5 (CRMP5), 387
anti-dipeptidyl-peptidase-like protein-6 (DPPX6), 385
anti-glial neuronal antibody (AGNA), 387
anti-glycine receptor (GlyR), 385
anti-LINGO-1, 141
anti-Ma. *See* dual Ma-1/M-2 positivity
antineuronal nuclear antibody type-1 (ANNA1), 386
antineuronal nuclear antibody type-2 (ANNA2), 387
anti-NMDAR encephalitis. *See* anti-N-methyl-D-aspartate receptor encephalitis
anti-N-methyl-D-aspartate receptor (NMDAR) encephalitis, 384
antinuclear antibody (ANA), 80
anti-ocrelizumab antibodies, 132
antioxidants, 290
anti-phospholipid antibodies (APLA), 326
anxiety disorders, 187
AON. *See* acute optic neuritis
APC. *See* advanced practice clinician
APLA. *See* anti-phospholipid antibodies
AQP4-IgG. *See* aquaporin-4 IgG
aquaporin-4 IgG (AQP4-IgG), 55

ARAT. *See* action research arm test
ARNMD. *See* Association for Research in Nervous and
　　Mental Disease
ARR. *See* annualized relapse rate
assistive devices, 274–275
Association for Research in Nervous and Mental Disease
　　(ARNMD), 2
Association for the Advancement of Research into Multiple
　　Sclerosis (AARMS), 9
Aubagio. *See* teriflunomide
autoantibodies
　　cytoplasmic antigens, 386–387
　　intracellular synaptic proteins, 388
　　neuronal nuclear, 386–387
autoimmune comorbidities, 326–328
autoimmune encephalitis (AE)
　　antibodies
　　　　anti-dipeptidyl-peptidase-like protein-6, 385
　　　　anti-glycine receptor, 385
　　　　extracellular plasma membrane antigens, 383–384
　　　　gamma-amino butyric acid B receptor, 385
　　　　intracellular antigens, 386–388
　　　　ionotropic glutamate receptor, 384–385
　　　　testing in, 388
　　　　tumor screening, 388–389
　　　　voltage-gated potassium channel complex, 383–384
　　anti-LGI1 encephalitis, 383
　　autoantibodies
　　　　cytoplasmic antigens, 386–387
　　　　intracellular synaptic proteins, 388
　　　　neuronal nuclear, 386–387
　　clinical syndromes, 382
　　cytoplasmic antibodies, 386
　　demyelinating disease, 388
　　immunopathogenic mechanisms, 381
　　neuronal nuclear, 386
　　overlap disease, 388
　　paraclinical biomarkers, 383
　　pathophysiology of, 380
　　suspect, 380–383
　　treatment
　　　　acute therapy, 389–391
　　　　long-term therapy, 391
autologous hematopoietic stem cell transplant
　　(aHSCT), 151
autonomic dysreflexia, 256
Avonex, 118, 119
axonal loss, 18–19
　　inflammatory axonopathy, 19
　　Wallerian degeneration, 19
azathioprine, 358–359

balance confidence scale, 269
balance impairment
　　assessment, 270
　　balance confidence scale, 269
　　exercise for, 270–271
　　rehabilitation, 270–271
BBS. *See* berg balance scale
BDI. *See* Beck Depression Inventory
Beck Depression Inventory (BDI), 185
bee venom therapy (BVT), 290

benign multiple sclerosis, 25–26, 98
benzodiazepines, 305
berg balance scale (BBS), 269–270
Betaseron, 118
BG-12. *See* dimethyl fumarate
biotin, 140, 153–154
bipolar disorder, 187
bladder dysfunction
　　evaluation and clinical findings, 244–249
　　factors, 245
　　pathophysiology, 244
　　symptoms, 50, 244
　　treatment, 244, 246–249
blindness, 339
blood tests, 79–81
body weight supported treadmill training
　　(BWSTT), 274
botulinum toxin (BTX), 305
　　bladder, 248
　　spasticity, 263
bowel dysfunction
　　constipation, 250
　　etiology, 249
　　evaluation and clinical findings, 249–250
　　exacerbate, 250
　　fecal incontinence treatment, 250
　　screening questions, 250
　　symptoms, 50
breastfeeding, 318–319
BTX. *See* botulinum toxin
BVT. *See* bee venom therapy
BWSTT. *See* body weight supported treadmill training

CAM. *See* complementary and alternative medicine
cannabinoids (CBs), 290–291
cardiovascular autonomic dysfunction, 256
caregiver
　　definition, 343
　　emotional support, 345–346
　　tips for, 347
　　trifecta, 345
　　wellness programs, 346–347
caregiver burden, 344
caregiving
　　description, 344
　　essentials, 346
　　stages, 344–345
CASPR2. *See* contactin-associated protein-2
causation theories, 3
caveat, 57
CBC. *See* complete blood count
CBs. *See* cannabinoids
CBT. *See* cognitive behavioral therapy
CDP. *See* confirmed disability progression
cell depletion, 101
cell trafficking, 101
cell-based therapies, 155
Center for Advancing Health, 171
Center for Neurologic Study-Lability Scale (CNS-LS), 188
central fatigue, 175
central nervous system (CNS), 130
central neuropathic pain (CNP), 226–228

cerebellum, 50
cerebrospinal fluid (CSF), 301
    IgG index derivation, 82
    red flags, 91
Charcot, Jean Marie, 53
chemokine receptors, 18
chemokines, 18
Chinese herbal medicine, 290
2-chlorodeoxyadenosine. *See* cladribine
chronic fatigue, 175
chronic stressors, 174
CIS. *See* clinically isolated syndrome
cladribine, 151
clinical red flags, 61, 88–89
clinical relapse management, 111
clinically isolated syndrome (CIS), 52, 56, 119, 302
CNP. *See* central neuropathic pain
CNS-LS. *See* Center for Neurologic Study-Lability Scale
COBRA. *See* Consolidated Omnibus Budget Reconciliation
        Act of 1985
cognition symptoms, 48
cognitive behavioral therapy (CBT), 185, 188
cognitive dysfunction
    disease-modifying medications, 193
    evaluation, 192–193
    indicators, 192
    minimal assessment, 193
    patient case study, 196
    symptomatic therapy, 193–196
cognitive impairment, 191
common disease-common variant hypothesis, 32
communication, 166, 167, 169
comorbid medical conditions, 174
comorbidities
    anti-phospholipid antibodies, 326
    autoimmune comorbidities, 326–328
    evidence, 327
    hyperlipidemia, 325–326
    mental, 325
    overview of, 324–325
    primary care issues, 279
    smoking, 326
    therapeutic decisions, 328
    vascular, 325
complementary and alternative medicine (CAM)
    definition, 290
    description, 289
    fatigue, 179
    NIH classification, 290
    therapies
        acupuncture, 290
        antioxidants, 290
        bee venom therapy, 290
        Chinese herbal medicine, 290
        cooling therapy, 291
        cranberry, 291
        echinacea, 291
        fish oil, 291–292
        ginkgo biloba, 292
        gluten sensitivity, 292
        immune-stimulating supplements, 291
        low dose naltrexone, 292–293

        marijuana, 290–291
        mindfulness, 293
        Swank diet, 291–292
        Tai Chi, 293
        traditional Chinese medicine, 290
        vitamin B$_{12}$, 293
        vitamin D, 293–294
        yoga, 294
complete blood count (CBC), 119, 127
comprehensive care center, 167, 168
    communication, 169
    enhanced access, 167–169
    patient reported outcomes, 169–170
    site research, 169–170
    in team, 168
comprehensive fatigue approach, 175
comprehensive symptom management, 163
confirmed disability progression (CDP), 130
Consolidated Omnibus Budget Reconciliation Act of 1985
        (COBRA), 337
constipation
    medications, 250
    treatment, 250
contactin-associated protein-2 (CASPR2), 383
cooling therapy, 291
Copaxone. *See* glatiramer acetate (GA)
corticobulbar symptoms, 218
corticosteroids
    placebo-controlled trials, 110
    side effects, 110–111
    symptomatic therapy, 112–113
    types/doses of, 111
cortisol, 127
cranberry therapy, 291
cranial nerves, 48–49
cranial neuropathy, 395
CRMP5. *See* anti-collapsin response mediator protein-5
CSF. *See* cerebrospinal fluid
cyclophosphamide, 313
Cytoxan. *See* cyclophosphamide

DAC. *See* daclizumab
daclizumab (DAC), 116, 117, 120
dalfampridine, 275
deconditioning, 174
demyelinating lesions, 374, 375
demyelinating optic neuritis (DON)
    alternative diagnoses, 210
    description, 208
    vision loss, 208–209
demyelination, 15–18
    afferent, 213–214
    efferent, 214–215
    retrochiasmatic, 215–216
depression, 48
    diagnosis, 183–185
    etiology, 185
    factors, 185
    fatigue, 174
    screening tools, 184
    treatment, 185–186
description, by Charcot, Jean Martin, 1–2

Devic's syndrome. *See* neuromyelitis optica (NMO)
dextromethorphan, 221–222
diagnosis
    aging in elderly patients, 330
    blood tests, 79–81
    clinical red flags, 61
    evolution of, 53–54
    future of, 61
    McDonald criteria
        clinically isolated syndromes, 52
        CSF-specific OCBs, 57
        diagnostic scheme, 54, 55
        MRI and clinical practice, 56–57
        primary progressive multiple sclerosis, 53, 57–58
        relapsing–remitting multiple sclerosis, 52, 55–56
        secondary progressive multiple sclerosis, 52–53
    neuromyelitis optica, 353–355
    neurosarcoidosis, 396–397
    pediatric multiple sclerosis, 302
    Poser criteria, 53
    primary progressive multiple sclerosis, 57–58
    pseudo-relapses, 59
    radiologically isolated syndrome, 59–60
    relapsing, 58–59
    Schumacher committee criteria, 53
diagnostic algorithm, 92
diagnostic red flags
    cerebrospinal fluid red flags, 91
    clinical red flags, 88–89
    imaging red flags, 89–91
differential diagnosis
    diagnostic algorithm, 92
    by disease category, 88
    mimics by disease category, 91–92
    pediatric multiple sclerosis, 302–303
diffusion tensor imaging (DTI), 376
dimethyl fumarate (DMF), 103
    mechanism, 122
    side effects, 123
    start-up, monitoring, and risk stratification, 123
    trial results, 122–123
    typical patients, 123
DIS. *See* dissemination in space
disability insurance, 338–339
disease activity free status, 98
disease modifying therapy (DMT), 116, 171
    administration, 102
    changing, 100–101
    comorbidities, 99
    convenience, 103
    cost and access, 103
    current treatment strategies, 98–99
    early treatment initiation, 97–98
    goals of, 97
    high-efficacy medications, 98
    induction, 98
    John Cunningham virus, 99–100
    long-term experience, 103–104
    mechanisms of action, 101–102
    monitoring, 100
    onset of action, 103
    patient case studies, 104–105

    patient's age, 99
    potency, 102–103
    prognosis in MS, 98
    progressive multifocal eukoencephalopathy, 99–100
    reproductive attributes, 104
    safety, 103
    stopping, 101
    tolerability, 103
disease-modifying medications, 193
disease-modifying therapy (DMT), 186
dissemination in space (DIS)
    clinical criteria for, 56
    MRI criteria for, 56–57
dissemination in time (DIT)
    clinical criteria for, 56
    MRI criteria for, 56–57
    paraclinical evidence for, 57
DIT. *See* dissemination in time
DMF. *See* dimethyl fumarate
DMT. *See* disease modifying therapy; disease-modifying therapy
DON. *See* demyelinating optic neuritis
DPPX6. *See* anti-dipeptidyl-peptidase-like protein-6
DTI. *See* diffusion tensor imaging
dual Ma-1/M-2 positivity (anti-Ma), 387
dynamic gait index, 272
dynamometry, 236
dysarthria, 220–221
    paroxysmal, 220
    types of, 220
dyschromatopsia, 209
dysphagia
    management options, 219
    neurogenic, 218

EAE. *See* experimental autoimmune encephalomyelitis
echinacea, 291
ECT. *See* electroconvulsive therapy
EDSS. *See* expanded disability status scale
educational sessions, 171
EEOC. *See* Equal Employment Opportunity Commission
efferent demyelination, 214–215
efferent pathology, 212–213
electroconvulsive therapy (ECT), 186
emotional abuse, 347
emotional disorders
    adjustment disorder, 186
    anxiety disorders, 187
    bipolar disorder, 187
    depression
        diagnosis, 183–185
        etiology, 185
        factors, 185
        screening tools, 184
        treatment, 185–186
    euphoria, 187
    pseudobulbar affect, 188
    psychiatric effects, 188
    psychotherapy, 188–189
    psychotic disorders, 187
    suicide, 186
emotional health, 283

emotional stress, 171
employment
    federal laws, 336–337
    vocational rehabilitation services, 336
enhanced access, comprehensive care centers, 167–169
environmental risk factors, 23–24
EP. *See* evoked potentials
epidemiology, 3–4
    epilepsy, 199
    neuromyelitis optica, 351–352
    neurosarcoidosis, 394
    transverse myelitis, 373
epilepsy
    clinical and paraclinical measures, 199–200
    epidemiology, 199
    seizures
        pathogenesis, 200
        treatment, 200–201
        types, 199
Equal Employment Opportunity Commission (EEOC), 336
escalation, 98
Escheria coli, 116
euphoria, 187
evoked potentials (EP), 82–83
exacerbate bowel dysfunction, 250
exacerbations, 163–164, 316
exercise
    ambulation, 273
    wellness, 281–282
exome sequencing, 37–38
expanded disability status scale (EDSS), 24–25, 98, 139, 191, 232, 238
experimental autoimmune encephalomyelitis (EAE), 119, 152
Extavia, 118

FA value. *See* fractional anisotropy value
facial nerve palsy, 395
familial aggregation, 28–29
Family and Medical Leave Act (FMLA), 336–337
fatigue, 339
    acute, 175
    complementary and alternative medicine, 179
    comprehensive symptom management, 163
    comprehensiveness, 175
    definition, 173
    factors, 174
    individual-centered approach, 175
    iterative process
        complementary and alternative methods, 179
        in-depth assessment, 176—177
        intervention, 178–179
        pharmacotherapy, 178
        problem identification, 175
        psychoeducation and behavioral programs, 178–179
        screen for severity, 175–176
    pathogenesis, 174–175
    principles, 175
    sensitive approach, 175
    systematic approach, 175
    types, 175
    wellness, 281
FCE. *See* functional capacity evaluation
fecal incontinence, 250

fertility, 313
FES. *See* functional electrical stimulation
financial abuse, 348
fine mapping studies, 39
fingolimod, 99, 102
    mechanism, 120
    side effects, 121
    start-up, monitoring, and risk stratification, 121
    trial results, 120–121
    typical patients, 121
first molecular markers, 29
fish oil therapy, 291–292
FLAIR. *See* fluid-attenuated inversion recovery
fluid-attenuated inversion recovery (FLAIR), 65–76
fluoxetine, 141
FMLA. *See* Family and Medical Leave Act
Food and Drug Administration (FDA), 104, 112, 127
    fish oil classification, 292
fractional anisotropy (FA) value, 376
FREEDOMS trial, fingolimod, 120, 121
functional capacity evaluation (FCE), 163, 339–340
functional electrical stimulation (FES), 236, 274

GA. *See* glatiramer acetate
$GABA_BR$. *See* gamma-amino butyric acid B receptor
gabapentin, 214, 305
GAD. *See* generalized anxiety disorder
gadolinium (Gd), 118
GALA. *See* Glatiramer Acetate Low-Frequency Administration
gamma-amino butyric acid B receptor ($GABA_BR$), 385
Gd. *See* gadolinium
generalized anxiety disorder (GAD), 187
genetics, 4
    exome sequencing, 37–38
    familial aggregation, 28–29
    familial risks, 29
    first molecular markers, 29
    genome sequencing, 37–38
    genome-wide association screen, 32–33
    human leukocyte antigen, 29
    limitations, 40
    linkage analysis, 29
    linkage screens, 31–32
    major histocompatibility complex, 33–36, 38–40
    missing heritability, 36
    primary progressive multiple sclerosis, 53, 57–58
    race and geography, 28
    susceptibility, 38–40
    twin studies, 29
    vitamin D, 36–37
genome sequencing, 37–38
genome-wide association screen (GWAS), 32–33
Gilenya. *See* fingolimod
ginkgo biloba, 292
glatiramer acetate (GA), 101, 104
    mechanism of action, 119
    side effects for, 119
    start-up, monitoring, and risk stratification, 119
    in therapy, 8–9
    trial results, 119
    typical patients, 120
Glatiramer Acetate Low-Frequency Administration (GALA), 119

gluten sensitivity, 292
GlyR. *See* anti-glycine receptor
GM. *See* gray matter
gray matter (GM)
   demyelination, 16
   inflammation, 18
GWAS. *See* genome-wide association screen

HADS. *See* hospital anxiety and depression scale
headache, 229
healing touch, 285
health insurance, 337–338
Health Insurance and Portability Act (HIPPA), 337
health practitioners, 281
health promotion, 280–281
hepatotoxicity, 99
high-dose corticosteroids, 110, 112
high-dose oral therapies, 110
high-efficacy medications, 98
HIPPA. *See* Health Insurance and Portability Act
HLA. *See* human leukocyte antigen
HLA-DRB1 allele, 300
HLA-DRB1*1501 allele, 300
HLA-DRB1*1501/1503 allele, 300
hospital anxiety and depression scale (HADS), 185
human leukocyte antigen (HLA), 29
hyoscyamine, 305
hyperlipidemia, 325–326
hypothalamic–pituitary dysfunction, 395

iatrogenic pain, 229
ibudilast, 140–141
ICAM-1. *See* intercellular adhesion molecule 1
IFN. *See* interferon
IgG index, 82
IM. *See* integrative medicine
imaging red flags, 89–91
immune-stimulating supplements, 291
immunological theory, 4–5
immunological therapy, 149–150
   autologous hematopoietic stem cell transplant, 151
   cladribine, 151
   further development of, 152
   laquinimod, 152
   sphingosine 1-phosphate receptors, 152
immunomodulation, 101
immunosuppressant therapy, 8, 101
IMSGC. *See* International Multiple Sclerosis Genetics Consortium
incontinence, 245
induction, 98
inflammation
   gray matter, 18
   white matter
      adhesion molecules, 18
      chemokines and its receptors, 18
      integrins, 18
inflammatory axonopathy, 19
infusion therapies, 126–127
   administration, 128–129
   alemtuzumab, 131–132
   characteristics, 128–129
   cyclophosphamide, 127, 130

   daclizumab, 120
   glatiramer acetate, 119–120
   interferon beta, 116, 118–119
   mitoxantrone, 127
   monitoring, 128–129
   natalizumab, 130–131
   ocrelizumab, 132–133
   patient case study, 123–124
   rituximab, 132
INR. *See* international normalized ratio
insurance
   disability, 338–339
   health, 337–338
   life, 340
   long-term care, 340
   sources, 337–338
   types, 337
integrative medicine (IM)
   healing touch, 285
   mind-body therapies, 285
   MS patients, 284
   nutritional issues, 284
   outcomes of studies, 284
   supplements, 285
   wellness recommendations, 280
integrins, 18
intercellular adhesion molecule 1 (ICAM-1), 18
interferon (IFN), 8, 188
interferon beta, 99, 100, 101, 103
   mechanism of action, 116, 118
   start-up, monitoring, and risk stratification, 118–119
   trial results, 118
   typical patients, 119
interferon beta-1a, 116, 118
interferon beta-1b, 116
International Multiple Sclerosis Genetics Consortium (IMSGC), 31, 33, 34, 37, 39
international normalized ratio (INR), 291
International Pediatric Multiple Sclerosis Study Group, 297, 299, 302, 303, 305
International Pediatric Multiple Sclerosis Study Group Consensus, 363
internet, 281
intraocular inflammation. *See* uveitis
intraparenchymal brain lesions, 395
intrathecal baclofen (ITB), 263
intravenous immunoglobulins (IVIGs), 112
intravenous methylprednisolone (IVMP), 110, 127
ionotropic glutamate receptor antibodies, 384–385
ischemic stroke, 395
ITB. *See* intrathecal baclofen
IVIGs. *See* intravenous immunoglobulins
IVMP. *See* intravenous methylprednisolone

JC virus. *See* John Cunningham virus
JCV PCR. *See* JCV polymerase chain reaction
JCV polymerase chain reaction (JCV PCR), 131
John Cunningham (JC) virus, 80, 99, 121, 130–131

KAFO. *See* knee ankle foot orthoses
Klein–Levin syndrome, 202
knee ankle foot orthoses (KAFO), 274

labor force participation factors, 335
laquinimod, 152
Late Life Function and Disability Inventory (LL-FDI), 161
LCLAT. *See* low contrast letter acuity test
LDN. *See* low dose naltrexone
left ventricular ejection fraction (LVEF), 127
LFA-1. *See* leukocyte function antigen
Lemtrada. *See* alemtuzumab
leptomeningeal inflammation. *See* meningitis
leucine-rich glioma inactivated-1 (LGI1), 383
leukocyte function antigen 1 (LFA-1), 18
LGI1. *See* leucine-rich glioma inactivated-1
Lhermitte's phenomenon, 56
Lhermitte's sign, 228–229
libido, factors affecting, 253
life insurance, 340
LL-FDI. *See* Late Life Function and Disability Inventory
long-term care insurance, 340
long-term therapy, 391
low contrast letter acuity test (LCLAT), 170
low dose naltrexone (LDN), 292–293
low-dose corticosteroids, 359
lumbar puncture, 81–82
LVEF. *See* left ventricular ejection fraction

magnetic resonance imaging (MRI)
  characteristics
    dissemination in space, 66
    dissemination in time, 66–67
    imaging sequences, 65
    morphology, 66
    neuromyelitis optica, 70–73
    nonspecific white matter disease, 68–70
  clinical applications, disease monitoring, 75–76
  and clinical practice
    dissemination in space, 56–57
    dissemination in time, 56–57
    optical coherence tomography, 57
    radiologically isolated syndrome, 59–60
    visual evoked potential, 57
  neurosarcoidosis
    dural thickening, 398
    intracranial parenchymal lesions, 398
    intramedullary spinal cord lesions, 398
    leptomeningeal enhancement, 397–398
    muscle involvement, 398
  pitfalls, 73–75
  relapse, 114
  safety issues, 76
  technical issues, 73–75
major histocompatibility complex (MHC), 33–36, 38–40, 101
Managing Fatigue: A Six-week Course for Energy Conservation, 179
manual dexterity test (MDT), 170
manual muscle testing (MMT), 235–236
marijuana therapy, 290–291
McDonald criteria
  clinically isolated syndromes, 52
  CSF-specific OCBs, 57
  diagnostic scheme, 54, 55
  MRI and clinical practice, 56–57
    dissemination in space, 56–57
    dissemination in time, 56–57

    optical coherence tomography, 57
    radiologically isolated syndrome, 59
    visual evoked potential, 57
  primary progressive multiple sclerosis, 53, 57–58
  relapsing–remitting multiple sclerosis, 52, 55–56
  secondary progressive multiple sclerosis, 52–53
MDC. *See* minimal detectable change
MDT. *See* manual dexterity test
Medicaid, 338
Medicare, 338
medication side effects, 174
meiotic recombination, 31
memantine, 214
meningitis, 395
menopause, 319–320
menstrual cycle, 313
mesenchymal stem cells (MSCs), 155
methylprednisolone. *See* corticosteroids
MH questionnaire. *See* MyHealth questionnaire
MHC. *See* major histocompatibility complex
mimics by disease category, 91–92
mind-body therapies, 285
mindfulness, 189, 293
Mini-Balance evaluation systems test (Mini-BEST), 269–270
Mini-BEST. *See* Mini-Balance evaluation systems test
minimal detectable change (MDC), 237
mitoxantrone, 102, 104, 127
  new developments in therapy, 9
MMT. *See* manual muscle testing
mobility
  balance impairment, 269–270
  definition of, 268
  imbalance and falls issue, 269
  limitations, 268–269
mobility impairments, 174–175
modified Rio Score, 98–99
MOG. *See* myelin oligodendrocyte glycoprotein
mood, 48
motor pathway symptoms, 49
MRI. *See* magnetic resonance imaging
MS. *See* multiple sclerosis
MS TOUCH program, 99
MSCs. *See* mesenchymal stem cells
MSFC. *See* Multiple Sclerosis Functional Composite
MSOAC. *See* Multiple Sclerosis Outcome Assessments Consortium
MSPT. *See* Multiple Sclerosis Performance Test
multidisciplinary medical team, 348–349
multiple sclerosis (MS)
  acute disseminated encephalomyelitis
    clinical features, 365–366
    definition, 297, 363
    differential diagnosis of, 365
    electrophysiologic studies, 368
    hallmark clinical presentation for, 363, 366
    imaging findings, 366
    incidence, 364
    infections, 365
    key features, 367
    laboratory findings, 366–368
    neuropathological findings, 368
    outcome and disability, 369
    risk for recurrent demyelinating attacks, 369

multiple sclerosis (MS) (*cont.*)
  treatment, 368–369
  variants, 368–369
 alcoholism, 280
 ambulation
  assessment tools, 271–273
  assistive devices, 274–275
  common gait abnormalities, 273
  exercise, 273–274
  interventions, 273–276
  limitations, 271, 274
  medications, 275
  orthoses, 274–275
  rehabilitation, 273–274
  surgical treatments, 275–276
  walking and falls, 271
 ARNMD report, 2–3
 axonal loss, 18–19
  chronic demyelination–related axonal transection, 18
  inflammatory axonopathy, 19
  Wallerian degeneration, 19
 balance impairment
  assessment, 270
  balance confidence scale, 269–270
  exercise for, 270–271
  rehabilitation, 270–271
 benign, 25–26
 bladder dysfunction
  evaluation and clinical findings, 244–249
  factors, 245
  pathophysiology, 244
  symptoms, 50, 244
  treatment, 244, 246–249
 blindness, 339
 bowel dysfunction
  constipation, 250
  etiology, 249
  evaluation and clinical findings, 249–250
  exacerbate, 250
  fecal incontinence treatment, 250
  screening questions, 249
  symptoms, 50
 caregiver
  definition, 343
  emotional support, 345–346
  tips for, 347
  trifecta, 345
  wellness programs, 346–347
 causation theories, 3
 cerebellum and cerebellar connections, 50
 clinical phenotypes of, 52–53
 clinical trial results, 117
 cognitive changes, 6
 cognitive dysfunction
  disease-modifying medications, 193
  evaluation, 192–193
  indicators, 192
  minimal assessment, 193
  patient case study, 196
  symptomatic therapy, 193–195
 cognitive impairment, 191
 comorbidities

  anti-phospholipid antibodies, 326
  evidence, 327
  hyperlipidemia, 325–326
  mental, 325
  other autoimmune, 326–328
  primary care issues, 279
  smoking, 326
  therapeutic decisions, 328
  vascular, 325
 complementary and alternative medicine
  acupuncture, 290
  antioxidants, 290
  bee venom therapy, 290
  Chinese herbal medicine, 290
  cooling therapy, 291
  cranberry, 291
  echinacea, 291
  fish oil, 291–292
  ginkgo biloba, 292
  gluten sensitivity, 292
  immune-stimulating supplements, 291
  low dose naltrexone, 292–293
  marijuana, 290–291
  mindfulness, 293
  Swank diet, 291–292
  Tai Chi, 293
  traditional Chinese medicine, 290
  vitamin B_{12}, 293
  vitamin D, 293–294
  yoga, 294
 as complex trait, 30–31
 demyelination, 16
 diagnosis
  characteristic of lesions, 53
  clinical red flags, 61
  evolution of, 53–54
  future of, 61
  new directions, 12
  Poser criteria, 53
  primary progressive MS, 57–58
  pseudo-relapses, 59
  radiologically isolated syndrome, 59–60
  relapsing, 58–59
  Schumacher committee criteria, 53
 differential diagnosis
  diagnostic algorithm, 92
  by disease category, 88
  mimics by disease category, 91–92
  red flags, 88–89
 differentiating definite, 53
 disease modifying therapy, 56
  administration, 102
  approved therapies, 102
  change/discontinuation, 101
  changing, 100–101
  comorbidities, 99
  convenience, 103
  cost and access, 103
  current treatment strategies, 98–99
  early treatment initiation, 97–98
  goals of, 97
  high-efficacy medications, 98

induction, 98
John Cunningham virus, 99–100
long-term experience, 103–104
mechanisms of action, 101–102
monitoring, 100
onset of action, 103
patient case studies, 104–105
patient's age, 99
potency, 102–103
prognosis in MS, 98
progressive multifocal eukoencephalopathy, 99–100
reproductive attributes, 101
safety, 103
side effects and safety considerations, 117–118
stopping, 101
tolerability, 103
drugs, side effects of, 212
early cases, 1
early description, 1–2
early monographs, 2
early reports, 2
emotional disorders
    adjustment disorder, 186
    anxiety disorders, 187
    bipolar disorder, 187
    depression, 183–186
    euphoria, 187
    pseudobulbar affect, 188
    psychiatric effects, 188
    psychotherapy, 188
    psychotic disorders, 187
    suicide, 186
emotional health, 283
environmental risk factors, 23–24
epidemiology, 22–23
epilepsy
    clinical and paraclinical measures, 199–200
    epidemiology, 199
    seizures, 199–200
exercise, 281–282
fatigue
    acute, 175
    complementary and alternative medicine, 179
    comprehensive symptom management, 163
    definition, 173
    factors, 174
    individual-centered approach, 175
    iterative process, 175–179
    pathogenesis, 174
    principles, 175
    sensitive approach, 175
    types, 175
fecal incontinence treatment, 250
functional capacity evaluation, 339–340
future promises, 14
genetics, 4
    exome sequencing, 37–38
    familial aggregation, 28–29
    familial risks, 29
    first molecular markers, 29
    genome sequencing, 37–38

genome-wide association screen, 32–33
    human leukocyte antigen, 29
    limitations, 40
    linkage analysis, 29
    linkage screens, 31–32
    major histocompatibility complex, 33–36, 38–40
    missing heritability, 36
    race and geography, 28
    susceptibility, 38–40
    twin studies, 29
    vitamin D, 36–37
health issues, 13–14
health promotion, 280–281
immunologic therapies, 149–150
    autologous hematopoietic stem cell transplant, 151
    cladribine, 151
    further development of, 152
    laquinimod, 152
    sphingosine 1-phosphate receptors, 152
immunological theory, 4–5
incidence, 22–23
infection search, 3
inflammatory mediators in, 17–18
infusion therapies, 126–127
    alemtuzumab, 131–132
    cyclophosphamide, 127, 130
    mitoxantrone, 127
    natalizumab, 130–131
    ocrelizumab, 132–133
    rituximab, 132
injectable therapies
    daclizumab, 120
    glatiramer acetate, 119–120
    interferon beta, 116, 118–119
    patient case study, 123–124
insurance
    disability, 338–339
    health, 337–338
    life, 340
    long-term care, 340
    sources, 337–338
    types, 337
integrative medicine
    healing touch, 285
    mind-body therapies, 285
    nutritional issues, 284
    outcomes of studies, 284
    supplements, 285
    wellness recommendations, 280
investigations, 5–6
magnetic resonance imaging
    characteristics, 65–73
    clinical applications, disease monitoring, 75–76
    dissemination in space, 56–57
    dissemination in time, 56–57
    optical coherence tomography, 57
    pitfalls, 73–75
    radiologically isolated syndrome, 59
    relapse, 114
    safety issues, 76
    technical issues, 73–75
    visual evoked potential, 57

multiple sclerosis (MS) (*cont.*)
  misdiagnosis of, 60–61
  mobility
    balance impairment, 269–270
    definition of, 268
    imbalance and falls issue, 269
    limitations, 268–269
  monitoring new directions, 12–13
  motor pathway, 49
  natalizumab
    new developments in therapy, 9
    relapse management, 109
  natural history, 24–25
  neuromyelitis optica
    clinical course, 356
    clinical features, 352–353
    diagnosis, 353–356
    epidemiology, 351–352
    imaging, 353–355
    laboratory studies, 355–356
    prognosis, 356
    treatment, 356–360
  neuronal degeneration mechanism, 18–19
  neuronal loss, 19
  neuroprotective therapies, 152–153
    biotin, 153–154
    further development of, 154–155
    sodium channel blockers, 154
    statins, 154
  nonpharmacological approaches, 238
  obesity, 283
  ongoing challenges, 14
  oral therapies
    dimethyl fumarate, 122–123
    fingolimod, 120–121
    patient case study, 123–124
    teriflunomide, 121–122
  osteoporosis, 282
  pain management
    assessment, 226
    central neuropathic pain, 226–228
    clinical presentation, 225–226
    headache, 229
    iatrogenic pain, 229
    impact, 225
    Lhermitte's sign, 228–229
    mechanism, 225–226
    musculoskeletal pain, 229
    patient case study, 230
    prevalence, 225
    pseudoradicular pain, 229
    trigeminal neuralgia, 228
    visceral pain, 229
  paroxysmal events in, 220
  pediatric multiple sclerosis
    acquired demyelinating syndromes, 297–298
    clinical features, 300–304
    demographics, 298–299
    incidence, 298
    management, 304–305
    patient case studies, 306–308
    prognosis, 305–306
    risk factors, 299–300

  phenotypes
    clinically isolated syndromes, 52
    primary progressive, 53
    relapsing–remitting, 52, 55–56
    secondary progressive, 52–53
  plaque, 5
  prevalence, 22–23
  primary progressive multiple sclerosis
    diagnosis of, 57–58
    prevalence, 23
  progressive phenotypes, 58
  pseudobulbar affect, 188, 221–222
  red flags, 60
  rehabilitation
    ambulation, 271
    assessment process, 161–162
    assessment tools, 161–162
    National Multiple Sclerosis Society, 159
    obstacles, 162
    professionals, 159–160
    purpose, 162–164
    referral process, 160
    specialized services, 160
    World Health Organization, 159
  relapse
    adrenocorticotropic hormone, 112
    clinical management, 111
    corticosteroids, 110–112
    definition of, 58–59
    intravenous immunoglobulins, 112
    McDonald Criteria, 53–54
    MRI, 114
    neuromyelitis optica spectrum disorder, 113
    patient case study, 114
    pediatric multiple sclerosis, 303–304
    plasmapheresis, 113
    red flags, 109
    symptomatic therapy, 113
  relationship-centered care, 166–167
    comprehensive care center, 167–170
    patient advisory councils and codesign, 170–171
    patient engagement, 171
  remyelinating/reparative therapies, 155, 156
    agents identified from cell-based screens, 155
    cell-based therapies, 155
    further development of, 156
    opicinumab, 155
  secondary progressive multiple sclerosis, 52–53
    natalizumab, 131
    prevalence, 23
    risk factors, 137
  sexual dysfunction
    assessment of, 254
    cardiovascular dysfunction, 256
    clinical management of, 255
    prevalence, 253
    symptoms, 254
    tertiary, 254
    treatment, 255
  sleep problems, 174
  smoking, 280, 283
  societies, 9
  spasticity

comprehensive symptom management, 163
definition, 259
evaluation, 259–261
management, 261–264
outcome measures, 260
patient case studies, 264–266
prevalence, 259
symptoms and signs, 260
treatment modalities, 261–262
survival, 22–23
symptoms and signs
  bowel and bladder pathways, 49
  case study, 45–46
  classic, 47
  cognition, 48
  cranial nerves, 48–49
  evaluation, 46–48
  mood, 48
  nonspecific *versus* specific, 49
  pattern recognition, 50
  pediatric multiple sclerosis, 300
  red flags, 46
  somatosensory pathways, 49
team approach, 14
therapy
  adrenocorticotropic hormone, 7
  alternative medicine, 9
  description, 6
  glatiramer acetate, 8–9
  immunosuppressant, 8
  interferon, 8
  new developments, 9
tools and tests
  blood tests, 79–81
  evoked potentials, 82–83
  lumbar puncture, 81–82
  optical coherence tomography, 83–85
  spinal fluid analysis, 81–82
transient neurological events
  case study, 203
  clinical description, 204–205
  description, 205
  pathophysiological concepts, 204
  tonic spasms, 205–206
transverse myelitis
  age, 374
  anatomical features, 375–376
  clinical features, 375–376
  diagnostic criteria for, 373
  diagnostic investigation, 376–377
  epidemiology of, 373
  incidence, 373
  management, 377
  nonpharmacological approaches, 377
  pathophysiology of, 373–375
  plasma exchange, 377
  prognosis, 377
  signs and symptoms, 376
  spinal cord pathology types, 375
  treatment for, 377
treatment of disease activity, 13
treatment of symptoms, 13

understanding new directions, 11–12
undiagnosing of, 60–61
upper extremity dysfunction
  action research arm test, 237
  Ai Chi therapy, 236
  complex multidimensional tasks, 232
  coordination problems, 237–238
  focal spasticity, 234
  iterative learning control methods, 236
  muscle weakness, 236–237
  nine hole peg test, 237
  occupational therapist, 238–239
  self-care deficits associated with, 238–239
  spasticity, 233–234
vascular theory, 4
vision problems in, 215
vitamin D, 282
walking scale-12, 271
wellness, 281–283
women
  breastfeeding, 318–319
  fertility, 313
  hormonal influence, 311–312
  menopause, 319–320
  menstrual cycle, 313
  oral contraceptive pills, 311, 312, 313
  pregnancy, 313–314
  sex differences, 311–312
  sex hormones, 312
Multiple Sclerosis Functional Composite (MSFC), 145
Multiple Sclerosis Outcome Assessments Consortium (MSOAC), 145
Multiple Sclerosis Performance Test (MSPT), 170
musculoskeletal pain, 229
mycophenolate mofetil, 359
myelin oligodendrocyte glycoprotein (MOG), 301
myelin protein phagocytosis, 16
myelopathy, 395
MyHealth (MH) questionnaire, 170

NAA. *See* N-acetyl aspartate
NAbs. *See* neutralizing antibodies
N-acetyl aspartate (NAA), 19
Nagi's disablement model, 161
narcolepsy, 202
NARCOMS. *See* North American Research Committee on Multiple Sclerosis
natalizumab, 99–100, 101
National Center for Medical Rehabilitation Research (NCMRR), 161
National Institutes of Health (NIH), 290
National Multiple Sclerosis Society (NMSS), 159, 336, 345–346
NCMRR. *See* National Center for Medical Rehabilitation Research
NEDA. *See* no evidence of disease activity
NEDA3, 98–99
NEDA4, 99
neurogenic dysphagia, 218
neuromyelitis optica (NMO), 80, 301
  clinical course, 356
  clinical features, 352–353
  diagnosis, 353–355
  epidemiology, 351–352
  imaging

neuromyelitis optica (NMO) (*cont.*)
 MRI brain, 353
 MRI spine, 353
 laboratory studies, 355–356
 magnetic resonance imaging, 70–73
 prognosis, 356
 relapse management, 112
 treatment
  acute relapse, 356–357
  azathioprine, 358–359
  low-dose corticosteroids, 359
  mycophenolate mofetil, 359
  novel investigational immunotherapies, 359–360
  recommendations, 360
  relapse prevention, 358
  rituximab, 358
neuromyelitis optica IgG antibody (NMO-IgG), 80
neuromyelitis optica spectrum disorder (NMOSD), 55, 113, 355
neuronal degeneration mechanism, 18–19
 axonal loss, 18–19
 energy failure, 19
 neuronal loss, 19
neuronal loss, 19
neuroprotective therapies, 152–153
 biotin, 153–154
 further development of, 154–155
 sodium channel blockers, 154
 statins, 154
Neuro-QoL (NQ) scale, 170
neurosarcoidosis
 biopsy, 397
 cerebrospinal fluid studies, 398–399
 cranial neuropathy, 395
 differential diagnosis of, 396–397
 epidemiology, 394
 hypothalamic-pituitary dysfunction, 395
 intraparenchymal brain lesions, 395
 ischemic stroke, 395
 magnetic resonance imaging, 397–398
 meningitis, 395
 myelopathy, 395
 myopathy, 396
 peripheral neuropathy, 395–396
 prognosis, 400
 systemic evaluation, 399–400
 therapies for, 401
 treatment
  corticosteroids, 400
  cyclophosphamide, 401
  rituximab, 401
  steroid-sparing agents, 400
  TNF-alpha antagonists, 400
  whole-brain radiation therapy, 401
neutralizing antibodies (NAbs), 119
NHPT. *See* nine hole peg test
NIH. *See* National Institutes of Health
nine hole peg test (NHPT), 237
NMO. *See* neuromyelitis optica
NMO-IgG. *See* neuromyelitis optica IgG antibody
NMOSD. *See* neuromyelitis optica spectrum disorder
NMSS. *See* National Multiple Sclerosis Society
no evidence of disease activity (NEDA), 98

nonprimary multiple sclerosis fatigue, 175
nonspecific *versus* specific symptoms, 50
nonspecific white matter disease (NSWMD), 68, 70
North American Research Committee on Multiple Sclerosis (NARCOMS), 238, 344
Novantrone. *See* mitoxantrone
NQ scale. *See* Neuro-QoL scale
NSWMD. *See* nonspecific white matter disease
Numeric Rating Scale, 233
nystagmus, 212

OAB. *See* overactive bladder
obesity, 283
OCB. *See* oligoclonal bands
OCP. *See* oral contraceptive pills
ocrelizumab, 102, 132–133, 139–140
Ocrevus. *See* ocrelizumab
OCT. *See* ocular coherence tomography; optical coherence tomography
ocular coherence tomography (OCT), 100
oligoclonal bands (OCB), 301
Ondine's curse, 202
ONTT. *See* optic neuritis treatment trial
opicinumab, 155
optic neuritis, 208
 treatment trial (ONTT), 110, 209
optic neuropathy, 395
optical coherence tomography (OCT), 57, 83–85
oral antispasticity agents, 262–263
oral contraceptive pills (OCP), 313
oral therapies, 116
 dimethyl fumarate, 122–123
 fingolimod, 120–121
 patient case study, 123–124
 teriflunomide, 121–122
osteoporosis, 282
overactive bladder (OAB), 244
oxybutynin, 305

Paced Auditory Serial Addition Test (PASAT), 100
pain management
 assessment, 226
 central neuropathic pain, 226–229
 clinical presentation, 225–226
 headache, 229
 iatrogenic pain, 229
 impact, 225
 Lhermitte's sign, 228–229
 mechanism, 225–226
 musculoskeletal pain, 229
 patient case study, 230
 prevalence, 225
 pseudoradicular pain, 229
 trigeminal neuralgia, 228
 visceral pain, 229
pain syndromes, 226
PAPLS. *See* primary anti-phospholipid antibody syndrome
Parkinson's disease, 236
paroxysmal dysarthria and ataxia (PDA), 220
paroxysmal events, 220. *See also* transient neurological events
paroxysmal symptoms, 46, 58
PASAT. *See* Paced Auditory Serial Addition Test

pathogenesis
    fatigue, 174–175
    relapsing–remitting MS, 136
    seizures, 200
pathological laughter and crying (PLC), 221
patient advisory council, 170–171
patient and caregiver multidisciplinary care model, 346
patient engagement, 171
Patient Health Questionnaire-9 (PHQ-9), 185
patient reported outcomes (PROs), 166, 169–170
patient-centered care, 166
patient-centeredness, 166
patient-directed education, 171
pattern recognition, 50
PBA. *See* pseudobulbar affect
PDA. *See* paroxysmal dysarthria and ataxia
pediatric multiple sclerosis
    acquired demyelinating syndromes, 297–298
    clinical features
        diagnosis, 302
        differential diagnosis, 302–303
        first demyelinating risk event, 303
        laboratory studies, 301
        MRI, 301–302
        relapses, 303–304
        signs and symptoms, 300
    demographics, 298–299
    incidence, 298
    management, 304–305
    patient case studies, 306–308
    prognosis, 305–306
    risk factors, 299–300
peripheral fatigue, 175
peripheral neuropathy, 395–396
pharmacotherapy, 144, 178
phenotypes, multiple sclerosis
    clinically isolated syndromes, 52
    primary progressive MS, 53
    relapsing–remitting MS, 52, 55–56
    secondary progressive MS, 52–53
PHQ-9. *See* Patient Health Questionnaire-9
physical abuse, 347
plasmapheresis (PLEX), 112, 113
PLC. *See* pathological laughter and crying
plegridy, 118, 119
PLEX. *See* plasmapheresis
PML. *See* progressive multifocal leukoencephalopathy
PMS. *See* progressive multiple sclerosis
polyunsaturated fatty acids (PUFAs), 291–292
Poser criteria, 53
PPMS. *See* primary progressive multiple sclerosis
pregabalin, 305
pregnancy
    delivery, 316–317
    description, 313–314
    disease-modifying therapies, 314–316
    exacerbations treatment, 316
    postpartum relapse and prevention, 317–318
    symptomatic treatment, 316
primary anti-phospholipid antibody syndrome (PAPLS), 326
primary care issues, 279–280
primary multiple sclerosis fatigue, 175
primary progressive multiple sclerosis (PPMS), 53, 132, 136

assessment of, 58
diagnosis of, 57–58
identification of, 136
ocrelizumab, 139–140
prevalence, 23
progression in, 57–58
primary sexual dysfunction, 255
Processing Speed Test (PST), 170
prognosis
    neuromyelitis optica, 356
    neurosarcoidosis, 400
    pediatric multiple sclerosis, 305–306
    transverse myelitis, 377
progressive multifocal leukoencephalopathy (PML),
    80, 99–100, 120, 121, 130
progressive multiple sclerosis (PMS), 136, 164, 194
    amiloride, 141
    classification of, 137
    clinical features, 136–138
    disease course, 136–138
    emerging therapeutics for, 140
        biotin, 140
        siponimod, 140
    fluoxetine, 141
    ibudilast, 140–141
    implications, 136–138
    pathogenesis and neurotherapeutic implications, 138–139
    patient case studies, 146
    placebo-controlled clinical trials, 138–139
    restorative therapies
        anti-LINGO-1, 141
        stem cell therapy, 141
    riluzole, 141
    simvastatin, 141
    symptom and disability management, 144–145
    treatment strategies, 145–146
prolonged lymphopenia, 100
PROs. *See* patient reported outcomes
pseudobulbar affect (PBA), 188, 221–222
    prevalence of, 221
    treatment options for, 222
pseudoradicular pain, 229
pseudo-relapses, 59, 109
PST. *See* Processing Speed Test
psychiatric effects, 188
psychopharmacology, 185
psychotherapy, 185, 188
psychotic disorders, 187
PUFAs. *See* polyunsaturated fatty acids

quinidine, 222

radiologically isolated syndrome (RIS), 53, 59–60
    diagnostic criteria, 60
randomized controlled trials (RCTs), 185
rapid eye movement (REM) behavior disorders, 202
RCC. *See* relationship-centered care
RCTs. *See* randomized controlled trials
Rebif, 118
red flags
    cerebrospinal fluid, 91
    clinical, 88–89
    imaging, 89–91

red flags (*cont.*)
    relapse, 109
    symptoms and signs, 46
rehabilitation, 159
    ambulation, 271
    assessment process, 161–162
    assessment tools, 161–162
    National Multiple Sclerosis Society, 159
    obstacles, 162
    professionals, 159–160
    purpose, 162–164
        comprehensive symptom management, 163
        education and teaching of home exercise program, 162–163
        evaluation and training, 163
        exacerbations, 163–164
        progressive multiple sclerosis, 164
        task-specific rehabilitation, 163
    referral process, 159–160
    specialized services, 160
    World Health Organization, 159
Rehabilitation Act of 1973, 336
Rehabilitation Services Administration, 336
relapse
    adrenocorticotropic hormone, 112
    clinical management, 111
    corticosteroids
        placebo-controlled trials, 110
        side effects, 110–111
        symptomatic therapy, 112–113
        types/doses of, 111
    intravenous immunoglobulins, 112
    MRI, 114
    neuromyelitis optica, 113
    patient case study, 114
    pediatric multiple sclerosis, 303–304
    plasmapheresis, 113
    red flags, 109
relapsing-remitting multiple sclerosis (RRMS), 52, 97, 136
    cyclophosphamide, 127
    diagnosis of, 55–56
    early treatment of, 97
    McDonald criteria for, 52
    mitoxantrone, 127
    monitoring guidelines for, 100
    ocrelizumab, 132–133
    pathogenesis and neurotherapeutic implications, 138–139
    prevalence, 23
    randomized clinical trials, disease-modifying medications, 194
    rituximab, 132
    smoking, 326
    symptoms, 144–145
    in women, 23
Relationship Matters (RM) program, 346
relationship-centered care (RCC), 166–167
    comprehensive care center, 167, 168
        communication, 169
        enhanced access, 167–169
        patient reported outcomes, 169–170
    patient advisory councils and codesign, 170–171
    patient engagement, 171
REM. *See* rapid eye movement disorders
REMS. *See* Risk Evaluation and Strategy program

remyelinating/reparative therapies, 155, 156
    agents identified from cell-based screens, 155
    cell-based therapies, 155
    further development of, 156
    opicinumab, 155
retinal nerve fiber layer (RNFL), 57, 154, 214
retrochiasmatic demyelination, 215–216
riluzole, 141
Rio Score, 98–99
RIS. *See* radiologically isolated syndrome
Risk Evaluation and Mitigation Strategy (REMS) program, 120
Rituxan. *See* rituximab
rituximab, 132, 358
RM. *See* Relationship Matters program
RNFL. *See* retinal nerve fiber layer
Romberg Test, 269
RRMS. *See* relapsing-remitting multiple sclerosis

saccadic dysmetria, 213
sacral neuromodulation system (SNS), 248
Schumacher committee criteria, 53
SD. *See* sexual dysfunction
SDM. *See* shared decision making
SDMT. *See* Symbol Digit Modalities Test
secondary fatigue, 175
secondary progressive multiple sclerosis (SPMS), 52–53, 127
    mitoxantrone, 127
    natalizumab, 131
    prevalence, 23
    risk factors, 137
secondary sexual dysfunction, 255
seizures
    pathogenesis, 200
    treatment, 200
    types, 199
selective serotonin reuptake inhibitors (SSRIs), 186, 187
serotonin norepinephrine reuptake inhibitors (SNRIs), 187
sex differences, 311–312
sex hormones, 312
sexual dysfunction (SD)
    assessment of, 254
    cardiovascular dysfunction, 256
        fatigue, 256
        impaired thermoregulation, 256
        orthostatic intolerance, 256
        patient case study, 257
        sleep disturbance, 256
    clinical management of, 255
    symptoms, 254
    tertiary, 254
    treatment, 255
shared decision making (SDM), 166
shared medical appointments (SMA), 167–168
shock, 171
simvastatin, 141
single nucleotide polymorphisms (SNPs), 32
single-photon emission computed tomography (SPECT), 376
siponimod, 140
6-minute walk (6MW), 272
6MW. *See* 6-minute walk
sleep disorders
    prevalence, 201
    rarer

Klein–Levin syndrome, 202
narcolepsy, 202
Ondine's curse, 202
rapid eye movement behavior disorders, 202
types, 202
sleep problems, 174
SMA. *See* shared medical appointments
smoking, 283, 326
SNPs. *See* single nucleotide polymorphisms
SNRIs. *See* selective serotonin reuptake inhibitors
SNS. *See* sacral neuromodulation system
Social Security Administration (SSA), 338
Social Security Disability Insurance (SSDI), 338
social workers, 334
sodium channel blockers, 154
somatosensory pathway symptoms, 49
S1P receptor modulators. *See* sphingosine 1-phosphate receptor modulators
spasticity
comprehensive symptom management, 163
definition, 259
evaluation, 259–261
management, 260–264
outcome measures, 260
patient case studies, 264–266
prevalence, 259
symptoms and signs, 260
treatment modalities, 261–262
SPECT. *See* single-photon emission computed tomography
sphingosine 1-phosphate (S1P) receptor modulators, 152
spinal fluid analysis, 81–82
SPMS. *See* secondary progressive multiple sclerosis
spontaneous bursting, 204
SSA. *See* Social Security Administration
SSDI. *See* Social Security Disability Insurance
SSRIs. *See* selective serotonin reuptake inhibitors
statins, 154
stem cell therapy, 141
stroke, 395
suicide, 186
supplements, 285
swallowing, 218
Swank diet, 291–292
Symbol Digit Modalities Test (SDMT), 339
symptomatic therapy, 112–113, 193–195
symptoms and signs
case study, 50
classic, 47
evaluation
examination confirmation, 48
history, 46–47
nonspecific *versus* specific, 50
pattern recognition, 50
pediatric multiple sclerosis, 300
red flags, 46
review by system
bowel and bladder pathways, 50
cerebellum and cerebellar connections, 50
cognition, 48
cranial nerves, 48–49
mood, 48

motor pathways, 49
somatosensory pathways, 49

Tai Chi therapy, 293
task-specific rehabilitation, 163
Tecfidera. *See* dimethyl fumarate
teriflunomide, 99, 102–104
mechanism, 121–122
side effects, 122
start-up, monitoring, and risk stratification, 122
trial results, 122
typical patients, 122
T25FW. *See* timed 25 foot walk
T-helper lymphocytes, 311
therapeutics
comorbidities, 328
window, 98
therapy
adrenocorticotropic hormone, 7
alternative medicine, 9
complementary and alternative medicine
acupuncture, 290
antioxidants, 290
bee venom therapy, 290
Chinese herbal medicine, 290
cooling therapy, 291
cranberry, 291
echinacea, 291
fish oil, 291–292
ginkgo biloba, 292
gluten sensitivity, 292
immune-stimulating supplements, 291
low dose naltrexone, 292–293
marijuana, 290–291
mindfulness, 293
Swank diet, 291–292
Tai Chi, 293
traditional Chinese medicine, 290
vitamin B_{12}, 293
vitamin D, 293–294
yoga, 294
description, 6
in development
daclizumab, 120
ocrelizumab, 132–133
glatiramer acetate, 8–9
immunosuppressant, 8
interferon, 8
last stage of developments
alemtuzumab, 139–140
dimethyl fumarate, 122–123
laquinimod, 152
teriflunomide, 121–122
new developments, 9
thyroid stimulating hormone (TSH), 131
timed 25 foot walk (T25FW), 271
T-lymphocyte activation, 101
TM. *See* transverse myelitis
TMS. *See* transcranial magnetic stimulation
TN. *See* trigeminal neuralgia
tolterodine, 305
tonic spasms, 205–206

tools and tests
    blood tests, 79–81
    evoked potentials, 82–83
    lumbar puncture, 81–82
    optical coherence tomography, 83–85
    spinal fluid analysis, 81–82
traditional Chinese medicine, 290
transcranial magnetic stimulation (TMS), 377
TRANSFORMS trial, fingolimod, 120, 121
transient neurological events
    case study, 203
    clinical description, 204–205
    description, 205
    pathophysiological concepts, 204
    tonic spasms, 205–206
transverse myelitis (TM)
    age, 374
    anatomical features, 375–376
    clinical features, 375–376
    diagnostic criteria for, 373
    diagnostic investigation, 376–377
    epidemiology of, 373
    incidence, 373
    management, 377
    nonpharmacological approaches, 377
    pathophysiology of, 373–375
    plasma exchange, 377
    prognosis, 377
    signs and symptoms, 376
    spinal cord pathology types, 375
    treatment for, 377
    United States, 374
treat to target approach, 98
trigeminal nerve, 395
trigeminal neuralgia (TN), 228
TSH. See thyroid stimulating hormone
Tysabri. See natalizumab

UE. See upper extremity dysfunction
Uhthoff's phenomenon, 58
UMN syndrome. See upper motor neuron syndrome
unconventional medicine. See complementary and alternative medicine (CAM)
upper extremity (UE) dysfunction
    action research arm test, 237
    complex multidimensional tasks, 232
    coordination problems
        assessment of, 237–238
        treatment of, 238
    focal spasticity, 234
    muscle weakness
        Ai Chi, 236
        assessment of, 235–236
        functional electrical stimulation, 236
        iterative learning control methods, 236
        secondary symptoms, 236
        treatment of, 236–237
    nine hole peg test, 237
    occupational therapist, 238–239
    self-care deficits associated with, 238–239
    spasticity
        assessment of, 233
        clinical evaluation measurement, 233

    definition of, 233
    treatment of, 233–234
upper motor neuron (UMN) syndrome, 233, 260
urgent/access appointments, 168
urinalysis, 131
urinary symptoms, 247
urinary tract infections (UTIs), 291
urodynamic testing, 246
UTIs. See urinary tract infections
uveitis, 216

varicella zoster virus (VZV), 121
vascular cell adhesion molecule 1 (VCAM-1), 18
vascular comorbidities, 325
vascular theory, 4
VCAM-1. See vascular cell adhesion molecule 1
VEP. See visual evoked potential
vestibulocochlear nerve, 395
VGKCs. See voltage-gated channels
virtual visits, 169
visceral pain, 229
visual evoked potential (VEP), 57
vitamin B_{12}, 293
vitamin D
    complementary and alternative medicine, 293–294
    genetics, 36–37
    risk factor, 23–24
    wellness, 282
vocational rehabilitation services, 336
voltage-gated channels (VGKCs), 383
voltage-gated potassium channel complex antibodies, 383–384
VZV. See varicella zoster virus

walking limitations, 271
Walking speed Test (WST), 170
Wallerian degeneration, 19
Welcome Trust Case Control Consortium 2 (WTCCC2), 34
wellness
    definition, 281
    emotional health, 283
    exercise, 281–282
    fatigue, 281
    integrative medicine, 284
    obesity, 283
    osteoporosis, 282
    smoking, 283
    vitamin D, 282
wellness programs, caregiver, 346–347
white matter (WM)
    active plaques, characterization of, 16
    characteristics of, 16
    demyelination, 15–16
    inflammation
        adhesion molecules, 17, 18
        chemokines and its receptors, 18
        integrins, 18
WHO. See World Health Organization
WM. See white matter
women
    breastfeeding, 318–319
    fertility, 313
    hormonal influence, 311–312
    menopause, 319–320

menstrual cycle, 313
oral contraceptive pills, 311, 312, 313
pregnancy, 313–314
    delivery, 316–317
    description, 313–314
    disease-modifying therapies, 314–316
    exacerbations treatment, 316
    postpartum relapse and prevention,
      317–318
    symptomatic treatment, 316

    sex differences, 311–312
    sex hormones, 312
World Health Organization (WHO), 159
WST. *See* Walking speed Test
WTCCC2. *See* Welcome Trust Case Control
    Consortium 2

yoga, 294

Zajicek criteria, 396